Praise for *Golden Holocaust*

"This is the most scientifically sophisticated, commandingly documented book ever addressed to the role of cigarettes in modern life."
David A. Hollinger, 2010–11 President, Organization of American Historians

"The great cause of global health is in Robert Proctor's debt. *Golden Holocaust* is a model of impassioned scholarly research and advocacy. As Proctor so powerfully demonstrates, the time has come to hold the tobacco industry accountable for the massive disease, debility, and death that they produce around the world."
Allan M. Brandt, author of *The Cigarette Century*

"Robert Proctor unpacks the sad history of an industrial fraud. His tightly reasoned exploration touches on all topics on which the tobacco makers lied repeatedly to Congress and the public."
Donald Kennedy, President Emeritus, Stanford University,
and former Editor, *Science*

"This book is a remarkable compendium of evil. It will keep you spinning from page one through the last with a detailed description of how one of the most notorious industries in American history deceived and manipulated the public, the politicians, and the scientific community into allowing an age-old toxin to be breathed directly into the lungs of millions of Americans. It is the type of book that makes you wonder how, in God's name, this could have happened."
David Rosner, author of *Deceit and Denial*

"Proctor powerfully documents how a small number of tobacco companies caused a tragic global epidemic."
Jonathan M. Samet, MD, MS, Director, Institute for Global Health,
University of Southern California

"Proctor weaves together the public historical record with inside details and insights from thousands of once-secret industry documents. Anyone who cares about health, deception, science, or politics will learn something new from this book."
Stanton A. Glantz, Professor of Medicine, UC San Francisco,
and author of *The Cigarette Papers*

"A powerful indictment of the world's deadliest industry."
John R. Seffrin, PhD, Chief Executive Officer, American Cancer Society

"Scholarly yet eminently readable, indeed gripping, this book asks us to consider what the end game for tobacco might look like. A must-read for policy makers and public health officials and for anyone struggling against the tobacco industry in the field."
Professor Judith Mackay, Senior Advisor, World Lung Foundation,
Hong Kong, China SAR

Golden Holocaust

The publisher gratefully acknowledges the generous
support of the Humanities Endowment fund
of the University of California Press Foundation.

Golden Holocaust

*Origins of the Cigarette Catastrophe
and the Case for Abolition*

———

Robert N. Proctor

UNIVERSITY OF CALIFORNIA PRESS

Berkeley   Los Angeles   London

University of California Press, one of the most distinguished university presses in the United States, enriches lives around the world by advancing scholarship in the humanities, social sciences, and natural sciences. Its activities are supported by the UC Press Foundation and by philanthropic contributions from individuals and institutions. For more information, visit www.ucpress.edu.

University of California Press
Berkeley and Los Angeles, California

University of California Press, Ltd.
London, England

© 2011 by The Regents of the University of California

Library of Congress Cataloging-in-Publication Data

Proctor, Robert, 1954– .
 Golden holocaust : origins of the cigarette catastrophe and the case for abolition / Robert N. Proctor.
  p. cm.
 Includes bibliographical references and index.
 ISBN 978-0-520-27016-9 (cloth : alk. paper)
 1. Tobacco industry—United States—History. 2. Tobacco use—Health aspects. 3. Smoking—Psychological aspects. I. Title.
 [DNLM: 1. Tobacco Industry—history—United States. 2. Government Regulation—history—United States. 3. History, 20th Century—United States. 4. Persuasive Communication—United States. 5. Smoking—adverse effects—United States. 6. Smoking—psychology—United States. 7. Tobacco Industry—economics—United States. HD 9135]
  HD9135.P76 2011
  362.29'60973—dc22   2011003825

Manufactured in the United States of America

20 19 18 17 16 15 14 13 12 11
10 9 8 7 6 5 4 3 2 1

To a world without tobacco, science without corruption, bodies free from disease

CONTENTS

ILLUSTRATIONS

PROLOGUE

It was 1970, and I was sixteen and a junior at Southwest High School in Kansas City. All the students were called into the auditorium to hear a guy from the tobacco industry tell us how bad it was for us to smoke. I don't remember much about the man, except that he was young and groovily dressed, with a striped shirt and white shoes. But his message was clear: smoking is not for children. "An adult choice" is what sticks in my mind. Smoking was like driving or drinking or having sex—things we weren't even supposed to be thinking about. We were supposed to wait.

I think of that guy whenever I hear people fret over "youth smoking," and I marvel at how Big Tobacco manages to keep a step or two ahead of everyone else. Mr. White Shoes's message was delicious advertising, merging the best of reverse psychology with the time-honored trick of tempting by forbidding fruit. Marketers know that no one smokes to look younger and that kids want what they cannot have, especially if it's "for adults"—which is also why school programs urging kids not to smoke tend to fail. Teenagers don't like to be infantilized or patronized, a fact the companies have long understood far better than their critics.

The tobacco makers are notorious masters of deception; they know how to manufacture ignorance and to rewrite history. They know the power of images and how to twist these to violate common sense and pulmonary civility. They also know how to engineer desire, and, of course, they'd like us to believe they don't want youngsters to smoke. Health advocates have a good rule of thumb: ask cigarette makers what should be done (say, to curb youth smoking), and whatever they say, do the opposite.

Time, though, has been surprisingly good to Big T. Cigarettes remain the world's single largest preventable cause of death—dwarfing all others—and most of that mortality lies in the future. Tobacco killed only about a hundred million people in the twentieth century, compared with the billion we can anticipate in the twenty-first—if things continue as they have in the past. Tobacco now kills about six million people every year, more than AIDS, malaria, and traffic accidents combined. Heart disease claims the largest number, but close behind are emphysema and lung cancer, followed by premature birth, gangrene, and cancers of the human bladder, pancreas, and cervix. Tobacco-induced fires kill a few tens of thousands—paltry when compared to the cardiopulmonary toll but still a lot compared with mortality from, say, plane crashes or terrorist attacks. Cigarette death in the United States alone is like two jumbo jets crashing *every day;* the global toll would be an entire fleet. Half of all lifelong smokers will die from their habit, and every cigarette takes seven minutes off a smoker's life.

But what do these numbers really mean? How much worse is it that tobacco kills six million per year rather than, say, six thousand?

"One death is a tragedy, a million is a statistic." Those are words attributed to Stalin, but they might as well be from the sellers of *Nicotiana.* Statistics certainly has its detractors but none with deeper pockets than the cigaretteers. The industry's archives, forced open by litigation, are full of jokes about how smoking is "the major cause of statistics" or how "sleep is to be avoided since most heart attacks occur then." More serious are charges that nico-nazis and tobacco fascists want to jack-boot us into a world where no one has any fun. Tobacco prevention is made to look like the priggish obsession of nanny-state naysayers, a backwater of the meddling, have-no-fun puritanical crowd. Smoking in the 1980s—when the hazards of secondhand smoke were finally nailed down—was actually declared a form of free speech, complete with threats of smokers becoming second-class citizens or stigmatized minorities. Brown & Williamson even whined about cigarettes being "brought to trial by lynch law."

Part of the industry's success must be traced to its mastery of the illustrated word and airwaves. "Be the media" was the plan in 1990, when Philip Morris pondered acquiring an entire news service, like Knight-Ridder or United Press International, to carry its message. Another goal, though, has been a kind of *invisibility:* to turn the tobacco story into "old news," basically dog-bites-man. Tobacco is imagined as a solved problem, a vanishing anachronism from our distant past. A great deal of effort has gone into having such nonsense fill our newspapers and magazines, while most of the industry's manufacturing remains invisible. *Incognito ergo sum.* The Herculean machines that drive today's cigarette mega-factories are kept far from public view, rendering the bowels (and brains) of the enterprise harder to access than even the Pentagon or the CIA.

The effect is a kind of mass blindness. Most people know that the industry's behavior has been less than honorable, but how many know that cigarette smoke contains arsenic, cyanide, and radioactive isotopes? How many know that 90 percent

of the world's licorice ends up in tobacco, or that cigarettes are freebased with ammonia to turn them into a kind of crack nicotine? How many know that only about
two-thirds of what goes into a cigarette is actually tobacco, with much of the rest
being a witches' brew of added sugars, burn accelerants, freebasing agents, bronchial
dilators, and moisteners like glycerine or diethylene glycol, the antifreeze contam-
inating all those deadly Chinese tubes of toothpaste? How many know about the
filth sometimes found in cigarettes—dirt and mold, of course, but also worms, wire,
and insect excrement?

There's an old saying in the world of smoke: a cigarette is no more tobacco than
the *New York Times* is a pine tree. The fact is that America's famous blends are more
juiced up and candified—and filthied up with nitrosamine stank—than what much
of the rest of the world smokes. But the rest of the world is catching up. With very
few exceptions, tobacco almost everywhere is essentially unregulated. French cigarettes must contain at least 85 percent tobacco, and Germans don't allow nicotine
to be freebased with ammonia, but most of the rest is the Wild West. Dog food has
been more tightly regulated; the stockyards in Upton Sinclair's *Jungle* were clean by
comparison. Try to imagine the inside of a cigarette factory, and if you can't, think
about why that might be so.

Almost as invisible is the political influence wielded by the tobacco lobby. Readers may be surprised to learn that President Lyndon Johnson refused to take on Big
Tobacco, fearing his party's loss of the presidency. Or that tobacco was a sizable part
of the Marshall Plan to rebuild Europe. I also don't think it's widely known that farmers in the United States are still paid *not* to grow tobacco or that tobacco industry
moles helped draft the 1964 Surgeon General's report. Less surprising perhaps, but
significant nonetheless, is the fact that global warming denialists cut their teeth on
tobacco tactics, fighting science with science, creating doubt, fostering ignorance.
The industry looks out onto the world as if through a one-way mirror; we see only
the final product and the marketeer's bluster, but the industry itself—its behemoth
factories and closely guarded formulas—remains cloaked, clandestine, opaque.

Then there is the cigarette itself, in the mind-boggling gargantuan aggregate. Six
trillion—that's 6,000,000,000,000—are smoked every year, enough to make a continuous chain from the earth to the sun and back, with enough left over for a couple of round trips to Mars (when the planet is in a near-earth orbit). Imagined as
one long rod, that would be a cigarette more than 300 million miles long. Cigarettes
are being extruded—and therefore smoked—at a breathtaking rate of over 300 million miles per year, which is about thirty-four thousand miles per hour, twenty-
four hours a day. Picture a never-ending shaft of cigarettes shooting out at fifty times
the speed of sound, faster even than the rate at which satellites orbit the earth.

Cigarette design doesn't get much attention, but we're talking about one of the
most carefully (and craftily) designed objects on the planet—and a bigger cause of
global death than bullets. Billions of dollars have been poured into the black arts

of cigarette science: "several tens of billions of dollars" in the United States alone by one industry estimate. Legions of chemists have crafted a kind of slow-motion killing machine, with the coup de grâce administered by the smoker him- or, increasingly, herself.

Self-administration is one of the hallmarks of modern torture—think of the wired Christ of Abu Ghraib—but it is also the sine qua non of modern addiction. A great deal of talent has gone into making the cigarette an instrument of chemical dependence: by artfully crafting its physical character and chemistry, industry scientists have managed to create an optimally addictive drug delivery device, one that virtually sells itself. "It costs a penny to make. Sell it for a dollar. It's addictive"— those are the words of the billionaire investment guru (and onetime Reynolds board member) Warren Buffett. Advertising bans make it easier for brand leaders to maintain their margins, and the same advantage can accrue from timid governmental regulation—which is one reason Philip Morris was so eager to obtain the Food and Drug Administration's (FDA's) blessing. The tobacco giant pushed for the passage of the Family Smoking Prevention and Tobacco Control Act, signed into law by President Barack Obama in June of 2009. After a century of resisting, the Marlboro men figured they could solidify their market dominance by agreeing to submit to (limited) federal oversight.

Cigarettes will now be regulated in the United States, though it remains to be seen with how much urgency and how much courage. The industry has long been expert in turning lemons into lemonade, and regulation may prove yet another victory for the cigarette makers, depending on whether certain key steps are taken. The FDA's new powers are limited—it cannot ban cigarettes, for example, or reduce their nicotine content to zero—but even within this narrow frame there is much that could be done. More than anything else, the newly empowered FDA should *reduce the maximum allowable nicotine content of cigarettes* and *require that no cigarette produce smoke with a pH lower than 8.* Lowering the nicotine content (not delivery!) of cigarettes will eliminate their addictive grip, and raising cigarette smoke pH to make it uninhalable will prevent most of the lung cancers caused by smoking. These two steps alone would probably do more to improve human health than any other single policy in the history of human civilization. What is astonishing is that simple steps such as these have never been taken seriously.

. . .

This is a book about the history of cigarette design, cigarette rhetoric, and cigarette science. My goal is to treat the cigarette as part of the ordinary history of technology—and a deeply political (and fraudulent) artifact. Our tour will be through secret archives, clandestine operations, and carefully lawyered marketing and chemical manipulations. It is also, though, a story of how smoking became not just sexy and "adult" (meaning "for kids") but also routine and *banal*. The banalization of smoking is one of the oddest aspects of modern history. How did we come into this world, where millions perish from smoking and most of those in power turn a blind eye? How did tobacco manage to capture the love of governments and the high rhetorical ground of liberty, leaving the lesser virtues of longevity to its critics? And what can we do to strengthen movements now afoot to prevent tobacco death?

Think again about the numbers: in the United States alone, 400,000 babies are born every year to mothers who smoke during pregnancy. Smoking is estimated to cause more than 20,000 spontaneous abortions—and perhaps as many as seven times that. Seven hundred Americans are killed every year by cigarette fires, and 150 million Chinese alive today will die from cigarette smoking. Tens of thousands of acres of tropical forest are destroyed every year to grow the leaves required to forge the nicotine bond.

If it is true that large numbers numb, that is only because we have allowed ourselves to think like Stalin. Likewise, if we believe that smoking really is a kind of "freedom," this is partly because the cigaretteers have spent billions to make us think this way. The propaganda machine is powerful and operates on so many levels—science, law, government, sports, entertainment—that it is hard to think outside the pack. Governments are entranced, hooked by the bounty of taxes brought in by selling cigarettes. (No single commodity brings in higher revenues.) The mainstream media are often inattentive, partly because the tobacco story is spun as "old news." So we are brainwashed, nicotinized, confused into equating fumery with freedom.

Healthy people tend to forget how crucial health is for other kinds of freedom. The tobacco industry wants us to think about smoking as an inalienable right of all free people, but how free is the amputee suffering from Buerger's disease, the cigarette-induced circulatory disorder expressed as gangrene of the feet? How free was my beloved grandmother, the once-lively South Texas flapper, rendered wheezing and immobile on her deathbed from the emphysema scarring her lungs? Health so deprived is surely a kind of violation, a slow robbery of the spirit to which the strong and healthy will never bear first-person witness. The industry sells this slow asphyxiation—and the unwary buy into it.

The smoke folk want us to believe that smoking is a "free choice," and it is true that no one puts a gun to your head. Sellers cannot sell without buyers. But cigarettes are addictive, and most people find it very hard to quit, often excruciatingly so. Nicotine rewires the brain, creating a pharmacologic dependency as strong as that from heroin or opium. The result for most users is a profound inability to quit—which is why some victims end up smoking through holes punched in their throats. Surveys show that most smokers *want* to quit and regret having ever started: tobacco is *not a recreational drug*, which makes it different from alcohol or even marijuana in this respect. Very few people who drink are addicted—only about 3 percent, compared with the 80 to 90 percent of smokers of cigarettes. Few people who have a beer or a glass of wine hate this part of their lives; they enjoy drinking. Cigarettes are different. Smokers usually dislike their habit and wish they could escape it. People who actually like smoking are so rare that the industry calls them "enjoyers." That is also why the comparison to 1920s-style Prohibition falls flat. Prohibition failed because most people who drink actually like it and can do so responsibly, whereas virtually all tobacco use is abuse. There is no "safe" smoking, and few users escape addiction.

Which brings us to two additional problems with the freedom argument. The first stems from the fact that smokers typically begin when they are thirteen or fourteen. Indeed it is rare for anyone to start smoking after their teen years: people become smokers as children, when they cannot make "an adult choice." Whatever choice they do make is then compromised by the grip of addiction. The freedom defense is further weakened by the fact that nonsmokers often suffer exposure to "second-" and even "thirdhand" smoke (*fumée passif* and *ultra passif* are the marvelous French expressions). An estimated fifty thousand Americans die from exposure to secondhand smoke every year, which is more even than from auto accidents. The global toll is unknown, but it must be upwards of half a million souls.

The hopeful fact is that we may well have already passed the point of "peak tobacco." Global consumption seems to have peaked at about six trillion cigarettes per year around the turn of the new millennium and may well have fallen somewhat since. And may keep on falling, once governments recognize the toll not just to human life but also to economic prosperity and environmental well-being. Smoking is a significant cause of world poverty and a nontrivial cause of global climate change (mainly from fires, deforestation for planting and curing, and heavy use of petrochemicals in growing and manufacturing). When people come to realize and act on this, the slide away from smoking will accelerate. What remains of the habit will have a ritual or furtive character as against the mass mindless fumery of today.

This hopeful glimmer of a downturn has lots of different causes, including the smoke-free legislation now spreading throughout the world. Bans on indoor and even outdoor smoking will likely render smoking an increasingly marginal behavior, bordering on the antisocial. Calls for additional restrictions are also prominent in the Framework Convention on Tobacco Control, the world's first public health treaty, adopted by the World Health Assembly in May 2003. As of 2011 some 174 nations had ratified this treaty, which commits member nations to reducing tobacco use via taxation, graphic warnings, bans on advertising, and policies to establish smoke-free public places. Article 5.3 requires that manufacturers be excluded from all decision-making aspects of tobacco control, and progress is being made to limit cross-border smuggling.

The Framework Convention does not as yet have strong means of enforcement, which helps explain why we have not yet seen a mass flight from fumery. More effective in the long run may be local acts of organized resistance, as citizens recognize their right to breathe clean air. Many cities, states, and entire nations are now going smoke-free, with outdoor air also coming under scrutiny. More than a hundred miles of California beaches are now smoke-free, and metropolitan centers such as New York are pondering smoke-free public parks. In some cities smoking has been banned in private apartments, to prevent smoke from traveling from one dwelling to another. These tend to be "ratchet laws"—they are rarely reversed—and we may soon start to see cascade effects whereby, once sufficiently marginalized, mass tobacco use could rapidly disintegrate. Few things are as consequential in the realm of public health: Do we all have a right to breathe clean air? Or do smokers have a more fundamental right to pollute?

Talk of "rights" may not be appropriate in many parts of the world, where preference may be given to talk of health, purity, or some other civic or moral virtue. The biggest political obstacle to change has been that governments still stuff their coffers from cigarette taxes. But even that is changing, as tobacco taxes account for diminishing fractions of total revenues. Governments are also starting to realize how much tobacco robs from public treasuries in the form of health care costs. Another hopeful change could come from a renewed appreciation of the value of the lives of our elderly. The fact that most people who die from smoking are older makes it easier to trivialize cigarette mortality: that is what old people do, they die, and young people may not appreciate the value of a life lived well to eighty or ninety over against a life lived sickly to sixty or seventy. Here we need a rethink, since it's not as if smoking strikes only the healthy elderly, who just suddenly drop dead. Smokers age prematurely—think wrinkles and sexual dysfunction—quite apart from cancer and cardiac arrest.

We also need to rethink the environmental costs of tobacco. Global warming may well become the final straw leading to smoke-free societies, once we realize how the manufacture of cigarettes contributes to global climate change. Cigarettes are a major resource hog and a significant cause of forest fires and deforestation.

Which leads me to a prediction: There will come a time, I am convinced, when people will no longer smoke tobacco, or at least not in the routine and obsessive manner of the present. Public smoking will come to be seen in the same way we now regard, say, the use of the spittoon or public urination. And as smoking is progressively denormalized, or even rendered anathema, global consumption will fall into the hundreds of billions of sticks per year and thence into the tens of billions—compared with the trillions of today. Readers of this book may some day even find it hard to believe that smoking was ever as widespread as it is and as deeply embedded in popular culture. The ubiquitous smoking in films, organized for over half a century by the industry, will become an amusing oddity. It is already strange to recall how recently smoking was allowed on buses, planes, and trains—and in elevators and doctors' offices—while kids made ashtrays in schools and scholars welcomed collaborations with the industry. Change will only come, though, when we properly honor our dead and realize that the world in which we live is not the world in which we have to live.

. . .

My goal, then, is to explore the cigarette as a cultural artifact, craftily designed, unloved by most smokers, and deadlier even than they need to be. As with other books I have written, my hope is to historicize the cigarette, making the familiar seem strange and the strange familiar. The presentation has four parts.

Part I traces the origins of the modern cigarette, including the deadly invention of flue-curing and the enabling roles of matches, mechanization, militarization, and mass marketing. Flue-curing, as we'll see, made cigarette smoke inhalable, matches made fire mobile, mechanization made cigarettes cheap, and mass marketing made them desirable. Also examined is the crucial role of wars in promoting (and sometimes curbing) tobacco use and how governments got hooked on cigarettes via the lure of taxes. Here also is traced the astonishing range of gimmicks used by the industry to sell cigarettes, from skywriting and comic books to fancy-sounding filters and richly funded sponsorship of sports, music, and the arts. And movie implants and medical endorsements and the curious case of candy cigarettes, characterized by one tobacco bigwig as "not too bad an advertisement" for youngsters learning the gestures of smoking. New media tricks also come into focus here ("Tobacco 2.0"), along with cultural exotica such as smoking porn.

Part II treats how tobacco cancer hazards were discovered, including the oft-neglected role of European scholars. Highlighted here are studies conducted during the Nazi era, including those showing Germans were the first to discover and nail down the lung cancer link. Here also, though, manufacturers in the Third Reich were powerful enough to resist the demands of public health authorities. We also encounter previously unknown studies conducted in secret by tobacco companies in the United States that give an even bigger lie to their early claims of innocence. We then look at what it means to say a "consensus" is established that cigarettes are killing large numbers of people, especially when powerful political forces have been trying to create and sustain ignorance.

Part III explores how tobacco tycoons in the United States organized a global conspiracy to hide the hazards of smoking. The conspiracy begins with a series of meetings at the Plaza Hotel in Manhattan in December of 1953 and is perfected through the establishment of bodies such as the Tobacco Industry Research Committee, which provided the industry with a "stable" of expertise and a facade through which they could call for endlessly more research. We then turn to some of the methods used by the industry to maintain ignorance—including techniques deliberately designed to keep the truth from its own labor force. Here we also open up the guts of the cigarette itself, exploring the many different ways cigarettes are supposed to have been made safer, from "toasting," "king sizing," and mentholation to filters, low tars, and lights—all of which are either frauds or follies. The point here is that duplicity has been built into the cigarette itself: filters don't really filter, for example, and the holes punched into the mouth ends of nearly all modern cigarettes (aka "ventilation") give falsely low tar and nicotine readings when measured on standardized smoking robots. We shall also see that "light" and "low tar" cigarettes turn out to be no less lethal than the regulars sold half a century ago; indeed on a gram-per-gram basis they are significantly *more* deadly. For all their talk of "improvements," cigarette manufacturers have really just managed to squeeze more death and disease from any given gram of tobacco—and ever more money. The companies make about a penny from each cigarette sold, and since one tobacco death results from every million smoked, this means that a human life is worth about $10,000 to your average cigarette maker. The companies talk a lot about "choice," and theirs is clearly that they'd rather make $10,000 in profits than save the life of one of their customers.

Part IV proposes certain paths of redemption. I look at the history of filth in cigarettes, from pesticides and flavorants to worm feces and insect parts. Radioactive polonium is a focus, along with arsenic and cyanide. I argue that the modern cigarette is deeply defective and should not be sold or manufactured; I also argue, though, that people should be free to grow and smoke whatever they like, so long as this is for personal use and does not contaminate others. Tobacco is not a vice or a sign of weak moral fiber; it is just too dangerous to be made for sale. But if people want to grow and cure their own for personal use, the state should have no say in this. I also argue that even short of a ban there are simple steps that can be taken by regulatory agencies to reduce the dangers of addiction, cancer, and heart disease.

On a methodologic note: There is a vast historiography of tobacco, most of which sings the praises of the golden leaf. Fortunately there is also a growing body of more critical work, including Richard Kluger's *Ashes to Ashes* (on Philip Morris) and Allan Brandt's *Cigarette Century*. The present text is different in taking more of a global view (even if America remains the centerpiece) but also by virtue of being almost entirely based on the industry's formerly secret archives, now (and only recently) available online in full-text searchable form. In this sense the book represents a new kind of historiography: history based on optical character recognition, allowing a rapid "combing" of the archives for historical gems (and fleas). Searching by optical character recognition works like a powerful magnet, allowing anyone with an Internet connection to pull out rhetorical needles from large and formidable document haystacks. (Try it—you need only go to http://legacy.library.ucsf.edu, and enter whatever search term you might fancy.) The Internet posting of documents in this form presents us with research opportunities that are largely unprobed. The advantage is largely one of speed, but it also means that entirely new kinds of topics can now be investigated—the history of single words or turns of phrase, for example. It is hard to say how this will transform historical writing, but we are likely to find new paths opening up that we have not even imagined.

In addition to novel source access methods, this book differs from previous works in its parting animus. Allan Brandt in his *Cigarette Century* writes that the tobacco industry "is here to stay." But we don't have to be so fatalistic. There is nothing timeless about cigarettes; they had a beginning and will have an end, as was true for lead paint and asbestos insulation. I believe that the manufacture and sale of cigarettes will eventually come to an end—and not just for health or even environmental reasons. Cigarettes will be snuffed out because smokers themselves don't like the fact they smoke. Most smokers come to abhor their addiction and will be happy to have help escaping from it.

So here are some key points, or "theses," that I would like the reader to come to appreciate in the course of reading this book:

1. Cigarettes are the *deadliest* artifacts in the history of human civilization. Most of these deaths lie in the future.
2. Cigarettes are *defective* in the legal sense, meaning designed in such a way that they end up killing far more people than they need to.
3. Cigarettes would kill far fewer people if manufacturers would simply raise the pH (alkalinity) of cigarette smoke back up to 8 or above, making the resulting smoke uninhalable.
4. Cigarettes would also kill fewer people if they were not *designed to create and sustain addiction*. Tobacco addiction could be largely eliminated if cigarettes were required by law to contain no more than one-tenth of one percent (by weight) of nicotine—meaning content in the actual rod.
5. Cigarettes are *environmentally unsustainable*. Cigarettes are a significant cause of resource depletion, fires, and global warming—not to mention poverty—and these will likely prove a factor in their prohibition.
6. Cigarettes are *not a recreational drug*. Most smokers dislike the fact that they smoke and regret having started. This means that many (if not most) smokers will welcome their disappearance.
7. Commercial cigarette manufacturing should be abolished, but people should be free to grow, cure, and smoke whatever kinds of substances they like, for personal or noncommercial use.
8. Globally the point of "peak cigarettes" is already passed—albeit only in recent years. That downhill slide will continue, until the cigarette exists only as a curiosity and an object of distant memory of a more foolish time.

A NOTE ON THE TITLE

I use the term *holocaust* with caution, primarily to draw attention to the magnitude of the tobacco catastrophe. Obviously there are significant differences between the murder of six million Jews at the hands of the Nazis and the sufferings of smokers. In both instances, though, we face a calamity of epic proportions, with too many willing to turn a blind eye, too many willing to let the horror unfold without intervention. Apathy rules.

I should also note that there is a long history of using this term with reference to cigarettes. Alan Blum in his 1985 *Cigarette Underworld* describes the tobacco toll as a holocaust, following a 1971 report by Britain's Royal College of Physicians denouncing "the present holocaust—a reasonable word to describe the annual death toll" from cigarettes. A *Journal of the American Medical Association (JAMA)* editorial from 1986 deplored the "tobaccoism holocaust," and Michael Rabinoff in his 2006 book, *Ending the Tobacco Holocaust,* highlights tobacco's unparalleled carnage while deploring complacency: "and yet we do nothing." Similar expressions can be found prior even to the Second World War, as when Max MacLevy in his 1916 *Tobacco Habit Easily Conquered* pointed to news reports of "fresh holocausts on the altar of the nicotine devil," referring to the many lives lost from fires caused by cigarettes (the Triangle Shirtwaist conflagration in New York City, just to name one example). The word *holocaust* means literally "total burning," with the added implication of catastrophe, malfeasance, and crimes against humanity. The death of one innocent is sometimes said to be the death of all humanity—and there is great truth in this—but *the* Holocaust also teaches us that ethics often has much to do with scale. And for sheer magnitude, it would be hard to exaggerate the misery caused by tobacco's energetic merchants of death. In polite society we tend to trade in euphemisms, but when the truth itself is outrageous, weak words can falsify the realities of needless, outrageous sufferings.

Introduction

Who Knew What and When?

Southern trees bear a strange fruit,
Blood on the leaves and blood at the root
ABEL MEEROPOL, 1936

Pisgah Forest in North Carolina's Transylvania County may seem like an odd place for human health fortunes to have pivoted, but there's something to be said for it. Here in the fall of 1953 an experiment was conducted that would change how tobacco companies viewed the world, demonstrating to their apparent satisfaction that cigarettes can cause cancer. The setting was the Ecusta Paper Corporation, the nation's leading supplier of rolling paper for the American tobacco industry. For more than ten years the company had been churning out the thin white papers that, when rolled into cylinders around chopped fermented tobacco leaf, got smoked in the form of cigarettes. Cigarette paper wasn't their only product: the company also produced paper for Bibles and financial forms.[1] Death and taxes in a Bible sandwich, good coverage, vertical integration.

Cigarette paper hasn't gotten much attention in the recent tobacco wars, though it is worth recalling that you can't smoke a cigarette without also inhaling the soot, tar, and gases released by burning paper. Unlike a pipe or a cigar. Today we know to blame the tobacco for the lion's share of cancers—thanks in part to Ecusta's experiments—but there was a time in the 1940s and early 1950s when some people blamed a pesticide (such as arsenic) sprayed on the leaf, or a chemical agent used in its manufacture, or the stems and ribs increasingly used from the leaf, or vapors released by lighters or safety matches, or outgassings from the burning paper. People didn't seem to be falling ill so much from smoking pipes and cigars—and clearly there weren't so many cancers of the lung in former years, when cigarettes had not yet come into fashion. What was causing this epidemic of malignancies? And if it was the tobacco, or its method of preparation, or even the paper, what could be done

13

to stop it? Was there a poison that could be identified and eliminated, giving to-bacco a clean bill of health? Could cigarettes be made safe?[2]

KNOWLEDGE, LIKE IGNORANCE, HAS A GEOGRAPHY

A great deal of attention has been given to when the tobacco industry could have—or at least should have—known that smoking was killing people. The question has become of substantial legal interest, given the many recent lawsuits in which the *timing* of such events takes center stage. Historians are being asked to testify to whether the industry acted properly in the 1950s, 1960s, 1970s, 1980s, and 1990s, when the Tobacco Institute, the Council for Tobacco Research, and other industry bodies routinely dismissed claims that cigarettes could cause cancer or any other malady. Historians are being asked to judge at what point it is reasonable to talk about a "consensus" or "state of the art" regarding knowledge of such hazards and by what time it was no longer legitimate to ignore or dismiss such hazards.[3]

These are not trivial questions, and it is often not even possible to say when a particular body of evidence becomes convincing or "indisputable" without also ask-ing, Convincing for whom? And to what level of certainty? Our answers will de-pend on the community whose knowledge pulse we are taking, and we shouldn't be surprised if discoveries are received differently in different parts of "the" scien-tific community—whose homogeneity is easy to exaggerate. Methods are not al-ways uniformly appreciated, and different disciplinary communities can have very different prejudices or investments. Why should we expect new scientific findings to permeate every discipline at precisely the same rate? The presumption of a sin-gular and well-defined state of the art is an ahistorical construct lawyers have to deal with, as part of their job of dividing the world into tidy packages of innocence and guilt. The law is more digital than analog, with nuance often the first casualty.

Judged from a historical distance, it makes sense that there must have been a time when the tobacco men didn't know (or believe) that cigarettes could cause can-cer. There must also have been a point by which they had come to recognize this fact, by which time we are justified in characterizing their protestations of igno-rance (as in "We need more research") as negligent or even duplicitous. How and when did this change take place? When did the industry recognize the reality of to-bacco hazards? When did they start lying?[4]

One way to approach such questions is to distinguish between *public* claims and *private* communications, with the former represented by, say, press releases and the latter by the millions of internal industry documents divulged in the course of lit-igation, most of which are now available online at http://legacy.library.ucsf.edu. This is an unparalleled historical archive—indeed a treasure—that scholars have only just begun to explore and from which we get a good sense of the changing status of knowledge within the industry (see the box on page 15).

THE "SECRET DOCUMENTS"

Much of what we know about the internal operations of the tobacco industry comes from documents released in the course of litigation. Documents of this sort have been produced since the first health-based trials against the industry in the 1950s, but the floodgates didn't really open until the late 1980s, when attorneys for Rose Cipollone forced thousands of formerly secret archives into the open. Whistle-blowers such as Merrell Williams, a paralegal working for Brown & Williamson lawyers, would later smuggle out documents revealing a complex history of targeting children, manipulating nicotine, and conspiring to defraud, but this was only the tip of a much larger iceberg.

The industry tried to keep such documents sealed under court order, but as early as 1981 a body of documents subpoenaed by the Federal Trade Commission was leaked to the press, including the notorious "doubt is our product" memo from 1969. In 1998, as part of the Master Settlement Agreement with the attorneys general of forty-seven states, the accumulated documents—especially an enormous treasure trove acquired in the discovery phase of *Minnesota et al. v. Philip Morris et al.*—were released to the public. (The release had been worked out earlier under the terms of a settlement with the state of Minnesota.) The industry was forced to pay for the establishment and maintenance of a website posting these documents, which by the year 2000 consisted of about 44 million pages—and today consists of over 70 million pages, following addition of documents from BAT's Guildford depository in the United Kingdom.

Now accessible at http://legacy.library.ucsf.edu, the Legacy Tobacco Documents Library is the largest business archive in the world. Most documents are full-text searchable, and searches for terms like "cancer" or "nicotine" turn up hundreds of thousands of documents. Searches for terms like "baseball" or "sports" yield many thousands of hits. Optical character recognition was introduced in 2007, which means you can now search for expressions like "please destroy" or "subjects to be avoided," with options to order the documents by date or by size; one can limit one's search to documents from a particular company or a particular year or author or a particular document type (consumer letters, for example). Full-text searchability means you can probe the rhetorical microstructure of the archives; the expression "need more research," for example, yields 666 documents, and there are hits for terms like "Nazis" and "Negroes" and "zealot." Some famous public health books are found complete in the industry's files, so it is possible to search the complete text of, say, Glantz et al.'s *Cigarette Papers* simply by going to Bates 524540205–0662.

The secret documents have helped spark additional lawsuits against the industry. Computer technology has also helped level the legal playing field to a certain extent: companies with deep pockets used to be able to respond to discovery demands by flooding plaintiffs with unwieldy dumps of documents (known as "papering"), drowning the recipient in paper. That strategy backfired with the rise of the Internet, however, since most of these documents can now be searched by anyone with an Internet connection. The industry built in a clause requiring the documents to disappear after 2012, but Federal Judge Gladys Kessler in 2006 extended the life of these archives to 2021 as part of her ruling in *USA v. Philip Morris*, where the industry was found to have violated the federal Racketeer Influenced and Corrupt Organizations (RICO) Act.

Historians have only just begun to work through these archives. They should not be regarded as complete, however. Many documents have been destroyed, and many of the most sensitive have been held back on grounds of attorney-client privilege. Hundreds of thousands of documents remain hidden from view, and those that we do possess—though they number in the millions—should be regarded as faint traces of the trail left by the industry. We are truly looking through a very small keyhole into a very large room, but only one of many in the industry's secret mansions.

Publicly, the industry is notorious for having refused, time and again, to admit the health hazards of cigarettes—until the final years of the twentieth century. As late as 1994 the CEOs of the nation's seven leading manufacturers—the "Seven Dwarfs"—all stood up before the U.S. Congress and swore they did not believe that cigarettes caused cancer or were addictive. Then again, in 1998, Philip Morris CEO Geoffrey Bible testified under oath, "I do not believe that cigarette smoking causes cancer." Bible conceded a "possible risk" but not a "proven cause," the distinction lying in a kind of legal having-it-both-ways: an admission strong enough to ward off accusations of having failed to warn, yet weak enough to exculpate from charges of having marketed a deadly product.[5]

Privately, however, the companies were already discussing tobacco as a potential carcinogen by the 1940s. Industry scientists were keenly interested in the evidence starting to show that smoking could cause cancer and took limited steps to identify and remove whatever offending agents could be found in cigarettes. The goal for a time (beginning already in the 1930s) was to create a "safe" or at least a "safer" cigarette—though this was rarely expressed in public, given the reluctance to admit that tobacco was at all unsafe. And once the decision had been made to deny *all* evidence of harms—in 1953—it was difficult (for legal reasons) to stray very far from this path. Management must have known that the sordid admissions would eventually have to be made, but the hope was that this could be delayed into the indefinite future, into someone else's watch. It's as if they were operating a gigantic—and deadly—oncologic Ponzi scheme.

So when did the industry realize it was killing people? That turns out to depend on what you mean by "the industry." Even if we restrict our attention to manufacturers in the United States, it is difficult to establish a uniform time scale for the acceptance or recognition of hazards, since we are talking about large and complex organizations with tens of thousands of employees. Did tobacco growers know as early as the chemists employed in the industry's research laboratories? (Surely not.) What about the workers mixing the flavorants, or the lawyers guarding against lawsuits, or the CEOs running the show?

The tobacco men eventually came to speak with a single voice, but this required painstaking planning by some of the best brains of American hucksterism. Coordination was not without certain risks, of course, since the industry had been reeling from charges of collusion since 1911, when "Buck" Duke's American Tobacco empire was broken up through exercise of the Sherman Anti-Trust Act.[6] Even after dismemberment the companies had to ward off charges of illegitimate consort— there are examples from the 1930s and 1940s—and the perennial threat of regulation. This was a clear and present danger into the 1950s, and the stakes must have been high for the companies to risk yet another charge of collusion, as they did on December 14, 1953, when CEOs from the nation's leading tobacco makers met at the Plaza Hotel in Manhattan to plan a response to escalating publicity of a cigarette–cancer link. Paul M. Hahn, president of the American Tobacco Company, had organized the meeting, knowing that the industry could well be fighting for its life. And it was here, with the aid of the public relations firm Hill & Knowlton, that the industry decided to launch its infamous "Not Yet Proven" campaign of distraction, false reassurance, and manufactured ignorance.[7]

We also have to recognize, though, that smoking causes myriad different kinds of disease and that evidence for these various links comes at different points in time. Attention is often focused on cancer, but that is partly for legal reasons, having to do with the fact that it is easier to litigate a relatively monocausal disease (like lung cancer) than a malady with varied and diverse causes (such as heart disease). Tobacco kills more people via cardiac arrest, but since a higher *fraction* of all lung cancers are traceable to smoking, it is easier to win a legal case on the cancer front than on the (messier) field of the cardiovascular. Ninety percent of all lung cancers are caused by smoking, compared with only about a third of all heart attacks. This also seems to have influenced tobacco historiography; there is much more written about tobacco cancer than tobacco heart disease. Or emphysema or chronic bronchitis.

The lung cancer focus, though, is not unjustified. Smoking causes many other kinds of tumors—lip, throat, esophagus, tongue, gums, jaw, even bladder and female breast[8]—but pulmonary malignancies are the quintessential calling card of smokers, killing about 160,000 Americans every year and more than ten times this globally.

So when was it realized that smoking *causes* lung cancer? The question is deceptively complex, and our answer will depend on what stage in the process of medical discovery we want to highlight. So we can talk about the first *hypothesis* of such a link (1898, by Rottmann in Germany);

the first *textbook mention* of such a link (1912, by Adler in the United States);

the first *statistical evidence* (1929, by Lickint in Germany);

the first *chemical identification of carcinogens in smoke* (1930s, by Roffo in Argentina);

the first *animal experimental evidence* (1930s, by Roffo);

the first *case-control epidemiology* (1939, by Müller in Germany);

the first *cohort studies* (1952–54, by Doll and Hill in England and by Hammond and Horn in the United States);

the first *experimental pathology at autopsy* (1955, by Auerbach in the United States);

the first *tumor-location exposure correlations* (1957, by Hilding in the United States);

the first *consensus reports* by public health agencies, medical editors, and blue-ribbon committees (1950s–1960s in Britain, the United States, and many other nations); and so forth.

All of this must be qualified, however, by recognizing certain ambiguities when we talk about "firsts." Galileo, using his improved telescope, was apparently the first to find craters on the moon and rings around Saturn, but how do we talk about discoveries where there is less of a distinct "Eureka!" moment, or where the meanings of words are shifting? Who first discovered that nicotine is addictive, for example? Concepts of addiction have changed over time, along with the nuances and emotions attached to that term.[9] Was Christopher Columbus aware of addiction when he complained about his men being reluctant to give up their newfound habit? Did Native Americans have any concept of addiction centuries before the golden leaf spread to Europe?

There is also the question of how and when a "discovery" is accepted by some larger community of scholars. Galileo clearly deserves credit for discovering mountains on the moon, the phases of Venus, and moons around Jupiter, but how long did it take for his colleagues to accept these as incontrovertible facts? And whom should we consider in coming to such a judgment? All scholars? All natural philosophers? All astronomers? What about astrologers—which would include Galileo himself—or physicians or the noblemen and noblewomen of the courts for whom he was working?

We often talk about *when* a discovery is made, but it is also important to talk about *where* it is made and its fate once found. Knowledge is like a plant that sprouts and can either grow and spread or wither and die; there is never any guarantee it will flourish and always the danger of being choked off or destroyed by pests and deprivations. Or we can use the analogy of a viscous fluid: knowledge flows from one community into another, and some nooks and crannies will take longer than others to fill—especially when "interested" parties obstruct the flow. Knowledge has this complex fluid dynamics, and obstacles will often impede its spread.

Crucial, therefore, is how knowledge ebbs and flows in different communities. Lawyers like to talk about the "state of the art," but it is misleading to consider this only in the singular. "States" of the art will change over time, as will levels of expertise in different parts of the world. Physicians in modern Greece have been embarrassingly slow to appreciate the lung cancer hazard, for example, but even where the reception was relatively fast, as in Nazi Germany or postwar Britain, different medical specialties were unevenly prepared to acknowledge the discovery. Epidemiologists were generally quick to come on board, whereas pathologists and pharmacologists seem to have been slower. Think also about the knowledge expressed in different media—in corporate memos versus articles published in academic journals, for example, or in popular magazines and etiquette guides versus medical textbooks and governmental reports.[10] Or the messages delivered by consumer advocacy groups or in cigarette ads or the industry's films shown in schools. This is irregular terrain, and surveyors will not find it easy to identify a well-defined time at which "the" tobacco hazard was recognized. Cancers of the lips and mouth were recognized before cancers of the lung, and recognition of the heart disease link came even later. Crucial to our inquiry is, therefore, *recognized by whom* (and why) and *denied by whom* (and for what reasons)?

If we use the language of *consensus,* for example, we can distinguish a "scientific" from an "administrative-bureaucratic" consensus on, say, when the lung cancer link was established, recognizing that *the science* was secure (in the 1940s and 1950s) before governmental panjandrums gave it their seal of approval (in the 1950s and 1960s). And both of these can be distinguished from popular understanding, or what some lawyers like to call "common knowledge," meaning broad public (majority?) acceptance by ordinary people that tobacco can kill, which doesn't begin to emerge in the United States until the 1970s and 1980s.

Even so, we have to realize that millions of people still cannot be considered terribly knowledgeable in this realm. How many people know that tobacco is a major cause of blindness, baldness, and bladder cancer, not to mention ankle fractures, cataracts, early onset menopause, ectopic pregnancy, spontaneous abortion, and erectile dysfunction? How many know that smoking in Hollywood films causes hundreds of thousands of Americans to take up the habit every year? Or that filters release plasticizers into the lungs of smokers? Or that hookah—the water pipe rage on today's college campuses—is no safer than cigarettes?[11]

Efforts have been made to quantify our ignorance. In 1989 the U.S. Surgeon General reported a residue of about 15 percent of all adult Americans still unconvinced of major health harms from smoking.[12] We shall probe this more deeply in Part III, but here let me simply note that much depends on the language used to ask such questions. As early as the 1950s a majority of Americans were "aware"—had "heard"—that smoking might cause cancer; far fewer, though, were convinced. In January 2007 I asked the freshmen in my World History of Science class at Stanford if they were "convinced" that smoking is "the major cause of lung cancer." Ninety-one said "yes," but forty-four said either "no" or "don't know." These were bright young scholars, most of whom had hopes for a career in science or engineering, and it is striking that nearly a third were unconvinced of this crucial fact, arguably the most important in the entire realm of public health.

Complicating this "common knowledge" business is the fact that many smokers suffer from mental disabilities of one sort or another. Estimates differ on the precise fraction, but a 2004 review in the *New England Journal of Medicine* reported that people with a diagnosable mental illness are about twice as likely to smoke as people without such a disorder, and more than two-thirds of Americans undergoing treatment for substance abuse are also tobacco dependent. Schizophrenics are about three times as likely to smoke as people in the general population, with smoking rates an astonishing 60 to 80 percent or even higher. There is some evidence even that the industry targets the mentally ill—through Project Scum, for example, a 1996 plan to market Camel cigarettes to San Francisco "head shops" and "street people." (What kind of business refers to its customers as "scum"?) Tobacco addiction afflicts an estimated 55 to 80 percent of all U.S. alcoholics, epitomized by the fact that both of the founders of Alcoholics Anonymous died from smoking-induced disease.[13]

The truth is that most people do not know much about what goes into cigarettes or the extent to which the industry has been fooling them. I have studied these companies for decades and still have to rub my eyes from time to time, marveling at some new revelation of malfeasance or chicanery.

We also have to recognize, though, that even when talking privately among themselves, the industry's advocates may not be expressing themselves with entire candor. Opinions expressed in the industry's documents cannot always be taken at face value, since some are written as if someone were looking over the author's shoulder, with the intended audience being a judge or jury in some future lawsuit. Tobacco talk often has this "eavescasting" aspect[14]—the kind of speech President Richard Nixon used when conferring with his cabinet about Watergate, postulating some devious course of action that he would then pause to qualify by saying, "But it would be wrong," knowing there were tapes of all this to which others might one day listen.

Medical speech often has an interestingly opposite problem: discoveries may be cloaked in ambiguities, through artless prose or rhetorical conservatism. Medical research papers are often written using a kind of ethic of understatement—the persuasive force of modesty—reflecting a desire to establish minimal baseline measures for some known toxic hazard. No one can honestly accuse a Surgeon General's report of virtuosity or overstatement, but understated rhetoric of this sort is often exploited by the industry in court, where cautious estimates of the magnitude of a particular hazard—say, in a 1950s published scientific paper—are used to defend the polluter's stance of "not yet proven."

ISLANDS OF DOUBT

When did scientists in the industry's laboratories learn about tobacco hazards? We shall see in a later chapter that this is territory often ignored by the historians hired to make the industry's case in court; they want us to focus more on medical doubts and "common knowledge," with the industry itself reduced to a vanishing observer on the sidelines. They want us to focus on popular knowledge of harms and weaknesses in the science nailing down the harms. The strategy has been to put the plaintiffs or even the plaintiffs' experts on trial, blaming the victim and those who would come to their assistance.

Of course in the courts, with their oddly narrowed scope, the requirement is for a certain simplification. Complexity is not always welcome, given the binary nature of innocence or guilt. Complexity can even become partisan, insofar as it is used as a smokescreen to distort large trends or simple truths. Courts often talk about a "standard of care" or "state of the art" at some particular point in time, but these are procrustean legal categories that do not always fit with how scientific facts are actually established. The presumption is that there is a certain body of knowledge accepted in some relevant community. But the reality is that islands of stable doubt can thrive and flourish, along with competing research traditions and communities of principled dissent or disinterest, especially on questions involving political controversy—such as what to do about cigarettes.

This can make it difficult to identify a noncontroversial community of expertise—especially if powerful economic forces have been working to magnify or manufacture dissent. In such cases it may be hard to fix a well-defined moment when a particular discovery became "state of the art." That may even be beside the point, if the question is whether the industry has been lying. We need to learn to think not just about common knowledge and the state of the art but also about common ignorance and the state of the deception. And how both of these can influence popular or even scholarly understanding.

We also need to think more about the forces operating to influence what people *don't know* about cigarettes. Crucial to the companies' defense in court has been a certain self-effacement; they'd like us to think they have never been more than a dumb instrument for extruding product. This allows them to represent themselves as a trivial link in the carcinogenic causal chain, so that nothing they ever did shaped expert or popular opinion—or people's desire to smoke. Recall that for decades it was their contention that while *everyone has always known* that tobacco is bad for you ("universal awareness"), *no one has ever been able to prove it* ("open controversy"). For decades these have been the twin pillars of the cartel's legal stance: everyone knew, but no one had proof. The industry by this account was simply being cautious in taking its "not yet proven" position: we needed to get to the bottom of this controversy and didn't want to rush to judgment; we owed it to those poor souls who suffer from this terrible scourge (cancer) to move cautiously and carefully, without the emotional hysteria of anti-tobacco zealots.[15]

Big Tobacco's manipulation of both public and expert knowledge is the stuff of legends. Among its tricks are a dizzying array of ways to cast doubt on the relevant science. Journalists have been hired to publish industry-friendly articles, and scientists have been bankrolled to research industry-friendly topics. Industry-financed articles have appeared without proper disclosure in peer-reviewed journals, and there are instances where company agents have ghostwritten articles that later appeared in published form. Popular science magazines have been founded by the industry,[16] along with technical journals of various sorts. Scientific congresses have been organized and new fields of (decoy and distraction) research opened up. Research has been suppressed, slanted, and skewed—with deadly consequences. More often, though, the industry funded sound, basic research only marginally related to "smoking and health," just to be able to say, "We are on top of this. We are taking it seriously." Research was funded that was not likely to come to any kind of inconvenient truths, allowing the industry to be able to say, "See how hard we have looked and how little we have found!" The move is an authoritarian one, with dollars thrown to science for the prestige rub-off: "Trust us, we're the experts."

END GAME

Of course, much more is at stake than just "who knew what when"; we also have to come to grips with "what should be done?" The pages that follow, I am hoping, will convince any fair-minded reader that we have not done nearly enough to stop this, the deadliest of scourges, now spreading across the globe. We cannot rest with treating the cigarette as a problem of notification, or "information," or labeling (even if graphic), and the like. Forcing smokers into refugia (think airports) is also only an interim solution. Tobacco is not like wine but is rather more like smallpox or heroin. Tobacco manufacturers are vectors spreading the world's worst communicable disease (by numbers afflicted) and the most commonly abused drug. And we are talking about not just a health catastrophe but also a cause of global poverty and a threat to environmental health and to scientific integrity. Stronger steps need to be taken not just to stop its consumption but (more important) also to stop its production. Smokers are addicted, and we cannot place all the burden of choice on their shoulders alone. Cigarette makers make cigarettes because there is money to be made thereby, and we need to start thinking about how to channel those productive energies into less lethal pursuits.[17]

But first, how did we come into this world, where every day a billion people will inhale soot and tar from a burning chemicalized leaf and find it too painful to give up? To fully grasp this oddity, we have to know a bit about the tobacco plant, its history and chemistry, and the means by which it is turned into cigarettes. We have to understand its social and symbolic significance and its service to governments as a cash cow. We have to understand the vast scope and impact of cigarette marketing and how the propaganda engines of the industry keep smoking afloat—generating ignorance, naturalizing smoking, making it all seem banal and ordinary, something we just have to accept. How did it all get going?

PART ONE

The Triumph of the Cigarette

There is little doubt that if it were not for the nicotine in tobacco smoke, people would be little more inclined to smoke than they are to blow bubbles or light sparklers.

MICHAEL A. H. RUSSELL, 1971, ECHOING STATEMENTS MADE
THIRTY YEARS EARLIER BY CIGARETTE MAKERS IN GERMANY

THE TOBACCO PLANT is an odd creature. Botanists figure there are about seventy different species in the genus *Nicotiana*—all native to the Americas—several of which have been smoked, chewed, snorted, and "drunk" for hundreds or even thousands of years. (The drinking metaphor is interesting: many people for many years seem to have thought the smoke entered not the lungs but the stomach.) Native Americans used several species, the most popular of which was *Nicotiana tabacum,* a plant first cultivated, we now believe, in the highlands of Peru and Ecuador, probably around three thousand to five thousand before the so-called common era.

People smoke for lots of reasons but principally to obtain nicotine, the psychoactive substance named after Jean Nicot, the French diplomat who in 1559 brought the plant back to France following a visit to Portugal. "Tobacco oil" was quickly recognized as a powerful toxin, but it was not until the nineteenth century that its chemistry began to be deciphered. European scientists eventually recognized the active ingredient as an *alkaloid*—an alkaline substance with chemical affinities to opium, heroin, and quinine. The compound forms in the roots of the tobacco plant, from where it flows up into the uppermost leaves, probably as an evolutionary response to herbivory (nicotine secretions increase in response to plant munchers). The plant is a member of the Solanacaea family, which includes tomatoes and eggplant, which means that you can graft a tomato plant onto tobacco root stock and smoke the resulting (nicotine-loaded tomato) leaves as you might a cigarette. The reverse— tobacco grafted onto tomato roots—doesn't work.

No one knows what kinds of ailments were caused by smoking in the pre-Columbian Americas. Surely some of those from which we now suffer, albeit with far less frequency, since the art of curing and blending had not yet made it easy for

tobacco smoke to be inhaled. Tobacco seems to have been used primarily for rit-
ualistic purposes and principally by the elite. Some users must have become addicts, but we don't have textual evidence on this point and perhaps never will. Hundreds of ancient Mayan glyphs depict the tobacco plant and smoking rituals of
various sorts (see Figure 1),[2] but there doesn't seem to have been any tradition of
depicting maladies of any kind—apart from the occasional ritual mutilations where
royalty would cut their lips or genitals to release sacrificial blood. Tobacco-caused
illness cannot have been terribly common, though, because (1) smoking was not
ubiquitous or continuous, (2) inhalation was not widely practiced, and (3) marketing professionals were not yet exhorting us to achieve ever greater "smoking
satisfaction."

The *cigarette* is often described as a nineteenth-century invention, but we also
know that the Maya smoked tiny rolled tubes of the precious leaf, which we might
as well call "little cigars" (cigarettes, literally). Paper wrapping is one thing that
distinguishes the modern fag from its fatter brown brethren, and the fashion seems
to have come about by accident, in the first half of the seventeenth century in
Seville, Spain, "the world's first tobacco manufacturing capital," where beggars
rolled *papaletes* from tobacco scraps. Early European cigarettes were thus "a poor-
man's by-product of the lordly cigar—scraps of discarded cigar butt wrapped in
a scrap of paper."[3] Other accounts have the crucial innovation coming much later.
In 1832, for example, during Egypt's siege of Acre (in what is now Israel), an Egyptian cannoneer had improved his rate of fire by prerolling his gunpowder in paper tubes. He and his crew were rewarded with a pound of tobacco. Having only
a broken pipe, they rolled their reward up in the paper tubes they'd been using
for gunpowder, and voila! The modern cigarette was born.[4] (See also the box on
page 29.)

Cigarettes were not terribly popular until the early decades of the twentieth century, however, and their triumph can be traced to eight crucial events:

1. The invention of *flue-curing,* which made it possible for cigarette smoke
   to be inhaled;
2. The invention of *matches,* which allowed the making of fire to become
   mobile, convenient, and ubiquitous;
3. *Mechanization* of cigarette manufacturing via the Bonsack machine and its
   successors, allowing cigarette making to be astonishingly fast and cheap;
4. *Taxation* by governments, which recognized in cigarettes an unprecedented
   source of revenue, producing a kind of "second addiction";
5. The provision of cigarettes with rations in the *First World War,* which caused
   millions of soldiers on both sides of the conflict to become addicted;
6. *Mass-marketing techniques,* which allowed the sale of uniform brands
   throughout the United States and eventually the world;

SLANG FOR CIGARETTES

Slang terms for cigarettes are numerous, with English expressions including ciggies, smokes, tabs, straights, fags, rollies, ronnies, baccie, snouts, tailies, doogans (or dugans), durries, rettes, butts, squares (from the shape of the box), loosies (single cigarettes), bogeys, boges, gaspers, darts, hairy rags, hausersticks, jacks, joes, and grits. Older expressions include cancer sticks, coffin nails, pimp sticks, and "little white slavers." More archaic (and generic) for tobacco in general would be witching weed, Lady Nicotine, hay, alfalfa, coffee, cabbage, rope, henbane of Peru, ambassador's herb, Queen's herb, American silver weed, Indian-weed, nicotiana, killikinnick, smokum, the panacaea, and drunkwort.

For hundreds of other examples, including Native American terms and sixteenth- through nineteenth-century expressions for snuff, chewing tobacco, and the act of smoking or smoking devices, see Katharine T. Kell, "Folk Names for Tobacco," *Journal of American Folklore* 79 (1966): 590–99. Covered here of course are only the English variants; many other languages show a similar linguistic efflorescence.

7. *Manipulation of knowledge* of hazards by the tobacco industry, including the manufacture and dissemination of doubt and the hiring of experts to present industry-friendly narratives in court; and

8. *Manipulation of tobacco chemistry* to increase the potency, kick, and addictiveness of tobacco.

I shall be dealing with each of these over the course of the next few chapters. I would like the reader to keep in mind that the modern cigarette is a highly engineered artifact, the result of over a century of design by armies of chemists, breeders, psychologists, lawyers, and Madison Avenue marketeers. There is no "natural cigarette," and it is certainly not a natural thing to become a slave to burning leaves. Such has been the genius of the industry, to turn an occasional indulgence into a global addiction. That took some doing, and let's now see how this came to pass.

The Flue-Curing Revolution

Fire guides all things. . . . The death of fire is the birth of air.
HERACLITUS

Few discoveries have been so consequential, and it all came about by accident. In 1839, or so the story goes, a Negro slave by the name of Stephen on Abisha Slade's farm in Caswell County, North Carolina, fell asleep while tending the fires inside a tobacco-curing barn. With the fire in danger of dying, the man rushed out and, failing to find any dry wood, gathered up some of the charcoal normally reserved for the blacksmith's forge and threw this onto the fire. Charcoal burns much *hotter* than wood, which caused the tobacco to cure in a way never before seen. The leaves turned a bright golden yellow and smoked much *milder* than expected. This was especially true when the method was applied to plants grown in the so-called Piedmont ("foot of the mountain"), a 150-mile sandy stretch of Appalachia from Virginia down through North Carolina, already famous as tobaccoland. This new, blond, bright-leaf, "colory" tobacco fetched a high price on the market and with the proselytizing efforts of Mr. Slade spread quickly through the barns of the Piedmont.[1]

Flue-curing has the name it does by virtue of how heat is transferred to the tobacco leaves during the fermentation process. Low brick chimneys with closed, iron-conduit pipes had been introduced to reduce the risk of fire earlier in the century, and it was through these metal "flues" that charcoal-heated air was pumped to warm the tobacco. Flue-curing was quickly recognized as having two principal advantages: (1) barns were much less likely to catch fire (a big plus in the days of building with wood), and (2) the tobacco would no longer be exposed to smoky fumes that could wreck the taste.[2] The most important consequence, however, was in the realm of smokability. Unlike other varieties prepared by other means, the smoke from flue-cured "bright" or "Virginia" tobacco was easily *inhalable*.

A CANDIED-UP CONTRAPTION

Now, I suspect some readers may be asking, what is the point of smoking if you don't inhale? The remarkable fact, however, is that for most of human history, or at least those parts when people have been smoking, tobacco was generally not drawn into the lungs but rather only into the mouth and nose—and the occasional alternate orifice, as when Native Americans administered tobacco enemas. (French police in Paris in the eighteenth century recommended reviving drowning victims by blowing tobacco smoke up the anus.)[3] Recall also that smoke from cigars and pipes was (and is) rarely inhaled: smoke is taken only into the mouth, from where the nicotine passes through the lining of the oral cavity and thence into the bloodstream. Cigarette smoke from flue-cured tobacco, by contrast, can be inhaled easily into the lungs because the smoke is *far less alkaline* and therefore less harsh, less irritating. Cigarette smoke is more neutral, triggering none of the coughing mechanisms of alkaline pipe or cigar smoke.

Deep inhalation is largely the product of the flue-curing revolution of the nineteenth century, though the change did not occur overnight. Measured in terms of pounds of tobacco consumed, cigarettes in the United States did not surpass pipes and cigars until 1923.[4] The First World War helped popularize cigarettes, but cigarettes were also cheaper and more easily lit (and kept burning) than either pipes or cigars and were sometimes even boosted as a "safer" form of smoking—because they were "milder." Cigarettes also didn't have the fat cat or fuddy-duddy image of the puffer on a stogie or a pipe. The stock market crash of 1929 put another dent in demand for fat cigars, to the cigarette's benefit. Cigarettes were also more like a snack than a meal and could often be consumed without taking a break from work, and in this sense were something like the fast food of the tobacco world.

Flue-curing made cigarettes inhalable—and far more deadly. Inhalation was not an easy habit to induce, however, and many smokers (even of cigarettes) as late as the 1930s and 1940s *did not* inhale. Cigarettes were often smoked like "little cigars"—without inhaling, in other words—and epidemiologists in the 1950s still sometimes asked on their survey forms, "Do you inhale?" The (plausible) theory had emerged that inhalation was a far more dangerous form of tobacco use: after all, if smoke doesn't enter your lungs you wouldn't seem to stand much chance of contracting lung cancer. Epidemiologists eventually stopped recording inhalation behavior since by the 1950s most smokers were inhaling, encouraged by the urgings of advertisers (see Figure 2). Scholars also found it hard to rely on smokers' own accounts of their behavior—and there was the complication that even noninhalers inhaled quite a bit of (their own) secondhand smoke. Gauging inhalation was therefore difficult, clouded by the proximity of secondhand smoke.

Why, though, was smoke from flue-cured tobacco so much easier to inhale? The answer has to do with the fact that flue-curing alters the basic chemistry of the leaf, increasing its natural *sugar* content. Green tobacco leaf starts off containing a great deal of starch, which converts into sugar in the initial "yellowing" stage of the curing process.[5] This yellowing is achieved through the application of gentle heat, with high humidity. In later stages, however—typically four days into the curing process—the heat is cranked up to about 72°C, which deactivates the enzymes that would otherwise degrade or ferment the sugars in tobacco (as happens with other methods of curing). The high sugar content of flue-cured leaf yields a smoke that is less harsh, *less alkaline,* and therefore much more easily inhaled without stimulating coughing. Cigarettes made from flue-cured leaf are also more addictive than pipes or cigars, because the lungs are far more effective conduits of nicotine than the tissues lining the mouth. That is mainly because our lungs have an enormous internal surface area—about the size of a tennis court—offering lots of opportunities for nicotine absorption. This huge surface area also offers a fertile field for injury, which is why inhalers of smoke become vulnerable to emphysema, bronchitis, and cancer.[6] Cancers typically begin as single mutant cells that multiply and spread, and with more cells exposed to carcinogenic tars the risk of any one turning traitorous grows proportionately.

This business of sugar in tobacco leaf is a fascinating one—and insufficiently appreciated outside the tobacco man's labs. Sugar and tobacco have a long and incestuous history, and as one leading insider put it in the 1940s, "Were it not for sugar, the American blended cigarette and with it the tobacco industry of the United States would not have achieved such tremendous development as it did in the first half of this century."[7] The American-blend cigarette launched by Reynolds just prior to the First World War was in fact a candied-up contraption, in two different ways.

First of all, there is the already mentioned fact that flue-curing yields a high sugar content in the finished leaf, typically around 20 percent by weight or even higher. Leaves with such a high sugar content produce a milder, less alkaline, smoke as the sugars convert to acids when burned, neutralizing the bases generated with the combustion of leaf proteins, amino acids, and the nicotine alkaloid itself (an alkaloid is literally an "alkaline body"). The important contrast here is with the *air-cured leaf* used in plug or chewing tobacco, usually a variety known as "burley," which has very little sugar left after curing—only about 2 percent. Manufacturers of plug or chew therefore typically sweetened air-cured burley leaf—which was porous in a spongy sort of way—by soaking it in honey, sugar, or licorice. An added advantage was that sweeteners of this sort were cheaper, pound for pound, than unadulterated tobacco leaves. Virginia tobacco interests denounced this process, decrying the "perverted taste of the Yankees" who cared little for tobacco "but dearly loved sweets." So apart from the sugar produced (and preserved) by flue-curing, cigarette tobacco was further sugared up by adding sweeteners to burley leaf, which when combined with flue-cured came to be known as the "American blend."

THE WORLD'S DEADLIEST INVENTION

R. J. Reynolds in 1913 changed the world by launching its Camel brand, the world's first "blended" cigarette. The marketing was a marvel, and mechanization certainly helped, but flue-curing chemistry was also key to the new cigarette's success. Cigarettes prior to this time had typically been made from unblended flue-cured Virginia (or Turkish) leaf; Camel's innovation was to combine the lower pH of flue-cured with the higher pH of sweet-flavored burley. The success of the enterprise in the United States was aided by the disruptions of the First World War, which limited access to Turkish (oriental) leaves and forced a turn to domestic varieties. In a nutshell: this new "American blend" had two distinct advantages over previous cigarettes. It was *sweet and flavorful* from its use of candied-up air-cured burley, and it was *mild and inhalable* by virtue of its incorporation of low pH flue-cured leaf.

Milder, more flavorful, and inhalable, the American blend would quickly take the world by storm. Cigarette production in North Carolina—the epicenter of this new combo (at Winston-Salem)—grew from 2 billion to 28 billion sticks per year over the course of the First World War. In the seven years after Camels were introduced, R. J. Reynolds went from making about 0.2 percent of the country's cigarettes to controlling roughly half the American trade. Flue-curing also conquered Europe, and with the same deadly consequences. German tobacco scientists by the 1930s were tracing the global lung cancer epidemic to the increasing use of inhalable cigarettes; and inhalability was being traced to the pH of the resultant tobacco smoke. German medical men recognized the significance of this novelty: the great Fritz Lickint, for example, noted the "decisive medical significance" of low pH cigarette smoke, commenting that "while most people are not able to inhale the smoke of tobaccos from the alkaline group (i.e., pipe and cigar tobaccos), they are able to do so with a large percentage of the acid group (i.e., cigarette tobacco)!" Low pH cigarette tobacco, with its nicotine in a milder, non-alkaline, form, "made inhalation possible." Lickint was also prescient enough, however, to suspect that pipe and cigar tobaccos were being made milder to emulate the inhalation made fashionable with cigarettes.[8]

Flue-curing may well be the deadliest invention in the history of modern manufacturing. Gunpowder and nuclear weapons have killed far fewer people, as has all the world of iron. The creation of the cigarette has been compared to the invention of the hypodermic needle, but the comparison underplays a crucial difference. Syringes can be used or abused, but the cigarette kills when used as directed. An estimated 100 million people died from smoking in the twentieth century, and hundreds of millions more will die in the twenty-first if the epidemic is not curbed.[9] The industry could easily have prevented many of these deaths—the majority of all lung cancers, for example—by making a cigarette that was difficult to inhale. (European black tobacco for many years had a higher smoke pH, and smokers were less in the habit of inhaling.) Inhalation was also encouraged by advertisements celebrating its sensuous pleasures. Deep inhalation by the 1930s was being given an aura of sexual gratification, with dreamy stars filling their lungs and sensuous smoke-play about the nose and mouth.

We'll return to advertising in a moment. But first some words on two other innovations crucial for the triumph of the cigarette.

Matches and Mechanization

The triumph of the cigarette over the cigar has been the triumph of machinery over handicraft.
CURRENT OPINION, 1924

We tend to take it for granted, but it is not so easy to make a fire without matches or some kind of petrochemical lighter. Humans have been doing it for tens of thousands of years, perhaps even hundreds of thousands, but a great deal of skill is involved, including knowledge of what kinds of wood or stones must be selected (for rubbing or striking) and what kinds of powders can be used as tinder. Stone Age peoples struck flaked flints against pyrites, for example, allowing the spark to fall on fine dry moss or sawdust cut by termites or the dust of certain fungi, all of which required a certain amount of nature lore. Many of these same techniques were being used as late as the eighteenth century, when starting and keeping the home fires burning was a vital necessity throughout the world. In England, stories were told of homes where fires had been kept alive for more than a hundred years.

Chemical means of kindling fires have been around for centuries, though elaborate preparation was sometimes necessary, and techniques were not always reliable. China's invention of gunpowder in the ninth century made it possible to make a fire by impact, but this was never very practical. The British philosopher Robert Boyle, better known for his invention of the air pump, by 1689 had found that phosphorus rubbed against sulfur could cause ignition, but there was not yet any good means of controlling the combustion. Not until the nineteenth century were matches with a controlled phosphorus burn devised. A key breakthrough took place in 1827 when John Walker, an English chemist and apothecary, affixed a mixture of antimony sulfide and potassium chlorate onto the end of a stick by means of certain gums and starches, which when rubbed against a suitable surface would catch fire. Walker never patented his "Congreves," as he called them (honoring the rocket recently invented), which were in fact the first practical friction matches. He was not much of a businessman, and it remained for a London druggist by the name of Samuel Jones to mass-produce Walker's invention, which, when rechristened Lucifers, became so popular that for many years all matches in much of the world were known by this name.

The world's first "Lucifers" were foul-smelling and not terribly safe. Accidental ignition was one big problem, but they were also poisonous to manufacture. In the 1830s and 1840s the white phosphorus commonly used caused a degenerative rotting of the mouth known as "phossy jaw" among the English women who labored in factories to make these luxuries. So searches were launched for safer means of fire making. A breakthrough came in 1844, when Gustaf Erik Pasch in Sweden patented a match using red instead of the more dangerous white or yellow forms of phosphorus. Crucial in his invention was the fact that "safety matches," as he called them, could be struck only on a specially prepared surface on the box, circumventing the danger of accidental ignition. Safety matches made lighting fires easier and safer and were essential to the rise of the cigarette. Fires could now be lit with speed and convenience, even by someone with little skill and while standing up—by military sentries, for example. Fire making no longer required concentration, or even much in the way of skill, and by the end of the century it would be rare for anyone in the urban parts of Europe or the Americas to know how to start a fire *without* matches.

Part of the attraction was that matches are easily produced en masse in factories. Match-making machines were invented in the 1860s, and by 1868, when the Vulcan AB Match Factory was founded in Tidaholm, Sweden, production was on the order of hundreds of thousands of sticks per day. So whereas a skilled worker in the 1830s could make only four thousand or five thousand per hour, by the 1870s match-making machines had increased this rate by more than an order of magnitude. Paper matchbooks were invented by Joshua Pusey in America in 1889, and by 1896 the Diamond Match Company (which bought the rights to his invention) was making more than 150,000 matchbooks a day. "Close cover before striking" was added to the front for safety and presumably legal reasons, and this eventually became one of the most widely printed phrases in the English language.[1]

The twentieth century sees the proliferation of fire-making devices, notably the liquid-fuel metallic lighter, many early examples of which were crafted in the high style of Art Nouveau or the Arts and Crafts movement. Hundreds of different commercial versions were available by World War I, most of which catered to the nascent cigarette habit. A consolidation of sorts took place with the invention of mass-market lighters, the most popular of which was the Zippo, developed by George G. Blaisdell in Bradford, Pennsylvania, in 1932. Blaisdell improved on an Austrian design with a windproof wick, reducing the size to fit the palm of the hand, while also incorporating a hinge to allow a cigarette to be lit with only one hand. He also offered a lifetime guarantee, one of the first such offers for any consumer product. (The name came from Blaisdell's fondness for the zipper, invented in a nearby Pennsylvania town.) A paltry eighty-two Zippos were sold in the first month of production, but it wasn't long before the Bradford plant was cranking out eighty thousand *per day*. By the dawn of the new millennium more than 400 million had been sold worldwide. Match-making also continues apace, with Swedish Match alone (in the tiny town of Tidaholm) churning out 90 billion sticks per year.

SIXTY MILLION KILOGRAMS OF TAR

Readers of this book will probably never have seen the inside of a tobacco factory; nor, I suspect, will many even be able to imagine what this might look like. And for good reason: the industry doesn't like to convey the *scale* on which its products are manufactured. The numbers are literally astronomical. Six trillion cigarettes are produced every year worldwide, a thousand for every man, woman, and child on the planet. Six trillion cigarettes is enough to stretch to the sun and back, but it is also enough to fill the Great Pyramid of Giza some 24 times or the Empire State Building in New York about 60 times. This number is enough to cover a football field up to about a mile high or to fill the Colosseum of Rome some 250 times. In China you could pave the entire Great Wall (6,000 kilometers long) with a tightly packed surface of cigarettes three meters wide and nearly four meters deep. We're talking about 60 million cubic meters of cigarettes, smoked year after year after year.

Of course, we can also think about how much soot, tar, ash, cyanide, and other crud is sucked into smokers' lungs. If an average cigarette brings 10 milligrams of tar into the lungs of a smoker (a conservative estimate), this means that 60 million kilograms of tar are drawn into the lungs of smokers every year. If a railroad boxcar holds 10,000 kilograms, this means that a train of 6,000 boxcars filled with tobacco tar is pulled into the lungs of smokers every year.

The cigarette mongers don't like us to think about such numbers, but this was not always the case. In the 1940s and 1950s the industry bragged about how big and modern its factories were—how fast it could churn out smokes, how hard its chemists were working to bring you quality products. Tobacco industry admen boasted of their contribution to the war, by generating taxes, for example (see Figure 3). The industry at this point was still willing to deploy what might be called the *rhetorics of gigantism*—a form of speech that would slowly shift over to tobacco's critics in subsequent decades. The turning point was the mid-1960s, following which it was rare for the industry to brag about its size. Internal bragging lasted somewhat longer: in 1973, on the sixtieth anniversary of Camels, a magazine published for Reynolds employees and their families announced that three trillion (3,000,000,000,000) Camels had been sold since the launch of the brand in 1913.[2] An American Tobacco newsletter in 1984 boasted that its Lucky Strike brand had sold 2.2 trillion units.[3]

This brobdingnagian productivity is the consequence of *mechanization*. The story here begins in 1880, when a young Virginia inventor submitted a "new and improved" design for a cigarette-making machine to the U.S. Patent Office, successfully awarded one year later. James Bonsack had basically modified a carding machine from his father's woolen mill, transforming it into a device capable of producing a continuous stream of cigarettes with "a capacity of one hundred thousand cigarettes per day of ten hours." The new contraption worked by feeding chopped-up tobacco into a tapered compressing tube, where it was matted into a long and continuous ropelike form. This was channeled into yet another tube, where a continuous roll of paper was made to curl around the tobacco cylinder. The result was a cigarette of quasi-infinite length, which could then be cut to appropriate size by powerful whirling shears.[4]

It would be hard to exaggerate the impact of mechanization on cigarette consumption. Bonsack machines were crucial to the success of James Buchanan "Buck" Duke's American Tobacco Company, which struck a special deal with the inventor to acquire his machines at a special discount rate. Duke had fifteen machines by 1886 and twenty-four three years later. One Bonsack could crank out a hundred thousand cigarettes per day, doing the work of about five hundred of the "cigarette girls" paid to roll by hand.[5] This was fast, but subsequent machines were even faster— by nearly two orders of magnitude (see Figures 4–6 and the box on page 40).

(The fastest known hand-roller in England seems to have been a certain Lily Lavender, "Queen of the hand-rollers," who in 1897 in a contest against England's fastest machines rolled 162 cigarettes in the space of thirty minutes. A contraption made by Bernhard Baron, a leading competitor of Bonsack, easily trounced Miss Lavender by cranking out this same quantity of cigarettes in only thirty seconds.)[6]

Bonsack's machines made cigarettes very cheap, allowing Buck Duke to sell them for pennies per pack while still turning a handsome profit. Costs of production fell from 80 *cents* per thousand in 1880 to about 8 *cents* per thousand in 1895. The situation was interestingly different for cigars, which resisted mechanization. Cigars had always been made from whole leaves, which are much harder to manipulate than the chopped-up product rolled into cigarettes. Cigars are also wrapped in (whole) tobacco leaves—rather than in paper—which was difficult for a machine to master. Cigarette companies in the 1930s joined with cigar makers to try to mechanize this leaf-wrapping process, hoping to use leaves instead of paper to wrap cigarettes, but never achieved much success. That was a great disappointment, since many experts at this time feared that some of the health harms of cigarettes might be coming from toxins (such as acrolein) produced by the burning paper. Paper-free cigarettes never materialized, and indeed much of the "tobacco" used in cigarettes came to be essentially a form of paper, consisting of flat sheets of dried, pressed, and rolled tobacco pulp known as "recon" (for "reconstituted tobacco")—about which I shall have more to say in later chapters.

Cigarette production surpassed the making of cigars in both Europe and America

THE MECHANIZATION REVOLUTION

Modern tobacco factories are gigantic, highly automated enterprises built around high-speed cigarette-making machines. Among the leading producers of such machines are American Machine and Foundry, the Hauni Corporation in Germany, Arenco-Decouflé in Paris, and the Molins Machine Company in London. These and a few other companies fabricate high-performance machines that strip, shred, roll, cut, and package tobacco into cigarettes at speeds that boggle the imagination. Here are some performance milestones for the big rollers.

Year	Machine	Rate of Cigarette Production
1850s–1880s	Hand rollers @ 500–1,500/day	~ 1 per minute
1867	Susini machine	60 per minute
1885	Bonsack machine	210 per minute
1895	Decouflé machine	37 per minute
1895	Munson machine	300 per minute
1898	Baron machine (the Elliot)	480 per minute
1898	Briggs-Winston machine	300 per minute
1899	Improved Bonsack	500 per minute
1899	BAT's Venners machine	480 per minute
1924	Molins packing machine	600 per minute
1924	Standard Triumph machine	700 per minute
1924	AMF machine	800 per minute
1926	Molins Mark I	1,000 per minute
1951	Molins Mark V	1,250 per minute
1955	Molins Mark VI	1,600 per minute
1970	AMF's Ypsilon Maker	4,000 per minute
1972	Molins Mark VIII	3,000 per minute
1976	Molins Mark 9	5,000 per minute
1991	MMDP-8000 (JTI)	8,000 per minute
1998	Lorillard's machines	14,000 per minute
2000	Gallaher's machines	16,400 per minute
2006	G.D. 121P maker	20,000 per minute
2008	Hauni PROTOS-M8	19,480 per minute

It should be realized, of course, that feed and packing devices of comparable speed must accompany the machines to avoid bottlenecks. Cigarette factories thus have high-throughput hoppers, spray guns, cutters, drying ovens, filter assemblers, and so forth. Behind these machines—and feeding them—stand companies such as American Filtrona and Celanese manufacturing filters, paper suppliers such as Ecusta, and makers of testing equipment such as Arenco of Swedish Match, plus of course chemical companies that supply flavorants and humectants and the like, not to mention suppliers of laboratory equipment such as microscopes, mass spectrometers, spectrophotometers, refractometers, polarimeters, precision analytical balances, puff profile plotters, and automatic smoking machines. Such operations are a nontrivial component of the global tobacco economy—though smokers never see this side of their habit. While cigarettes are nearly ubiquitous, the means by which they are made are essentially invisible.

around World War I, and by 1924 it was realized that "the triumph of the cigarette over the cigar has been the triumph of machinery over handicraft."[7] Many of the world's most expensive cigars are still rolled by hand—though none I assume on the inner thighs of Cuban virgins, as was once mythologized. Most mass-market cigars nowadays are actually machine-made, with tobacco-paper recon wrappers making them very much like fat brown cigarettes. Some cigar manufacturers even use flue-cured tobaccos, making them nearly as inhalable as their whiter counterparts.

TWENTY THOUSAND CIGARETTES PER MINUTE

Bonsack's machine took the United States by storm—but it would be wrong to end our history of mechanization here. Britain's leading manufacturer, W. D. & H. O. Wills, contracted an exclusive agreement with Bonsack, which is one reason they were able to resist the American onslaught as effectively as they did. British manufacturers in the 1890s were using several different kinds of high-speed cigarette-making machines: Gallaher & Company in Belfast was supplied by the American Luddington Machine Company, which could manufacture cigarettes in different sizes; John Player & Sons in Nottingham used a machine called "the Elliott" made by Bernhard Baron in the United States; and the tobacco shops run by Salmon & Gluckstein installed a machine known as "the Munson," which could produce an estimated eighteen thousand cigarettes per hour. Other machines used in Britain included the Briggs, imported from North Carolina by J. S. Molins.[8] The net effect of mechanization was to consolidate cigarette manufacturing into an ever tinier clique of companies, forging oligopolistic dynasties that would dominate global manufacturing for much of subsequent history.

The French of course were not to be outdone, and by end of the nineteenth century Decouflé and Allegnon in Paris were making machines that rivaled Bonsack's both for productivity and reliability. The Italians and Germans also entered vigorously into this arena. The German case is particularly interesting, given that by 1930 the state of the art was such that *cigars* were also starting to be made by machines. German hand-rollers raised quite a big fuss about this, protesting that workers in the trade were in danger of being thrown out of work. Sellers of cigars advertised their products as "handmade," and one company even called itself "the enemy of machines" *(Maschinenfeind)*. The Nazi government responded with a law banning the use of machinery in cigar manufacture, hoping to ease the unemployment crisis. Cigar makers were grateful and returned the favor by supporting Hitler's regime. Even the storm troopers' own brand of cigarette, the Sturmzigarette, the chief source of income for the Brownshirts, was rolled by hand, eschewing mechanization to keep hand-rollers on the job.[9]

Machine speeds continued to increase throughout the twentieth century, and by 1956 the Mark VIII equipment made by the Molins company of London could crank out two thousand cigarettes per minute. (Philip Morris bought ten such devices in 1959.) The industry has never said much publicly about its machines, but from their internal archives we know that by 1973 Philip Morris in its new Richmond plant had 200 Molins Mark IX machines, allowing it to produce about a quarter of the cigarettes smoked in the United States. None of this came cheap: a Molins Mark VIII cost the British American Tobacco Company (BATCo) 16,200 pounds in 1971. Some tobacco authorities predicted a never-ending acceleration of manufacturing speed: in 1953, for example, Brown & Williamson executives envisioned a machine of the future that would roll, flavor, and finish cigarettes at a rate of ten thousand per minute. This turned out to be an underestimate, as we now have machines about twice that fast, shooting out about a mile of cigarettes—twenty thousand sticks— in any given minute of operation (see again the box on page 40). Packing machines were developed to keep up with the rollers, and by the 1980s Reynolds had machines that could fill and seal 205 packs per minute, with twenty cigarettes per pack. Filter makers had to be just as fast, and in 1981 the Hauni Corporation's KDF-2 Filter Maker spat out filters for the Reynolds company at the rate of "450 rod meters per minute."[10]

As important as speed, however, has been the reduction in costs associated with mechanization. Cigarettes today are as cheap as they are—far too cheap, in fact— largely because these indefatigable beast-machines are doing most of the work. In 1998, mechanization allowed Reynolds factories in Turkey to produce 2,847,000 packs of cigarettes per employee. That's more than a thousandfold increase in productivity compared to the hand labor of the nineteenth century. Mechanization and addiction are the two principal reasons cigarettes are among the most lucrative products ever sold. Hence again that famous comment from Warren Buffett, defending his takeover of R. J. Reynolds: "I'll tell you why I like the cigarette business. It costs a penny to make. Sell it for a dollar. It's addictive."[11]

Speed and lowered costs, though, are not the only consequences of mechanization. Increased machine speeds require careful control of the cigarette leaf: left to get too dry it will crumble, for example, and allowed to get too moist it will develop mold. Solving these problems required adding fumigants and humectants (moisteners) to the leaf. The modern cigarette is as adulterated as it is partly as a consequence of mechanization. Humectants such as glycerine are added to make the leaf pliable, to prolong shelf life, and to keep those chopped little bits from falling out of the cigarette. Hand-rolled cigarettes didn't need such additives, because they were finished with a little twist at either end to keep the tobacco in. Pre-Bonsack machines—those made by Susini and Sons in Cuba in the 1850s, for example—had churned out cigarettes with little paper twists at each end, but continuous process machines such as Bonsack's extruded cigarettes in one long column, which meant that at least one end had to be exposed (or both, if the cigarette didn't have a filter). These open-cut cigarettes lost their moisture faster, which was yet another reason for the use of wetting agents. Mechanization thus degraded the product in ways rarely appreciated outside a narrow circle of industry insiders.

Not that this mattered terribly much from a public health point of view. Quality control for the cigarette industry has always been something of an oxymoron, since the product itself is so toxic. Many of the industry's additives can be regarded as diluting a poison with yet another poison, which means that "quality control" with regard to cigarette manufacturing is sort of like a high code of ethics inside a criminal gang of thieves.

What is astonishing, though, is how little attention these machines have received from historians, policy makers, or even tobacco control experts. It is a rare tobacco control scholar who has ever heard of Hauni, G. D. (Generate Differences), or the Molins company. That is part of the larger conceptual bias we face: scholars study smoking *behavior* ad nauseum, describing in exquisite detail how cigarettes are consumed, but no one ever talks about how they are *produced*. That, of course, is precisely how the industry wants it: all the burden of "choice" is put on the smoker, with none on the manufacturer. Only consumers have "choices" in this scheme, with the industry itself left to its own devices and invisible. As if cigarettes were some natural and inherent part of human custom, a fact of nature or gift of God that we cannot refuse.

3
___

War Likes Tobacco, Tobacco Likes War

Wars greatly stimulate smoking in all forms.
HARRY M. WOOTTEN, INVESTMENT ADVISORY DIVISION,
REYNOLDS & CO., 1942

It makes sense when you think about it: why should anyone worry about cancer or emphysema thirty years down the road, when bullets are whizzing overhead? That's basically how tobacco's critics were silenced during the First World War, when the moralistic prohibitionism that had led to tobacco bans in fifteen U.S. states was brought to its knees. Fine young army boys may die tomorrow, so who are we to deny them the comfort of a smoke? The medical case against tobacco was not yet strong enough to resist the onslaught, and so the YMCA, the Red Cross, and other charities reversed their earlier opposition and started distributing smokes to the fighting men abroad. Cigarettes were included with military rations, and government commanders stressed the vitality of cigarettes for the war. General John J. Pershing, commander of the American forces in France, once quipped, "You asked me what we need to win this war. I answer tobacco as much as bullets!" General Douglas MacArthur would make a similar request from his Pacific theater of operations during World War II. Tobacco propagandists are fond of citing such comments, along with George Washington's 1776 appeal for aid for his beleaguered troops: "If you can't send money, send tobacco."[1] Patriotic charities during the Great War of 1914–18 rose mightily to the occasion, shipping 425 million cigarettes to dough-boys on the front in France every month in the peak years of the conflict.

CIGARETTES AS PATRIOTS

War has been important for smoking in several respects. War moves men and materiel around, transfecting fashions from one part of the world to another. The Crimean War of 1853–56 is notorious for having exposed Western fighting men to

44

Eastern cigarettes; the French, English, and Turks (Ottomans) were united against the Russians in this contest, so Turkish tastes flowed westward. Then again in the U.S. Civil War of 1861–65, northerners were introduced to southern tobacco habits—partly by theft, partly by dislocation. General Sherman raided the stocks of several tobacconists in his famous march to the sea, and when northerners came to like what they'd smoked, requests were sent down south for further supplies. Tobacco manufacturing shifted northward as a result, especially to New York, where dandies were eager to try new cultural fashions.

World War I was another crucial turning point in the rise of the cigarette. The fighting dragged on for years, and many a long night in the trenches was warmed by the friendly fire of fags.[2] Cigarettes were also a distinctly war-friendly form of smoke. Easy to light and quick to finish, they were conveniently smoked while standing, marching, or even (sometimes) shooting. And they didn't require that extra burden or distraction of the pipe. Thousands of soldiers etched their enthusiasm for smoke into ornately carved tobacco boxes and lighters, born from boredom in the trenches. The net effect: millions of soldiers returned home from the war addicted to this new form of smoking, spreading the habit in the peacetime world. The "war to end all wars" turned smoking from a marginal indulgence of questionable morality to an unobjectionable mark of stalwart manhood. More dryly put: war legitimized cigarettes. The numbers say it all: per capita consumption of manufactured cigarettes in the United States *nearly tripled* from 1914 to 1919, from 155 per year to 505 per year.[3] This is one of the most rapid increases in smoking ever recorded.

Cigarettes have been popular in subsequent wars, however. In World War II American cigarette manufacturers were required to turn 18 percent of their total output over to the military—by order of the War Production Board. And advertisers capitalized on the opportunity by linking smoking with patriotism, hygiene, and homespun virtues. The American Tobacco Company in 1942 eliminated the green from its Lucky Strike pack, claiming that the color had "gone to war" with the troops. (The pretense was to save on copper, but the green actually came from a chromium compound.) Smoking Luckies was equated with patriotic fidelity and "national intelligence," and cigarettes were even made to march in military formation in some of the world's first animated ads. Lucky commercials suggested military prowess but also a certain sensuality: "so round, so firm, so fully packed," as one animated series put it.

War works for cigarettes because it *distracts* from distant health effects, but cigarettes have served in other ways. In 1942 in the Philippines, native resisters of Japanese occupation were alerted to the impending American invasion by air-dropped packs on which American and Philippine flags had been printed, along with a signed message from General Douglas MacArthur, commander in chief of the Southwest Pacific Theater, announcing, "I shall return." The Tobacco Institute, the industry's chief propaganda oracle, would later sprinkle such stories into the popular press, along with pledges that tobacco would be ready to help in any future conflict, given its value as a "morale booster to fighting men."[4]

War has often been good for consumption, especially on the winning side. American consumption of cigarettes nearly doubled between 1935 and 1945, while smoking rates declined in many other countries. In Germany, for example, consumption fell by about half from 1940 to 1950, a decline only partly traceable to the Nazi campaign against tobacco and more directly a consequence of the impoverishment and dislocation (and death) of millions of people. Many European cigarette factories were destroyed, along with much of the continent's agricultural capacity. There weren't a lot of cigarettes to go around in Europe in 1945 and 1946—which is one reason America could step in with its mild, sweet "American blend" to readdict the Continent.[5]

THE MARSHALL PLAN

Most people will be surprised to learn that tobacco was a large part of the Marshall Plan to rebuild Europe. The total value of all goods shipped to Europe from 1947 through 1951 was about $13 billion, about $1 billion of which was tobacco. Nearly a third (!) of all "food-related" funding in the plan went for tobacco. In 1947 alone the European Recovery Administration shipped ninety thousand tons of tobacco free of charge to Europe. Critics at the time objected to tax dollars being used to support a frivolous or even dangerous habit: George Seldes, a New York consumer advocate who published In Fact, a kind of Naderite broadsheet avant la lettre, was vocal on this point, lambasting this "most amazing" feature of the plan, according to which "the hungry people of Europe, whether they like it or not, will have to take almost half as much in tobacco as in bread and other foodstuffs, because there is an unsaleable surplus of tobacco in the U.S." Seldes reported speculations that American tobacco interests were hoping to use the plan to spread the demand for American-style cigarettes into Europe; tobacco was supposed to be part of an effort to halt the expansion of communism. In 1948 Seldes published an article titled "Tobacco vs. Communism," quoting Virginia Congressman John W. Flannagan's assurance that tobacco gifts to Europe "will aid in eliminating or retarding the spread of ideologies antagonistic to democracy and to world peace."[6]

The origins of this tobacco bonanza are interesting. Tobacco was not originally considered for inclusion in the Marshall Plan. It was not mentioned in the speech delivered by George C. Marshall to Harvard's graduating class on June 5, 1947, in Sanders Theater, where such a plan was first called for. And it did not figure prominently in the plan drawn up in Paris six weeks later by the seventeen nations considered for inclusion in the program. It was not until southern legislators got hold of the plan that tobacco was included. The key figure here, interestingly, was Senator A. Willis Robertson from Virginia, father of the televangelist Pat Robertson, who insisted on having tobacco figure big in the shipments. There is a certain irony in this demand, given that the elder Robertson was an ardent opponent of alcohol, which he railed against from time to time on the floor of the U.S. Senate. Robertson knew where his bread was buttered, however, and tobacco farmers appreciated his support.[7]

Here is a good place to honor the life and work of George Seldes, the first American journalist of any note to realize that tobacco was causing an epidemic of lung cancer, based on work being done in both Germany and the United States. Seldes was one of the first journalists to publicize Raymond Pearl's 1938 discovery that cigarettes were cutting the lives of smokers short by nearly a decade and one of the first to report that magazines and newspapers were reluctant to challenge the industry by virtue of their dependence on tobacco ad revenues.[8] Seldes is often ignored by cigarette historians, and one reason is that his crusade came before the time was ripe. There was not yet much of an audience for left-leaning cigarette criticism in the 1940s and 1950s. Anti-tobacco fervor had dwindled from its peak in the early years of Prohibition (1919–33), and surviving pockets often had a pungent puritanical odor. German physicians were railing hard against the demon weed, but German science had lost much of its prestige overseas since the persecution of the Jews and withdrawal from the international scientific community. (Seldes never comments on Nazi anti-tobacco work—though he does reveal that while posted as a journalist in Berlin he had been advised not to smoke by a certain Dr. Johann Plesch, a professor of medicine at the University of Berlin.) Even in the United States, though, anti-tobacco rhetoric usually came from more conservative quarters—such as *Reader's Digest*, which tended to regard tobacco as an insult to the temple of the body and a flight from traditional American values.

Tobacco control really wasn't an issue for progressives in the 1950s, despite fears along these lines from some corporate heavies. (William Randolph Hearst Jr., the publishing magnate, in 1954 expressed his fear that "anti–big business fanatics" might turn the cigarette–health angle into "another means of attack on American business.")[9] The fact, though, is that the political left was conspicuously silent on smoke during this period, and most liberals smoked—with Seldes being rather exceptional in both respects (he had quit in 1931 following his encounter with Professor Plesch). And even Seldes's voice was pretty much silenced after 1950, when his beloved *In Fact* newsletter, subtitled *An Antidote for Falsehood in the Daily Press,* was forced to halt publication. The closure was largely for financial reasons, as his subscription list shrank with the lurch to the right in American culture. McCarthyism was just beginning to rear its ugly head, and Seldes himself was soon thereafter (in 1950) called to appear before the House Committee on Un-American Activities to answer charges of Communist sympathies—which were quickly dropped. (He had never been a member of the Communist Party and carried on an oddly intimate correspondence with FBI chief J. Edgar Hoover about this.) By the time the lung cancer–tobacco link was rediscovered in the early 1950s, with study after study confirming the connection, Seldes was no longer in a position to rally anti-tobacco forces. And though he went on to live another forty-five years—departing only in 1995 at the age of 104—his courageous tackling of tobacco was largely forgotten. Today his life and work should serve as a reminder that history is often a tale of forgetfulness and that being right and being early are no guarantees of glory.

As for the Marshall Plan: global tobacco charity continued long after its formal demise, through successor programs such as Food for Peace. The U.S. Department of Agriculture (USDA) continued to unload surplus tobacco in the Third World for decades thereafter, with American farmers dutifully compensated. In 1964 the USDA had an estimated $500 million worth of tobacco leaf in storage, with allotments going to friendly governments at rock bottom prices the world over. Which even the conservative *Barron's* magazine deplored as making Washington a kind of international Typhoid Mary.[10]

Taxation

The Second Addiction

All governments love money much more than your life.
THE SCRIBE, ANONYMOUS BLOG, 2009

It is strange when you think about it: millions of people are killed every year by tobacco, but governments don't seem to mind very much. Worse, they bend over backwards to encourage it. Governments throughout the world promote the cultivation and manufacture of tobacco via subsidies to farmers, price supports, and agricultural training. Agricultural field stations help farmers learn how to plant, fertilize, and harvest the golden leaf, and most nations have incentives to promote its cultivation. Why do governments encourage the growing and manufacture of such a dangerous consumer "good"?

The simple answer is revenues from taxation. Tobacco is easily taxed, thanks to several key features of its cultivation and manufacture. For one thing, cigarettes are fairly homogeneous. Packages are standardized for convenience of sale and manufacture, which also renders them easily monitored for taxation purposes. Taxation is also facilitated by the fact that months or even years are required to bring the finished product to market. A tobacco leaf harvested in the fall is typically not smoked until two or even three years later, with the intervening time devoted to curing, cutting, blending, "casing" (i.e., flavoring), reconstituting, rolling, and packaging, plus, of course, distribution, display, and sale. The final product also has a relatively long shelf life, which makes it easy to come under the surveillance of taxation authorities. Imagine, by contrast, taxing bread or broccoli: each loaf or head is different and cannot be stored for more than a week or two (without freezing), the packaging is not uniform, and profit margins are low. People also are not addicted to bread or broccoli, which means that if prices go too high they can always turn to substitutes. Tobacco, by contrast, has a fiercely loyal clientele: most smokers say they want to quit but can't, which translates into a low price elasticity. A 10 percent rise in prices means roughly a 4 percent decline in consumption, though this will fluctuate according to how wealthy a society is and how deeply addicted.

Summarizing, then: tobacco taxation is facilitated by the long time delay between harvest and use, by centralized distribution of the finished product, by the high and inflexible demand, by durable packaging and a long shelf life, and by the homogeneity of the finished article. Addiction adds the final touch: most people find it hard to quit smoking, harder even than to give up heroin or cocaine. Smokers are therefore a "captive market" and may be willing to pay five, ten, or even twenty times what it costs to make cigarettes because they cannot do without.

CASH COW

Tobacco has been taxed at least since the seventeenth century, and perhaps even earlier by Native American elites, whom we know to have used the cured leaf as a form of tribute. The big push to tax didn't come until the nineteenth century, however, when governments started to rely on pipe and cigar taxes as a source of revenue. Tobacco taxes accounted for nearly a third of the U.S. government's entire income by the 1880s, by which time many nations had recognized "the golden leaf" as a cash cow. Spain had established a tobacco monopoly in 1636, and France followed suit in 1674.[1] Britain's was actually the first, established by King James I in 1619. Austria's tobacco monopoly was established in 1784, Poland's in 1924. Japan Tobacco monopolized the production of cigarettes in that country for most of the twentieth century, and though many of these monopolies have been eroded by privatization and the iron arm of global trade—aided by the cigarette transnationals and their allies—they still rule the roost in many countries.

Even when tobacco has not been monopolized, however, national governments have profited greatly from tobacco taxes. In the United States in the mid-1930s, tobacco taxes brought the federal government nearly as much (73 percent) as the income taxes paid by individual earners. Yugoslavia in the 1930s got more than 22 percent of its governmental income from tobacco taxes. A 1935 estimate figured that European governments *on average* obtained about 15 percent of their income from tobacco taxes. Those numbers diminished in the postwar era, as affluence expanded the tax base. In 1950, however, tobacco taxes still supplied Britain with 20 percent of its state revenue. And in the mid-1960s tobacco monopolies provided 5 percent of the national budget in France, 10 percent in Italy, and 15 percent in Taiwan. China as recently as the 1990s was getting more than 10 percent of its entire governmental income from tobacco taxes. Zimbabwe is highly dependent on tobacco; it used to produce about 230,000 metric tons per year, though the chaos in that country under Mugabe has shifted some of that business to its neighbors, notably Malawi and South Africa.[2]

Germany is an interesting case, since the Nazi government received about 10 percent of its income from tobacco taxes, and some Nazi party organizations depended heavily on cigarette revenues. Hitler's notorious Brownshirts (also known as the *Sturmabteilung,* or Storm Troopers) received about two-thirds of its income from tobacco taxes, an arresting fact overlooked in most histories of the Third Reich. Several of Germany's leading political parties had their own brands of cigarettes, which they used to generate income. The Brownshirts produced a "Storm Cigarette," for example, which provided handsome revenue even though Hitler was always grumpy about smoking.[3]

China is also remarkable, given that it was a relatively minor consumer until the Revolution of 1949 that brought Chairman Mao to power. From about 80 billion that year cigarette consumption grew to 200 billion in 1960, 300 billion in 1970, and 1200 billion in 1990. By the mid-1990s the Chinese were smoking a whopping 1.7 trillion (1,700,000,000,000) cigarettes per year, nearly a third of the world's total. The Middle Kingdom by this time had 180 cigarette factories and 500,000 people working to produce nearly a thousand different brands. The Communist Party has promoted the farming and manufacture of tobacco as a source of revenue for the Chinese state, but at what cost? Deng Xiao Peng's vision of "socialism with a Chinese face" has this ghoulish aspect, that hundreds of millions of Chinese alive today will die from smoking even if this policy is reversed (since many of the health effects won't be felt until decades hence). Beijing's leaders are mostly nonsmoking engineers who need to realize that China is going to face a health catastrophe over the next few decades—my colleague Matthew Kohrman calls it "an extermination"—unless steps are taken to curtail smoking.

Today, though, the Chinese government is still doing far more to promote tobacco than to limit it. Coercive means are being used to induce farmers to grow tobacco; farmers get only about 2 percent of the value of the finished manufactured product and often don't even want to grow tobacco but have no choice. Many foreign companies are trying to get a foothold in China, but so far the government remains the largest single producer. The Chinese army owns a number of cigarette factories, and the government did not issue a formal statement on health hazards until 1979.[4] And the China National Tobacco Corporation (CNTC) paints a rosy view of the golden leaf. In 2005 the CNTC website crowed, "Smoking removes your troubles and worries," quoting a thirty-seven-year-old magazine editor's words, "Holding a cigarette is like having a walking stick in your hand, giving you support. Quitting smoking would bring you misery, shortening your life." The government sells the Longlife brand of cigarette with these same reassurances.

Privatization has been a double-edged sword when it comes to health impacts. It generally leads to increased competition, which allows foreign manufacturers to penetrate domestic markets, bringing their aggressive tactics. In most cases this means an increased sale of Japanese, British, and American cigarettes, which tend to be less harsh and therefore easier to inhale; they also tend to be doctored with additives and chemically manipulated to maintain addiction. Keeping a state monopoly has risks of its own, however. Monopolies typically don't have to submit to independent regulation, they are often harder to tax (because the taxer is the taxee), and their cozy relationship with the government often makes them immune to litigation or other forms of social accountability.

Tobacco taxes are now very high in many European countries. In 2008 a pack of twenty premium cigarettes in the United Kingdom cost nearly £6, or about U.S.$10. France, Germany, Ireland, and all the Scandinavian countries have very high taxes. Norway may well have the highest in Europe, with a pack of twenty costing 70 krone, which is about $12. About 90 percent of this is tax—which is why smokes in other parts of Europe can be bought for less than one-tenth this amount. Cigarettes in most parts of the Balkans (Serbia, Montenegro, Albania, etc.) still cost less than a dollar a pack. Cigarettes are even cheaper in certain parts of Asia.

The United States has some of the world's lowest national cigarette taxes, measured as a fraction of retail price (currently less than 10 percent). Taxes are also imposed at the state level, however, which means that cigarettes vary widely in price. Kentucky, for example, was taxing cigarettes at a rate of only 3 cents per pack as late as 2005, when the state legislature raised it to 30 cents. South Carolina still taxes at the rate of only 7 cents per pack, and Missouri charges only 17 cents. Rhode Island currently has the highest state tax ($3.46 per pack in 2009). New York State has allowed the city of New York to levy an additional amount, bringing state and local taxes in Manhattan and the other boroughs to nearly six bucks. (A pack of Marlboros can now cost upwards of $11, and singles are being sold—illegally—for a dollar apiece.) Residents of Indian lands are still able to buy cigarettes tax-free, though efforts have been made to close this loophole. In most states, though, taxes do not make up even half the retail price, a legacy of the power of the industry to suppress all challenges to its rule.[5]

WHO'S TO BLAME FOR SMUGGLING?

Taxation is potentially one of the most powerful means of tobacco control. It has be done with care, however, since it also creates an incentive for smuggling wherever tax rates are uneven ("buttlegging" is what some like to call it). Criminal and terrorist gangs are sometimes involved, and the industry itself has not exactly remained neutral. In the 1990s more than 70 billion cigarettes were shipped every year from the United States to Antwerp, even though few of these were smoked in Belgium. Most ended up on the black market: Winstons were trucked to Spain and Marlboros to Italy, with the origin disguised to evade taxation.[6]

The companies say they don't like smuggling, but they are also known to have aided and abetted it. In 1994, for example, Canada was forced to lower its federal cigarette tax in consequence of cross-border smuggling from the United States;

Canadian manufacturers had helped organize the illegal transport of Canadian brands into New York State, from where they were routed via Akwesasne Indian lands back into Canada. By 1995 an estimated one in three cigarettes in Canada's eastern provinces was being sold illegally. Tobacco manufacturers then used this to demand a rollback in tobacco taxes (to stop smuggling!), and the plan succeeded: taxes were reduced, and smoking rates rose in response. The same thing happened in 1999 in Sweden, where some of the world's highest tobacco taxes were abandoned in response to smuggling from Estonia and Poland. Smokers were also able to evade local taxes by ordering cigarettes by mail from tobacco-friendly places like Greece. Buttlegging became such a problem in the United Kingdom in the 1990s that the country's dominant manufacturer, Imperial Tobacco, was sued for having conspired to aid and abet illegal distribution. Philip Morris was likewise sued in November 2000 for helping to organize the U.S.-Antwerp ring. Philip Morris and BAT also benefited from massive smuggling operations organized in Colombia, which caused many local farmers to shift from tobacco to coca (for cocaine) as illegal imports undercut local brands.[7]

Internal documents from British American Tobacco reveal the company collaborating with its Argentine subsidiary, Nobleza-Piccardo, to exploit smuggling opportunities in northeastern Argentina. The company used the term *duty not paid* (D.N.P.) to designate this illegal trade, described as a "significant market yet to be satisfied." One element in this plan was to introduce the Jockey Club brand as a D.N.P. cigarette in Posadas, a town on the border with Paraguay notorious as a crossroads for illegal transit. BAT already had "long-standing strength in the D.N.P. region" and was hoping to leverage this strength with the goal of "maximizing group profit from the D.N.P. trade." BAT knew that the Argentine government would eventually move to close this opportunity and emphasized being prepared "to vacate the D.N.P. segment completely without leaving a vacuum which our competitors are better placed to fill." Plans were also made to introduce similar products legally into Brazil "to protect N-P [Nobleza-Piccardo] from accusations of complicity."[8]

Smuggling has long been a global phenomenon. An internal industry report from 1980 conceded that roughly 30 percent of all Italian cigarettes were smuggled, and during the peak years of the 1990s as much as a quarter of the world's entire cigarette trade was illicit. Clamp-downs in the new millennium—including self-policing by companies worried about their image as criminal co-conspirators—seem to have cut this illicit trade by about half. Even so, smuggling still involves hundreds of billions of sticks every year, with $40 billion to $50 billion lost in revenue to governments.[9]

In some parts of the world, however, smuggling has been and remains more the rule than the exception. In the Ukraine in 1999 President Leonid Kuchma announced that three quarters of the cigarettes sold in his country were either smuggled or produced illegally. For many years cigarette makers did little to combat illegal trade or even encouraged it—and not just in Canada, Sweden, or Britain. In

2001, for example, documents came to light showing that British American Tobacco had organized a smuggling ring involving the illegal shipment of hundreds of millions of cigarettes into Somalia, Afghanistan, India, and Pakistan. One corporate document from 1987 notes that "transit to Sudan will be supplied via Kental [a Cypriot trading company] and Somalia via Easa Gurg," Dubai's ambassador to London. *Transit* was another code word used by the multinationals for smuggling, as revealed by BAT's internal admission that "opportunities for legal imports need to be fully investigated before we seek transit opportunities." Cyprus has long been a crossroads for contraband, though the problem exists wherever there are inequalities in tax rates. New York's Chinatown even today is awash in illegal cigarettes, mainly knockoffs of Marlboro and other popular brands counterfeited in the People's Republic.[10]

Prosecutions for smuggling have increased in recent years, partly as a result of increased global port vigilance in the wake of the attacks of September 11, 2001. More diligent searching of containers has cut out part of this illicit trade, but police and customs officials have also become more vigilant. In January 2003, for example, two hundred German customs officials raided the Hamburg offices of Reemtsma, a subsidiary of Imperial and the maker of West and Davidoff cigarettes, arresting several board members, including the company's sales and marketing director, for smuggling. Imperial became the world's fourth biggest tobacco company following its acquisition of Reemtsma in 1998 and is thought to have been making half of the cigarettes smuggled into England.[11] The World Health Organization's Framework Convention on Tobacco Control has called for more careful product tracking across international borders, to help put an end to illicit trade.

Taxation inequalities can of course open opportunities for illegal transit, but usually only if the industry cooperates and local law enforcement is weak. Crucial to keep in mind, though, is that smuggling fosters smoking. Smuggled cigarettes are usually cheaper than the legal variety, but smuggling can also help to popularize a new brand, giving it a kind of "street cred." Smuggling also has the effect of undermining market restrictions (bans on imports, for example), which serves to undermine local monopolies. And since smuggling is illegal, the companies can even argue that taxation leads to illegal activity—that is, smuggling—which can then be used to argue for lowering taxes. Which is precisely what happened in Canada and in Sweden.

The industry claims that taxes cause smuggling, but the fact is that smuggling tends to be low where taxes are high—because those tend to be places (like Norway or Sweden) where the rule of law is respected. Versus, say, Albania, where nearly three quarters of the market is illicit, even though cigarettes cost only about 31 cents per pack.[12] And penalties are generally weaker if you are caught smuggling a legal product than some other form of contraband (cocaine or weapons, for example). It is bizarre that ordinary packages shipped by UPS or Federal Express have electronic tracking while crates and cartons of cigarettes do not. Nor do we yet have the kind of high-tech tax stamps that would help prevent counterfeiting. Smuggling could easily be reduced if the problem were taken seriously.

A THIRD ADDICTION?

I've spoken about taxes as the "second addiction," but in the United States there is arguably a *third* addiction insofar as states that successfully sued the industry in the 1990s now rely on the health of the tobacco trade to guarantee an uninterrupted flow of litigation payments. The Master Settlement Agreement (MSA) of 1998, forged to compensate state governments for medical costs from smoking, required the companies to pay $250 billion to the states over a period of twenty-five years, but the tobacco men were clever enough to include riders that allow them to *stop* making payments if revenues fall below a certain point. And in the new millennium, when judges and juries began considering awards to plaintiffs in other cases, some state attorneys general sent industry-friendly letters to the courts supporting limits on such claims. The fear has been that high-price awards will hurt the companies' ability to make their payments to the states. That is one reason the MSA has been viewed as a sellout,[13] a kind of joint embrace with the cancer mongers. The MSA can be thought of as an excise tax, with lawyers taking part of the proceeds and a side benefit for the companies in the form of informal guarantees of financial stability. Which is also why tobacco stock prices have skyrocketed in the intervening years.

Governments throughout the world are now addicted to the continued sale of cigarettes. Taxing the industry can be a great way to reduce smoking, but since taxes are more often seen as a way to fill state coffers, it is hardly surprising that most successful politicians remain soft on tobacco. It is easy to blame smokers for their foolish habits, but governments must also shoulder part of this blame, both for what they do and for what they fail to do. It is a callous calculus, but governments are likely to do the right thing only when they realize that the cost of *paying* for smoking-caused diseases cuts perilously deep into the benefits derived from taxation. And this doesn't even count lost productivity from premature death and disease and costs from environmental damage and fires. Considered as a whole, we are talking about a habit that exacts a far greater toll than what is derived from taxation.

Marketing Genius Unleashed

More doctors smoke Camels than any other cigarette.

Come to where the flavor is, come to Marlboro Country!

CIGARETTE SLOGANS

We tend to take it for granted, and find it hard to imagine a world without, but *branding* on a broad scale is an invention of the nineteenth century. And the grand curse and creation of the Americas. Ivory soap was one of the first: Procter and Gamble launched its campaign to market a "99.44 percent pure" mix of lye and fat in 1882, by which time there were only a few other branded consumer products sold nationwide. Americans in different parts of the country could buy Uneeda Biscuits, Paine's Vegetable Compound, Royal Baking Powder, and the like, but widely advertised and standardized consumables were just beginning to emerge—along with coast-to-coast marketing.

Advertising grew with the spread of newspapers and (later) popular magazines, as new packaging and transport technologies made it possible to attach name brands to common household goods. Coca-Cola was invented in 1886 and by the end of the century was available from Atlanta to Los Angeles. W. K. Kellogg launched his first national cereal in 1906 (in *Ladies' Home Journal*), and R. J. Reynolds began marketing Prince Albert (roll-your-own) tobacco nationwide one year later.[1] And though many such brands were destined to fail, several of the winners had spectacular careers. A 1920 study of the most popular revealed a host of names still familiar today: Kodak cameras, Singer sewing machines, Campbell's soup, Wrigley's chewing gum, Colgate toothpaste, and Welch's grape juice, for example.[2]

And Camel cigarettes.

Camel cigarettes were unveiled by the R. J. Reynolds Company in 1913, following a billboard and newspaper blitz announcing "the Camels are coming." Oriental themes were already common in the trade, with prized brands having names like Sultan, Omar, Fatima, Mecca, Murad, and Mogul, advertised with tropical or

U.S. CIGARETTE CONSUMPTION AND LUNG CANCER DEATHS, 1900–2010

Year	Billions Smoked	Cigarettes Smoked per Capita (adults)	Lung Cancer Deaths
1900	2.5	54	Extremely rare[a]
1905	3.6	70	Extremely rare
1910	9	151	Extremely rare
1915	18	285	400[b]
1920	45	665	n.a.
1925	80	1,085	n.a.
1930	119	1,485	2,837
1935	134	1,564	5,049
1940	182	1,976	8,086
1945	341	3,449	12,130
1950	370	3,522	18,313
1955	396	3,597	26,826
1960	484	4,171	36,420
1965	529	4,259	48,483
1970	537	3,985	65,927
1975	607	4,123	82,799
1980	632	3,851	104,456
1985	594	3,461	123,146
1990	525	2,827	141,963
1995	487	2,515	161,815
2000	430	2,092	155,967
2005	389	1,777	163,500
2010	340	1,500	157,300

Sources: Tobacco Outlook Report, Economic Research Service, U.S. Dept. of Agriculture; NCI, ACS, USDA. Includes cancers of the trachea, lung, bronchus, and pleura.
[a]Only 140 known cases recorded worldwide prior to 1900.
[b]Number is from 1914, the first year lung cancer was listed as a cause of death in the United States.

desert backgrounds and sultry women in suggestive poses. Cigarettes were not yet as popular as pipes or even cigars, but the trend was clearly upward: only 2.5 billion cigarettes were smoked in the United States at the turn of the century, but by the end of the "war to end all wars" Camels *alone* would be selling ten times that (see the box on this page).

And with this came the great "shakeout," as local trademarks succumbed to the onslaught of standard brands. A German manufacturer has estimated there were thirty thousand different brands of cigarettes by World War I, with some of this efflorescence stemming from efforts to discourage counterfeiting (Susini and Sons in Cuba, for example, routinely changed its wrappers to stymie European fakers.) Cigarettes were locally rolled and playful by design, with odd and curious brand names like Fire Cracker, Freckled Squaw, and Sour Grapes. Some were flagrantly libertine or even comic, thumbing their noses at fuddy-duddy prohibitionists: so we have fin-de-siècle cigarettes with names like Christian Comfort, Coffin Nail, and Forbidden Fruit. Cigarettes were often considered an effete or sissy smoke by comparison with cigars or pipes, whence macho brands like Police Club, Carrie's Hatchet, and Scalping Knife.[3] R. J. Reynolds's nationally advertised Camel brand forced many of these smaller marks out of business; some were bought up by the bigger boys, but most just vanished without a trace.

SHEEP DIP AND SKYWRITING

Hungry for the same kind of success as Reynolds, the companies reborn from the Duke empire breakup established their own flagship brands. Liggett & Myers rolled out Chesterfields in 1912, and three years later began a Camels-style national campaign. The American Tobacco Company launched its Lucky Strike brand in 1917, crafting it to appeal to women as well as men. Camels, Luckies, and Chesterfields would dominate for decades, capturing 88 percent of the U.S. market by 1930, though Lorillard did pretty well with its rejuvenated Old Gold, transformed into a "standard brand" in 1926. Brown & Williamson broke into the majors in 1933 with its menthol-flavored Kool, a cigarette later popular with—because of deliberate marketing to—African Americans.[4] The explosive growth of smoking didn't lift all boats, but it did mean that brands selling less than a billion per year were no longer considered "significant."

Slogans.   Key for these early brands were carefully crafted slogans. Smokers were said to be willing to "walk a mile for a Camel," a catchphrase developed in 1921 for Reynolds by the Ayer Advertising Agency, already famous for coining Morton Salt's: "When It Rains It Pours." (The same company later won with de Beers's "A diamond is forever" and the U.S. Army's "Be all you can be.") Luckies' signature was, "It's toasted," joined later by its "Reach for a Lucky instead of a sweet!"—which irritated candy makers to no end.[5] (One might even wonder whether candy cigarettes were a kind of compensation to candy makers for the "Reach . . . sweet" slight.) Chesterfield's was originally "They do satisfy," later condensed (in 1915) to "They satisfy."

Some slogans make you want to scratch your head, they sound so odd. The American Tobacco Company in 1931, for example, ran a series of ads boasting that its "toasting" process expelled the "sheep-dip base naturally present in every tobacco leaf." The background here is convoluted and has to be understood in terms of how tobacco leaves were processed. The crucial fact is that in the process of steam heating prior to manufacture ("toasting"), some pretty awful gases are released. This was taken as evidence that toasting "purified" the leaves used in Lucky Strike cigarettes. Tobacco manufacturers collected and condensed these foul, acrid gases and sold them in liquid form to farmers as an insecticide for livestock: "sheep dip." Sheep would then be driven into large vats of this smelly stuff, usually with a jump-off from a platform of some sort to make sure their heads got submerged. This "sheep dip" from "toasting" killed whatever lice, ticks, or fleas might be on the animals— which certainly was better, or so we were led to believe, than inhaling that same stuff with our favorite cigarette. Whence the value of "toasting" and its sheep-dip defense.

Advertisers eventually realized that positive images sell better than negative, though the lesson has never been perfectly learned. R. J. Reynolds as recently as 1973 praised its Focus cigarettes for delivering "no more plastic taste"—which helps explain why nothing much came of this clumsily handled brand. Philip Morris fared much better with its "Call for Philip Morris," rung out by a diminutive hotel bellhop named Johnny Roventini. A charming four-foot gentleman, Roventini was "discovered" by an adman in the New Yorker Hotel in 1933, whereupon he was hired to croon his signature "Call for Philip Maw-ree-ass" on radio shows beamed to every corner of the nation. As "the world's first living trademark," Roventini eventually traveled the country for his cigarette superiors, dining with President Eisenhower and talking politics with Richard Nixon, all the while smoking Marlboros. He has often been called a "dwarf" but was actually a midget—and referred to himself as a "Lilliputian." Roventini didn't seem to mind being turned into a kind of one-man tobacco-ad freak show; with his image on countless billboards, magazine ads, and cardboard cutouts, Philip Morris credited him with supplanting the cigar store Indian, the once-ubiquitous ornament of the smoke shop.[6]

Tobacco makers have always been careful to match up slogans with popular sentiments: patriotism in times of war, feminism in times of emancipation, savings in times of hardship, medical reassurance in eras of "health scares," and so forth. Cigarettes are equated with "risk" when they want to capture the imagination of masculine youth, with slimness or "diets" or glamour to capture the female cigarette "vote." Whatever will sell—and by whatever means.

Indeed it is probably fair to say that the industry *invented* much of modern marketing. Tobacco manufacturers were the first to advertise using color lithography (in the 1850s) and among the first to use coupons and photo inserts (cigarette cards) to attract customers. Cigarettes were the first items advertised by skywriting and also the first products sold using billboard panel photolithography (in the 1970s). Tobacco mongers pioneered animated cartoons (for use in movie theaters) along with product placements in Hollywood films, "impulse buying" in grocery stores (by clever shelf placement), human trademarks such as Roventini, "graphic branding" on towels and the like, brand-linked merchandising of items such as T-shirts and coats (in Marlboro stores) and even product-linked vacations and "expeditions" (Marlboro Adventure Teams and Camel Expeditions, as we shall see). Cigarette paper makers got into this act: the Rizla company, a subsidiary of Imperial Tobacco Ltd., in 1996 launched "Rizlaware," a line of clothing intended to promote its roll-your-own cigarette papers. It also created Rizla Suzuki, a road bike racing team. In 2005 alone Rizla sold enough rolling paper to circle the earth some fifty-two times, or to make a continuous path from the earth to the moon and back three times.[7]

Tobacco cards.   Tobacco cards were an early triumph from the middle decades of the nineteenth century. Stiff cardboard inserts had been used to keep cigarette packs from being crushed; manufacturers eventually realized these were ideal surfaces for ads and that if the designs were fine enough people would collect them. By the 1870s manufacturers were printing thematic series onto such cards—famous Indian chiefs or pin-up queens, for example, or dog breeds or presidents or heroes of baseball or boxing or some other sport. These were popular in a nascent era of collecting and indeed must have helped spawn such crazes, judging from the plethora now offered at any given moment on eBay. The gimmick soon spread into Europe, with cards eventually featuring "the German army" and "pictures of the Führer" and hundreds of other themes. The world's first baseball cards were actually stiffeners in cigarette packs; a recent history of the topic notes, "The tobacco industry is responsible for baseball cards as we know them today."[8]

Skywriting and Skycasting.   Another innovation was introduced in 1923, when a state-of-the-art biplane flew over Times Square in New York City, spelling out "Lucky Strike" in giant, mile-high letters. Major Jack Savage from Britain was paid a thousand dollars for each six-minute flight, but the American Tobacco Company apparently judged it worth the expense, given the sensational press coverage. The campaign was quickly extended nationwide, with 122 cities covered in 1923 alone. Lorillard was not to be outdone and in 1928 introduced "skycasting," a technique by which a professional radio announcer would fly three thousand feet above Manhattan in a three-prop Fokker, urging (by massively amplified voice) the smoking of Old Gold cigarettes. According to a (preposterous) report in the *New York Times,* the voice was amplified "a hundred million times." Skycasting did not last very long, but other kinds of gargantuan gimmicks would persist: Allan Brandt in his *Cigarette Century* recalls the huge smoke rings blown by the Camel Man on Times Square, torn down in 1966 only to be replaced (twenty-three years later) by an even larger neon Joe Camel, erected as part of the Winston-Salem company's plan to "youthen" its image to compete with Marlboro.[9] Nostalgia for such grandiose ads has been featured in many films, and the industry itself has tried to capitalize on nostalgia by reintroducing "classic" or "anniversary" brands with retro imagery.

Comic strips.   As a vehicle for selling cigarettes, the earliest comic strip ads date from the 1930s, drawing flak from publishers worried by this flagrant move to target children. In 1935 newspaper mogul William Randolph Hearst asked Reynolds to shift its cigarette ads from the comics pages to the adult sections of his papers, accusing the tobacco manufacturer of engaging in "a direct effort to teach the children to smoke cigarettes." Reynolds by this time was spending 15 percent of its advertising budget on Sunday comics, reaching 23 million readers in 149 different newspapers. Hearst's protest drew a polite but firm riposte from S. Clay Williams, Reynolds's chairman of the board, who claimed that comic strip adverts were in no way designed to attract children; the comics (he said) were principally for adults.[10]

Billboard photolithography.   Yet another invention of the tobacconists followed the 1970 federal ban on tobacco advertising on television. Manufacturers were desperate to find new ways to reach customers, to fill the void from the broadcast ban. Billboards had been a common advertising edifice prior to the Second World War, though television had caused something of a demotion in the 1950s and 1960s. Most people today will have forgotten that large-format billboards used to be painted by hand, according to a kind of mega paint-by-number process. This was tedious and time-consuming, and Philip Morris contracted with Kodak to develop a new process by which large-format images of, say, the Marlboro man on the open range could be printed on prefabricated sheets. Billboard painting soon thereafter became an obsolete trade, replaced by on-the-spot assembly and pasting of outsized photographic panels. American cigarette makers spent many millions of dollars on billboards prior to their disappearance as part of the 1998 Master Settlement Agreement, though advertising by such means is still quite common in many parts of the world.

Radio broadcasts.   Tobacco sponsorship of radio began in the 1920s, with popular comedians such as Jack Benny hosting and hawking cigarettes. American Tobacco's *Lucky Strike Radio Hour* entertained millions with its Lucky Strike Dance Orchestra; transcripts of shows from the late 1920s contain thousands of ads for Luckies, touted as "the healthy cigarette" and "a splendid alternative to fattening sweets." Famous personalities were invoked to hammer home this "health in Luckies" theme: the actress Irene Bordoni smoked Luckies "to keep petite"; George Gershwin smoked them to keep "physically fit and mentally alert"; and Al Jolson smoked them to keep "peppy" but also because Luckies were "as sweet and soothing as the best 'Mammy' song ever written."[11] Toasting was boosted as a "mouth disinfectant" and "the most modern step in cigarette manufacture." And we learn that visitors to the Lucky Strike factory in Reidsville, North Carolina, left "with a sense of sweetness, with a sense of cleanliness, with a sense of efficiency." Transcripts of such shows reveal the announcers' words being very carefully chosen: in one such set wherein

Luckies get more than 1,800 plugs, the word *throat* crops up 98 times, but *lungs* are not mentioned even once.[12] Such omissions are revealing; this is true even for the industry's private internal speech. So among the thousands of named secret projects, there are projects for every sign of the zodiac save one; I'll leave it to the reader to guess which (clue: it has to do with crabs).

Films and television.   Cigarettes are among the very first products advertised on film. The oldest movie ads date from the 1890s; Thomas Edison's charming ad for Admiral cigarettes is from 1897, for example, which may well be the world's first "commercial" (it can now be seen on YouTube).[13] Tobacco ads were common in movie theaters by the 1920s and on television by the 1940s. State-of-the-art animation was used in several of these, as in 1948, when American Tobacco aired its famous "dancing cigarettes," using stop-motion photography techniques first developed by animators working for French tobacco manufacturers (George Pal's famous "puppetoon" from 1932, shown in European theaters, featured dancing cigarettes). Ads of this sort were a big hit with the public, but they also showed how valuable television could be as an advertising medium. Cigarette makers were avid early sponsors of TV, from news and sports to sitcoms and dramas. Philip Morris sponsored *I Love Lucy*, the nation's number one show for most of the 1950s, with extra pay going to Lucille Ball and Desi Arnaz for endorsing Philip Morris cigarettes in magazine ads. (*I Love Lucy* when it first aired in 1951 featured animated matchstick figures of Lucy and Ricky climbing down an oversized pack of Philip Morris cigarettes.) Even lesser shows like *Public Defender*, with heavy Marlboro plugging, captured 12 million viewers per week. Lorillard started sponsoring televised baseball in 1948, which is also about when Brown & Williamson started sponsoring televised college basketball. Careful studies were made of the reception of such broadcasts, and by 1948 Kool's makers knew that 3.5 people per TV set were watching on any given evening, with a sponsored-brand recall (one day later) of about 68 percent.[14] These were exceptionally good results, prompting a mad rush to the medium. And by the 1960s 45 percent of *all* television shows in the United States were being brought to you by cigarette manufacturers.[15] Cigarettes remained the most widely advertised product on television until 1971, when ads were banned from the airwaves by an act of Congress.

CIGARETTES ON THE SILVER SCREEN

Cigarettes owe more to film than is commonly realized. In a calculated effort begun more than a century ago, tobacco was brought to many remote parts of the world using movies as an enticement. British American Tobacco introduced cigarettes into China, for example, by showing films to village crowds and then offering cigarettes for sale or as free samples. Other parts of the world started smoking by similar means. The first "moving pictures" ever shown in Korea were screened in the final decade of the nineteenth century, when British cigarette agents rented a barracks to show a series of French film shorts for the Korean Tobacco Company. Free admission was granted to anyone with an empty box of the company's cigarettes. British American continued this practice of using film to spur cigarette sales when it set up its first manufacturing plants in Korea in 1906. Here again, free admission was offered to anyone who could produce ten or twenty empty boxes of a BAT brand.[16] Similar techniques are still being used in poorer parts of the world: in Pakistan, for example, Philip Morris subsidiary, Lakson, makers of Diplomat cigarettes, as recently as 2008 was running a "mobile cinema" luxury truck through remote parts of the Karakoram mountains, showing films while enticing young viewers to smoke.[17]

Hollywood's romance with cigarettes began in the 1920s, when the industry landed on the idea of paying actors and studios for brand endorsements ("testimonials"). Studios benefited from the massive budgets allocated for such ads, which lined the pockets of literally hundreds of actors, not to mention singers, sportsmen, and at least ten U.S. senators. The tobacco archives contain contracts signed by some of the world's most beloved stars of the silver screen—people like Clark Gable, Spencer Tracy, Joan Crawford, and Claudette Colbert. From the very first feature-length "talkie" of 1927 *(The Jazz Singer)* through 1951, at least 195 Hollywood stars endorsed cigarettes. Studios brokered cigarette contracts, and the tobacco companies "spent more to advertise Hollywood than Hollywood spent to advertise itself."[18] And that was just the beginning.

Product placement was banned by the studios as early as 1931, but there wasn't yet much of a need for tricks of this sort, given how easily the actors themselves could be bought. Television also later became such a wildly successful vehicle for cigarettes that little thought was given to surreptitious branding. Much of that changed with the broadcast ban of 1970, however, and the rush to create new ways to advertise. Reynolds in its 1971 Management Plan recognized the value of "sponsored films," noting that short subjects (travelogues, sports highlights, musicals) and full-length features showing company brands could be used as "subtle forms of advertising to the cinema audience." The plan was to explore both short subject and feature-length film "plugs" as advertising opportunities, with test programs planned for 1971 that would include "opportunities in ethnic cinema."[19] Reynolds's budgets from the 1970s already show thousands of dollars allocated for "movie plugs" or "brand plugs."

The golden age of implants began in the 1980s, when tobacco companies started paying high-profile actors to smoke or flash a particular brand on screen. Sylvester Stallone in 1983, for example, agreed to smoke Brown & Williamson brands (such as Kool and Bel Air) in five of his forthcoming movies, for which he signed an agreement to receive $500,000.[20] Stallone's sweatshirted jogging up the steps of

Philadelphia's Museum of Art to prepare for his fights-against-all-odds has become a film icon—a life-size statue of Rocky erected for one of the scenes still stands nearby—but today's viewers may find it odd to see the "Italian Stallion" or his co-stars smoking in such flicks.

In the real world of athletics, of course, smoking-while-in-training was already an anachronism long before Stallone started puffing for cash. In 1941 Gene Tunney, the former heavyweight champion, had attacked the use of athletes to sell cigarettes in an article for *Reader's Digest*. Tunney was then in charge of physical training for the U.S. Navy, and to emphasize the strength of his convictions issued a challenge to world heavyweight champion Joe Louis: "If Joe Louis will start smoking, and promise to inhale a couple of packages of cigarettes every day for six months, I'll engage to lick him in fifteen rounds!" Tunney added that Louis would surely refuse, since he too knew that "No boxer, no athlete in training smokes. He knows that whenever nerves, muscles, heart, and brain are called upon for a supreme effort, the tobacco user is the first to fold."[21] Tunney while preparing for a previous fight (with Jack Dempsey) had been offered and refused $15,000 to endorse a certain brand of cigarettes, citing Ty Cobb's view that cigarette smoking "stupefies the brain, saps vitality, undermines health, and weakens moral fiber."

(Prior to World War I Ty Cobb had allowed his name to be used on tobacco cards—as "King of the Smoking Tobacco World"—to market Sweet Caporal and Polar Bear cigarettes; the baseball star had also appeared in ads for American's Tuxedo brand.[22] His biographers note his fondness for briar pipes, so his doubts about cigarettes seem not to have extended to other forms of tobacco. In 1928 he appeared in ads for Old Gold cigarettes, and in 1954 he was paid again to endorse Luckies.)

Stallone's agreement to smoke-for-pay in films is not unique. Dozens of Hollywood stars have taken such payments, including Paul Newman, Sean Connery, and Clint Eastwood. Brown & Williamson gave Newman a car worth $42,307 for placements in *Harry and Son;* Connery received $12,715 in jewelry for placements in *Never Say Never Again;* Eastwood got a car worth $22,000 for *Killing Ground,* and so forth. Product placement was common by the 1980s, when more than fifty different companies specialized in brokering such deals. Philip Morris paid $350,000 to have Lark cigarettes featured in the James Bond thriller *Licence to Kill,* for example, and *Superman II* had twenty-two distinct Marlboro implants, including a gigantic Marlboro billboard on the side of a truck that Christopher Reeve (as Superman) bursts through during the film's final climax. Philip Morris paid 20,000 British pounds to get its famous red-roof chevron (code-named "the Material") into the movie, which also featured a chain-smoking Lois Lane—a first for her since her debut in comics in the 1930s. In 1987 and 1988 alone Philip Morris provided free cigarettes and other props (including Marlboro signs) for fifty-six films. There was no shortage of opportunities, as the tobacco giant was being sent 150 scripts per year by this time—which amounted to about a third of all Hollywood films being made. Twentieth Century-Fox and several other studios had special merchandising divisions for handling product placement.[23]

Reading how smoking was incorporated into such scripts can be amusing. A 1989 Charlton Heston film titled *Solar Crisis*, for example, lists the following "Storyline" and "Potential Exposure":

> *STORYLINE:* "The sun has gone haywire and we have to go to the sun to fix it". It's a heck of a job, and Captain Steve Keslo leads the group of astronauts and scientists on a mission to save the world. With his father, Admiral Keslo, and his son Mike, Steve is motivated even more to save the lives of those below. One of the masterminds of the mission, Alex Noffe, makes great sacrifices for the success of the project, but will that be enough . . . ?"
> *POTENTIAL EXPOSURE:* LUCKY STRIKES, PALL MALL and CARLTON CIGARETTES will be seen in the bar. Steve Keslo will smoke LUCKY STRIKES throughout the film.[24]

Fifty other films are described in this same memo, and for each an "exposure" opportunity is offered. For *White Palace,* starring Susan Sarandon, "Nora will smoke Pall Mall Cigarettes throughout the film." For *3000,* starring Julia Roberts, "Vivian's friend, Kit (Laura San Giacomo) will smoke Carlton Cigarettes throughout the movie." (This was released in 1990 as *Pretty Woman.*) For *Harlem Nights,* starring Eddie Murphy, "Lucky Strike & Pall Mall Period Packaging will be seen in the Night Club on the bar counter and being smoked by the patrons."

Marketing and PR agents often specialized in arranging cinematic implants. In 1981, for example, the firm of Rogers & Cowan in Beverly Hills recapped its work for Reynolds over the past twelve months, during which cigarettes had been successfully placed in *The Jazz Singer* (the remake, with Neil Diamond), *Backroads* (Sally Field), *Cannonball Run* (Burt Reynolds), *Pennies from Heaven* (with Steve Martin), *Blowout* (John Travolta), *Rich and Famous* (Candice Bergen and Jacqueline Bisset) and "many, many others." The company also scripted cigarette-friendly spots for television—on *Good Morning America,* for example, where Paul Newman was shown practicing lighting two cigarettes at once for his remake of *Now Voyager.* Rogers & Cowan also supplied cigarettes to TV talk show "green rooms" (where guests wait when not on stage), worked with fashion photographers to make sure models smoked, distributed photos of smoking celebrities, and placed a story about Mikhail Baryshnikov smoking four packs a day as part of his ballet routine.[25]

The use of smoke in film is often defended on grounds of historical realism, but more often than not we are talking about a falsification of history. Stanton Glantz and his colleagues at the University of California, San Francisco (UCSF) have shown that Hollywood actors are more likely to smoke on film than their counterparts in real life.[26] And no society has ever smoked as much as we find in, say, Randal Kleiser's *Grease* or *The Edge of Love* with Keira Knightly and her friends. Emilio Estevez's 2006 *Bobby* is a particularly egregious affront, given that Robert F. Kennedy was one of only a handful of U.S. senators brave enough to stand up to the tobacco cartel. As if to mock the man, this award-winning dramatization of RFK's assassination features Demi Moore awkwardly brandishing a pack of Marlboros center-screen for a full thirty seconds. Kennedy would have been horrified, albeit perhaps unsurprised given his recognition of the industry's perfidy. As a champion of the move to ban tobacco ads on TV, he was forceful on this point: "The industry we seek to negate is powerful and resourceful. Each new effort to regulate will bring new ways to evade. Still, we must be equal to the task. For the stakes involved are nothing less than the lives and health of millions all over the world."[27]

Realism is actually a poor excuse for depicting smoking in movies. In the 1930s, when smoking was all the rage on the silver screen, smoking was nowhere near as popular as it would later become. Americans smoked only 134 billion cigarettes in 1935, compared with 630 billion in 1980. Smoking was not so common in the films of 1980, even though that was close to the peak year for total U.S. consumption. And film implants from that point on increased, even as smoking rates declined. The big push for implants—and payoffs—came in the late 1980s and 1990s, when film was turned into one of the industry's favorite advertising vehicles. And as recently as 2005 one in six box office leaders in the United States featured specific cigarette brands. Children's movies have been targeted, with implants appearing in films such as *Bad News Bears, The Muppet Movie,* and *Men in Black.* Old movies also get recirculated, extending the life of the ad as no other medium can. Many film classics have become immortal cigarette ads. Epidemiologists have suggested that half of all new smokers start as a result of exposure to smoking in Hollywood films.[28] Disney, Warner Brothers, and Universal have all recently announced policies to limit or discontinue such displays, but most of the other studios—Sony, Fox, and others—continue to portray smoking as an attractive and ordinary part of life.[29] And as for realism: how realistic was it when *Avatar's* exobiologist (played by Sigourney Weaver), working in a closed oxygen environment on an alien planet in the year 2154, has as her very first line, "Who's got my goddamn cigarette?" Moviemakers need to appreciate—and challenge—the advice Philip Morris got in 1989 from its marketing experts, who reported that "most of the strong, positive images for cigarettes and smoking are created and perpetuated by cinema and television."[30]

MORE DOCTORS SMOKE CAMELS

One curious aspect of early magazine and newspaper ads is how often doctors were used to sell cigarettes. (Robert and Laurie Jackler and I have created a website with some of the most astonishing images—search "Not a Cough in a Carload.") Ciga-

rettes in the nineteenth century had been touted as a cure-all—vintage "asthma cigarettes" can occasionally be found for sale on eBay—and regular cigarettes were
sometimes smoked to treat lung ailments of one sort or another. Parents are even
known to have forced their children to smoke to treat a lung infection. But it was
not really until the 1930s that medical endorsements became big business. Liggett
& Myers began placing cigarette ads in medical journals in 1933; the company that
year paid the *New York State Journal of Medicine* to hawk its Chesterfield brand
("pure as the water you drink . . . and practically untouched by human hands"), and
dozens of medical journals began running tobacco ads soon thereafter.

The American Tobacco Company paved part of this way by using doctors to celebrate its "secret toasting" process. Tobacco had long been thought to have certain
"disinfecting powers"—just as fire cleaned medical instruments—and the hope was
to associate "toasting" with health protection. As hype, toasting was buoyed by contemporary obsessions with germs, with the idea being that heat applied during the
curing process might kill microbes lurking in the leaf. Some people smoked as a
treatment for colds, and some at least seem to have imagined that fumigation might
effect a kind of cauterization of the lungs. Heat sanitized tobacco (and your lungs)
just as cooking (or smoking) made meats safe. Marketers capitalized on such fantasies, with ads from the 1920s claiming that "20,679 physicians" found Luckies "less
irritating to the throat" or that Luckies could help smokers keep "a slender figure,"
and so forth. Another series compared the discovery of toasting to Columbus's discovery of America, Fulton's invention of steam navigation, Franklin's discovery of
electricity, and a dozen-odd other heroic exploits—all likened to the miracle of
Lucky Strikes.[31]

The Reynolds company was angered by this and launched a counterattack, reminding smokers that while it was "fun to be fooled" (by silly claims for toasting)
it was "better to know." The William Esty Advertising Agency unrolled its "magic
campaign" for Camels in 1933, exposing the secrets of the conjurer's art (disappearing elephants, women sawed in half, etc.) to boost the Reynolds brand over
Lucky Strikes. Reynolds also published a book on how to perform magic tricks, featuring tricks with cigarettes.[32] The company's "healthy nerves" campaign ("Camels
never jangle your nerves!") followed shortly thereafter, with ads promising that
Camels would "give you a lift" or never "get your wind."[33] Testimonials from athletes appear in countless ads from this era, with substantial payments going to baseball, golf, and football stars along with heroes from perhaps a dozen other sports.
All for a price: baseball fans may recall Babe Ruth's tearful good-bye from Yankee
Stadium, looking emaciated and with a harsh, raspy voice from the throat cancer
that would soon take his life.

Medico-tobacco hype culminated in R. J. Reynolds's "More Doctors Smoke
Camels" campaign, another William Esty brainchild featuring idealized physicians
reassuring smokers they would experience "not one single case of throat irritation"

so long as they kept to Reynolds's flagship brand. Surveys were said to have generated these ridiculous statistics. The method was textbook bias: free cigarettes were handed out at medical conventions, following which doctors would be stopped and asked, "What brand do you smoke, Doctor?" Since many were carrying their newly acquired Camels, the admen used this to claim that Camels were preferred by medical men. Similar campaigns were run in Europe: 1,004 doctors were said to have found Kensitas cigarettes less irritating, for example, in consequence of the use of ultraviolet rays in manufacturing.

Ads in the 1930s and 1940s often featured endorsements by nurses or medical students, and the American Tobacco Company had a string of ads in which "Scientific Tests" touted Lucky Strikes as "milder than any other brand." Smokers were also invited to conduct their own "taste tests," which Martha Gardner and Allan Brandt have identified as a means by which manufacturers undermined the growing medical evidence of hazards.[34] Cigarette makers at this point were still competing with one another in the realm of health—so when American Tobacco claimed that "toasting" made its cigarettes less irritating, Reynolds countered that "over-cooking" would degrade the natural taste of tobacco. Mentholated cigarettes such as Kool, introduced in 1933, were supposed to protect you from colds, and Philip Morris advertised in medical journals throughout the United States that "3 out of every 4 cases" of smoker's cough disappeared after smoking the Philip Morris brand.[35]

At the height of all this medical hoopla in the 1940s and early 1950s, cigarette makers often set up booths at medical meetings to bolster the fortunes of one brand or another. Free cigarettes were handed out,[36] and in at least one instance giant photo-murals showed Reynolds scientists dutifully at work in the lab. Explicit medical endorsements disappeared in the mid-1950s with the nailing down of the cancer consensus (see below), but it is important to realize that tobacco advertising continued, surprisingly late, in many state and local medical journals. Journals of state medical associations in Virginia, Massachusetts, Nebraska, Arizona, and more than two dozen other states carried cigarette ads into the mid-1960s. As late as 1969 ads for Tareytons were still being published in the *Delaware Medical Journal,* the *Journal of the Louisiana State Medical Society,* the *Journal of the Mississippi State Medical Association,* and the *Virginia Medical Monthly.*[37]

IF NEWPORT WERE A WOMAN . . .

Oddly enough, the tobacco industry has maintained for decades that advertising causes no one to smoke (or to start smoking); ads are just supposed to make people who already smoke *switch* from one brand to another. Scholars investigating this question, however, have shown that advertising causes not just switching but initiation, and that young people tend to smoke brands that are most aggressively advertised. The industry admits as much in memos intended purely for internal use. It also makes sense, given that cigarette makers advertise even when competition from other brands is absent (in countries where the production and sale of tobacco are monopolized by the state, for example). The idea that advertising won't cause anyone to try smoking is a bizarre violation of common sense—and has drawn ridicule even from advertisers who have worked with the industry. Here is the view of Emerson Foote, a former CEO of McCann-Erickson, a global advertising agency with millions of dollars in tobacco accounts:

> The cigarette industry has been artfully maintaining that cigarette advertising has nothing to do with total sales. This is complete and utter nonsense. The industry knows it is nonsense. I am always amused by the suggestion that advertising, a function that has been shown to increase consumption of virtually every other product, somehow miraculously fails to work for tobacco products.[38]

The industry privately admits that advertising for other products—including nicotine patches—causes an increase in demand, so again: why should this be any different for cigarettes? Robert K. Heimann, executive vice president of American Tobacco, put the matter nicely in a 1966 talk to his sales force; the purpose of advertising was "simple: to get more triers."[39]

The fact is that tobacco marketeers have worked very hard to find out what kinds of ads work best, spending enormous sums on marketing psychology, focus groups, and every imaginable state-of-the art technique for tracking desire and persuading to buy. Focus groups are asked questions like, "What kind of car would a Marlboro smoker drive?" or "If Newport were a woman, what kind of woman would that be?" A 1997 study comparing brand imagery of Marlboro, Marlboro Lights, and Newports found that smokers of Marlboro Reds "have often overcome difficulties" and remain "slightly angry, resentful, bitter, judgmental," with "feminist leanings." Smokers of Marlboro Lights, by contrast, were more likely to "enjoy the social scene, find a significant other, marry, own a beautiful home, [and] have healthy, happy children." Smokers of Reds, Lights, or Newports were distinguished by their preferred cars, clothing, and music; favorite actresses and role models; and political attitudes—even preferences in the realm of tattoo types and piercings. This same study looked at how smokers of one kind of cigarette regarded smokers of other brands: so whereas urban young adult female Newport smokers regarded smokers of Marlboro Lights as "white girls who have to look perfect all the time," smokers of Marlboro Lights regarded Newport smokers as "slutty girls" who "think they're tough" but are really "immature" and "ignorant."[40]

Cigarette marketers have also quantified the number of advertising images to which people are exposed. In 1954, for example, Philip Morris revealed that Americans had been exposed to 3.2 billion cigarette "messages" over the past year. *I Love Lucy* alone—a show owned by Philip Morris at one point—reached an audience of

41 million people per week.[41] Philip Morris was still only a minor player in the cigarette business, which means that if their advertising budget was typical there must have been over 37 billion "messages" broadcast by the industry in that one year. The industry later measured advertising impact in terms of "Commercial Minute Impressions," defined as one person viewing one minute of advertising. In January of 1961, for example, Americans watched a total of 2,567,085,000 minutes of cigarette advertising on television.[42] That's about 30 billion person-minutes of cigarette ads per annum—or about fifty hours per person. And that was only for TV. Radio accounted for an additional chunk, as did advertising via billboards, newspapers, point-of-sale posters, and various other media. Millions of Americans got catchy cigarette jingles stuck in their heads before 1970, when the airwaves were finally cleared of such rubbish. Most Americans from my generation have creases in our brains where ditties like "Winston tastes good like a [clap clap] cigarette should!" are indelibly seared. Ask your parents (or grandparents).

Tobacco advertising also "works" more indirectly, however, to create allies in the form of editors and producers who want to maintain the tobacco money pipeline. Advertising dollars for many years were a major source of income for newspapers, radio, television, and magazines—and for athletes, artists, musicians, and others hooked on cigarette sponsorship. Commentary to this effect can often be found in the industry's archives, as when Philip Morris cautioned that loss of advertising could mean a loss of the industry's "political clout": "If you take away advertising and sponsorship, you lose most, if not all, of your media and political allies."[43]

One interesting aspect of magazine advertising is the portrayal of tobacco as an icon around which opposites could unite. Tobacco ads from the 1930s and 1940s depicted cigarettes or cigars as uniting North and South, Lee and Grant, Yankees and Red Sox, Democrats and Republicans, and rivals in other realms. "Brothers under the cellophane," is how Bob Hope and Bing Crosby were cast in Chesterfield ads: rivals in golf and baseball but united in their chosen brand of smoke. "Unity" and "accommodation" were also themes in the industry's global "Courtesy of Choice" campaign of the 1990s and 2000s, crafted to secure rights for smokers to the air of restaurants, bars, and cafés. Spearheaded by Philip Morris, and using the International Hotel Association as a front, this ambitious campaign popularized a yin-yang symbol to express this fantasy of smokers and nonsmokers eating, working, and puffing away together in blissful harmony. Philip Morris ran a similar "Accommodation Program" in the United States, establishing front groups in the hospitality industry to combat any effort to prohibit smoking in restaurants or public spaces. The yin-yang design was supposed to convey this theme of uniting opposites, basically: Can't we all just be friends and get along, smokers and nonsmokers alike? Presumably all sharing each others' exhaled and sidestream particulates.[44]

CANDY CIGARETTES

Cigarette marketing budgets grew dramatically in the 1930s, 1940s, and 1950s, though some kinds of advertising came at little or no cost to the companies. One of the less obvious techniques involved marketing to children via candy cigarettes. We can't yet tell whether the industry ever directly sponsored such products, but we do know that for many years the companies turned a blind eye to brand infringements of this sort, as confectioners churned out candy sticks with names like "Winston," "L&M," "Lucky Strike," "Chesterfield," and "Philip Morris." Cigarette manufacturers claim never to have encouraged such practices, but they clearly welcomed the infringement. Addison Yeaman, a top lawyer at Brown & Williamson, in 1946 wrote to one candy manufacturer, "We have never raised any objection to the use of our labels feeling, for your more or less private information, that it is not too bad an advertisement." Philip Morris coordinated the sale of candy cigarettes with its Johnny (Roventini) Jr. Operation, the goal of which was to "create Philip Morris in the minds of our future smokers."[45]

Candy cigarettes first appeared in the nineteenth century, when the Hershey Corporation in Pennsylvania began marketing a Hershey's brand chocolate cigarette for children. Brand infringements had begun by the 1920s and were not at first welcomed by the industry. In 1928 the American Tobacco Company filed suit to prohibit the sale of a candy cigarette known as "Lucky Smokes," and Lorillard one year later sued a candy manufacturer for using its Old Gold name and font.[46] By the late 1930s, however, the more common attitude had turned to a quieter kind of accommodation. American Tobacco had offended candy makers in the late 1920s with its exhortation to "Reach for a Lucky Instead of a Sweet," and when that campaign was curtailed (in 1930, when the last four words were jettisoned) the path was smoothed for friendlier collaborations. Joint candy and tobacco labor unions were established, along with combined tobacco and confectionery journals. And smoking itself eventually came to be more like a candified luxury treat, with fruity-sweet flavorings added to appeal to starters and learners.

By the 1940s and 1950s candy simulations were available for most leading brands—packaged to look like near-perfect copies of the original article. Candy cigarettes came to be seen as gateways to the smoking habit, a kind of training in gestures cigarette makers were quite willing to tolerate. Addison Yeaman at Brown & Williamson had regarded chocolates imitating the company's Raleigh brand as "not too bad an advertisement"; he elaborated on this view every now and again, commenting on his company's belief that "the simulation of one of our trade marked cigarette package labels does not constitute any threat to our trade mark rights" so long as there was no "cheapening" of its design. The company had therefore "not made any objection to candy manufacturers using copies of our labels for their products."[47]

Yeaman's comments are significant, given his subsequent denial of having ever tolerated such infringements. In 1967 the administrator of the industry's Cigarette Advertising Code wrote to ask if his company had ever had anything to do with the many kinds of bubble gum and candy packaged to look like cigarettes. The administrator observed that while the code did not explicitly cover candy cigarettes, "its spirit is certainly offended by them." Yeaman responded that his company did not manufacture or sell candy cigarettes and that "certainly for the length of my recollection as General Counsel to Brown & Williamson, we have never authorized nor consented to the use of our marks by candy manufacturers."[48] Yeaman must have been playing word games, however, since he clearly *had* endorsed this practice two decades earlier. Yeaman at the time (1940s) had not yet risen to the rank of general counsel, which may have allowed him this rather disingenuous and misleading denial.

The fact is that in the 1940s and 1950s at least, Brown & Williamson had regarded infringements of this sort as fine, so long as the quality of the candy was up to par and the likeness of the package sufficiently close to the company's real cigarettes. Yeaman had written to many candy manufacturers to express his desire for quality control and an exact pack-art likeness; he had also implemented a policy whereby the granting of permission to use the company's trademarked brands was made contingent on the production of quality candy and packaging—to ensure that a particular brand be "faithfully reproduced so as to do justice to it." Brown & Williamson was not alone in this respect: Lorillard also allowed candy brand imitations in cases where "the candy and the reproduction of our labels and trade-marks are of high quality." We also have examples in which if a candy company's labels or packages deviated sufficiently from those of the actual cigarette, Brown & Williamson would demand that the candies be made to more closely resemble the tobacco originals. And to facilitate compliance, Yeaman often included samples of the relevant cigarette packaging labels in his letters granting permission.[49]

Philip Morris employees also recognized the value of using candy cigarettes to attract youthful sympathies. Gus Wayne, one of four "Johnny Juniors" used when Roventini wasn't available, made this clear in a 1953 proposal to his handlers:

> In my travels I've noticed that "Johnny" is more readily recoginized [sic] by the children than the adults. Children, being very impressionable, remember things they see and hear, long after they've occurred. Here now, I further feel, based on my observations, that the Philip Morris trade mark "Johnny" has fallen into the same category as Hop-a-long Cassidy, Howdy-Doody, etc.
>
> Due to these facts, I've found it necessary to, when I'm making appearance in supermarkets, drug stores, etc., to buy and hand out to the children bars of candy, chocolates, lolly pops etc.
>
> Now then, here's my idea: we could, if you feel it has merit, have chocolate cigarettes made up in Philip Morris wrappers, and in the process of handing guest pack-

ages out to the adults, we could give the children a replica of our Philip Morris guest package containing chocolate cigarettes. I feel that the gesture, in conjunction with "Johnny" personally handing them to the children will remain in their minds for years to come.[50]

Candy cigarettes continued to be made throughout the 1960s, albeit increasingly with names slightly skewed from those of genuine cigarettes: Viceray instead of Viceroy, Marlbro instead of Marlboro, Winstun instead of Winston, Cool instead of Kool, and so forth. Hundreds of candy "brands" of this sort were sold, with names like Lucky Stripes, Lucky Stride, Lucky Spike or Bucky Strike, or Camales, Camols, Cammels, Camals, Kamel, Kamols, Kemel, Pamel, and so on. And if cigarette makers relished this cost-free advertising, candy makers for their part were happy to profit from the tie-in.[51] Candy makers capitalized on the desires of kids to be like adults, sometimes explicitly. The American Nut and Chocolate Company of Boston, for example, sold "Harvard Brand" candy cigarettes in twenty-four-pack cartons, with cover art featuring a cheerful young boy holding a (smoldering?) candy cigarette and trying to be "Just Like Daddy!" (see Figures 7 and 8).

Concerns also began to grow, however, that candy cigarettes might be creating bad PR for tobacco makers. A 1963 letter published in Britain's *Medical Officer* complained about the "very early age at which smoking is being presented as an attractive habit," and some tobacco manufacturers started publicly declaring their opposition to candy brand infringements. Lorillard in 1969 put World Candies on notice that it would not tolerate the "counterfeiting" of its True brand; R. J. Reynolds threatened to sue the same company in 1980; and other tobacco manufacturers sought to distance themselves from candy imitations.[52] Some of these protests were just for show, however. Lorillard, for example—just as it was putting World Candies on notice—pondered and then quietly endorsed the use of its Kent brand imagery in candy cigarettes made in Holland and Italy. The company decided that while no formal permission would be granted, back channels would be used to indicate the company's approval of such infringements: "We would also like to be included in the selection [of cigarette brands chosen for candy modeling], without giving our written approval but letting it be known to the people involved that we would not object if they did."[53]

Tobacco companies continued to view candy cigarette manufacturers as "friends," partly by virtue of sharing a common enemy. In 1983 the chief of New York State's Tobacco Action Network (TAN)—an industry group—wrote to his fellow TAN activists "to call your attention to several other issues which could also rear their ugly heads," including a proposed ban on sampling, a bill requiring disclosure of cigarette ingredients, and a bill to prohibit the sale of candy cigarettes. Lobbying efforts were organized to stop such bills: in 1971, for example, the New York State Association of Tobacco and Candy Distributors mounted a campaign to defeat a law that would have banned all candies in the form of pipes, cigars, or cigarettes. The association warned that "even a Tootsie Roll" might fall under the law (for appearing in the shape of a cigarette) and circulated to legislators an expert report from a psychologist denying any causal link between candy cigarettes and youth smoking. The Association managed to turn a 134-to-14 majority for the ban into a slight minority, and the bill was defeated. The organizer had earlier been active in the tobacco industry's efforts to block tobacco taxes in New York, through a group calling itself the Committee Against Unjust Cigarette Taxes.[54]

Candy distributors have played a little-appreciated role in the industry's lobbying and propaganda efforts, including its myriad denialist campaigns. California's Association of Tobacco and Candy Distributors, for example, in the late 1970s distributed leaflets with titles like "Is Tobacco Smoke a Health Hazard to Nonsmokers?" and "Today's Anti-Smoking Prohibitionists Follow Path Blazed by Carry Nation." Candy wholesalers have often been called upon to help defeat tobacco control legislation. In 1985, for example, Minnesota's Senate Finance Committee approved an amendment banning the sale of candy cigarettes, but the measure failed in the state senate, following lobbying by the state's Tobacco and Candy Distributors Association and other industry groups. As late as 1995 Philip Morris was still including World Candies and NECCO, two leading manufacturers of candy cigarettes, on its list of "Tobacco-Related Web Addresses." That list included more than a hundred friends of the industry—and no opponents.[55]

When tobacco companies finally began taking stronger steps to discourage candy cigarettes—responding to public pressure—they usually allowed candy makers to continue using such labels until inventories were exhausted. In 1985, for example, Brown & Williamson's Kendrick Wells wrote to the president of World Candies, Samuel Cohen, asking him to discontinue the use of the Barclay name with candy cigarettes. The letter stated that the "American public has formed a firm consensus that the marketing of candy cigarettes bearing real cigarette brand names could stimulate children's interest in real cigarettes and, therefore, is improper." The language here is carefully crafted: the company doesn't admit that candy cigarettes contribute to youth smoking but only that "the American public" believed this to be true. Wells later thanked Cohen for agreeing to discontinue the label, but he also granted him permission to use up whatever inventories he might have on hand.[56] So despite acknowledging the public's sense of a danger of stimulating children's interest in smoking, Brown & Williamson remained unconcerned about the existence of unsold candy cigarettes. The company could have purchased existing stocks from warehouses and retailers, for example, but no such steps were ever taken.

Similar apathy is apparent in correspondence from 1990, when the Stark Candy Co. of Pewaukee, Wisconsin, wrote to Brown & Williamson regarding a letter the tobacco manufacturer had sent concerning Viceroy brand candy cigarettes. Stark Candy noted that it had changed the name of its Viceroy candy cigarettes to "VICE-

RAY Candy Cigarettes" and that the artwork had been changed "to have our candy cigarette box be as dissimilar to your trademark item as possible." But the company also admitted to having a year's supply of packaging in the older style and announced that it would use these to "run out the packaging that we own."[57] As with the Barclays, Brown & Williamson agreed to allow Stark to continue using its brand name until its supplies ran out—with no offer to compensate the company for destruction of the labels. The financial cost of such a solution would have been trivial, but it would have diminished Brown & Williamson's brand contact with children.

CIGGIES FOR KIDDIES

Marketing to children has drawn a lot of heat for the industry, but we should also recall that intensive targeting of teens is actually fairly recent. The Joe Camel campaign launched in 1987 is notorious, and the 1970s are full of calls for youth marketing, but young teen targeting is not really a strong priority prior to this time. There are, however, some exceptions. In the 1920s and 1930s, for example, R. J. Reynolds targeted elite preparatory schools in the United States, hoping to capture this pre-college market. One breathless missive sent to all sales division managers in 1927 announced, "School days are here. And that means BIG TOBACCO BUSINESS for somebody. Let's get it.—and start after it RIGHT NOW." Ads were placed in college newspapers, posters were posted on campus, and free samples were handed out. George Seldes in 1947 caught wind of this trend and cautioned that with the market for men nearly saturated, the only direction for expansion was to women and children. That was also the view of "most cigaret experts," according to the advertising weekly *Tide*.[58]

The big push to target teens doesn't really come until the 1970s, as a result of increased competition for the crucial—and relatively new—middle teen market. American smokers in the 1950s had tended to start in their late teens, whereas by the end of the 1960s they were starting in their mid- to early teens. Cigarette makers recognized this and actively competed to hook into this market—and not just in the United States. Philip Morris included teenagers in its marketing plans for Japan, for example, and in Argentina, British American Tobacco collaborated with Nobleza-Piccardo to position Kent cigarettes as the "International Smoker Reassurance brand" for males and females aged fifteen to nineteen.[59]

Tobacco manufacturers have used many different expressions to characterize this young smoker segment. *Starters, learners,* and *first* or *beginning smokers* are terms we commonly find in the archives, along with *rookie smokers, new smokers, presmokers, new starters, new triers, trend-setters,* the *young adult franchise,* and *tomorrow's cigarette business.* A more general term used by the marketing department at Reynolds was *replacement smokers,* envisioned as needed to offset the "attrition" coming at the terminal end of a lifetime of smoking. Reynolds documents from the

1970s talk about the *young adult market aged 14–21* and the *starter smoker segment;* Brown & Williamson's "Viceroy strategy" targeted *young starters* for whom cigarettes—along with beer, first-time sex, and courtship—served as "the initiation into the adult world." The companies talk about *entry level users* and the value of marketing to *Generation Y (13–19)*, and so forth. A 1970 Roper report to Philip Morris identified the primary market for Marlboros as teenagers and suggested a plan to measure the smoking habits of soldiers and college students but also "young people in the 14 to 17 age group." Philip Morris researchers in 1981 identified "today's teenager" as "tomorrow's potential regular customer," noting also that Marlboro was as successful as it was partly because it had become "*the* brand of choice among teenagers who then stuck with it as they grew older." Children in the 1970s were explicitly regarded as "prospective smokers" in Philip Morris's Nicotine Psychopharmacology Program, which produced internal research reports with titles like "Aggressive Monkeys" and "Hyperkinetic Child as a Prospective Smoker."[60]

Children have also been targeted in other parts of the world. Philip Morris's marketing plan for Holland in 1982 included "starting and current smokers" as part of its "prime target group," and the same company sponsored Chinese professional soccer because of its appeal "among YAMS" (young adult male smokers). "Starters" were also important in Philip Morris's 1992–94 "Three Year Plan" for Europe. ("Marlboro's leadership in the foreign full flavor segment is reflected in continued gains in its share among starters and among young adult smokers.") Canadian manufacturers targeted youngsters: Imperial Tobacco in 1979, for example, constructed a "media plan" to advertise du Maurier and Player's cigarettes, both of which had high "starter numbers," meaning they were attractive to beginning smokers. The plan distinguished four different "target groups" by age: 12 to 17, 18 to 24, 25 to 34, and the geezer crowd at 35 and older. Each of these groups was assigned a different numerical "weight," according to its importance for the advertising campaign. In the plan for Player's, for example, the youngest group (12- to 17-year-olds) was given a weight of 1.0, whereas the group aged 25 to 34 was given a weight of .7, and the 35-and-over crowd was ignored altogether (with a weighting of 0.0). Teenagers were clearly a prime target for Imperial, a priority also expressed in the expectation that while most new users would be "switchers," some nontrivial percentage would be "starters"—people who had never before smoked.[61]

Marketing to what Roper called "the very young" presented certain challenges, however, given that this was "the most fickle group of customers." Young smokers are not so fixed in their brand loyalty, which is one reason pitching to this group has been so earnest. Marlboro in the late 1960s was becoming the nation's leading cigarette (according to Roper Research) "almost solely because of its great popularity among young people"; even so, there was always the danger that "should another brand catch the attention of young smokers and become the 'in' brand, Marlboro could face a severe problem."[62]

That of course was the hope of brand managers at every other company. High school students became one of the most highly prized targets, which is why a 1978 Lorillard memo (to the company's president) identified high schoolers as "the base of our business": "The success of NEWPORT has been fantastic during the past few years. Our profile taken locally shows this brand being purchased by black people (all ages), young adults (usually college age), but the base of our business is the high school student."[63] Newport by this time accounted for nearly a third of Lorillard's total cigarette sales, and though the brand was still presumed to have "plenty of room to grow," there was also the danger that some of these younger smokers might start quitting. In strategy planning documents developed for its five-year plan from 1981, the company commented on the threat posed to the company if this "under 18" crowd (and African Americans) were ever to quit the habit: "The easiest is to keep riding with Newport. However, I think we must continually keep in mind that Newport is being heavily supported by blacks and the under 18 smokers. We are on somewhat thin ice should either of these two groups decide to shift their smoking habits."[64]

The danger ("thin ice") was not that high schoolers were smoking Lorillard brands; the danger was that they might stop. Capturing kids was key given the high brand loyalty in this business—which is also why Claude E. Teague, Reynolds's powerful assistant director of research, recommended a search through high school American history textbooks to find brand names or images that would resonate with rookie smokers.[65]

Reynolds was particularly eager to market to youngsters, with the goal of regaining some of the market share lost to Marlboro. A 1973 memo by Claude Teague noted, "Realistically, if our Company is to survive and prosper, over the long term, we must get our share of the youth market." Cigarettes were to be deliberately designed with this young smoker in mind—by making them long and (therefore) easy to handle and to light, for example. A 1975 Reynolds update on its "Meet the Turk" campaign, stamped "Secret," concluded that "To ensure increased and longer-term growth for Camel Filter, the brand must increase its share penetration among the 14–24 age group which have a new set of more liberal values and which represent tomorrow's cigarette business." Reynolds sponsored supercross (off-road motorcycle racing) because its 575,000 fans constituted "perfect Camel demographics": four out of five were males aged sixteen to thirty-four, most were beer drinkers, and more than a third were smokers. Market profilers often tried to estimate how a particular brand would appeal to this crucial teenage market; the companies knew that most new smokers were now starting in their mid- or early teens and that brands chosen early on were likely to have staying power. This was also true in Europe: in Sweden in the 1990s, for example, a series of interviews conducted for Philip Morris found that "almost all the people interviewed started smoking when they were still at school; between the ages of 14 and 16."[66]

Marketing to kids has sometimes been more indirect, as when cigarettes are sold in vending machines to which children often have access. Or even via special designs in packaging. Sale of singles ("loosies") has been banned in many parts of the world for precisely this reason—to limit youth access. Sale of cigarettes in packets of two or four has been halted for similar reasons, though the industry has used some interesting tricks to get around such laws. In the Philippines, when the government banned the sale of cigarettes in anything smaller than a twenty-pack, Philip Morris responded by producing cigarettes in a folding, tear-off, accordion-like package consisting of four conjoined mini-packs housing five cigarettes each and the whole tied into a folded bundle. The tied-up bundle follows the letter of the law since it contains twenty cigarettes, but the mini-packs are easily detached and sold separately, violating the spirit of the law (see Figure 9).

The industry has always denied marketing to children and has long tried to appear not to condone such sales. The paper trail reveals a more cynical opportunism, however. A 1970 document in Lorillard's files talks about the value of packaging that would be "attractive to kids (young adults)"; the Kicks brand planned by the company was to be sold in packages of ten (vs. the standard twenty) to be more affordable to teens. This same memo cautions that the company should not be "obvious" in its efforts to market to youngsters, lest it arouse suspicions; the point was "to attract the youthful eye . . . not the ever-watchful eye of the Federal Government." We can also ask, though: if the companies didn't want to market to youth, why did they advertise in comics? Why did they fantasize about incorporating "video game imagery into pack design," using motifs of Pac-man and Space Invaders and the like to capitalize on "the video game craze"?[67]

ACCEPTABLE REBELLION

I've mentioned my own personal experience of being told—in high school—that kids weren't supposed to smoke; smoking was an "adult choice" like skydiving or drinking or having sex or riding a motorcycle, things that, of course, no teenager would ever want. The industry's effort to define smoking as an "adult" indulgence has this convenient backdraft: if it is only for adults, kids are pretty sure to want it. Brown & Williamson in 1975 talked privately about smoking as an "illicit pleasure" and "the entrance ticket" to the halls of adult society; "starters" were therefore to be reached by presenting cigarettes as "one of a few initiations into the adult world":

> In the young smoker's mind a cigarette falls into the same category with wine, beer, shaving, wearing a bra (or *purposely* not wearing one), declaration of independence and striving for self-identity. For the young starter, a cigarette is associated with introduction to sex life, with courtship, with smoking "pot" and keeping late studying hours. For the young smoker, the cigarette is a clean/socially acceptable (to a degree at least), communication symbol of maturity, sophistication and adulthood. The cigarette is the entrance ticket to the hall of the adult society.

For anyone wanting to sell cigarettes to "young starters," the imperatives were clear. Sellers would have to convey the allure of maturity, the veneer of rebellion, and the illusion that new smokers know what they are doing:

- Present the cigarette as one of a few initiations into the adult world.
- Present the cigarette as a part of the illicit pleasure category of products and activities.
- Don't force your brand on the starters. They don't take orders. They are not yet as tame as the "liberated" adult society. *Suggest* a cigarette.
- Consider a sampling technique to allow the young starters to actually try your brand. (They have very little ability to really compare, but they would like to see themselves as having this ability.)[68]

And so forth.

The Tobacco Institute's public face was somewhat more subtle, claiming, "We don't think our kids should smoke. . . . As with many of life's pleasures, smoking, drinking and driving a car require a knowledge of oneself and a sense of moderation that come only with age." Most of the programs organized by the industry to "discourage" youth smoking have been ineffective, however, or worse. Some look more like de facto ads for smoking. In fall 2000, for example, Philip Morris sent 13 million schoolbook covers to high schools throughout the United States—with plans for another 13 million—instructing youngsters, "Think. Don't Smoke." The colorful image featured a snowboarder soaring over snow-topped mountains (tobacco leaves?) with "Don't Wipe Out" emblazoned over a loner standing apart from the crowd. School board authorities quickly realized this was not much of an anti-tobacco ad, no more than Lorillard's 2002 "Tobacco is whacko if you're a teen" or Reynolds's "Support the Law." Scholars have shown that the industry's professed efforts to discourage teen smoking have little or no effect and may even encourage the kinds of rebellion that stimulate experimentation. California schools refused the book covers, and even the industry-friendly *Advertising Age* observed that the Philip Morris ad looked "alarmingly like a colorful pack of cigarettes."[69] (See Figures 10 and 12.)

Studies have shown that ads of this sort make kids less likely to regard cigarette companies as duplicitous, and less likely to want them to go out of business. This isn't hard to understand, once you see how feeble most such ads are. Early in the new millennium, for example, Philip Morris produced a series of brochures titled "Raising Kids Who Don't Smoke." Nominally intended for parents, the advice in these brochures was basically: "talk to your kids about smoking." The series was produced with the help of an advisory board headed by Lawrence Kutner of Harvard Medical School, and neither he nor the other members of the board seems to have thought it worth mentioning that parents who smoke should set an example by trying to quit. Parents are advised, "Encourage your child to talk with her doctor," "Talk with a guidance counselor" about cessation, and "Call up local chapters of national organizations like the American Lung Association" for further advice. One brochure reassures the worried (smoking) parent: "You may feel guilty. You may think that because your child has told you again and again not to smoke, he would never try it. Or you might feel like a hypocrite telling him not to smoke when it's something he knows you do. . . . But you're still the parent. You set the rules."[70]

Philip Morris is basically advising parents to keep on smoking, even if they feel like hypocrites for asking their kids not to. The parent is not supposed to set an example but rather just to "set the rules." It might be hard to imagine a better recipe for rebellion—and noncompliance—which may well be one of the goals of such ads. "Acceptable rebellion" is one way the industry defines youth smoking.[71] The industry wants us to think they don't want kids to smoke, when the reality is that young people are crucial for their business. We should hardly be surprised to find, then, that smoking prevention brochures put out by the industry tend to be lame to the nth degree, a kind of rhetorical double-speak, with parents and kids being led to hear the same literal message in very different ways.

Parents are supposed to think the industry is talking straight about how "whacko" it is for kids to smoke, for example, when the ads have actually been carefully designed to deliver very different messages to parents and to kids. The industry's "youth smoking prevention" campaigns often use this trick, which involves a calculated misuse of slang. The strategy has been to use slang that will sound "kid-like" to parents while being alien to contemporary youth (how many kids say "whacko"?). Ads of this sort also typically infantilize the nonsmoking "crowd" from which the kid is supposed to distance him- or herself. In one Reynolds ad from 1994, the smoking teen is told, "If you think smoking makes you fit in . . . think again." The nonsmoking kids in the image—playing a game—are infantilized and definitely not cool: all are younger than the smoker; one sports a flattop; one even has to stand on tiptoe to reach the game. And one is wearing suspenders. How many cool kids wear suspenders? (See Figure 11.)

The utility of such a dual-rhetorical strategy was anticipated by the industry some twenty years earlier: Claude Teague in his memo calling for new brands "tailored to the youth market" had also called for "a careful study of the current youth jargon" to better appeal to the younger mind-set. Teague proposed that names for new youth appeal brands should ideally have a kind of double meaning, saying one thing to the young and something else to older folks—just as Marlboro suggested both independence to youngsters and hard-work virtues from "the good old days" to old-timers. Teague advised a search of "currently used high school American history books" to find good brand names and images for new cigarette brands. All for the purpose of developing "novel, useful cigarette systems."[72]

LAZY GREENS AND VIRILE FEMALES

Marketing to children has been notoriously successful. A 1991 study by the Medical College of Georgia found that by the age of six over 90 percent of American kids were able to recognize Joe Camel; nearly a third were able to do so *by the age of three.* Smokin' Joe had about the same name (and face) recognition as Mickey Mouse. Joe Camel was one of the most successful ad campaigns in history: from the beginning of the blitz in 1987, Camel's share of the under-eighteen market jumped from 0.5 to a whopping 33 percent in just three years. A *Wall Street Journal* article covering the story headlined, "Joe Camel Is Also Pied Piper."[73]

Of course, one doesn't have to market *directly* to children to entice them. Kids after all want to become adults, and we can hardly expect marketing to "young adults" not to influence people trying to act like adults. Reynolds realized this when it designed its Joe Camel campaign, which ended up capturing much of the young teen crowd while nominally appealing only to the eighteen and older set. Philip Morris quickly recognized this as a threat to its cowboy brand and tried to youthen its image in response. Here is how the company contrasted the appeal of Marlboro with that of Camel in 1992:

Marlboro Man	*Joe Camel*
HARD	EASY
SERIOUS	FUNNY
OUTDOORS	URBAN
WORK ETHIC	PARTYING
THEN—DELAYED GRATIFIATION [SIC]	NOW
UNCOMMUNICATIVE	SOCIABLE
OLDER	YOUNGER
THE BEST; ONLY A SELECT FEW	EASY TO BELONG
HANDSOME	NON THREATENING
A LOOK	A PERSONALITY
NEVER SMILES	SMIRKS
RESPECT	SPONTANEOUS
AN IDEAL	REALITY
CLASSIC	COMMON
LONG LASTING	HERE TODAY
OLD FASHIONED	NEW
STABLE	EVER CHANGING
INDIVIDUAL	GROUP ORIENTED
COUNTRY WOMEN	TRENDY WOMEN
SETTLED; MARRIED	WILD; PLAYBOY
MR. RIGHT	MR. TONIGHT

Bruce Willis, Jack Nicholson, Mickey Rourke, Dana Carvey, Warren Beatty, and Mick Jagger ("of his times") were listed as embodying this Camel image, whereas Marlboro was more in the character of John Wayne, Charles Bronson, Clint Eastwood, Chuck Norris, and Steven Segal.[74]

We should certainly not imagine, though, that every form of advertising involves youth marketing. The industry has marketed to women, children, and blacks—as we so often hear in patronizing tones—but also to Jews, the homeless, blue-collar workers, military men and women, gays and lesbians, physicians, nurses, hospital workers, the elderly, and dozens of other "segments." Marketing targets (or proposed targets) have included affluent extroverts, "lazy greens," "slackers," "drifters," "new traditionalists/nesters," "the rich who need the extra nicotine," "upscale intellectuals," "middle tar downshifters," "yuppie rejectors," and "the breath conscious." Reynolds has also targeted what it calls the "virile segment"—meaning younger males and notably military men but also "virile females." Project Virile Female, for example, was a Reynolds effort developed by Promotional Marketing of Chicago to target blue-collar women with its Dakota brand, embracing the kind of girls who might like tractor pulls, hot-rod shows, and cruising and for whom "work is a job, not a career." A 1995 Philip Morris marketing plan included Asians as "a viable audience to pursue" (and "previously untapped") but also highlighted behavioral and "psychographic" indicators such as whether people owned pets, cooked for fun, dyed their hair, or wore gold jewelry. Segments are often broken down into subsegments, so Reynolds in the 1980s divided its youth market into Goody Goodies, Preps, GQs, DISCOs, Rockers, Party Parties, Punkers, and Burnouts. Monkeys and the dead would no doubt be targeted, if they were somehow able to cough up the cash. "They got lips, we want 'em," is how the Marlboro Men once put it.[75]

Individual companies have spent a great deal of time deciding how to divide and conquer this territory. In Britain in the 1990s, for example, the Gallaher Group (makers of Silk Cut and Benson & Hedges) divided its market into "slobs" (27 percent), "aspiring sophisticates" (20 percent), "conservatives" (28 percent), and "worriers" (25 percent). RJR McDonald in Canada distinguished "Experimenters, Latent Quitters, Unselective Habituals, Selective Habituals and Ostriches." R. J. Reynolds in the United States has distinguished Traditional, Virile, Refreshment (or Coolness), Stylish, Concerned, and Moderation segments. Reynolds and Philip Morris in the 1980s were considered dominant in the Virile market, with Reynolds playing second fiddle to Brown & Williamson in Coolness (Salem vs. Kool) and to Philip Morris in Moderation (Merit vs. Vantage). Philip Morris and Lorillard were strongest in the Stylish category, while Lorillard and American led in the Concerned segment (with Kent and Carlton, respectively). American Tobacco brought up the rear with its "Traditional" brands, Pall Mall and Luckies.[76]

A lot of psychology has gone into finding out how to sell cigarettes in different parts of the world. Researchers have explored the meaning of Marlboro for Arabs and how best to market cigarettes in postcommunist Poland or post-Mao China. Brand plans are often adjusted by geographic region—which is why we get gender-bender oddities like the fact that in South Korea Virginia Slims are smoked almost exclusively by men. BAT in the mid-1990s organized "a highly focused attack on student organisations with American Nights" (to recapture the Dutch student market from Gauloises Blondes). Studies have been done to explore the kinds of images that appeal to "value conscious" smokers, and scales have been developed to quantify the extent to which a particular product is judged acceptable—with "Hedonic Ratings" applied to fine-tune the system. Marketing segmentation is a much-studied science, which takes into account myriad different demo-, geo-, and psychographic variables. Reynolds in the 1990s defined "loyalty groups," with "Camel Loyal Segments" ranging from "Committed" and "Frequent" to "Occasional," "Non-Rejector," and "Rejector." The same company's president in 1983 claimed to be able to segment its market "geographically, demographically, by brand style, even to the extent of the type of packaging preferred"—which in his view was why Camels were "on the verge of becoming a truly global power brand."[77]

We also have instances in which the impact of specific promotions has been quantified. In 1974, for example, BAT reported on a campaign by its affiliate, Ceylon Tobacco, to promote its Bristol brand during the Esala Perahera, a religious festival held annually in Sri Lanka's capital city of Kandy to honor the Sacred Tooth Relic of the Buddha, an object of veneration carried in a golden casket on the back of an elephant. BAT's *Marketing News* described a campaign to market to the 1.5 million people crowded into the city to celebrate the festival as "an excellent opportunity for Ceylon Tobacco to promote its brands." Traffic signs were installed featuring large and enticing images of Bristol cigarettes, and Rover Scouts—comparable to our Boy Scouts—sold the brand from handheld trays ("the only salesmen permitted by the authorities"). Prizes were awarded in the form of cigarettes and branded ashtrays, and refreshments were delivered to local police by vans in Bristol colors. Advertising was supposed to be barred from the event, but "the authorities allowed a BRISTOL spot to be broadcast at regular intervals," along with the signage. The impact is expressed in BAT's internal documents: "Total sales showed an increase of 22.5% over the previous year, with sales of BRISTOL over 100% better than a year before." Not to mention value accrued in the form of goodwill toward the company and its products.[78]

NIGGER HAIR AND THE NEGRO DOLLAR

Targeting opportunities have changed over time, of course. In the United States the industry was slow to exploit what it called the "Negro market," for example, and in the 1940s was actually encouraged to cultivate this clientele as part of an effort to reduce juvenile delinquency. This odd suggestion was put forward by a PR firm specializing in Negro consumerism, a firm having as its motto, "Court the Negro Market—And Count the Results." Reynolds was not impressed, responding that "Negroes read magazines we use and listen to radio programs—They are part of the general public and not a group set apart." This may well have been a sensitive issue within the company, which had suffered racial turmoil following a series of labor uprisings in the early postwar era, blamed by the company on communist agitators. The civil rights movement soon thereafter made it hard (or easy?) to imagine how companies could have marketed brands with names like Nigger Head or Nigger Hair, products that ended up part of the American Tobacco empire in the early years of the twentieth century (originally manufactured by William Kimball and the Leidersdorf Co., respectively). Nigger Head cigarettes apparently didn't survive the federally ordered trust bust of 1911, but Nigger Hair tobacco was selling at a robust rate of 425,000 pounds per year in Milwaukee in 1936,[79] and survived for a disturbingly long time—into the 1960s, in fact, under the brand name Bigger Hair. (See Figure 13.)

Racism was common in the tobacco industry, especially in the Jim Crow South. Manufacturing tasks were typically segregated by race, with the dirtier jobs like stemming being assigned to African Americans while higher-paying jobs were reserved for whites. Racism can also be found in the language used in company documents: American Tobacco's "Sold American" plan from the mid-1940s was supposed to instill employee pride in "the glories of the South, the glories of the southern planter and the glories of the southern plantation culture . . . all part of the 'heritage' of even the most ignorant negro."[80]

Money is money, though, and beginning in the 1950s, and especially after the onset of the civil rights movement, a great deal of energy was put into capturing the Negro dollar (or "southern Negro market"). Not without some resistance, however. Ads were placed on African American radio and in African American magazines, drawing the odd ire of white supremacists who protested Philip Morris's support for the Urban League and efforts to make Philip Morris the "negro cigarette." Philip Morris was already strong in this niche, with 27 percent of the African American market, making it second only to Camel's 29 percent—and we should recall that Philip Morris was a much smaller company back then. The Ku Klux Klan managed to have its voice heard in this realm, judging from a *New York Post* report that "at a cross-burning ceremony in a field near Charlotte, an unidentified grand klaliff exhorted his white-robed listeners to refuse to buy from 'nigger lovers.'" The boycott was supposed to include the Ford Motor Company, Carnation Milk, and Philip Morris, all of whom had contributed to the NAACP.[81] (Times change, and it is worth noting that Philip Morris in 1936 had registered and sold a Clansman brand, which apparently was not much of a success.)

Menthol brands became popular with African Americans in the 1960s, though sales to blacks lagged behind sales to whites up until the 1970s. A Reynolds docu-

ment from 1966 talks about "Negro problem markets," meaning areas in which purchases by blacks trailed those in other parts of the country. Philip Morris in the
1970s puzzled over why its Marlboro Greens (menthols) were selling so well in
Grand Rapids, Michigan; a study found that "almost all Marlboro Green was being
purchased by teenagers" (especially at convenience stores near high schools) but
also that whites in at least one high school were denigrating Kools as the "nigger
cigarette."[82]

It is not entirely clear why menthol brands became so popular with African
Americans. The argument has been made that menthols joined a longer list of traditional Negro cold remedies, but it's not clear how much evidence there is for this.
We do know that the industry by the late 1950s was starting to market menthols to
blacks: Lorillard targeted African Americans with its Newport brand, for example,
distributing cigarettes free of charge from trucks that would roll into urban housing projects, sort of like the old ice-cream trucks. We also know that the industry
had some bizarre notions about why blacks liked menthols. The strangest may be
the one a Lorillard employee came up with, preserved for eternity in a 1970 marketing document titled "Why Menthols?" in which we're told that the menthol attraction might have something to do with a "mythical" Negro body odor:

> Negroes, as the story goes, are said to be possessed by an almost genetic body odor.
>   Now whether or not this is real is irrelevant. More importantly, Negroes recognize
> the existence of this "myth." And they realize that "Whitey" does, too.
>
>   Now what does this have to do with menthol cigarettes? Here's the theory.
>   *Negroes smoke menthols to make their breath feel fresh. To mask this real/mythical
> odor.*
>
>   Let's examine this theory a little. First . . . [83]

And off we go into racist fantasyland. This same document notes that African Americans at this time were slightly more likely to smoke than whites, that 30 percent of
all smokers of Kool were African Americans, and that peppermint candies were especially popular in Harlem—with Mason Mints selling "as if they were being endorsed by Adam Clayton Powell" (the popular Harlem congressman). There is no
mention of the fact that blacks were more likely than whites to die from smoking
or that magazines such as *Ebony* and *Jet* earned a higher fraction of their advertising revenue from cigarettes than did comparable white publications.

Code words or shorthand was often used when referring to distinct segments.
Companies talked about the "BHM" (Black + Hispanic market), "ethnic" markets,
and the like. Camel cigarettes in the 1960s and 1970s were supposed to be for "NFF
smokers," meaning "normal full flavor" smokers. Cigarettes were also designed in
such a way as to be more attractive to specific targets. Project BIG BOY, for example, was a Brown & Williamson campaign to market a "larger circumference ciga-

rette" to smokers who needed "macho/assertive image enhancement," especially "blue collar, adult male smokers likely to work in construction or similar jobs." A great deal of attention was paid to military markets, since by the 1980s military personnel on average smoked about twice as many cigarettes as the civilian population. Brown & Williamson at this time had an entire "Special Markets Department"—with about fifty account managers—devoted exclusively to military sales. Lorillard was also enthralled by the military market, especially for its black-attract Newport brand. A 1983 Lorillard memo outlined a program of aggressive face-to-face promotions targeting military personnel, commenting that "the plums are here to be plucked."[84]

Much of this marketing literature deals in rather coarse stereotypes. Blacks and Hispanics are treated as falling into the "Coolness" and "Virile" segments, for example, whereas Jews were said to prefer brands that "most successfully reinforce independence, confidence and upward mobility" (Vantage, Salem, and Now were considered "priority brands in the Jewish market"). R. J. Reynolds in a 1982 management summary observed that the "Virile" segment was "the largest among Hispanics, accounting for 45 percent of Hispanic smoker's usership." Younger adult males were the target, with the archetypal occupation being the construction foreman. The "Stylish" segment was more likely to respond to images of fashion models and Cadillacs, a lifestyle especially appealing to Hispanics, "who tend to operate more on a 'fantasy' level." Gender was often a focus: tobacco researchers in the 1970s found that Winstons were seen as more feminine (Doris Day), whereas Marlboros were more masculine (Clint Eastwood).[85]

Other groups were shoehorned into such schemes. Jewish smokers, for example, according to a 1984 market survey, "tend to gravitate towards lower tar brands," explaining why, for Hebrews at least, brands in the "Moderation and Concerned segments" had the highest market share, whereas "the fuller flavored Virile and Traditional brands don't fare as well." Jews thus chose Camels over Marlboros, Vantage over Merit, and (among the women) Mores over Virginia Slims. Philip Morris, with its focus on sociability and "having fun," was faring poorly in this Jewish market. Reynolds concluded that it should continue its special promotions in the New York metropolitan area, while "other areas with high Jewish populations should be investigated for similar programs." The company had earlier scored against Jews with its Winston brand, which in 1962 radio ads was deliberately pushed to the *Yiddishen taam* (Jewish taste) segment.[86]

STEREOTYPE THREAT

We need to think more about how advertising images of this sort may have helped to reinforce stereotypes of race, class, and gender, or even what it means to be cool, gritty, sexy, rebellious, or avant-garde. Billions of dollars have gone into campaigns

to identify specific types of cigarettes with particular kinds of people. "Stylish" cigarettes were "long in length and high in tar with a fashion model, elegant, high
class image"; "moderation" and "concerned" cigarettes were generally short, non-
mentholated, and "low in tar with a doctor, career woman, sensible, in control image." Coolness was typically conveyed through menthol—especially to African
Americans—whereas traditional and virile cigarettes were high-tar regulars with
"a tough, rugged male image." And "short in length." The kinds of jobs and clothing preferred by smokers of particular kinds of cigarettes were detailed, along with
cigarette-specific political affiliations—as in cigarettes that would be popular with
liberals, conservatives, or "worriers." Reynolds according to one 1976 survey was
weak among liberals, "slightly above average among conservatives," and "strong
among the smaller worrier segment." Young males were targeted by glorifying risk
(hang gliding, mountain climbing); young females were promised a slim physique
and sham political parity: "You've come a long way, baby." Lorillard in 1973 distinguished eight different segments in its female market, along a sliding scale from
"Emotional Bra-Burning Extremists" and "Blatant Lesbians" to "Traditional Women"
and "Anti-Libbers."[87]

. . .

Smoking has been called "a wordless but eloquent form of expression . . . fully coded,
rhetorically complex . . . with a vast repertoire of well-understood conventions."[88] But
if that is so, it is largely because marketing professionals have made it so, to augment sales. Admen skilled in the arts have managed to take an essentially homogeneous product—blindfolded tests show you really can't distinguish one brand
from another—and imbue it with elaborately differentiated symbolic powers. It is
not a natural thing to smoke; people start when young because they have been led
to believe it is fashionable or rebellious, and they continue because they become
addicted. Marketing joins with psychopharmacology to transform a rare or ritual
indulgence into brain-rewiring mega-morbidity. The imperative is alkaloid, but the
fantasies are cloaked in illusion and the product of human craft.

Sponsoring Sports to Sell Smoke

We're in the cigarette business. We're not in the sports business. We use sports as an avenue for advertising our products. . . . We can go into an area where we're marketing an event, measure sales during the event and measure sales after the event, and see an increase in sales.

T. WAYNE ROBERTSON, R. J. REYNOLDS, 1989

From Formula One Dominance to world class football. From horse racing to world class tennis. From cycling to windsurfing and virtually everywhere in between, Marlboro has demonstrated its leadership and earned its place as the world's number one sponsor of international sporting events. And what better arena could we possibly be in to enhance the young, dynamic, masculine image of our brand?

"NEW PRODUCTS MEETING" FOR MARLBORO, 1990

Big Tobacco has been using sports to sell smoke (and chew) since the nineteenth century. Baseball (= cigarette) cards we've already encountered, but tobacco sponsorship of teams also dates from this era, as when Buck Duke paid a roller-skating polo team—christened the "Cross Cut Polo Club of Durham, North Carolina"—to tour the United States for his Cross Cut cigarettes. Cigarettes would later often be sold with athletic endorsements: American newspapers and magazines from the 1930s and 1940s are full of athletic endorsements, as when New York Giants fans were told that "21 out of 31 Giants smoke Camel cigarettes" or that "America's champion athletes choose Viceroy." Stars from more than a dozen sports had contracts with the majors: in baseball, for example, Stan Musial and Ted Williams were paid to plug Chesterfields, while Lou Gehrig, Joe DiMaggio, and Mickey Mantle plugged Camels. Cigarettes were touted as performance-enhancing drugs that calmed your nerves, eased tension, and readied you for the big game. One of the few baseball greats to refuse such collaboration was Honus Wagner, the Pittsburgh Pirate shortstop, who in 1911 revoked his contract with American Tobacco fearing that circulation of his card "would influence children to purchase tobacco products."[1] Only a few dozen were ever distributed, which is one reason the Wagner T206 has become the Holy Grail or Mona Lisa of baseball cards. A 2007 sale fetched $2.8 million for the rarity.

CIGARETTE LEAGUES

New media open up new opportunities, and by the 1930s sporting events were often "brought to you by" cigarette manufacturers, exploiting the persuasive powers of radio. Imperial Tobacco sponsored the first Canadian football radio broadcasts, and Liggett & Myers in the United States sponsored baseball on radio and soon thereafter on TV. Liggett in 1946, for example, was arranging the televised broadcast of baseball games on behalf of its Chesterfield brands. And by 1949 Chesterfield (i.e., Liggett & Myers) was sponsoring radio broadcasts of games played by the New York Giants and the Washington Senators, plus televised airings of both teams' hometown games. One year later the company added the Chicago Cubs and Cleveland Indians to its broadcast roster. Liggett also had what it called the "Cigarette League," a team of Chesterfield-smoking ballplayers assembled purely for advertising purposes, starring pitcher Robin Roberts of the Phillies and other baseball greats. For the *Perry Como Show* and newspaper dailies, Liggett named a "Chesterfield Star Team" with Yogi Berra as catcher and Stan Musial, Joe DiMaggio, and Ted Williams in the outfield. "They're all great ball players, and they all agree Chesterfield is a great cigarette."[2]

Substantial sums were paid to teams for such purposes. Liggett in 1950, for example, paid the New York Giants $291,368 for the privilege of airing its games on the radio, plus another $214,829 for TV rights. This was a tiny fraction of the company's Chesterfield contract advertising for that year (roughly 4 percent, since the total was about $14 million),[3] but that would grow substantially over time.

Baseball also figured in the ads entertainers were paid to announce (or sing) on the radio. Lounge lizard Perry Como—the "Chesterfield Star of Song"—wrote cigarettes into his show, as in this croon from 1951:

> Chesterfield salutes the Yanks
> There's plenty of power within their ranks
> They made a great fight, that Bomber crowd
> So sing their praises long and loud
> Sound Off for the Yankee team
> Sound Off for the Yankee team
> The Yankee fans they've satisfied like Chesterfield!
> The Yanks at bat, and in the field
> are Champions like Chesterfield [etc.]

By 1953 Liggett was broadcasting sporting events in Philadelphia on the Chesterfield Baseball Network, part of a larger marketing plan involving sponsored musical broadcasts and free public tours through Liggett's factories in Richmond and Durham. The Chesterfield orchestra in the mid-1940s was accompanied by a group of singers called the Satisfiers, who did backup for Perry Como on NBC's *Chesterfield Supper Club* ("music that satisfies"), one of thirty-seven radio programs sponsored by Chesterfield from 1921 to 1953. The same cigarette also sponsored nine different television shows.[4] Tobacco companies targeted specific regions and specific teams, creating strong local brand allegiances. Alan Blum, founder of the pioneering Doctors Ought to Care, describes this nicely: "So close was the identity of a brand to the baseball team it sponsored that it is no exaggeration to note that in New York a Giant fan invariably smoked Chesterfields, a Yankee fan Camels (later Winston when the filter was introduced . . .), and a Dodger fan Luckies."[5]

Explicit athletic endorsements came largely to an end in the United States in the 1950s, when "the health scare" made it harder to believe that Camels would never "cut your wind" or "jangle your nerves." Sports sponsorship was revived in the late 1960s, however, when it became clear that television ads were going to be banned. Television had become the principal vehicle for selling cigarettes, and the loss was a grievous one, triggering a scramble to other venues. Billboards and movie implants were exploited, but sponsorship of athletic events, the arts, and eventually fashion shows and spring break bashes became an astonishingly successful way of selling cigarettes. And one with global reach.

BINGO AND BOBSLEDDING

It is difficult to summarize tobacco sports sponsorship in the peak years of the 1970s, 1980s, and 1990s—the scope and scale was so vast. In Britain alone, according to a 1978 report by that nation's (corporate) Tobacco Advisory Council, member companies had sponsored

> Angling, Archery, Athletics, Aviation, Aerobatics, Backgammon, Badminton, Basketball, Billiards, Crown Green Bowls, Indoor Bowls, Boxing, Canoeing, Car Rallying, Chess, Coaching, Cricket, Curling, Cycling, Darts, Eventing, Fencing, Football, Gliding, Golf (professional and amateur), Grass Skiing, Greyhound Racing, Hang Gliding, Highland Pentathlon, Hill Rallying, Horse Racing, Hockey (Indoor and Field), Lacrosse, Motor Cycle Scrambling, Motor Racing, Mountaineering, Parachuting, Polo, Pool, Powerboat Racing, Rowing, Rugby (League and Union), Sand and Land Yachting, Sailing, Sheepdog Trials, Shooting (clays), Shooting (N.R.A.), Shove-Halfpenny, Show Jumping, Skittles, Snooker, Speedway, Squash, Surfing, Swimming, Tennis (professional and amateur), Ten-Pin Bowling, Water Polo, and Water Skiing.[6]

Several of these I had to look up—"shove-halfpenny," for example, which turns out to be a kind of miniature shuffleboard in which coins are pushed across a slate or wooden grid. No sport seems to have been too small or obscure for the industry's blessing (see the box on page 92). Thousands of events were sponsored, from bingo and bobsled to skittles and extreme skiing. Philip Morris in a 1980 internal memo noted that "virtually every sporting activity has, at some time, benefited from tobacco company help."[7] And vice versa, of course.

How, though, did this post-1960s collaboration get going? What has the industry gained from such relationships, and how has sport been transformed?

The short answer to the first question is TV—or rather its loss as a medium of advertising. In the United States Liggett & Myers and Philip Morris began sponsoring racing competitions in the 1960s, anticipating the "forthcoming problem with television." (Reference is to the broadcast ban that went into effect on January 2, 1971, following a "deferment" to allow one final barrage of ads on Super Bowl Sunday.)[8] The industry realized this was a huge loss and pondered other advertising venues. Magazines were an obvious alternative, and in fact the amount spent on magazine ads nearly doubled in the space of a single year (in the United States). But many other outlets were investigated. Reynolds explored "transit ads" on the side panels of trucks, commercial broadcasts in supermarkets, feature-film plugs, and even talking vending machines.[9] Lorillard bought time for Kent on closed-circuit television at seventy horse racing tracks, and American Tobacco sold water filters to boost its Tareyton cigarette with the charcoal tip. Philip Morris about this same time—1971—gave away 7.3 million copies of a sixteen-page cookbook, *Chuckwagon Cooking from Marlboro Country*, with another 1.5 million handed out in supermarkets. Dozens of other promotions were put in place but none with more success than those involving sports.

European manufacturers had begun racing sponsorships somewhat earlier— and for similar reasons. Television advertising of cigarettes was banned in Britain in 1965, prompting the shift to novel conduits. (Italy had banned ads even earlier, in 1962, and was also early to sponsor sports.) W. D. & H. O. Wills, maker of Embassy cigarettes, was an early sponsor of British powerboat racing and rallycross (cross-country auto racing) and by the early 1970s was sponsoring "boxing, brass band championships, professional cycling, fishing, flying (Air Tattoo), golf, horse racing, rallycross, polo, powerboat racing, rugby league, showjumping, speedway and the Welsh National Eisteddfod."[10] Wills eventually (in 1975) created its Sponsored Events Department to coordinate such activities, as did Reynolds and several other firms.

Reynolds for its part established a new business unit, RJRN Golf, rechristened Sports Marketing Enterprises, Inc., in 1988, by which time the company was spending more than $80 million a year on sports, including licensing and promotions. Sports Marketing Enterprises in its first year of operations oversaw 1,600 different events, with a full-time staff of ninety-four and a payroll of $4 million.[11] Sponsored events included thirty NASCAR Winston Cup events, eighteen Camel GT sports-car races, seventeen Winston Drag Racing events, and golf tournaments all over

SPORTING EVENTS SPONSORED BY CIGARETTE MAKERS, 1960–2000

Event	Date Launched	Sponsoring Corporation
W. D. & H. O. Wills Masters (golf, Australia)	1960	W. D. & H. O. Wills
Players 200 (auto racing, Canada)	1961	Imperial Tobacco Products
Rothmans July (horse racing, South Africa)	1963	Rembrandt
John Player Special Trophy (rugby league, U.K.)	1966	Imperial
Regal Trophy (rugby league, U.K.)	1967	Imperial
Rallycross (open-road auto racing, U.K.)	1967	W. D. & H. O. Wills
Players Grand Prix (auto racing, Canada)	1967	Imperial Tobacco Products
John Player Tournament (tennis, UK, later Sri Lanka, etc.)	1968	Imperial
John Player Special League (cricket, U.K.)	1968	Imperial
All India Wills 99 Kite Flying Tournament (Lucknow)	1968	W. D. & H. O. Wills
Benson & Hedges 500 (auto racing, Auckland, NZ)	1968	W. D. & H. O. Wills
Player's County League (cricket, U.K.)	1969	Imperial
Canadian Olympic Training Regatta	1969	Rothmans Pall Mall Canada
Gunston 500 (surfing, Durban)	1969	Rembrandt
Malaysian Open Championship (golf, Kuala Lumpur)	1969	BAT, Malayan Tobacco
Benson & Hedges Open Tennis Tournament (New Zealand)	1969	W. D. & H. O. Wills
Marlboro Trans Am 200 (auto racing, U.S.)	1970	Philip Morris
Wills Open (golf, U.K.)	1970	Imperial
Marlboro Trans Am 200 (auto racing, U.S.)	1970	Philip Morris
Marlboro Open Championship (tennis, U.S.)	1970	Philip Morris
Marlboro Championship Trail (auto racing, U.S.)	1970	Philip Morris
L&M Continental Championship (Formula 5000 racing)	1970	Liggett & Myers
W. D. & H. O. Wills Open Tennis Championship (Bristol, U.K.)	1970	Imperial
Virginia Slims Invitational (tennis, U.S.)	1970	Philip Morris
Virginia Slims Women's Open Tennis Tournament (U.S.)	1970	Philip Morris
Virginia Slims National Indoor Tennis Championship (U.S.)	1970	Philip Morris

Benson & Hedges International Open (golf, Fulford, U.K.)	1970	Gallaher
Jockey Club Int'l Grand Prix (sand dune racing, Argentina)	1971	Nobleza de Tabacos
Player's No. 6 Trophy (rugby league, U.K.)	1971	Imperial
NASCAR Winston Cup (stock car racing, U.S.)	1971	Reynolds
Winston TransContinental Series (NASCAR)	1971	Reynolds
Powder Puff Derby (women's aeronautics, U.S.)	1971	Philip Morris
Winston-Salem Bowling Classic (U.S.)	1971	Reynolds
Eve LPGA Championship Tournament (women's golf)	1971	Liggett & Myers
National Match Play Championship (golf, U.S.)	1971	Liggett & Myers
Winston 500 (NASCAR, Talladega, Alabama)	1971	Reynolds
Marlboro PGA Golf Tournament (U.S.)	1971	Philip Morris
Benson & Hedges Cup (international professional skiing)	1971	Philip Morris
Doral Ski Club (recreational skiing competition, U.S.)	1971	Reynolds
Camel GT Challenge Series (auto racing, U.S.)	1971	Reynolds
Doral Citizen Series (amateur skiing, U.S.)	1972	Reynolds
Doral Club Council Series (amateur skiing, U.S.)	1972	Reynolds
Benson & Hedges Grand Prix of Skiing (Vermont)	1972	Philip Morris
John Player 125 Motor Cycle Championship (U.K.)	1972	Imperial
Embassy European Rallycross Championship (U.K.)	1972	Imperial
Embassy Sprint Championships (boat racing, U.K.)	1972	W. D. & H. O. Wills
Embassy Grand Prix (powerboat racing, U.K.)	1972	W. D. & H. O. Wills
John Player Race of the Year (U.K.)	1972	Imperial
Embassy Air Tattoo (aeronautic acrobatics, U.K.)	1972	W. D. & H. O. Wills
Embassy World Indoor Bowls Championship (U.K.)	1972	Imperial
Embassy Short Circuit Championship (sportscar racing)	1972	Imperial

Winston Championship Rodeo (U.S.)	1972	Reynolds
Benson & Hedges Cup (cricket, U.K. at Lords)	1972	Gallaher
Benson & Hedges Gold Cup (horse racing, York, U.K.)	1972	Gallaher
Winston-Salem Most Improved Bowler Trophy (U.S.)	1973	Reynolds
L&M Hydroplane Boat Racing (Owensboro Regatta, KY)	1973	Liggett & Myers
Marlboro Cup (thoroughbred horse racing, Belmont Park, NY)	1973	Philip Morris
Marlboro Australian Open Tennis Championships	1973	Philip Morris
Camel Pro Series (dirt track motorcycle racing)	1974	Reynolds
Benson & Hedges Masters (snooker, Wembley, U.K.)	1975	Gallaher
Benson & Hedges Open (tennis, Christchurch, U.K.)	1975	Gallaher
Camel Challenge (world championship motocross, Europe)	1975	Reynolds
Delta Rally (auto racing, El Salvador)	1975	Cigarerria Morazan
Winston Drag Racing (U.S.)	1975	Reynolds
John Player Special Cup (rugby union, Twickenham, U.K.)	1975	Imperial
Raleigh Bowling Spectacular (U.S.)	1976	Brown & Williamson
Embassy World Cup (professional snooker, Sheffield, U.K.)	1976	Imperial
Benson & Hedges Indoor Championship (tennis, Wembley, U.K.)	1976	Gallaher
Rothmans Grand Prix (snooker, Reading, U.K.)	1976	Rothmans
John Player Trophy (rugby league, U.K.)	1977	Imperial
Embassy World Cup (darts, Stoke on Trent, U.K.)	1977	Imperial
State Express Pro-Am Challenge (golf, U.K.)	1978	BAT
Embassy World Professional Darts Championship (U.K.)	1978	Imperial
Benson & Hedges Championship (curling, U.K.)	1978	Gallaher
Delta Grand Prix (auto racing, El Salvador)	1979	Cigarerria Morazan
State Express of London 555 Sky Extravaganza (parachuting)	1979	Malaysian Tobacco
Marlboro Aerobatic Team (U.K.)	1979	Philip Morris

Marlboro International Trophy (auto racing, U.K.)	1979	Philip Morris
John Player Special Colombian Open (golf, Colombia)	1979	BAT
Malayan Tobacco Open Golf (Malaysia)	1979	Malaysian Tobacco
State Express Challenge Cup (snooker, U.K.)	1979	BAT
Embassy World Cup (indoor bowls, Coatbridge, U.K.)	1980	Imperial
Camel Trophy (off-road driving competition, Germany)	1980	Reynolds
Wills Cup Cricket (Pakistan)	1980	W. D. & H.. Wills
Winston Pro Series (motorcycle racing, U.S.)	1981	Reynolds
State Express Classic (tennis, U.K.)	1981	BAT
Kent South China Open Tennis Championship (Hong Kong)	1981	BWIT
Marlboro British Formula Three Championship (U.K.)	1981	Philip Morris
National Greyhound Racing Derby (Australia)	1982	BAT
Regal Championship (motorcycle racing, U.K.)	1982	Imperial
Winston Hispanic Amateur Soccer (U.S.)	1982	Reynolds
Silk Cut Amateur Tennis Challenge (U.K.)	1982	Gallaher
Silk Cut Derby (show jumping, Hickstead, U.K.)	1982	Gallaher
Benson & Hedges Fly Fishing Championship (U.K.)	1982	Gallaher
Lucky Strikes Again American Dream Classic (bowling, U.S.)	1982	American Tobacco
Lucky Strike Classic (bowling, U.S.)	1982	American Tobacco
Winfield Cup (rugby league, Australia, Papua New Guinea)	1982	BAT
Camel Professional World Speed Skiing Championships	1982	Reynolds
Camel Trophy (off-road competition, Papua New Guinea)	1982	Reynolds
Regal Motorcycle Championship (U.K.)	1982	Imperial
Lucky Strikes Again Pool Championships (New York)	1983	American Tobacco
Camel Supercross (motorcycle racing, U.S.)	1983	Reynolds
Camel Challenge Motocross (U.K., Portugal)	1983	Reynolds
World of Outlaws Skoal Bandits Shootout (auto racing, U.S.)	1983	U.S. Tobacco
Winston Team America (soccer)	1983	Reynolds

Lucky Strike Day at the Beach (boardsailing, U.S.)	1983	American Tobacco
Lucky Strike Filters Classic (bowling, U.S.)	1983	American Tobacco
World Windsurfing Championships (Kingston, Canada)	1983	Reynolds-Macdonald
Silk Cut Masters (European PGA golf)	1983	Gallaher
Silk Cut Inter-Club Tennis Championship (U.K.)	1983	Gallaher
Camel Sprint Series (amateur speed skiing, U.S.)	1984	Reynolds
Export "A" Cup (ski racing and jumping, Canada)	1984	RJR-Macdonald
Silk Cut Challenge Cup (rugby league, U.K.)	1984	Gallaher
Silk Cut Dominoes Tournament (U.K.)	1984	Gallaher
Dunhill British Masters (golf, Woburn, U.K.)	1985	Rothmans
Embassy Premier Chase Series (horse racing, U.K.)	1982	Imperial
Camel MX Motocross (South Africa)	1985	Reynolds
Windsurfer International Export A Cup (Canada)	1985	RJR-Macdonald
Marlboro 500 (auto racing, U.S.)	1986	Philip Morris
Marlboro Dynasty Cup (soccer, Korea, Japan, China)	1986	Philip Morris
Camel World Cup (soccer, Mexico City)	1986	Reynolds
Camel Trophy (off-road driving adventure, Madagascar)	1987	Reynolds
Vantage Cup Golf (Vantage Aces, Vantage Classics, etc.)	1987	Reynolds
Vantage Championships (Senior PGA Tour)	1987	Reynolds
Marlboro Soccer Cup (U.S.)	1987	Philip Morris
Marlboro Ski Challenge (U.S.)	1987	Philip Morris
Bristol Cup (soccer, Sri Lanka)	1987	Ceylon Tobacco Co.
Cambridge Bowling (U.S.)	1988	Philip Morris
Benson & Hedges on Ice (U.S.)	1988	Philip Morris
Camel Challenge Cup (soccer)	1988	Reynolds
Salem ProSail Racing	1988	Reynolds
Air Camel Warbirds series (air racing, Reno, U.S.)	1988	Reynolds
Marlboro Tennis Championship (Hong Kong)	1988	Philip Morris
Premier Cup (Senior PGA Tour, U.S.)	1989	Reynolds
Embassy Gold Cup (darts, U.K.)	1989	Imperial
Regal Masters (snooker, U.K.)	1989	Imperial
RJR Cup Series (professional golf)	1989	Reynolds

Philip Morris World Championship of Golf	1989	Philip Morris
Red & White Latif Masters Snooker Tournament (Pakistan)	1990	BAT
Camel Mud & Monster Series (truck racing)	1990	Reynolds
555 Hong Kong–Beijing Rally (auto racing)	1990	BAT
Embassy Challenge (angling, U.K.)	1991	Imperial
Regal Welsh (snooker, U.K.)	1991	Imperial
Hungarian women's soccer	1992	BAT Pecsi Dohánygyar
Camel Striper Series (fishing, U.S.)	1992	Reynolds
Malaysian Cup (soccer)	1993	BAT, Dunhill
Marlboro Cycling Tour (bicycling, Philippines)	1993	Philip Morris
Marlboro PBA Basketball Showdown (Philippines)	1993	Philip Morris
Pittsburgh Three Rivers Regatta	1993	Marlboro
Merit Bowling Pro/Am Championship Event	1994	Philip Morris
Marlboro Cup (soccer, Hong Kong and China)	1994	Philip Morris
Winston Select (stock car racing)	1994	Reynolds
Davidoff Swiss Indoors (tennis)	1994	Reemtsma, Imperial
Kent Tour (bicycle racing, China)	1995	BAT
Camel 8-Ball Classic (pool)	1995	Reynolds
Camel Pro Exhibition Tour (pool)	1995	Reynolds
Virginia Slims Legends Tour (U.S.)	1995	Philip Morris
Camel Pro Billiards	1996	Reynolds
Salem Open Tennis (Hong Kong)	1996	Reynolds
Jordan Grand Prix (auto racing)	1996	Benson & Hedges
Alley-Cats Scramble (bike courier racing, Toronto and Vancouver)	1997	Dunhill
Rothmans Cup (soccer, South Africa)	1997	Rothmans
Philip Morris Golf Classic (Manila, Philippines)	1998	Philip Morris
Benson & Hedges Malaysian Open (golf)	2000	BAT
Sportsman Kakungulu Cup (soccer, Uganda)	2000	BAT

the United States, yielding an estimated 15-billion-plus "brand mentions," counting only print media. Sports Marketing Enterprises made it clear to Reynolds's PR department that sponsorship was well worth the effort:

> Research over the past decade demonstrates that sports marketing pays excellent returns. The sponsoring brand's share of market among a given target group is always

significantly higher. Winston Cup racing and NHRA Winston Drag racing shows an eight to one return on dollars invested.

Sports marketing has the ability to target a certain segment of a brand's potential franchise more efficiently than virtually any other advertising medium. It hits the consumer when he is most susceptible [sic] to reacting positively to the message—when he is enjoying a leisure activity that ensure[s] a positive frame of mind.[12]

PRODUCT MYTHOLOGY AND THE COST OF CONVERTS

One key principle of tobacco sponsorship was to cultivate events that had not gained much respect as spectator sports. The companies would basically take a marginal or obscure sport and transform it into a high-profile vehicle for a line of tobacco products. NASCAR, for example, was not a big spectator sport prior to the 1970s; cigarette sponsorship changed that. The Alabama 500 in Talladega attracted a modest twenty thousand fans in 1970, but Reynolds sponsorship and promotion boosted that to forty thousand within the space of a single year. Similar gains were reported for tobacco-sponsored tennis, rodeo, and many other sports, with even larger gains coming from television viewerships.

The goal, of course, was to increase sales of a particular brand of smoke. This is explicit in the industry's archives. So when Reynolds sponsored Doral skiing in 1970 the goal was "to establish DORAL as the cigarette for skiers." Sponsorship was planned to give skiers "more of a propensity to smoke DORAL," a process referred to as "conversion"—meaning conversion to the company's brand. Doral sponsorship of skiing, as expressed in the company's internal documents, was to help "increase brand awareness, trial and conversion."[13]

We actually have some of the records kept of conversion rates—and even of costs per convert. In 1995, for example, Reynolds measured conversion rates for eight of its leading sponsorships: the Camel Biker Rally, Winston Cup NASCAR, NHR Drag Racing, Unlimited Hydroplane, AMA Superbike, Camel Pool, and Winston Racing and Simulator/Show Car. Bikers showed the highest conversion rate (10.1 percent), followed by devotees of drag racing, NASCAR, pool (billiards), superbike, and hydroplane, all of which averaged between 5 percent and 10 percent. Reynolds had special "conversion teams" for these events. For its Camel Pool Tournaments in the fall of 1996, for example, the company had seven "conversion personnel" whose job was to attend and convert as many people as possible. The company's archives are full of elaborate tabulations of conversion rates for different Camel events, defined as the percentage of smokers who, following a trial or promotion of some sort, devoted at least 80 percent of their new smoking volume to the target brand. Similar calculations were done for direct mail, with conversion rates distinguished according to how the company obtained the smoker's name—from Camel Cash Players, for example, or "bounce-back" offers in which smokers returned address cards to obtain brand-themed merchandise. A promotion known as "Camel Genuine Taste Mission" converted 15,600 smokers to Camels via a staged sequence of free pack offers, sign-ups, and exposure to what the company liked to call its *product mythology*. Converts joined a Camel VIP Club, apparently requiring little more than a preference for that particular brand. The company's Genuine Taste Mission promotion, according to a 1995 assessment involving a "Convert-Meter," anticipated 18,000 to 36,000 converts from a targeted mailing to 480,000 smokers at a cost of $5.4 million—or about $150 to $300 per convert.[14]

This may seem like a lot, but since smokers tend to be a faithful bunch—brand-wise I mean, even with conversion efforts in full swing—the rewards to a company from a lifetime of brand fidelity can be great. And Reynolds found that different promotions produced converts at very different rates—and costs. The cost per convert for motorsports, for example, was $1,064, whereas biker events generated converts for about $779 each. Sponsorship of pool cost nearly $2,000 per convert. The cost was not so much in the cigarettes handed out but rather in the purchase of advertising rights and hiring of "conversion specialists" to conduct video simulations and role-playing to propagate the company's "product mythology." In 1994 the cost to Reynolds for conversion efforts at sixteen Reynolds-sponsored events was $576,000. The industry calculated both conversion rates and cost per smoker for different promotions, with the "learning" being that different techniques generated different rates of return. Personal "intercepts"—typically by young and attractive samplers—produced some of the highest conversion rates, but high rates were also obtained through the company's Camel Cash program, which allowed smokers of non-Camel brands to redeem coupons for merchandise. Many other methods were proposed—as in 1994, when Reynolds entertained the idea of hiring strippers to smoke and display Camels at strip joints. The document unveiling this plan, drawn up by the company's Cultural Initiator Task Force, referred to these strippers as "Camel ambassadors."[15]

I have focused on Reynolds, but every company seems to have performed such calculations. British American Tobacco calculated the benefit of sponsorships in terms of "total branded value exposure"; so in 1993, in preparation for the 1996 Cricket World Cup, the value of sponsoring that contest (for its Benson & Hedges brand) in Australia, New Zealand, and South Africa was figured to be 5,985,000 British pounds.[16] Calculations were also made of the value of television coverage, through viewer exposure to the Benson & Hedges logo. The advertising value of "signage exposure" through telecasts in Australia and New Zealand was assumed to be $150 for each three-second visual display. Surveys indicated forty such exposures per broadcast hour, so for the combined total of 270 broadcast hours for Australia and New Zealand, this meant televised signage worth $150 × 40 × 270 = $1,620,000, with added value from other media. In Australia alone, the twenty matches of the Cup were expected to have a "reach" of 80 million (4 million people watching twenty matches), with forty three-second signage exposures per match yielding a total of 10 billion personal seconds of brand logo exposure. Separate calculations were made for exposures from opening- and closing-ceremony billboards, posters, cards, and so forth.[17]

EQUAL OPPORTUNITY CANCER

Women's tennis is one of the more dramatic examples of the industry promoting—and redesigning—a sport to sell cigarettes. Philip Morris established the Virginia Slims (VS) tournaments in 1970 to stimulate demand for its fresh-off-the-press "female" cigarette ("It's a woman thing"). The "first cigarette created specifically for women" had been unveiled in the summer of 1968, and VS tournaments drew attention to the brand while also boosting the popularity of women's tennis. According to a 1994 assessment, sponsorship helped transform the game "from little more than a sideshow into one of the premier sporting events today."[18] So whereas virtually no one watched women's tennis prior to 1970, by 1990 the $3.5 million Virginia Slims Championships at Madison Square Garden were drawing over a hundred thousand fans and far larger TV viewerships.

This was not the first time Big Tobacco had hooked up with tennis. Philip Morris had sponsored the first broadcast of the U.S. Open in 1968, and for decades prior even to the Second World War the companies had paid tennis stars—not to mention movie stars and opera singers and U.S. senators—to endorse some favored brand. Women's tennis in the 1970s offered a new opportunity, insofar as females were an untapped market and had (supposedly) never had "their own cigarette." Every part of this plug was a myth. Salome cigarettes, made by the Rosedor Cigarette Company of New York in 1915, were expressly meant for women, as were Benson & Hedges's Debs cigarettes of the 1930s, "rose tipped for the well groomed woman," as it said on the back of every pack. First Lady cigarettes were meant for females, as were Fems, both of which had red tips to hide lipstick marks. German manufacturers had targeted women, prompting Nazi authorities to ban any advertising use of the term *Damen-Zigarette* (women's cigarette). And Bulgaria circa 1960 sold a Femina brand. Marlboro itself, prior to its sex change into a cowboy brand in 1955, was expressly pitched to females, who were offered a choice of ivory or crimson "beauty tips" to hide unwanted lipstick marks.

Philip Morris's hope, however, was to exploit new waves of women's liberation to capture (and augment) the female cigarette "vote." All contestants in Virginia Slims events were given sweaters with neckbands in brand colors and instructed to wear these during warm-ups and after play. A designer by the name of Teddy Tinling was hired to create the outfits, along with a broader line of Slimswear—including jogging suits—sold at Slimshops. Philip Morris wanted its players to wear as many VS logo items as possible, since "tournament merchandise sales increase when spectators see players wearing licensed clothing items." The goal, of course, was to turn tennis fashions into cigarette sales: "Used to be a woman couldn't wear fun clothes, much less smoke a cigarette. Things have changed. Now you've got a cigarette all your own, along with a nifty new collection of Virginia Slimswear designed just for you."[19]

The tobacco giant also played a crucial role in founding the Women's Tennis Association—in 1973—and even helped finance the "junior version" of the sport through the Maureen Connolly Brinker Tennis Foundation (MCBF). Brinker had been a tennis superstar in the 1950s, and the foundation established following her death from stomach cancer in 1969 supported tournaments for female players aged fourteen to eighteen. By the 1980s, however, the MCBF had joined with Philip Morris to promote tennis for teenage girls. Foundation officers used Virginia Slims stationery (featuring the "smoking Ginny") and professed their "loyalty and support" to the tobacco giant while helping to develop "secondary markets for Virginia Slims in Denver, Colorado; Wichita, Kansas; and Little Rock, Arkansas." (The reference is presumably to the games and not the cigarette, but the ambiguity is telling.) Players as young as eleven wrote to the foundation, thanking it for help and for tickets to Virginia Slims tournaments. The logo of the MCBF featured the already mentioned "Ginny" brandishing a cigarette, and ads for the tennis/tobacco tourneys carried the Surgeon General's warning.[20]

Philip Morris sponsorship radically transformed women's tennis. New in the VS era was an increase in the number of players, higher-paying prizes, new clothes worn by the contestants, and a dramatically enlarged audience, including the first televised broadcasts. Rankings were also transformed. Philip Morris early on introduced the Virginia Slims SlimStat, a computerized record-keeping system designed to provide newsmakers with rankings, biographies of players, match results, attendance records, and so forth. The grip of Philip Morris was such that when the Women's International Tennis Council debated whether to break its relationship with the company (in 1989), the cigarette maker was able to force a continuance by pressuring Procter and Gamble to withdraw from the competition.

By which time other companies had started sponsoring the sport. Salem sponsored the 1994 Tennis Open in Beijing and Hong Kong, for example, and State Express sponsored a Far East Tennis Classic. Canadian manufacturers went to great lengths to keep their names associated with the Canadian Open: Sport Canada in 1985 had implemented a policy denying federal funding to bodies that take tobacco money, and Canada's Tobacco Act of 1988 banned tobacco advertising, but Imperial Tobacco responded by setting up shell companies carrying the names of company brands (Players Ltd. and du Maurier Ltd., for example) to circumnavigate the ban. The 1993 Canadian Open, for example, was advertised as the "Matinee Ltd International" as part of an Imperial plan to target women with its Matinee brand.[21] London's Imperial likewise stretched the limits of advertising bans by having its Davidoff brand sponsor the Basel International Tennis Tournament ("Swiss Indoors"). Davidoff has sponsored the event since 1994, splashing its cigarette logo all over the courts to encourage TV transmission. Davidoff has also had the tennis superstar Roger Federer appear on event brochures and postures. The Davidoff brand may not be as widely recognized as Marlboro or Camel, but its association with a major tennis name should raise eyebrows. (Federer did not respond in 2007 when a group of public health advocates led by Pascal A. Diethelm sent him a petition with nearly six hundred signatures protesting his tobacco collaboration. Swiss Indoors finally bowed to the pressure, vowing that the November 2010 event would be the last to have a cigarette sponsor.)

What is remarkable is how eagerly athletes have welcomed such collaborations,[22] even players who were politically astute in other respects. Billie Jean King, for example, was one of the industry's most ardent supporters. King started working with Philip Morris in 1971, the same year she became the first woman ever to earn $100,000 as a professional athlete. King was looking for ways to enlarge the profile of women's tennis, and Philip Morris was looking for new ways to market its "female cigarette." The match was perfect, and King over the next couple of decades became a big defender of Virginia Slims, while Philip Morris became the main bankroller of women's tennis. King appeared in ads for Virginia Slims tournaments and signed rackets for use as prizes in VS sweepstakes. Sponsorship provided an opportunity for the cigarette maker to champion "equality" for women in the form of equal rights to smoke: "You've come a long way, baby," was a slogan in both the tennis and the tobacco ads, with the insignia of the Virginia Slims World Championship featuring a flamboyant cartoon flapper holding a tennis racket and lit cigarette, complete with a svelte cigarette holder. Umpires wore official badges with this same "smoking Ginny" insignia.[23] (See Figure 14.) Billie Jean King encouraged this collaboration, helping Virginia Slims to become "virtually synonymous with women and tennis." Thomas R. Keim, director of brand management for Philip Morris, celebrated the relationship as helping to make Virginia Slims "the leading cigarette made expressly for women."[24]

Tennis was attractive to Big Tobacco because, as unpublished industry surveys showed, about a quarter of all viewers of televised matches—and a third of all amateur players—were under the age of eighteen. King's endorsements were highly valued, especially after her victory over Bobby Riggs, the aging male star, whom she trounced in 1973 in a match dubbed "The Battle of the Sexes" (for which King wore an outfit in Virginia Slims colors). King would become one of the most famous women of the decade, much to the delight of the PR men at Philip Morris, who listed her appearance at tennis/cigarette events as "brand activity." King welcomed cigarette advertising in the magazine she founded, explaining that she would be "a hypocrite to accept their help in sport events and turn it down in *WomenSports*."[25]

And King was nothing if not loyal to her benefactor. In 1975 and 1976 thirty-four of the thirty-five ads for cigarettes in her *WomenSports* magazine were for Philip

Morris brands.[26] King let Philip Morris run its (unimpressive) "Youth Smoking Prevention" program through her Women's Sports Foundation and routinely defended the firm in public forums. In a 1993 letter to the *New York Times* she characterized Philip Morris executives as "enlightened people who understand and acknowledge the possible hazards of smoking." *Possible hazards?*[27] King continued to work for the cigarette maker and in 1999 joined its board of directors, by which time she had become a virtual trademark for the firm. Philip Morris in her view had gotten "a bad rap" since the company had "probably done more charitable things for people than anybody." A 1999 Philip Morris report observed that King had proved "time and again that she can deliver results for the brand."[28] As recently as 2001 she was allowing her signature to appear on Philip Morris coupons offering free packs of cigarettes.

One of the odd things about Billie Jean King's collaboration is that she considered herself a feminist and social activist. King founded the Women's Tennis Association in 1973, shortly after having helped to push through Congress the Equal Opportunity in Education Act, with its groundbreaking Title IX, forcing universities to fund women's athletics on a par with men's. King won numerous awards from progressive and charitable organizations, and *Life* magazine in 1990 named her one of the "100 most important Americans of the 20th century." Her pioneering work for women's equality in sports, however, was compromised by her collaboration with the deadliest industrial enterprise on the planet. History will have to judge whether this devil's dance was worth it.

STRATEGIC PHILANTHROPY

Bowling was another area of heavy investment. By 1973 Reynolds was funding two Winston-Salem Classics and three Winston-Salem Opens, plus a Hawaiian contest and the National Championship Pro-Am. Efforts were under way to market to female fans and to African American bowlers ("a market we need to penetrate.") Philip Morris sponsored Merit Bowling teams in Holland (in the early 1980s) and the Merit Bowling Pro/Am Championship in the United States (in the early 1990s). Reynolds, though, remained the most ardent supporter, consistent with its lower-class slant. The company delivered thousands of branded wall clocks to bowling alleys throughout the U.S. and in 1974 alone distributed 11 million score- and record-keeping books at 8,200 American bowling centers. Sponsorship was envisioned as helping Reynolds to keep its "brand names in front of millions of bowlers," with the ultimate goal of making Winston and Salem "the preeminent cigarette for bowlers."[29]

Bowling was typical of many other collaborations in that sponsorship was approved at the highest levels of the sport. Raleigh's sponsorship in the United States, for example, was endorsed by the National Bowling Council. Ten different bowling proprietors' associations expressed their support for Philip Morris's "Accommodation Program"—a useful political payback for the tobacco giant's munificence. (The Accommodation Program was an elaborate effort from 1994 to oppose smoke-free indoor policies—by encouraging separate sections for smokers in hotels, restaurants, and recreational facilities; the campaign also allowed the industry to create alliances within the hospitality industry.)[30] Philip Morris continued its Merit Bowling marriage until 1998, when the Master Settlement Agreement forced its discontinuance, along with most other sports sponsorships. Banning of sports sponsorships was one of the few good things to come out of the settlement, which on the whole must be regarded as a modest (and inefficient) tax of about 40 cents per pack stretched over a quarter of a century. (The "tax" is inefficient because it took a lengthy court battle to obtain, and a portion of these funds went to law firms involved in the suit. Very little went to public health: in recent years, in fact, more settlement money has gone to tobacco farmers than to tobacco control.)

Sponsorships of this sort were almost always announced not through a particular *company* but rather through a particular *brand*. So Raleigh (the cigarette) sponsored the Raleigh Bowling Spectacular in 1976, with Brown & Williamson (the company) keeping a low profile behind the scenes.[31] That was the pattern: the brand, not the company, bankrolled promotions. So Kool (not Brown & Williamson) sponsored bowling and ballooning, Regal and Silk Cut (rather than Gallaher) sponsored rugby, Winston (rather than Reynolds) sponsored drag racing and softball, and Camel (not Reynolds) sponsored speed skiing, trophy fishing, and snowboarding.[32] The brand and the company sometimes had the same name: so L&M sponsored hydroplane boating, Rothmans sponsored microlight flying and snooker, and so forth. The featured brand would appear on posters, tickets, and ticket stubs but also on scoreboards, banners, and playbooks, plus of course giveaways or buyables on which a logo could be printed—T-shirts and toy cars, for example—to generate multiplier effects.

An interesting contrast here is with higher-brow sponsorships, where the *company* and not the brand was on display. So when a company wanted to sell *cigarettes,* attention was drawn to the *brand.* When the hope was to spread *goodwill* or *political influence,* attention was drawn to the *company* putting up the money. The rich are needed to influence policy or legislation; the poor are needed to move product. In recent years the wealthy have been less likely to smoke in any event, so there hasn't been much point in pitching cigarettes to them. The rich are needed to impress through acts of corporate benevolence, which is also why so much effort has been put into displays of "corporate responsibility" and "goodwill."[33]

Strategic philanthropy became a priority for Big Tobacco in the 1980s and 1990s, following moves by universities, foundations, churches, synagogues, and pension funds to divest themselves of tobacco stocks. The industry responded by reinventing itself as a "good corporate citizen," endorsing recycling and charity and other visible causes green and eco-friendly. A 2003 report of the World Health Organization described tobacco industry sponsorship of programs for "small business development in Kenya, crime prevention in South Africa, business education in China, folk culture preservation in Venezuela, and medical treatment and flood relief in Pakistan." Philip Morris in 2008 donated two million pesos to the Philippine National Red Cross, to associate its name with disaster relief (see Figure 15). The sham nature of such stunts should be apparent, but it is also worth highlighting some of the devious means by which "social responsibility" has been sought. In 1984, for example, the "Final Report on Research" for R. J. Reynolds's Social Responsibility Program, prepared by the PR firm of Rogers & Cowan, began by noting the deception used to conduct its research:

> To maintain the utmost confidentiality throughout, we identified ourselves in all contacts as either (a) freelance writers preparing materials on the smoking issue, or (b) students writing dissertations on the subject. In some contacts with potential academic or professional supporters, we indicated the Rogers & Cowan affiliation, but said that we were seeking third-party assistance on social issues for a range of clients. At no time did we mention that we were researching on behalf of RJR.[34]

Of course what really makes this pretense of "corporate and social responsibility" ring hollow is the brute fact of needless megadeaths. One might as well (again) talk about the high ethics of a criminal gang, or the quality of construction at some Potemkin village.

USEFUL ALLIES, DEAR FRIENDS

What is the point of sports sponsorships? The companies get good advertising, of course, and therefore increased profits ("positive sales 'ruboff'") but also good PR and political allies. Philip Morris defended its bowling program, for example, by noting that Merit cigarettes were helping to build awareness of the sport in "a smoker-friendly environment." Sponsorship also created useful allies among facilities owners, as when the Bowling Centers Association of Michigan urged the Bowling Proprietors' Association "to take a neutral stance on the smoking issue." Alley owners had come to depend on the Merit Bowling program and didn't relish the idea of having the funding faucet turned off. Not everyone went blindly down this alley; there are some notable voices of protest. In 1984, for example, the Olympic medalist Steve Podborski refused to accept the Export "A" championship cup in skiing at Rossland in British Columbia, protesting, "I don't want to be associated with a tobacco company."[35] And some sports escaped almost entirely—track and field, for example, which in the United States at least eschewed tobacco sponsorships. The same with swimming and gymnastics, perhaps for no other reason than their failure to attract a sufficiently large and "convertible" audience.

In most other sports, however, the tobacco companies found no shortage of athletes (and organizers) willing to serve. Arnold Palmer praised Brown & Williamson's Viceroy Rich Lights for sponsoring Florida's 1981 Bay Hill Golf Classic, and Paul Fitzpatrick of Britain's Rugby League claimed that without the industry's money "the game would be struggling to stay alive." Peter Lawson, secretary of England's Central Council for Physical Recreation, commented, "When cricket was on the wane, it was tobacco sponsorship that revived it and brought it back to public attention: they did a superb job." Douglas Bunn, master of Hickstead, the equestrian show-jumping venue, offered this observation: "There are a few lunatics around who think that sports can survive without tobacco companies. That is not so." Tradesmen from less effete sports were equally gratified. Charlie Mancuso, president of the U.S. Hot Rod Association, felt "honored" when Reynolds agreed to sponsor the "electrifying sport" of mud and monster truck competitions. Mancuso added—as if this were not self-evident—that tobacco money would help create "a foundation of excellence in Mud and Monster Truck motorsports."[36]

The archives preserve many examples of athletic organizations writing to request sponsorship from tobacco manufacturers. In 1990 alone Philip Morris received requests for sponsorship from Cates Brothers Offshore Racing; the National Wrestling League; an AA/Fuel Funny Car firm; an offshore powerboat racing team; the "First Poker Team Championship of the World"; the Antioch Speedway in Glen Alpine, North Carolina; the United States Sports Academy; Rattler Racing Enterprises; and the World Congress on Fitness, Nutrition, and Sports. Reynolds that same year received—and rejected—a proposal to sponsor the Jamaican Bobsled Federation. Universities sometimes requested support: in 1982 Lacy Lee Rose from Stanford University's Department of Athletics wrote to Philip Morris ("Dear Friend"), inviting the firm to advertise in a forthcoming series of promotional brochures. Rose was putting together brochures for the university's 1982–83 season and offered to help Philip Morris increase its business by advertising in either the brochures or one of the tabloid-size inserts planned for the *Peninsula Times Tribune*. Rose pointed out that the maker of Virginia Slims cigarettes had "a chance to help Stanford sports, but also an opportunity to increase your business."[37]

GLOBAL PENETRATION

Searching the industry's archives, we find that most parts of the world have been targets of sports sponsorship. In Australia alone Philip Morris by 1971 was sponsoring the Marlboro Rodeo in Wagga, a four-year-old trotting race for Viscounts, a footrace in Wangaratta, state surf championships in New South Wales, night baseball in Newcastle, an alpine automobile rally, the South Pacific Bowls Carnival in Windang, and the International Fireball sailing championship for the Marlboro Trophy.[38] Other companies caught (or created) the wave: Silk Cut sponsored the island nation's 1986 Silk Cut Dominoes Tournament; Winfield sponsored rugby; and Benson & Hedges sponsored cricket (and ballet). The list of sponsoring brands is long: Craven Filter sponsored trotting, Peter Jackson sponsored darts, Ardath sponsored greyhound racing, and so forth.

And we are talking about substantial funds. In 1991 the four largest tobacco companies in Australia spent an estimated $20 to $25 million on sports sponsorships on the continent. Medical studies from the time showed that teenagers attending such events tended to smoke the sponsoring company's brand: so Winfield cigarettes were preferred in New South Wales, Peter Jackson brands in Victoria, and Escort cigarettes in South Australia. In each case those were also the sponsoring brands of the local rugby or football teams. Britain's Cancer Research Campaign in 1997 found race-car fans twice as likely to become regular smokers, with the direct and immediate cause being industry sponsorship.[39]

Cigarette sponsorship eventually became a global phenomenon, with all the transnationals having a hand in the action. Reynolds sponsored motocross and rallycross in France, motorcycle trials in Greece, Jeep Jamborees in Japan, World Cup soccer in Mexico, a Camel-Peugeot racing team in Paris, show jumping in Spain, and badminton and breakdancing in various parts of Asia.[40] British American sponsored the Cricket World Cup in India, golf in East Africa, deep sea fishing in Honduras, ice racing in Russia, Kent snooker in Beijing, and Kent beach volleyball in Guangzhou. BAT had sponsored motorsports since the 1960s[41] and had its own Lucky Strike Formula One racing team until 2006, when the European Union barred such hookups. Local manufacturers were often involved: Gudang Garam in Indonesia, a manufacturer of clove cigarettes, sponsored Grand Prix racing and owned one of that country's leading badminton teams. Nobleza-Piccardo sponsored sand dune racing in Argentina, Wills sponsored kite flying in India, Djarum Super sponsored soccer and off-road biking in Indonesia, and 555 sponsored badminton in Beijing. State monopolies got into the act: France's Société Nationale d'Exploitation Industrielle des Tabacs et des Allumettes (SEITA), for example, sponsored sailboat racing in the 1970s and 1980s as part of its effort to boost sales of its Royale brands.

Philip Morris was not the first to enter this realm but eventually became its most aggressive. In 1971 the company sponsored a Marlboro bridge tournament under the auspices of the Venezuelan Bridge Federation and by the 1980s was sponsoring aerobatics, racing, and show jumping in the United Kingdom, along with bridge, bowling, and backgammon in Holland. Soccer was supported in Nigeria, as part of the company's African penetration plan. Asia became a priority in the 1990s, with Koreans for the first time being able to enjoy Marlboro Motor Sports, a Marlboro ski challenge, Marlboro tae kwon do, a Marlboro disco promotion, Marlboro championship tennis, and Marlboro Dynasty Cup soccer. By 1997 Philip Morris had spent an estimated $77 million on Formula One racing sponsorships. We don't have global totals, but Marlboro in the 1990s was advertising itself as "the world's leading corporate sponsor of sporting events."[42]

Funding of such events was often orchestrated with efforts to enlarge them. In 1994, for example, as part of its sponsorship of China's National Football League, Philip Morris helped to increase the roster of teams from twelve to eighteen, to merge with the Hong Kong Football League, and to increase the annual number of matches from 132 to 306. The plan was also to bring in foreign coaches and players and to raise the quality of play to enable the Chinese to participate in World Cup Finals.[43] Philip Morris sponsored Chinese soccer from 1994 to 1999, attracting two million spectators and a much larger television audience in the first year of sponsorship. The grand plan was to undermine the dominance of Japan Tobacco (JT) in the region; JT had already sewn up sponsorships for pan-Asian play with its Mild Seven brand, just as BAT had captured Malaysian sports with Dunhill. The "sponsorship package" drafted by Philip Morris guaranteed television, radio, and newspaper coverage on a very large scale. (The Chinese-language *Soccer* magazine alone reached a million fans twice weekly.) All participants in the Marlboro Chinese Football League were required to wear Marlboro logos on their team shirts. The cost to Marlboro's maker was surprisingly low: only $2 million for 1994, scheduled to rise to $4 million by 1996. China came pretty cheap.

Trademarking such events was important, to prevent encroachments. A 1994 document lists the following registered trademarks for United States Tobacco, a maker of oral snuff and chew: Copenhagen Racing, the Copenhagen/Skoal Shootout, the Copenhagen/Skoal Crusher (a demolition derby), Skoal Bandit Racing, Skoal Bandit Monster Truck, and more than a dozen others. U.S. Tobacco was one of the smaller American firms but by 1987 was sponsoring some seven hundred racing and other events each year "to raise brand awareness." Louis Bantle, the company's president, explained the target market: "The racing enthusiast there is the type of person we're looking for—young, the outdoor type, involved in sports. And it's worked."[44] Which also helps to explain why, in spring 2008, during her run for the presidency, Senator Hillary Clinton allowed herself to be photographed under a large Skoal banner.

Clinton was never a friend of Big Tobacco, which is more than one can say for many other politicians. Prime Minister Tony Blair, for example, in 1997 cut a secret deal with Britain's leading racing tycoon, exempting Formula One racing from the country's planned ban on tobacco sponsorship of sport. London's *Sunday Telegraph* revealed the depth of this scandal in October 2008, noting that Blair had "personally ordered" the exemption after accepting a secret £1 million donation to the Labour Party from Bernie Ecclestone, the Formula One boss and billionaire who stood very much to gain from the special treatment. The new documents show that Blair demanded this "derogation"—against the protests and better judgment of his health secretary—within hours of a meeting with Ecclestone on October 16, 1997. The *Telegraph* also made public a Whitehall memo showing that the prime minister wished to see "a permanent exemption for Formula One" advertising.[45] The

Labour Party returned the money when parts of the deal were leaked but not before a seven-figure sum of Britain's currency came to be known (in racing circles at least) as "a Bernie." And tobacco sponsorship continued far longer than it should have, thanks to some rather sleazy backdoor dealing. Even for a million pounds sterling Britain, too, came pretty cheap.

China was somewhat late to enter the sponsorship game but has recently caught up with help from foreign bodies. Philip Morris scored big with its Marlboro Chinese Football League (soccer in American parlance), but other companies have since become players. BAT's Kent, for example, sponsored the Tour of China bicycle race in 1995, and the same company sponsored the 555 Hong Kong–Beijing Rally, watched by an estimated 750 million Chinese on TV that same year. Reynolds, meanwhile, put on the Salem Beijing Open tennis tournament. Philip Morris has more recently sponsored Grand Prix motorcycle racing and an "American Music Hour." Marlboros were widely advertised on Chinese television in the 1990s, and advertising—especially of local brands—has continued in more oblique forms even after tobacco ads were formally banned in 1995. The Shanghai Tobacco Company's popular Chunghwa brand, for example, posts billboards with slogans like "Love Our Chunghwa," which translates as "Love Our China." Soccer clubs are still being financed by tobacco magnates, albeit now more often with a Chinese face. The Yunnan Hongta Group funds the local Hongta Soccer Club, for example, and in 2003 sponsored David Beckham's Real Madrid soccer team during its visit to Kunming.[46] Japan Tobacco has been trying to enter the Chinese market but so far has had more success in Taiwan, where its Mild Seven brand has been promoted through Mild Seven Karaoke, a Mild Seven Young Female Concert, and a Mild Seven Film Festival. The brand is not well known in Europe or the Americas but is in fact the most popular cigarette in many parts of Asia and the world's second most smoked brand after Marlboro.

Russia has become an attractive transnational target, but even during the Cold War the Soviet tobacco monopoly pushed cigarettes with a youth-oriented academic twist. In 1973, for example, the state-owned tobacco monopoly brought out a new cigarette, the Universiade-73, timed to coincide with the World Student Games in Moscow. Russia since the fall of communism has become a paradise for the global Bigs: whereas one in ten women smoked in the Gorbachev era, ten years after perestroika this had climbed to one in three. Two in ten men smoked in 1985, compared to two in three by 2000. With an annual smokeage soon to reach 400 billion cigarettes, Russia now faces a public health catastrophe of First World proportions. Transnational corporations bear much of the blame: Philip Morris now makes about a third of all cigarettes smoked in the country, and most of the rest is BAT and smaller Russian companies such as Nevo-Tabak, Tabakprom, and Donskoy Tabak. This is quite a recent shift: Philip Morris entered Russia only in 1993 but within a decade controlled nearly a quarter of the entire market.[47]

CHANGING THE GAME

One interesting fact about cigarette sponsorships is that sporting events have often been rejiggered to make them more visible carriers of the sponsor's message. In 1972, for example, Reynolds established its Winston "Rodeo Awards," providing $105,000 in prize money for the best performance in several categories for "top members of the Rodeo Cowboys Association [RCA]." Rodeo had not had much of a television presence, however, until Reynolds invented a "Rodeo Scoreboard" for use at RCA events—bull riding, calf roping, steer wrestling, and the like—allowing brand display. Scoreboards had been unknown at such events, but Reynolds came up with the idea and managed to have them designed and installed—with the Winston name prominently displayed—creating a new advertising platform. A 1979 review concluded that the scoreboards were helping to create brand exposure: "Boards are provided to rodeos at no cost. In addition to the exposure the WINSTON brand receives, it has provided considerable leverage with rodeo committees. Last year scoreboards were viewed at 194 rodeos throughout the nation with exposure to 4 million people."[48] Rodeo was not an easy ride for Reynolds, however, since the popular identification of cowboys with its nemesis Marlboro was already so strong as to prove nearly insurmountable.

Cricket was another sport transformed by tobacco sponsorship. Proud but "sometimes stuffy" was the image Benson & Hedges wanted to overcome in South Africa, which is why the company basically took over South African cricket, infusing a measure of "glitter and entertainment" into the sport to make it more exciting and television-friendly. New and colorful uniforms were designed for the teams, along with new colors for the wickets and sightscreens and substantial prize and travel money for players and staff. Time limits for each side to bat were also established, to prevent overly long games. Stadiums throughout the country were upgraded—by installing powerful electric lights, for example—to facilitate television transmission. Cricket had always been a daytime sport, but the cigarette maker got the South African Cricket Union to approve a "totally new competition" in the form of *night cricket,* which would enable the sport to compete with "more traditional forms of evening entertainment such as the cinema, discos and restaurants." Audience participation was encouraged through events like the Benson & Hedges Throwing the Ball Competition, in which spectators competed to see who could throw a cricket ball the farthest. Cigarette manufacturers judged the new facilities and special events, combined with the live television coverage, "of inestimable benefit in a country where cigarette advertising on the national television channel is not permitted."[49]

Sponsorships of this sort were most often a response to the disappearance of tobacco ads from the airwaves. Sponsorships had another advantage, however, insofar as images of a sponsor's brand could still show up on TV or in newspaper coverage, if carefully positioned. Marlboro and Winston logos often appeared as back-drops for sports stories even in media that didn't take (paid) advertising. Sponsors would typically plan an event to maximize brand visibility—by plastering a logo where it could be seen by cameras. So a Marlboro sign might be glimpsed each time a car passed a certain point on the track, or cameras might catch Martina Navratilova wearing a Kim brand logo during Wimbledon play. (BAT in Britain in 1983 pleaded not guilty to charges of trying to evade that country's advert ban, even though the Kim logo and cigarette pack had identical designs.) At the Winston 500 in Talladega, an oversized Winston pack was parked directly behind the winner's circle "to show up good in photographs and TV coverage." The cars themselves were often painted in vivid Marlboro or Silk Cut colors, and several companies sponsored (or bought up) racing teams. Philip Morris paid millions to acquire the McLaren Formula One team, for example, and McLaren cars even today (and ever since 1981) carry chassis designations of the form "MP4/x," with the MP4 standing for "Marlboro Project 4." So while the event itself might be named for a certain brand, the company could also buy rights to a particular driver, along with the car and gear worn by the crew. Model cars in full Silk Cut or Marlboro regalia were made available for purchase, and hundreds of such "collectibles"—essentially tobacco ads on wheels—can now be found at any given moment on eBay. Judging from the numbers still in circulation, millions of such toys must have been cranked out in the heyday of sponsorships. Some of course must have made their way into the hands of children, and some of those sold in Britain—emblazoned with John Player Special insignia, for example—came with instructions cautioning that "modeling skills" were helpful "if under 10 years of age."[50]

That of course was the whole point: to keep the brand in the public eye. It didn't really matter what sport was being sponsored, or even whether it really *was* a sport, so long as cigarettes entered the hearts and hands of the right kinds of people. Which increasingly in the 1970s and 1980s meant the young and your average blue- and pink-collar working stiff. We don't normally think of auto shows as a sport, for example, but R. J. Reynolds in 1982 started sponsoring Winston Championship Auto Shows, which it took over and renamed from the International Championship Auto Shows. Three million people were expected to attend these two hundred annual events, where 730,000 free packs of cigarettes were to be handed out by "attractive sampling girls." The script by then was familiar: auto shows provided Winston "with a vehicle to reach their prime prospect (blue & white collar) in a recreation activity which is a living execution of the Brand's copy strategy."[51]

Reporting on such events was not left to chance. Reynolds was particularly creative in this respect, inventing a Camel Scoreboard for newspapers inside which scores from the previous day's contests would be printed in agate-font type. Ad-framed information of this sort appeared in hundreds of U.S. newspapers in the mid-1980s. The same company also introduced a Winston Sports Connection Telephone Service, which you could call to get the latest scores (somewhat like Philip Morris's SlimStat). Sports-themed "advertorials" were also placed in newspapers, as when Lorillard (in 1982) convinced the *Wall Street Journal* to run a weekly Kent Sports Business column, creating "an editorial environment within which the Kent family of cigarettes can be promoted." Readers were supposed to think they were getting genuine news ("the content should be perceived as reporting") when the reality was that information was being organized as "an advertising vehicle."[52] *Money* magazine printed similar advertorials for the cigarette maker.

SPECIAL OLYMPICS, ROLLING BILLBOARDS

Most sports sponsorships involved giving away free cigarettes, also known as "sampling." Sampling has a long history: free cigarettes were handed out to patients in hospitals in the 1950s and to passengers on commercial airline flights from the 1940s on (Brown & Williamson had a special arrangement with TWA for this purpose, a practice known as "third party sampling"). Lorillard even handed out free samples to children in the housing projects of urban Boston, prior to the prohibition of this practice by city ordinance in the 1980s. Young men and women dressed in brand-colored outfits would drive trucks into such neighborhoods and hand out mini-packs containing four Newport menthol cigarettes, a practice reminiscent of (and perhaps intentionally designed to emulate) the arrival of the ice-cream man. Sampling was also coordinated with medical conventions—as in 1962, when African American physicians attending the annual meeting of the National Medical Association in Chicago received free Kent cigarettes in attractive plastic flat-packs specially designed for the occasion (see Figure 16). Tobacco companies often sent African American company reps to such meetings (to give away free cigarettes) to make a good impression.[53]

In the 1990s Reynolds sampled at gun shows, swap meets, and flea markets and at car shows, country fairs, and cruising strips. Motorcycle shops were targeted, along with tractor pulls and demolition derbies. Camel sampling was even done in junkyards. Brand themes were sometimes taken into consideration, which is why Brown & Williamson gave away Kool cigarettes at Michigan ice fishing festivals, snowmobile races, and ice sculpture contests. Reynolds in the 1980s was trying hard to attract male smokers of lower socioeconomic status, which is why Camel events were supposed to recognize the "primary interests" of target smokers as "cars, parties, women and music." In the peak years of the 1980s and 1990s, plans for Reynolds promotions included Camel bowling nights, Camel boxing nights, Camel surfing contests, Camel fishing tournaments, Camel bikini contests, a Camel comedy showcase, a Camelcade of sports, a Camel joke book, a Camelfest '89, and a "Camelfornia dreamin'" program "to make Camel synonymous with California lifestyle."[54]

Planning for such events was always kept confidential. One set of instructions

("For Managers Only") detailing plans for Reynolds's 1981 motorcycle racing program had the following caution on its cover:

> UNDER NO CIRCUMSTANCES WHATSOEVER IS ANY OF THIS MATERIAL TO BE SEEN BY TRACK, PRESS, OR CONCESSIONAIRE PERSONNEL. IT WOULD RESULT IN A DISASTER FOR THE PROGRAM. THEREFORE, ALL OF THIS MATERIAL SHOULD BE LEFT AT THE OFFICE WHEN CALLING ON TRACKS, ETC.
> *DO NOT REPRODUCE*[55]

The companies were also careful to make sure sponsored events wouldn't be scheduled in such a way as to draw attention to tobacco's seamier side—say, a breast cancer charity drive taking place in the same hotel as a Virginia Slims Fashion Spree.[56] American Tobacco did sponsor a Lucky Strike Darts for Diabetes tournament in Seattle in 1983, thinking perhaps that the diabetes-smoking link was not strong enough to prompt any recall of tobacco realities. Philip Morris sponsored a number of AIDS charities, principally through its tennis events, though tournaments in Chicago, New York, and Florida in 1992 and 1993 raised only a paltry $70,000. Philip Morris's director of event marketing nonetheless explained to the press why AIDS was important for the company: "We are trying to create an awareness in every market we are in. And, second, we want to raise money."

Philip Morris archives reveal a third benefit in the form of media attention for the sponsoring brand. Media monitors hired by the company in 1993 recorded 126,899,040 "Total Impressions" from recent press coverage of Virginia Slims events, including press releases heralding its charity support. A thick Philip Morris file of press clippings contains 666 mentions of Virginia Slims (or just "Slims") while cancer is mentioned only once, and nowhere in connection with tobacco. Philip Morris summarized the impact of its event marketing for 1993–97, recording 6,158 separate stories in the press with a total circulation of two billion and a readership of five billion—just in the United States. That was five billion opportunities for drawing attention to a Virginia Slims tournament, Merit Bowling, Marlboro Grand Prix, Marlboro dance or music, or Club Benson & Hedges. Press reports were categorized according to whether they were "sports," "lifestyle," "grassroots," or "protest"—though protests were in fact quite rare. In Tampa in 1997 among 135 stories mentioning Philip Morris sponsorships there was only one protest story. Protest reports were consistently below one percent, showing the seductive efficacy of sponsorship but also the moral myopia of the media.[57]

I've mentioned Philip Morris's support for AIDS charities, but the tobacco giant has also given money to shelter the homeless and feed the hungry—and to help battered women.[58] Lorillard and Philip Morris both donated money to the Special Olympics and to the National Theatre for the Handicapped. Imperial Tobacco sponsored a chess tournament for the blind. Altogether between 1995 and 1999 the five largest U.S. tobacco companies spent more than $365 million to sponsor 2,733 distinct events or causes. Sports consumed the largest share, but hunger charities were in second place, receiving more than $100 million. By 2003 the Marlboro men were giving nearly $10 million per year to 295 separate arts and cultural organizations, including children's groups such as the Big Apple Circus.[59]

There was no point in sponsoring such activity without being able to brag about it, however, which is why Philip Morris advertised its support for "innovative initiatives in hunger and nutrition, the arts, education, the environment, domestic violence and the battle against AIDS—around the corner, and across the nation. Providing meals to needy seniors, victims of domestic violence, and people living with AIDS. Preserving American farmlands. Supporting extraordinary dance companies. Promoting diversity among educators throughout the country."[60] Tobacco philanthropy was eventually extended to many different parts of the world. In 1998, for example, Philip Morris published a Spanish-language brochure boasting of its support for a series of environmental initiatives in Latin America, encompassing watershed protection and the teaching of "ecologically sound farming methods." Philip Morris insiders described the brochure as "a beautiful record of our environmental sponsorship," bragging about partnerships forged with the Nature Conservancy, the Audubon Society, the World Wildlife Fund, and the Resource Foundation, all of which had supposedly come to recognize Philip Morris as exemplifying "corporate responsibility toward the environment."[61] And all at "a relatively modest" cost—to the company.

Fortunately, some of our better journalists have challenged such blustering. Bob Herbert in the *New York Times* in 1993 chided Philip Morris for funding the NAACP, the Urban League, the United Negro College Fund, the Harlem YMCA, and other African American charities. Herbert also reported on his interview with David Goerlitz, the jut-jawed Winston Man model, who had once asked whether he could take home some of the cigarettes used in a photo shoot. "Sure, take them all," was the answer from the Reynolds man in charge. Goerlitz then asked whether any of the company's executives smoke and got this answer: "Are you kidding? We reserve that right for the poor, the young, the black and the stupid." Goerlitz was also once told that his job was to be a "live version of a G.I. Joe action figure" and to help the industry get four thousand kids per day to start smoking.[62]

Pushing the envelope, some companies have even used sponsorships to link their products with safety. BAT Germany, maker of that country's popular HB brand, targeted young German drivers by issuing a special monthly *HB Bulletin* containing articles on automotive safety from the *Deutsche Automobil Revue*. In 1982 each of Germany's eight thousand registered driving schools received twenty to twenty-five copies per month of these bulletins, adorned with prominent ads wishing the country's new drivers "safe driving." HB diaries, stickers, and other cigarette-themed goodies were distributed at such schools, along with raffle tickets for substantial prizes. The campaign was coordinated with discotheque sampling and

Windsurfing Fascination shows, as part of the company's effort to target "young adults and people just starting to smoke." In one night of this operation 350 different discos were sampled twice each by the company, during which 105,000 HB three-packs were given away. All part of an effort to address this perennial worry within the industry: "Where will the starter smokers come from?"[63]

THE POWER OF NAMING

Cigarette makers have often been accused of violating broadcast bans, but when the sporting event itself was named for a particular brand it was hard even to talk about without serving up a kind of advertisement. Reynolds events were sometimes held in the North Carolina town of Winston-Salem—corporate headquarters for the tobacco giant—which turned even the venue into a (double) branded ad. Television commentators sometimes tried to avoid mentioning where such contests were taking place, but this was awkward, to say the least. Brand visibility was the whole point, and to maximize impact sponsors often required an event to change its name. When Reynolds took over the Alabama Cup (in Talladega), for example, the race was rechristened the Winston Cup. The Houston Invitational became the Virginia Slims Invitational; the Australian Open (tennis) became the Marlboro Australian Open; Team Yoshimura Suzuki became Team Viceroy Suzuki; the National Singles (Pool) Championship became the Camel 8-Ball Classic; the Grand National Championships (motorcycling) became the Winston Pro Series; the National Volleyball League became the Winston Volleyball League—there are dozens if not hundreds of examples. The cost to the companies was often surprisingly low: Philip Morris in 1970 paid only $2,500 to get its name on the Virginia Slims Invitational, for example, surely one of the best deals ever in the history of marketing.

The companies defended such sponsorships by claiming they were helping to bring neglected sports into the limelight. But the goal was clearly to sell cigarettes. T. Wayne Robertson, director of sports marketing at Reynolds, admitted as much in 1989, noting, "We use sports as an avenue for advertising our products. We can go into an area where we're marketing an event, measure sales during the event and measure sales after the event, and see an increase in sales."[64] This is hardly surprising, given that many of these events were turned into veritable smokefests. Cars at NASCAR races were transformed into rolling billboards, with brand names splashed across every conceivable surface. "Miss Camel girls" posed for publicity shots and handed out awards to drivers or samples to prospective converts. Added value came from a "Smoking Joe" race car and Miss Winston beauty queen. A 1993 estimate put the value of TV exposure accrued to the Winston brand from NASCAR at $20.7 million for that one year. The Winston Cup that season had been the subject of seventy separate telecasts on ABC, CBS, ESPN, and other networks, during which the brand received some 1,707 mentions or images. Reynolds by this time had a 20 percent stake in ESPN, the cable sports network, which helped facilitate such transmissions. For Reynolds too, then, the hope was to "be the media!"

There was also of course the less tangible political support generated from people who ran the tracks or sold concessions or otherwise profited from ticket sales, television coverage, hotel rooms, and other spillovers from the tobacco trade—all of which made sponsorships attractive to the organizers and local merchants. Tobacco money paid for hundreds of thousands of gallons of paint to refurbish decaying stadiums (in brand colors, of course), with money going also to install rest rooms and concession stands. Costs in the form of damage to human organs from augmented cigarette sales remained comfortably invisible and uncalculated, distant in both time and space.

ALIBI BRANDING

Sports sponsorship was banned in the United States under the Master Settlement Agreement in 1998, and other countries are slowly following suit. Germany and France had never allowed much in the way of sports sponsorship, and in 2005 the European Union barred all such sponsorships, along with all print and radio advertising. If the past is any guide to the present, however, we can expect creative ways to get around such bans. The Framework Convention on Tobacco Control calls for an end to all sports sponsorships, but quasi-ads of one sort or another keep cropping up in many parts of the world, even by signatories to the convention. In China, which ratified in 2005, the Olympic gold medalist hurdler Liu Xiang has been paid by the Baisha Tobacco Company to endorse that brand of cigarettes: a 2008 booklet celebrating his life, titled *My Heart Is Flying: A Liu Xiang Photobook,* included more than fifty images of flying cranes, the brand logo of Baisha cigarettes. Profits from the book were supposed to go to charity, but values also accrued to the company from the publicity given its logo.

Sponsors of Formula One cars have also tried to evoke a particular brand using novel cues and subliminal tricks. When tobacco ads were barred on cars at the French Grand Prix, for example, manufacturers came up with surrogate images: Benson & Hedges painted its cars with "Buzzards and Hornets" or "Buzzing Hornets"—and sometimes "Bitten Hisses" or "Bitten Heroes" or "Be On Edge"—hoping to evoke the B&H brand. Britain's Gallaher for many years was able to evoke its Silk Cut brand simply by showing sheets of purple silk cut, pierced, or otherwise ripped in one fashion or another; Israeli manufacturers circumnavigated laws barring the use of human images by turning cigarette packs into human figures—in risqué poses (see Figures 17 and 18). Recall also Scuderia Ferrari's F1 2008 "livery" emulating the bright red of Marlboro while incorporating also a bar code design that looks remarkably like the tall-font lettering of "Marlboro" (Figure 19). Philip Morris has labored hard to have its red chevron "roof" design—and where possible the color red itself—identified with its flagship global brand. The plan of course is to have such shapes and colors trigger brand recall, with no words required. Pavlov would be proud.

Tricks of this sort are known as *alibi branding*, defined by BAT as "a creative execution which does not carry the normal brand name and/or mark," even though it "carries the same likeness."[65] Deployed where advertising is illegal, this is consistent with the industry's long-standing practice of following the letter of the law while violating its spirit. These are after all nimble, agile entrepreneurs, with years of experience turning lemons into lemonade.

Parties, the Arts, and Extreme Expeditions

The unlit cigarette was a tease, the cigarette held near a flame was a provo-cation, the cigarette stuck behind an ear was a promissory note, the cigarette held aloft was a sheathed knife, the cigarette held laterally was a broken ar-row, the cigarette stubbed out was an ultimatum. It was like the language of flowers, or postage stamps. . . . It all resided in the beholder and the beheld, of course.

LUC SANTE, *NO SMOKING*, 2000

Sport has long been a tobacco target, but the same holds true for many other kinds of events where people gather—especially the young. Which is why a decision was made to sponsor festivals and parties, beginning especially in the 1970s and 1980s. The goal here was to identify where a coveted market target might congregate— college students at spring break hot spots, for example—and then to stage elabo-rately branded club events. South Padre Island in Texas and Florida's Fort Laud-erdale and Daytona Beach were prime early prospects, though the practice has since been globalized. Philip Morris has sponsored Marlboro "Red Zone" parties at For-mula One racing events in Malaysia, and Vietnam's National Tobacco Corporation has sponsored the Cambodian Water Festival to drum up support for its Golden Eagle brand. BAT stages similar events in Africa and in other parts of the world.

Marlboro parties seem to have emerged from Philip Morris's Marlboro Resort Program, established in 1977 to target summer vacation spots frequented by young people. By 1990 the program was operating in eighteen cities for the July 4, Me-morial Day, and Labor Day holidays. Marlboro's 1989 Spring Break Program for South Padre Island included "pool deck parties" and a Marlboro Racing Sweep-stakes, featuring as first prize a 1990 Camaro Z-28 convertible. Events of this sort were typically coordinated with local clubs—Charlie's Paradise Bar and Country Club on South Padre Island, for example, which hooked up with Philip Morris by hosting a weeklong promotion of Virginia Slims during the 1987 spring break sea-son. Charlie's hosted the 1989 Marlboro Sweepstakes for which a total of ten thou-sand Marlboro items were distributed, including tank tops, beach towels, fanny packs, koozies, sunglasses, key rings, mugs, and lighters. Places like Charlie's were happy to get the business and knew they could deliver, judging from the promise of club president Charles Lewis to Philip Morris for the 1990 season: "Charlie's can guarantee exposure for your product [from] a minimum of 60,000 to a maximum of 100,000 college students between the ages of 18 and 25. This number of students will be paid admissions to our facility and represents an estimated 20%–25% of the total students at South Padre Island for Spring Break."[1] Bands were often hired for events, but party promotions also included amateur singing nights, dances, drinking parties, and other events where "performance" wasn't really even in the cards. Philip Morris's "Bar Promotions" in the 1990s, for example, included Marlboro Bar Nights, Party at the Ranch, Marlboro Country Dance, Marlboro Latin Dance, Parliament Party Zone (featuring games and sweepstakes), Virginia Slims Dueling Divas, Club Benson & Hedges (music), and a Merit Comedy series.[2]

GOLDCLUB PARTIES AND ETHNIC FESTIVALS

Promotions of the sort described above have sometimes been characterized as *contact sponsorships,* a form of marketing especially popular from the 1980s onward. I've mentioned the spring break bashes at Daytona Beach and South Padre Island, but "club events" and less formal parties have also been staged. In Canada from 2000 to 2003, for example, Rothmans sponsored a series of "Goldclub" parties in the Kitchener-Waterloo area to push its Benson & Hedges brand. Goldclub events featured superstar deejays like Bad Boy Bill, go-go dancers in cages, circus performances, prizes of various sorts, and dancing girls dressed in B&H colors (gold and black) offering cigarettes for sale. The industry would sometimes also pay "cool people" to smoke in select bars and clubs; the technique is known as *viral advertising* or *influential seeding,* with the idea being that people will copy this fashion, which would then spread as if by infection.[3]

Party sponsorships from early on included "ethnic" festivals. Reynolds led with its Winston San Juan Fiesta in 1976 and then used its Salem Summer Street Scenes in 1981 "as a means of penetrating the Black Market." Philip Morris organized competing Marlboro events at Carnival in Miami, Cinco de Mayo and Mexican Independence Day in Los Angeles, the Fiesta Del Sol in Chicago, the Fiesta de San Juan in New York, the Tejano Superfest in Houston, Charro Days and Calle Ocho in Miami, and so forth. Marlboro Hispanic Festivals typically involved a mix of entertainment, auto racing, Marlboro booths, banners, posters, sweepstakes, and distribution of "incentive items" such as lighters and caps, more than a hundred thousand of which were given out in 1982 alone. Spanish-language media were paid to cover the festivities—with the goal of making Marlboro "the primary focus of the festival." Entertainment was carefully planned to provide "brand visibility to Marlboro while giving the audience the impression that Marlboro had discovered and presented the talent for everybody's enjoyment." Such sponsorships grew throughout the 1980s, and in 1988 alone Philip Morris added eighteen new events, plus a "Marlboro Menthol Inner City Bar Night Program for African Americans. Brown & Williamson sponsored Kool Jazz Festivals, which targeted blacks with cosponsorship from Kentucky Fried Chicken, Stroh's Beer, and Exception black hair care products. Reynolds in 1982 predicted an increased opportunity in the form of "ethnic markets"—especially blacks and Hispanics—because of the "phenomenal growth rates" of such groups relative to the population as a whole. Blacks and Hispanics were also attractive because this market was "younger than the population as a whole," with more than 40 percent of Hispanics being under eighteen years of age.[4]

MUSEUMGOERS VERSUS NASCAR FANS

Tobacco-wise, *sponsorship of the arts* has never been much different from sponsoring sports, though the markets are somewhat different. Museumgoers and NASCAR fans tend not to smoke the same brands of cigarettes, but smoking by the 1970s was also becoming more of a lower-class phenomenon, meaning a lower payoff (in terms of sales) for a dollar spent promoting the arts compared with a dollar spent on sports. The difficulty was expressed in a 1978 Philip Morris discussion of the "problem." As one author put it, "The most important problem I see with sponsorship of the arts is that it reaches the wrong target group. In the main the arts are more of interest to the A/B class than to the lower social classes C and D. Smoking is becoming more and more a C/D class habit." This same tobacconist concluded that "sport sponsorship fits the class and mass exposure criteria much better, and therefore sells more cigarettes per $ spent."[5]

Quite apart from short-term sales, however, sponsorship of the arts was judged to have a certain "commercial value" by virtue of its impact on public relations. Sponsorship created an attractive image for a company but also a certain useful dependency—and not just for connoisseurs or performers. Promoters and organizers were in effect "hooked," making it hard to refuse tobacco money or hard even to perform without. In a 1994 exposé for the *Village Voice* Alisa Solomon dubbed this "The Other Nicotine Addiction," asking what by now should sound like a very strange question, "Can there be art without tobacco?"[6]

Big Tobacco has sponsored hundreds if not thousands of art exhibits, dance performances, museum shows, and concerts.[7] The goal has generally been less to attract smokers than to gain good feeling among the cultural elite. Sponsorship buys a kind of silence or, if need be, political support. Dozens of the world's leading theaters and museums have taken tobacco money—in New York alone this includes the Museum of Modern Art, the American Folk Art Museum, the Brooklyn Academy of Music, the Guggenheim Museum, the American Ballet Theatre, the American Museum of Natural History, the Dance Theater of Harlem, and quite a few others. BAT has supported the London Symphony Orchestra; Imperial and Gallaher have supported Glyrodeboume and Covent Garden; Benson & Hedges (BAT) has put on the Australian Ballet; Philip Morris has sponsored Pavarotti.

The tobacco companies defend such acts as philanthropy, but of course they want something in return: "innocence by association," as one watchdog website puts it. Or as Peter Taylor writes in his *Smoke Ring*, BAT sponsors the Philharmonia to get us to associate cigarettes with "Elgar and Tchaikovsky, instead of cancer and bronchitis." As in sports, though, there is no point to sponsorship if the company's name cannot be made *visible*. The sponsoring corporation is identified on tickets and programs—and sometimes even in the title of the event. When Philip Morris sponsored the Marlboro Country Music Festival at New York's Lincoln Center, the name of the world's most popular cigarette was splashed across the marquee. The juxtaposition may seem odd, but ads for the festival came with a Surgeon General's warning.[8]

Sampling is not unknown at such events. In 1994, when the Metropolitan Museum of Art sponsored an exhibit on the origins of Impressionism, a journalist at the opening remarked on how the smoking of free cigarettes had led to the Temple of Dendur being "enveloped in a cloud of smoke." Art-oriented sponsorships have prompted spiritual benedictions, as in 1987, at the Met's *Treasures of the Vatican,* when the Catholic archbishop of New York led a prayer for George Weissman, president of the sponsoring corporation. A Philip Morris vice president later remarked that his was probably "the only cigarette company on this earth to be blessed by a cardinal." Payback more often takes less spiritual forms—as in 1990, when the artistic director of the Alvin Ailey American Dance Theater (Judith Jamison) allowed her name to be used in ads for Philip Morris—wherein smoking was defended essentially as a form of free speech. The dance company testified in support of the industry before the U.S. Congress that same year, following which (in 1991) the dancers accepted half a million dollars from the Marlboro maker.

Not all such sponsorships are for adults. In 2005 Altria—the new name for Philip Morris as of 2002—sponsored a string of performances of Maurice Sendak's *Brundibar* at Berkeley's Repertory Theatre. I once asked the producers how they felt about having a cigarette maker sponsor a play for children, and their sheepish defense was basically that money has to be taken wherever it can be found. That is part of the problem: we live in a world where funding for the arts is not easy to come by. Tobacco companies in the United States helped fill a void created by Ronald Reagan's withdrawal of support for the arts in the 1980s—making collaborations of this sort more attractive. Performance Space 122 artistic director, Mark Russell, when asked what he thought about such sponsorships replied, "Of course they're using us. We're using them too."[9]

JAZZ VERSUS CLASSICAL AND ROCK MUSIC

Music has been another solid tobacco platform, and for many of the same reasons. Collaborations of this sort date back to the 1920s and 1930s, when popular radio shows were sponsored by cigarette makers: the *Lucky Strike Radio Hour,* the *Lucky Strike Hit Parade,* the *Al Pearce Show for Camel Cigarettes,* the *Chesterfield Supper Club,* and so forth. Sponsorships continued into the television era, until the broadcast ban of 1971 forced the industry to seek other outlets.

Philip Morris in 1982, for example, began its "Marlboro Music" program, sponsoring the gamut of genres from rock and classical to folk, Latin, and rhythm & blues. Country music was the focus for the first seven years, as Philip Morris filled one arena after another with shows featuring Alabama, Hank Williams Jr., Randy Travis, George Strait, Reba McEntire, Merle Haggard, Dolly Parton, and countless others, all of whom became veterans of the Marlboro circuit. Marlboro Music was broadened to include rock and roll in 1990, by which time sponsorships had been extended to state and county fairs. Military bases became a target in 1989, when Latin shows and "top names from the genres of Rock, Country and/or R&B" were incorporated. Industry-sponsored concerts were often innovative: Marlboro's country music events, for example, were among the first to use video displays to augment spectacular sound and lights.[10]

Brown & Williamson focused more on jazz than on country or rock, no doubt because it already had a strong African American base with its menthol-flavored Kools. The Kool Jazz Festivals—launched in 1975—were part of the company's "Kool Brand Strategic Plan," designed to maintain the current "Kool ethnic franchise" but also to entice "young adult starting smokers and non-menthol switchers."[11] Millions of dollars went into acquiring top musical talent for these events, with performers including Aretha Franklin, B. B. King, the Isley Brothers, Smokey Robinson, the Pointer Sisters, the Temptations, and numerous others. By 1982 the company was running twenty events in twenty different cities, using jazz as a means of reaching young blacks and Hispanics. Here again the plan was to expropriate an already existing cultural icon: the Newport Jazz Festival had been founded by jazz maverick George Wein in 1954 (with financial support from Elaine Lorillard, heiress of the Lorillard tobacco fortune), and all Brown & Williamson did was to (dramatically) expand the event while also changing the name to highlight its flagship menthol brand.

The beauty of this scoop was that "Newport" was also the name of the leading competitive threat to Kool. Lorillard's Newport brand had been growing in popularity among African Americans since the 1950s, and by attaching the Kool name to the festival Brown & Williamson achieved a kind of marketing double whammy. (For a while, though, the Newport event had the oddly chimerical title "Kool Newport Jazz Festival"—odd by virtue of the fact that Kool and Newport were cigarette

brands made by separate companies.) Kool Jazz Festivals drew millions of afi-
cionados, but the cigarette brand was made further visible via Kool Jazz Records,
Kool City Jams (in fifteen cities), Kool Super Nights at military installations, and
the Kool Newport Jazz Festival scholarship for jazz musicians at the Juilliard School
of Music. Brown & Williamson commissioned detailed studies of the perception of
such events and found that people who had heard about the concerts were significantly more likely to have "quality and satisfaction perceptions of the KOOL brand."
They were also more than twice as likely to buy Kool cigarettes. People who knew
about the concerts were also far more likely to think highly of the company doing
the sponsoring.[12]

Musicians usually appreciated this support. George Wein, producer of the New-
port/Kool events, once characterized Brown & Williamson's support as "incredi-
ble[,] . . . a great bonanza for jazz," and "like a dream come true." Wein seems not
to have recognized (or cared about) sponsorships as a vehicle for selling cigarettes.
Jazz clubs have been notoriously smoky over the years, which is no doubt one reason so many jazz greats have succumbed to lung cancer (see the box on page 124).
Marketers at Brown & Williamson were quite pleased with the fact that its Kool
Jazz Festivals had become "an excellent, if not the best, way to reach over half a million Blacks directly and create awareness of Kool among many more."[13]

Interesting in all of this, again, is the distinction between advertising the *brand*
and advertising the *company*: the brand was featured when an event was designed
to sell cigarettes; the company was featured when the event was supposed to spread
goodwill. So "Marlboro" typically didn't sponsor events at the Met or the Guggenheim; that was the job of Philip Morris. Reynolds funded academic appointments;
Winston sponsored racing. Recall also that "sponsoring" an artistic or musical event
rarely meant just giving someone money. Signage and sampling rights were usually part of the deal, and the sponsoring company typically got exclusive rights to
set up banners and booths for distributing brand-themed merchandise. All of these
were involved in Philip Morris's 1990 sponsorship of the Summer Lights Festival
in Nashville, Tennessee,[14] as in most other industry-financed happenings.

Not all musicians agreed to take tobacco money. In the summer of 1983, when
James Taylor and Peter, Paul, and Mary learned that a concert for which they had
been scheduled (on the Boston Commons) was sponsored by R. J. Reynolds, they
refused to perform. The cigarette maker was eliminated as a sponsor, and the show
went on as planned—absent the cigarette pitch. Hall and Oates have turned down
tobacco money, as have the Oak Ridge Boys and a number of other groups. Pete
Seeger resigned from the Weavers (in 1958) when the group decided to make a cigarette jingle. Not everyone will do anything for a buck.

Collaboration seems to have been more common than resistance, however. Thousands of musicians have performed at events organized by the industry. Barbara
Mandrell was supported by Marlboro, and Juice Newton and Alabama's tour of 1983

AMERICAN JAZZ GREATS KNOWN TO HAVE DIED FROM LUNG CANCER

Kenny Rankin, vocalist	d. 2009
Haydain Neale, member Jacksoul	d. 2009
Joe Beck, guitarist	d. 2008
Dave McKenna, pianist	d. 2008
Leroy Jenkins, violinist	d. 2007
George Melly, vocalist	d. 2007
Albert Timothy Eyermann, instrumentalist	d. 2007
Lou Rawls, soul singer	d. 2006
Clarence "Gatemouth" Brown, fiddle and guitar	d. 2005
Preston Love, saxophone, Count Basie's band	d. 2004
Walter Perkins, Chicago drummer	d. 2004
Ruby Braff, trumpet	d. 2003
Rosemary Clooney, singer	d. 2002
Marion Montgomery, singer	d. 2002
Billy Mitchell, tenor saxophone, Count Basie's band	d. 2001
Donald Tecumseh "Tee" Carson, Count Basie's band	d. 2000
Lee Allen, saxophone	d. 1994
Eric Gale, guitar	d. 1994
John Carter, clarinet	d. 1991
Art Blakey, drummer and band leader	d. 1990
Sarah Vaughan, singer	d. 1990
Paul Desmond, alto saxophone, with Dave Brubeck	d. 1977
Duke Ellington, bandleader	d. 1974
Don Byas, saxophone, Count Basie's band	d. 1972
Ike Quebec, saxophone	d. 1963
Jimmy Dorsey, bandleader	d. 1957
Vic Berton, drummer	d. 1951

was sponsored by Salem. Philip Morris used to keep a list of talent for use in such events, as did most of the other companies. Artists have always been carefully chosen to match the target audience: so when Reynolds organized the Salem Harlem Week Music Festival in New York, artists were chosen to appeal to the target black community. The goal in each case has been to reach "a highly targeted mass audience at an event which is associated with the brand."[15] Which is also why cigarette makers have encouraged public involvement in music as performers in company-sponsored competitions.

In 1989, for example, Philip Morris launched a "grassroots" promotional scheme with its Marlboro Music Talent Roundup. Amateurs were invited to fill out a form and send in a cassette, from which a select few were chosen to move on to regional and national tryouts—something like an early version of *American Idol*. The winner of the 1989 competition, a group called Angel Train, toured military bases ("selected by military sales to meet their sale objectives") together with Poco and .38 Special. The industry has a long history of encouraging mass participation: Allan Brandt in his *Cigarette Century* recounts how in the 1930s two million Americans filled out elaborate forms for a chance to win a $100,000 prize from Lorillard, makers of Old Gold cigarettes.[16] "Contesticians" spent an average of 80 hours researching and writing their answers, which means that something on the order of 160 million hours were squandered on such nonsense. Philip Morris continues such tricks in the new millennium, asking people to send in their favorite chili recipes as part of a Marlboro promotion. "50 Winning Chili Recipes" were published in 2002—from a pool of some 25,000 recipes submitted.

ADVENTURE TRAVEL

Another ploy from the 1980s was to sponsor "adventure travel" to remote parts of the world where "the man or woman who wants a challenge, not a snapshot," would raft, climb, or trek through spectacular hostile/lush terrain as part of a brand-themed extravaganza. Reynolds was the pioneer here, sponsoring Camel Expeditions to exotic locales that could then be filmed and broadcast as branded bravado posing as frontier sport. Extreme sports management was in fine form in the Camel Expeditions, which in 1981 included a rafting trip on the Allagash in Maine, a two-week trek through Ecuador, and a ten-day sailing and diving adventure in the Caribbean. Thomas Cook Travel helped Reynolds plan and run these junkets, for which seventeen thousand brochures were sent out to agents. Subsequent Camel Expeditions included the Great Borneo Traverse of 1983, a Camel Ski Adventure, and a Camel Mount Everest Circumnavigation. A million-dollar advertising blitz invited participants to take one of these "rugged, demanding, memorable" adventures "into the unknown and unexpected"; applicants were assured that the experience would leave them "forever changed."

> For there is an adventurer's heart in millions of us. No matter how comfortable, civilized or sophisticated we become, we share a deep and natural yearning for the primitive.
>
> As the wilderness calls to us, it shrinks. It retreats even as we treasure it, becoming less and less accessible. Still, common knowledge tells us there is no mass market for adventure travel.
>
> Perhaps that was so.
>
> Until now.
>
> Until Thomas Cook and R. J. Reynolds combined to create and promote The Camel Expeditions.
>
> Never before has adventure travel—or any group travel package—received such massive promotion.[17]

The ultimate goal, as revealed in unpublished corporate correspondence, was somewhat less breathtaking. Camel Expeditions were envisioned as "an excellent way to build the perception of Camel cigarettes among its target smoker audience." Film crews were hired to "document" the adventure for use in subsequent publicity, as was done for the 1982 Camel International Speed Skiing Championship. The idea was to associate the Camel name with noble risks and epic masculinity—and to have this reported in the popular press. Which seems to have worked rather well. The 1982 Camel Expeditions program generated "nearly 60 million print impressions and more than 15 million television and 6 million radio impressions," including stories in the *New York Times* and other major news outlets, along with coverage by newswire services and network television.[18] Similar coverage was given to a "Winston Recovery Team" trip to Greenland, a trek through Borneo and Papua New Guinea, the circumnavigation of Everest, and a Camel Arapahoe race. Cigarette companies in other parts of the world sponsored similar events: Export "A" (RJR-Macdonald's Canadian brand) sponsored men's downhill ski racing in Canada, for example, and other extreme sports. The point was to associate smoking with pushing the limits, living fearlessly on the edge; smokers were to be imagined as intrepid adventurers, people who are willing to take chances. Extreme cowboys, one could say, who won't let the "Big C" drag them down (as John Wayne used to say before he succumbed).

Not every effort along these lines was successful. Philip Morris in 1995 made a big deal of its Marlboro Unlimited Sweepstakes, offering two thousand Marlboro smokers an opportunity to travel on a specially outfitted luxury train, a third of a mile long, through America's remote western mountains and basins. Fanfare for the gimmick lasted for a couple of heavily promoted years, but by 1997, with the industry facing PR problems and onerous litigation, the plan was scrapped. Eighteen finished luxury cars were dismantled by Denver's Rader Railcar, and Philip Morris took a $50 million bath on the botched project.

FASHION SHOWS AND DISASTER RELIEF

Since the 1980s the tobacco industry has found many new ways to advertise. Companies pay retailers to guarantee product placement and pay bartenders to flash target brands in high-status social clubs. Event sponsorship has spun off into support for film festivals and fashion shows—with fashion in particular conceived as a way to reach female smokers.

Fashion has been a cigarette hook since the 1920s, when American Tobacco organized green gown fund-raising balls and "Green Fashion Fall" luncheons to promote colors that would match the (green) Lucky Strike pack. The 1970s incarnations, however, were nationwide in scope and directed at a more diverse audience. R. J. Reynolds sponsored all 158 Ebony Fashion Fairs in the 1975–76 season, for example, with the goal of popularizing More cigarettes among African Americans. In the 1980s this same company sponsored the More Bloomingdale's Program to reach upscale smokers. More-brand Ebony Fashion Fairs involved sampling, door prizes, models with wardrobes selected by the cigarette maker, plus of course ads in local media. Philip Morris piled on with extravagant, two-week Virginia Slims Fashion Fun Fairs incorporating beauty makeovers, hair styling, color analysis, wardrobe coordination, antique jewelry appraisal, and showings of the film *You've Come a Long Way, Baby.* Lorillard for its part ran Newport swimwear shows and body art exhibitions featuring "Newport inspired" pseudo-tattoos on models hired for that purpose.[19]

Disaster relief has also been used to boost corporate images. Philip Morris in 1989, for example, capitalized on Hurricane Hugo by helping to finance cleanup operations. "Our corporate-wide disaster relief made a series of splendid hits in the aftermath of Hurricane Hugo," is how Corporate Affairs put it, when it thought no one would be listening. The cleanup and surrounding publicity yielded "solid and positive reaction to our activity from Puerto Rican and South Carolina officials," the company claimed.[20] No calamity seems too big, judging from Japan Tobacco's 2009 sponsorship of a memorial (in Vienna) to the victims of Hiroshima—with no mention of the inconvenient truth that smokers are exposed to more deadly radiation from cigarettes than from any other source.

New techniques have also been devised to get around advertising bans. Philip Morris developed its Marlboro Classics line of clothing and camping gear, for example, to keep the brand name in circulation. The same purpose was served by the company's Marlboro Country Store, established as a mail order catalog in 1972 for cowboy items such as belts, boots, and Stetson hats. One advantage of advertising in this form is that manufacturers don't have to affix warning labels of any kind—and brand names can end up circulating long after their initial purchase. Search "Marlboro" on eBay, for example, and you'll find hundreds of items for sale, mostly clothing, cookbooks, camping gear, and other products designed to keep that hallmark brand on display.

BRAND STRETCHING

The trick is known as *brand stretching, indirect advertising, alibi advertising, co-advertising,* or *trademark diversification,* and has been deliberately developed to get around advertising bans. A 1979 internal document from BAT explained how the company could keep its brands in view, even with a total ban on advertising: "Opportunities should be explored by all companies so as to find non-tobacco products, and other services which can be used to communicate the brand or house name, together with their essential visual identifiers. This is likely to be a long-term and costly operation, but the principal way nevertheless to ensure that cigarette brands can be effectively publicised when all direct forms of communication are denied."[21] BAT followed this recommendation when it unveiled its Lucky Strike Leisure Wear in 1991, but the technique has been deployed all over the globe. In Hong Kong, for example, RJR Nabisco established a Salem Attitude line of clothing "to extend the Trademark beyond tobacco category restrictions."[22] Marlboro Classics stores have been set up in more than a dozen countries to sell jeans, belts, boots, jackets, wallets, and sundry forms of outdoor gear. Reynolds has done the same with its Camel Trophy Clothing, Camel Adventure Gear, Camel Music, Camel Planet (a nightclub promotion), Camel Party Zone CDs, and so forth. The brand name is insinuated into popular culture by attaching it to items that have only fantasy associations with smoking. Brand stretching has been widely deployed in Asia, especially for items likely to be used by teenagers. So in Thailand cigarette logos have appeared on notebooks, kites, pants, earrings, and chewing gum. In Romania Reynolds somehow got its Camel brand name emblazoned onto traffic lights—the actual parts that turn green or red. And in the Czech Republic Camel has even sponsored weddings.[23] The scale and scope of such activities is impressive. By the mid-1990s more than a thousand Marlboro Classics stores had been established in Europe and Asia. R. J. Reynolds had fifteen Camel clothing stores in Thailand and Malaysia alone. The idea is that people will walk around displaying branded merchandise, becoming mobile ads for the brand. Reynolds for many years had a special merchandising division to handle such sales, which in 1975 topped more than a million items in the United States alone. The company's marketers celebrated this as a million " 'walking billboards' for our brand."[24]

Malaysia has become a proving ground for many such efforts, following the banning of more traditional forms of advertising (television, magazines, billboards, etc.) in the early 1990s. BAT established a chain of Benson & Hedges Bistros in the capital city of Kuala Lumpur in 1998, with menus, sugar packs, staff outfits, and the eatery itself decked out in the cigarette's trademark golden colors. Salem Cool Planet had seven outlets in Malaysia by the end of the 1990s and further spread the cigarette via brand-themed concerts. BAT for a time used the locally popular brand Perilly's to sponsor movies in the country, and the Peter Stuyvesant Travel Agency was established by Rothmans to push that brand. Reynolds drew criticism in the early 1990s when it advertised Salem High Country tours—which apparently existed in name only. The company was using this fictional entity simply to keep the Salem name on television, contra the broadcast ban.[25] Similar tricks were tried in Thailand, where ads appeared for luxurious "Kent Leisure Holidays." Is it fraud to advertise a product that does not exist?

Coffee has been another advertising vehicle in Malaysia. In 1996 BAT started a line of Benson & Hedges Quality Blend Coffee to capitalize on—and reinforce—rituals linking coffee and cigarettes. One shop manager in Kuala Lumpur was quite open about the purpose behind such endeavors: "Of course this is all about keeping the Benson & Hedges brand name to the front. We advertise the Benson & Hedges Bistro on television and in the newspapers. The idea is to be smoker-friendly. Smokers associate a coffee with a cigarette. They are both drugs of a type." BAT about this time confirmed that it had set up a subsidiary to look into Lucky Strike clothing, John Player special whiskey, and a Kent travel agency: "Yes, these products share the trademarks of our tobacco products—luxury products have done that for years—but they should not be caught by any marketing restrictions because we are not selling cigarettes with them. The [advertising] regulators could rightly be suspicious if the products do not stand on their own feet but as serious revenue-generating products then I think the regulators do not have a case." A BAT official close to the campaign observed that such products were "a logical step" for cigarette makers: "They are running out of markets in which they can openly advertise. So the thinking is, well 'Okay, if we can't advertise cigarettes we will advertise another product which will have a halo effect on the cigarette brand.'"[26]

Efforts to establish similar "halo effects" can be found in Romania, where the transnationals have come up with schemes to circumvent a 2000 law banning ads in the vicinity of schools and medical facilities. BAT can no longer advertise cigarettes directly, but it has managed to put up banners bearing Kent cigarette slogans such as "Smooth Transmission" and "True: Performance." Philip Morris has banners for L&M announcing, "Get Smooth and Get Going." Both companies' banners were on display at the Agronomy Faculty in Bucharest as recently as 2006.[27] Romania joined the European Union in 2007, and it remains to be seen what trickery will be tried when EU-wide regulations are enforced. The stakes are high, given that Romanian teens have one of the highest smoking rates in Europe.

The Chinese have come up with equally clever ways to circumvent that country's 1995 ad ban. One trick has been to advertise not the cigarette but rather the cigarette *factory*—which often has the same name as the brand. So billboards splash the words "Honghe Cigarette Factory" across a bright red background with a fast car or motorcycle front and center. Manufacturers also use the names of famous temples or monuments to sell cigarettes. Huanghelou, for example, is both a brand of cigarette and a famous temple in Hubei; and the Ningbo Factory's Dahongying brand captures the cultural panache of China's most beloved Neolithic site (from where rice is said to have originated). The country's much-smoked Chunghwa brand has China itself as its name and the famous cloud-winged marble pillar of Tiananmen Square—the Huabiao—right on the pack. The point is to identify cigarette brands with beloved sites or sacred icons, as if we here in the United States had, say, "Liberty" or "Christ" cigarettes festooned with the Liberty Bell or a crucifix—or a cowboy for that matter. The packs are designed to entice in the manner of a miniature ad, but the sites themselves can be harnessed to carry the manufacturer's message.

This *hijacking of symbols* has become quite widespread. The Virgin Mary is used to sell cigarettes in the Philippines, just as Shakespeare is used for this purpose in Great Britain (Benson & Hedges once sold a Hamlet brand, though I have also seen a Romeo y Julieta brand from Havana). Angkor cigarettes are sold in Cambodia, Great Wall cigarettes in Hong Kong, Red Star cigarettes in North Korea, Taj Mahal cigarettes in India, and Sumer cigarettes in Iraq. The hope of course is that the referenced place or object will evoke the cigarette, so that when you think about pandas or cowboys or some temple in China your thoughts may drift to that faraway place—and the cigarette bearing its name. The use of symbols in this manner also has a certain political value: in China, for example, one argument against graphic warnings has been that these would deface venerated national symbols. In reality, though, it is the tobacco factories that are abusing Chinese life and symbols.

Perhaps even more disturbing in the Chinese context is that *schools* are being used to promote tobacco. The Ningbo Cigarette Factory has been building libraries for schools in many parts of China and naming these after its popular Dahongying brand. Tobacco companies helped rebuild schools after the Wenchuan earthquake in 2008, in exchange for which they were allowed to place gigantic ads on the schools' walls. Sichuan Tobacco Hope Primary School in the Wenchuan area has huge permanent wall lettering instructing students, "Genius comes from hard work; Tobacco helps you to be successful." There are at least seventeen "Hope Primary Schools" named after sponsoring tobacco firms, all in poorer parts of the country. China is home to the youngest known person ever to have been taught to smoke (a two-year-old from Chongqing—though an Indonesian kid about the same age—Ardi Rizal—has recently become an Internet sensation), and efforts to advertise even in elementary schools show the callous shortsightedness of the country's state-run Tobacco Monopoly Administration.[28]

PACK ART AND POWER WALLS

Tobacco-pack art presents us with a kind of micro-advertising, and it is important to realize how diverse such images have been in the century since the rise of the modern cigarette. I have seen Boy Scout cigarettes, Eros cigarettes, and Sport cigarettes; and in Japan we have Hope and Peace smokes, both with name brands in English, interestingly. The Tong Nam Tobacco Company in Singapore for a time manufactured My Dear cigarettes, and Nanyang Brothers in China used to sell a Double Happiness brand. Cigarette names are sometimes politically charged: China in its early Communist era had a Liberation cigarette, for example, while the Soviets had a Sputnik brand celebrating the world's first artificial satellite and a Laika brand honoring the first dog in space—both of which boasted hammer and sickle designs on the pack (Laika didn't make it back to earth alive, a fact not mentioned in Soviet-era ads). German political parties in the 1920s and 1930s made and sold cigarettes to generate income: the Nazi Party's Brownshirts had their own brands—Sturm, Alarm, and Front, for example—and some cigarette companies incorporated swastikas into their cigarette pack art (Nortag, for example). Some such associations are ironic: in China a number of lung cancer victims live in a Kunming housing project called Red Pagoda Gardens, named for the tobacco company (Red Pagoda) that supplied the funds for it to be built. Several countries in Asia have had Long Life or Longevity brands.

Health has long been a theme in naming brands. The Axton-Fisher Company in Kentucky in the 1930s sold a Listerine brand cigarette (Figure 20)—marketed as a remedy for colds—and a Greek company more recently evoked health with its Santé brand. (Denmark also used to have a brand by this name.) Health has been implied in many Asian brands: herbal cigarettes are commonly smoked in China, for example, and you often find brands with names like Ginseng or Hong Gou Qi, with the healing root or herb featured prominently on the pack. Some generics in the United States are named for the pharmacy chains that sell them—which is why we find Rite Aid Quality Seal Cigarettes and the like. In 2011 Safeway still sells cigarettes, violating the assurance in the supermarket chain's very name.

Sport has long been a theme of cigarette pack art. Canadians in the 1890s smoked an Athlete brand, for example, and early American brands had names like Home Run, Knockout, and Hole-in-One Golf. Europeans jumped on this same bandwagon. A Dutch company in the 1930s sold a Sport brand featuring a big soccer ball on the front of the pack; BATCo Amsterdam sold Race Cigarettes featuring a revved-up hot rod; and Swedes in the 1960s smoked a Chessman cigarette. A Singapore company used to sell a Golfer pack, and as late as the 1970s Liggett sold its nostalgic Home Run brand with images of vintage baseball players on the pack. Sport itself has been a cigarette in many parts of the world; the Wiki-site Cigarettespedia in 2009 listed eighteen different brands with this name.

What trick has *not* been tried? High fashion is evoked in brands such as Ritz, Cartier Vendome, and Pierre Cardin, but brand names have also included Love (1968), Space (1958), and Sex Bomb (1912). I myself own a pack of Texas brand cigarettes from Rhodesia, some Harley Davidsons made by Lorillard, and a Revelation brand tobacco tin from Philip Morris's Factory No. 15 in Virginia. The Swiss in the 1920s sold Nadir cigarettes, and Germany's A. Batschari about this time sold a Radium brand—which may or may not have contained the precious isotope. Some brands are jokes: witness Horse Shit cigarettes ("stable blended . . . not a fart in a car load") or the same company's Go to Hell brand ("I like 'em and I'm going to smoke 'em . . . Cheaper than psychiatry, better than a nervous breakdown"). Some of these humor packs are morbid: Black Death cigarettes, for example, come with a top-hatted skull on the front and a Jolly Roger on the back. More serious are the packs specially made for distribution during presidential campaigns. I have seen Bush, Nixon, Dukakis, and Eisenhower cigarettes, but surely there are others. Special cigarettes have also been made for the presidential retreat at Camp David (by Liggett) and the presidential yacht Sequoia (by Philip Morris).

With opportunities for traditional advertising curtailed, new ways to keep the product in view are constantly being devised. One avenue has been to build more advertising into the packaging itself. *Cigarette pack art* has become one of the final frontiers of advertising, a "media vehicle" in Philip Morris-speak: "As media restrictions increase, the brand pack should become a media vehicle. The 'book pack' objective is to transform the pack from a 'passive container' into an 'active means of communication,' an object that projects an image and a lifestyle by itself."[29] Marketers have been creative in fashioning point-of-sale and specifically *point-of-pack* marketing. When tobacco ads were banned in Canada in 2003, cigarette marketers responded by setting up "power walls" in retail stores consisting of huge stacks of packs that function more or less as billboard ads. Cigarette makers pay a premium for retail display space close to checkout counters, realizing that this will encourage impulse buying. Impulse buying is a big part of cigarette sales, which makes sense when we consider the deeply irrational nature of the habit. Smoking is not a rational act: witness the force of symbolic goading and affect-rich promotions. Smoking is also increasingly an affliction of the poor and mentally infirm, which helps explain why cigarettes are one of the most commonly shoplifted items in many parts of the world.

Point-of-pack advertising has blossomed as a result of macro-advertising bans, as cigarette makers capitalize on the fact that cigarettes are objects of intimacy for smokers. Smokers who reach for a cigarette, say, twenty times a day will end up fondling those packs some 7,300 times per year—whence the incentive to exploit this intimacy. Reynolds has developed special "series" or "collectors' editions" packs, some of which sport graphics by up-and-coming artists. Reynolds in the mid-1990s put NASCAR scenes on its Winston Cup packs to celebrate the twenty-fifth anniversary of racing sponsorship, and in the new millennium introduced packs featuring the signed designs of well-known tattoo artists. The artists get good exposure, and Reynolds gets its cigarettes linked to a popular teenage fashion. Which is also why tobacco control advocates call for banning all brand imagery (and color) on all cigarette packs—and graphic warnings covering some large fraction of any pack's surface. The world leader here is Uruguay, which now requires all cigarettes sold in that country to have graphic warnings covering at least 80 percent of the pack—front and back. Australia has also recently passed a law allowing no brand art whatsoever on any cigarette packaging, with a target onset date of 2012.

. . .

It would be impossible to list *all* of the ways the industry has marketed its products; there are simply too many.[30] In a sense everything they do is a form of marketing, just as everything is done with an eye to the threat of litigation. Marketing is not inherently a black art, but that is what the smoke folk have turned it into. And since cigarettes are the world's leading preventable cause of death, marketers are complicit in that mortality. We need to think more broadly about these myriad causal links chaining us to smoking, insofar as these are links that might be broken. We also have to keep in mind that if cigarettes cause cancer, then so does everything that causes cigarettes to be made and people to smoke them. We don't think often and hard enough about the "causes of causes," which is crucial for understanding how we might free ourselves from this deadly bond.[31]

8

Clouding the Web

Tobacco 2.0

The Internet will help achieve "friction free capitalism."
BILL GATES

Welcome to Cigarettes Cheaper. Save Money, Save Time.
ADVERTISEMENT FOR CIGARETTES ONLINE

Cigarettes are one of the most carefully designed small objects on the planet. But it was not an easy thing to get people to smoke. To make smoking as ordinary as, say, eating carrots or drinking orange juice, you needed an elaborate marketing and promoting apparatus, the likes of which the world had never seen. People also had to learn how to smoke. And while this is easy enough in a world of ubiquitous smoking peers and visual models (just look at today's Hollywood films), there was a time when people had to be taught how to smoke. In the 1930s the American Tobacco Company organized classes for such purposes, directed principally at women. Company reps used dolls to demonstrate the proper way of holding, lighting, and smoking a cigarette, and some of these manikins can be found on display in tobacco museums. The saturation of film and virtually every other medium with smoking has to be seen in this light: smoking had to be made socially acceptable, and huge budgets were devoted to this cause.

Anthropologists like to talk about "material culture," meaning the diverse ways physical objects are built into the daily life of a people. The material culture of smoking has a long and complex history, appreciated best perhaps by the collectors of *tobacciana,* comprising the endless variety of pipes, cards, silks, lighters, humidors, matchbooks and cigar boxes, wooden Indians, tobacco tins, posters, advertisements, and other paraphernalia that now fill the world's (mostly industry-run) tobacco museums. Collectors prize the well-made meerschaum pipe, the lighter carved in a World War I trench, the agate snuff box cut for the European aristocrat, the minstrel-era matchbox or tobacco tin.[1]

But cigarettes have been built into life in many other ways. The front shirt pocket that now adorns the dress of virtually every American male, for example, was born from an effort to make a place to park your cigarette pack.[2] Alternate uses of course have become common—just as we now plug electronic devices into holes once meant for lighters—but the fossil function testifies to the intrusive power of the cigarette and to how easily we overlook the origins of everyday objects. There are many other examples. Germans still talk about male formal wear as a "Smoking" (jacket), and in many parts of Europe you get your newspaper from "Le Tabac." My vote for the creepiest goes to the U.S. military, which in the wake of the Korean War outfitted war-wounded veterans with artificial arms housing built-in cigarette lighters.

VENDING MACHINES AND ASHTRAYS

Vending machines may already seem like an anachronism, but for more than sixty years they were a prime source of cigarettes in the United States, especially for young people, who could get their fix of sticks in perfect anonymity by simply dropping in a few coins (see Figure 21). Early vending machines dispensed gum and other novelties—the *Oxford English Dictionary (OED)* gives 1895 as the first known use of the expression—but prior even to its breakup in 1911 American Tobacco owned a controlling share in the Garson Vending Machine Company, part of its effort to control all links in the cigar and cigarette supply chain. Patents for the automatic dispensing of cigarettes and cigars date from the 1880s,[3] but serious exploitation of such devices doesn't really begin until after the First World War, when skyrocketing consumption and standardization of packaging led to new commercial opportunities. An American by the name of William Rowe invented an improved cigarette vending machine in 1926, and by 1938 the Rowe Cigarette Service Company of New York was operating 14,000 dispensers in twenty-two U.S. cities.[4] Coin-operated sales grew steadily up through the late 1970s, when 875,000 machines in the United States were bringing in $2.7 billion in annual cigarette business.[5] This was an effective way to move product, and companies paid a premium to place their brands in favored spots inside the machines (center column was best) and in high-traffic areas of a store or a city. Nothing was left to chance; the industry's archives preserve detailed calculations of how placement or on-the-machine advertising would affect sales.[6] Cigarette companies also paid for lobbyists to defend such machines when efforts arose to have them banned.

Vending machines were often criticized for making it too easy for children to get cigarettes, and in 1988 Surgeon General C. Everett Koop urged a ban on all such devices. Trade associations fought back, with the Amusement and Music Operators Association distributing brochures with titles like "A Responsible Program for Cigarette Vending Machines," recommending ways to block youth access. The whole point of these machines was to automate sales, however, which is why kids were so easily enticed. A number of U.S. states enacted bans in the 1990s, though automated cigarette dispensers remain legal in many parts of the world. Japan may have more than any other nation and has come up with some high-tech—and ridiculous—ways to bar access from underaged smokers, such as optical scans and software for detecting facial wrinkles. Clever teens can apparently game the system by simply making a contorted face.

Ashtrays are another example of the insinuation of cigarettes into everyday life. It is hard to imagine a world without, but ashtrays were not a common part of life until about a century ago. The word we most often use (and spell) did not even exist: until the twentieth century *ash-tray* was typically spelled as either two separate words or a hyphenated compound, and the *OED* records the first single-word spelling (with no hyphen) in 1926.

Louis Kyriakoudes, director of the Oral History Project at the University of Southern Mississippi, has shown that cigarette makers spent a great deal of time and effort getting ashtrays into American consumer products. Automakers were cajoled into putting one into every car, and anyone who flew in a commercial plane in the 1960s, 1970s, or 1980s will remember ashtrays in the armrests of their seats—later stuffed with trash or gum after the smoking bans of the 1990s. Ashtrays were ubiquitous in offices and restaurants, hospitals and doctors' offices, trains and taxis, and for a time it was hard to get very far from one without hiking into the woods. Movie theaters and university lecture halls had ashtrays built into the seats, and ashtrays were built into barber chairs. I have seen (Japanese-made) slot machines with built-in ashtrays and "smokeless" ashtrays powered by batteries or USB cables. Bridge tables had clip-on ashtrays, and Kyriakoudes tells how Edward Bernays, the marketing genius for American Tobacco, approached furniture makers in the 1930s to get them to build ashtrays into kitchen cabinets. Designers threw themselves into the art, fashioning ashtrays in the shapes of pianos, shoes, turtles, toilets, tires, and naked ladies. I have seen ashtrays celebrating Walt Disney World, Penn Central Station, the 1980 Olympics, and every state in the Union.

My all-time favorite, though, is the ashtray built into the U.S. military's SAGE computer, a digital brain behemoth designed in the 1950s to protect U.S. airspace against a Soviet nuclear attack. SAGE—Semi-Automatic Ground Environment—was the world's most advanced electronic brain, linking hundreds of radar stations in the United States as "the first large-scale computer communications network."[7] The charming part of this doomsday machine, now on display at the Computer History Museum in Mountain View, California, is the cigarette lighter and ashtray built into the console, just to the left of the radar screen intended to reveal enemy aircraft or missiles penetrating our airspace. One can imagine these guardians of our national security, stoic in their morbid duties, carefully extinguishing their cigarettes as the world descends into Armageddon . . .

Kyriakoudes has also shown that for decades, teachers in American schools taught industrious young kids how to make ashtrays. Ashtray making was part of the curriculum in many public schools, and teachers were encouraged to assign such projects as a useful pedagogic activity. Well into the 1970s American schoolboard-issue textbooks encouraged middle- and even grade-school teachers to instruct children in how to craft an ashtray out of clay, glass, ceramic, stone, or metal. (I have even seen precious stones—even agates—turned into receptacles of this sort.) Many kids from my generation and even later were taught how to make such objects—and there may be parts of the world where children are still being taught such skills.

Ashtrays have always been important for cigarette makers; they realize the danger of smoking becoming inconvenient and for many years worked hard to place receptacles wherever possible. The document trail is not what it should be (because subpoenas have not targeted this realm), but the industry has fought to keep ashtrays in public parks, hospitals, planes, trains, and automobiles. Ashtrays became a kind of de rigueur furniture for several generations of Americans, as they remain in many parts of the world today. With the gradual extinction of smoking, however, we can expect these to glide into antiquity. Readers of these pages in the not too distant future will probably find the ashtray as much of a curiosity as public urination or the spittoon.

(Spittoons were ubiquitous in nineteenth-century America because of the widespread use of chewing tobacco. The chaw in the cheek generated spittle, which admen sometimes offered as proof that tobacco "aided digestion." Oscar Wilde in 1882 described the nation as "one long expectoration"; other visitors were astonished to find Americans spitting inside theaters, streetcars, and seemingly every other public place. Spittoons were introduced to prevent the spread of germs, and some states barred spitting anywhere but into a spittoon. In courtrooms a lawyer might have his own brass pot, as would the judge and jury. Spittoons bit the dust with the broader triumph of the germ theory of disease and fears of spreading microbes, though not without some protest. The governor of Pennsylvania in 1905 characterized spitting as "a gentleman's constitutional right" and its banishment "an infringement of liberty."[8] Ashtrays will eventually suffer the same fate; they are already an anachronism in richer parts of the world.)

Ashtrays may not seem like rocket science, but readers might be surprised to learn how many patents have been awarded for innovative designs. A search of Google Patents turns up thousands of claims for ashtrays, from the "Snuf A Rette" of 1937 to the battery-powered "smokeless" receptacle (with USB port) of our own millennium. Ashtrays have been designed to protect against fires, to stand up steady in an office, and to attach to the dash of your car. There are patents for windproof ashtrays and safety ashtrays and illuminated ashtrays; also for ashtrays that are self-cleaning or attached to thermometers or double as coasters or containers for napkins, coins, poker chips, or food. Patents describe ashtrays that can be folded for carrying or are stackable, portable, or disposable. There are ashtrays that sound an alarm (to prevent fires) or look like human lungs (to help you stop smoking). Others are specially made for urinals, sportsmen, the female smoker, or the disabled. Cigarette makers have even researched the cigarette–ashtray "fit": Brown & Williamson in the 1980s, for example, asked test panels of smokers to evaluate how easy a particular brand was to handle "with respect to placement in an ashtray."[9]

The tobacco industry has also tried to design ashtrays that will absorb secondhand smoke or allow a smoker to dispose of ashes when under way. Philip Morris in the 1990s, for example, worked with Royal Philips Electronics to create an ashtray that would absorb smoke; "active ashtrays" of this sort had a little fan inside and an electrostatic filter to scrub the smoke from a fuming cigarette.[10] The industry had already spent a great deal of time designing cigarettes that would emit less or less visible smoke along with a whiter, firmer ash, and these newfangled ashtrays were part of this push to shore up the "social acceptability" of smoking, a high priority since the late 1970s. Portable ashtrays were developed for similar reasons: the idea was that smokers would carry around little boxes or pouches into which ashes could be discreetly tapped. A Google Patents search for "ashtray" and "portable" in 2010 returned more than two hundred items.

SYRINGES FOR KIDS?

There are other ways, of course, that cigarettes have been insinuated into everyday life. I've mentioned candy cigarettes, but we also find smoking toys and dolls of various sorts, including toy cigarette packs, spring-loaded cigarette pranks, smoking toy animals, even miniature cigarettes and ashtrays for your child's dollhouse or toy soldier (Figure 22). Rarely were such toys produced as generic brands; most are faithful renderings of commercially popular cigarettes. It is not yet clear whether the makers of such playthings obtained permission from cigarette manufacturers to make them; it could well be that, as with candy cigarettes, the industry turned a blind eye or even welcomed such infringements as nice advertising for the novice.

What is remarkable, though, is how many different kinds of infringements can be found. Apart from those already mentioned, a short list would include gag or trick packs for use in magic shows, exploding cigarettes in name-brand packs, and battery-powered cigarette pack "smokey amps" ("the world's smallest and least expensive guitar amplifier") used supposedly by "artists like The Rolling Stones, The Foo Fighters, Mike Watt, The Red Hot Chili Peppers, and many, many others!" I have seen novelty prank packs that deliver an electric shock, wind-up packs that jump around on the table, cigarette trick (magic) books, cigarette-pack squirt guns, cigarette-pack spy cameras, cigarette-pack radios, cigarette-pack peep shows, and cigarette-pack measuring tapes—all in popular name-brand packaging. I myself own a Kent cigarette solar-powered calculator, a Marlboro disappearing cigarette pack for use in magic acts, a Basic (Philip Morris brand) tape measure, and a set of art-fully crafted buttons (from the 1930s) made to look like Camel, Lucky Strike, and Old Gold cigarette packs—only smaller. The phenomenon is not purely American: miniature lighters, ashtrays, and cigarettes were made in England in the 1960s by a company called Kiddicraft, which sold reduced-size packs of brands like Players Navy Cut for use as toys. Novelty shops in the United States still sell toy cigarettes of various sorts—some of which emit puffs of pretend smoke ("not recommended for children under the age of 8 years"). One might wonder why we don't have toy syringes for kids to pretend to shoot up heroin, or toy hash or crack pipes.

So much for Tobacco 1.0. What is new, tobacco-wise, in the virtual world?

INTERNET SAVVY

Cigarette makers have always been technically adroit and by the 1960s had com-puterized many of their operations. British American Tobacco had established a kind of Internet by the early 1980s: the INTERBAT linked seven leading European tobacco makers via an early version of email, and by the end of that decade every major cigarette company was Internet savvy. BAT held its first INTERBAT Work-shop in 1982, by which time it had already developed a series of computerized data-bases containing product information, direct mail addresses of customers, and so forth. By 1966 Britain's Tobacco Documentation Centre was compiling annotated reviews of dozens of Internet tobacco sites—both pro and con. In one such com-pilation, "Anti Tobacco" websites included those put out by the World Health Or-ganization and the American Cancer Society.[11] BAT by this time was effusing over the Internet, pointing out that while 95 percent was "rubbish, puerile, imitative, self-indulgent, irksome, tedious," or even "ranting commercial rubbish," the remaining 5 percent was "innovative, fascinating, quirky, profound, enlightening, mischievous, anarchic and stimulating," and above all else a great opportunity, a place where you could advocate the need for "tolerance and harmony between smokers and non-smokers, and all of this theoretically without censorship (commercial or moral) or vast expense."[12]

Early tobacco websites were mostly directed at the investment community, but it wasn't long before advertising opportunities were exploited. By the mid-1990s Rothmans in Canada had a Rothmans Williams Renault Formula One site, BAT had a site selling T-shirts and toasters sporting its Lucky Strike logo, Reynolds had a site for Camels, and Burrus in Switzerland had a site for its brands. Reemtsma in Germany had one of the most ambitious sites, communicating the virtues of its West brand in a manner consistent with its avant garde self-image: "We were the first to integrate gays into our brand, to have a dominatrix, the first to show naked breasts on a billboard, and we've always addressed sexist issues. Not just to point out focal points but to be provocative."[13] Reemtsma's Westcyte, launched in October 1995, offered flashing brand graphics, techno-friendly music, competitions to win a trip to Russia's "space city" for training to be an astronaut, and other freebies. "Image gain" by means of brand exposure has been the most common goal, but companies have also used the Internet to discredit evidence of health harms and to forestall regulation. By the mid-1990s pro-smoking "astroturf" groups like the American Smokers Alliance, FORCES (Fight Ordinances and Restrictions to Control and Eliminate Smoking), and the Fair Cigarette Tax Campaign (funded by Philip Morris) had their own websites, as did a number of tobacco prevention organizations—notably Globalink, organized and operated by the International Union Against Cancer.

Since this time, despite some success in curtailing web-based advertising, the Internet has become a major source for cigarette sales. A Prudential Securities report cited by the Campaign for Tobacco-Free Kids in 2005 estimated that in the United States alone cigarettes were available from more than five hundred different websites. Internet transactions accounted for an estimated 14 percent of all cigarette sales, with the percentage steadily growing.[14] For the industry this is like manna from heaven: smokers can order cigarettes and have them delivered by mail, and there is the added (and substantial) allure of avoiding sales tax—which for in-state traffic is illegal but quite hard to police. A 2002 U.S. General Accounting Office study found three quarters of all Internet sales avoiding sales tax.[15] Online buyers also don't have to face the shame of a public display of their addiction. And shoddy age verification systems make it easy for computer-savvy minors to get cigarettes online: a 2003 study published in *JAMA* found that children as young as eleven were able to get cigarettes 90 percent of the times they tried.[16]

Cigarette manufacturers have responded with a number of technical fixes to try to catch such "cheaters." (Recall those Japanese efforts to verify age by means of optical scanners programmed to detect facial wrinkles.) State governments in the United States are trying to recoup revenues lost to Internet sales: New York State loses an estimated $75 million annually down this drain and has started billing people found to be evading taxes, sometimes to the tune of several thousand dollars.[17] Many states ban Internet tobacco purchases, but enforcement is lax and difficult, especially for small-scale buyers and sellers. Credit card companies have pledged to help curtail online sales,[18] though it remains to be seen how effective this will be. Flying below the radar, the clever and persistent buyer can usually get through.

DRAGGIN LADY AND SMOKINGBABE

Internet sales are only one of several ways tobacco circulates in the virtual world. The companies have their own websites, but smoking is also promoted through auction sites, cigarette rating clubs, "smokers' rights" organizations, and clubs with specialty interests in cigars, smokeless tobacco, hookah, or even cigarette pack art.[19] Tobacco manufacturers have started seeking input from users to design tobacco ads: *Playboy* magazine in 2008, for example, launched its "Skoal Builds Playboy" promotion in which Skoal fans were invited to help design the content of a twelve-page Skoal-themed spread for the January 2009 issue of the magazine.[20]

Pornography sites catering to smoking fetishists have also become popular. A 2008 Google search returned 1,950,000 hits for "smoking fetish" and 139,000 for "smoking porn." There are tens of thousands of such sites, with names like "MSInhale" and "Dirty Smokers," featuring artists such as "Draggin Lady" or "Smoking-Babe" and others with names less fit to print. There are even websites to help you rank and evaluate such sites, rating ease of navigation and image and video quality (of course) but also models, locations, frequency of image updates, number of brands displayed, inclusion of "subfetishes," and originality. One such site (www.smoking fetishsites.com) asks, "Are the photos & videos completely original and shot specifically for the site, or are they bought from a broker as non-exclusive content, which means they could be on any number of other sites out there? Was the content shot by a smoking fetishist or is the site run by a faceless company who buy the content in and have it shot by a photographer who doesn't understand the ins and outs of the fetish?"[21] Cigarettes also figure in various forms of online role-playing games. There are several dozen smoking groups in "Second Life," for example, which also has "smoke shops" that offer virtual cigarettes for sale for Linden dollars. Ashtrays and smoking gear can be purchased at Second Life Classifieds sites, where you can also find ads for virtual cigarettes, cigars, and ashtrays. It is not yet clear how much of this—if any—has been organized by the industry.

More politicized are the "smokers' rights" groups coordinated through websites such as CLASH (Citizens Lobbying Against Smoker Harassment), which features prominent links to groups like FORCES, FOREST (U.K.), Smokers of the World Unite, Minnesotans Against Smoking Bans, and several dozen others. CLASH also directs smokers to several sites where discount cigarettes can be purchased online and to OLTRA (Online Tobacco Rights Association), a trade association formed to defend the sale of cigarettes online.[22] CLASH also links to numerous online pro-smoking newsletters and political contact sites like Congress.com, where users are instructed in how to create pro-smoking "Video Advocacy Messages" for uploading on YouTube.

Facebook and MySpace are also sites where smoking is being promoted. As of March 2008 there were 311 groups for "smokeless tobacco" on Facebook, with one or two new sites being added every week. Some of these groups are quite large: one called "Actually, I DID know that cigarettes are bad for me! NOW SHUT THE F**K UP" had more than 12,000 members and 124 discussion boards, with hundreds of people contributing opinions on topics such as "most annoying time that someone bitched about smoking." This site is linked to others with equally heartwarming ti-

tles, such as "I Secretly Want to Punch Slow Walking People in the Back of the Head."
Some tobacco companies also have Facebook sites: British American Tobacco has
several closed sites (membership by invitation only), the largest of which has nearly
seven hundred members.

Yahoo as of 2008 had 1,200 "smoker" groups and 5,300 "smoking" groups; My-
Space also has lots of people with smoking network friends. "I ♥ Smoking" as of
June 2008 had 487 friends, virtually all of which were smoke-themed. Many of these
MySpace sites post smoking video clips, and many are linked to smoking fetish sites.
It is hard to monitor or even get an overview of such sites, however, given how rapidly they change. Already by September 2006 YouTube had 65,000 new videos
uploaded *daily* and by March 2008 was growing by more than 150,000 per day.
A YouTube search of "tobacco" gets over 30,000 hits, with "smoking" returning
177,000 separate videos, split roughly equal pro and con. And hundreds of ads from
cigarette manufacturers. A Ruyan ad for its electric cigarette had been viewed over
320,000 times as of November 2008, and many of the larger companies have widely
watched YouTube ads. MySpace also has lots of smoking-themed uploads: my search
in June 2008 using the search term "smoking" yielded over a thousand MySpace
videos, from smoking chimps (and dogs) to smoking kids (as young as eight), a lot
of sensual/seductive smoking (with females way outnumbering males), smoking
comedians, a rock group called Smoking Presidents, and Fred Flintstone's famous
smoking cartoon from 1960 in which he and Barney sneak out (!) behind a rock to
savor a Winston, hiding from their wives.

SMOKING PASSIONS, CIGARETTE GEAR

Internet dating services for smokers are a relatively new phenomenon; sites like www
.smokerdatelink.com and www.smokingpassions.com have thousands of smoker
profiles online, with hundreds added daily. Simon Chapman of the University of
Sydney documents a growing trend to indicate a preference for nonsmoking partners on Internet dating sites, signaling in Australia at least an increasing denor-
malization of smoking. These sites may be somewhat upscale, but people everywhere are starting to demand smoke-free hotel rooms, apartments, rental cars, and
roommates. The stigma attached to smoking is growing in many parts of the world,
though it is easy to exaggerate the extent to which we have already transcended
the habit.

Readers may find it surprising, for example, that at any given moment on eBay
there are upwards of a thousand items plugging the Marlboro brand. A March 2008
search returned Marlboro-branded Swiss army knives, toy trucks, lighters, canteens,
jogging suits, cookbooks, sweatpants, jeans, jackets, playing cards, photo frames,
suitcases, belt buckles, money clips, and dozens of other items. Similar returns are
obtained by searching "Camel," "Silk Cut," and other leading cigarette brands. Judg-

ing by availability on eBay, it would seem that much of the world is awash in cigarette gear. A search of "cigarette" returns tens of thousands of items, with pro smoking offerings outnumbering antis by more than fifty to one. Most of these are things
like cigarette cards (or silks), lighters, magazine ads, or antique cigarette packs and
cases, but many are items designed originally to spread the name of a particular
brand of cigarette. A search of "tobacco" yields this same material asymmetry. "Ashtray" returns about 10,000 items on eBay—which could well be an index of their
disappearance. Smoking rates are falling in many parts of the world, though even
in a state like California, with its aggressive smoke-free laws, there are still about
eight hundred cigarettes smoked per person per year—which is not much lower
than average for the earth as a whole.

There are of course other kinds of tricks being used to penetrate web and net-
working culture. One has been to collaborate with manufacturers of nontobacco
products to create cigarette synergies. Food and clothing are often involved, but electronic communications have recently joined these ranks. British American Tobacco,
for example, has been bragging about its use of a Neverfail BlackBerry network to
keep its global workforce in touch ("Neverfail keeps that heart beating"). BlackBerry
and BAT have both been celebrating their newfound alliance, but why such a fuss
about a system that presumably all large corporations have in place? The company's
repeated "announcements," press releases, videos, and so on, about its use of global
communications seem designed to keep the BAT name in view. YouTube even has
a puff piece on BAT's BlackBerry network (at http://www.youtube.com/watch?v=
MOTaTQ8-dbc), which is hard to see as anything but an ad for both companies.
The clip does not allow any commentary, presumably to keep up the illusion of honest communication. A BlackBerry newsletter on the web reveals that the devices
were supplied to top BAT personnel as part of a plan to "seduce your users." BAT's
Information Technology director, David Sampson, explains that use of such devices
"is really a matter of personal choice,"[23] like cigarettes, presumably.

Another trick has been to buy up potentially embarrassing web domains, making it harder for critics to organize advocacy. In 2010 Lorillard, makers of America's most widely smoked menthol brand (Newport), bought up over fifty different
web domain names, including MentholKillsMinorities.com, KillerMenthol.com,
MentholAddictsYouth.com, and FDAMustBanMenthol.com. Lorillard here followed a path blazed by Philip Morris in 2001, when the Marlboro giant bought up
dozens of domains with names like AltriaSucks, AltriaLies, AltriaKills, AltriaEquals
Death, and AltriaStinks, each in suffixed variations of .com, .net, and .org, anticipating its rebirth as "Altria." The company even bought up misspellings of its new
moniker: Altreea.com, Alltreya.com, and so forth.

A very different kind of web presence has emerged in the form of chat groups
and message boards, which let us hear the protest voices of a few courageous former smokers. The "WhyQuit" site, for example, allows former smokers dying from

their addiction to share stories and forge alliances: "I'm Deborah and Smoking Has Smoked this Body."[24] This lived, and dying, cancer presence is more often invisible, though, until it is too late. Most people who contract lung cancer regret ever having smoked; and the sad reality is that when people start smoking at age thirteen or fourteen they have no idea what lies in store for them. Physical suffering is not an image conveyed through tobacco advertising, which is one reason health advocates call for graphic pictures of diseased bodies on all packs of cigarettes.[25]

No image, though, can convey the real terminal horror of smoking, with all its bodily torment and social aftershocks. How do you capture the smell of a gangrenous foot, or the torture of a sleepless wheezing night rent by cough? How do you convey the lost years of life, or the indignities of medical impoverishment, or the intangibles of familial loss and dependence? Marketing effaces all this, giving a false front to suffering that, in the end, leaves no living memory.

PART TWO

Discovering the Cancer Hazard

Knowledge is Power.
FRANCIS BACON

Ignorance is Power.
GEORGE ORWELL

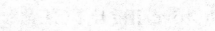

HERE WE DROP BACK deeper into the past, to revisit "who knew what and when?" about tobacco cancer in the crucial years leading up to the January 1954 launch of the industry's multidecade campaign of denying and distracting from the evidence linking lung cancer to cigarettes. The topic is a broad one, and I'll focus primarily on what the industry knew based on animal experiments, including a series of heretofore hidden experiments carried out by the Ecusta Paper Corporation in the summer and fall of 1953—at the request of the American Tobacco Company. These experiments are significant in a number of different respects.

For one thing, they are apparently the first conducted by a tobacco manufacturer showing tobacco tars as carcinogenic agents. Previous experiments—notably American Tobacco's 1941–42 efforts to induce lung cancer in mice by having them *breathe* cigarette smoke—had failed to produce cancers.[1] Ecusta's experiments are also notable in that "whole tobacco *smoke*" was *blown* onto the backs of animals. Previous experiments had most often *painted* tobacco *tars* onto the backs of mice or the ears of rabbits.

The experiments are also significant in that they have been kept pretty much under wraps for more than fifty years. Even now they are little known outside a narrow circle of litigation attorneys—and might never have come to light if plaintiffs' lawyers had not forced their disclosure through subpoena.[2] For many years the industry denied having ever conducted such experiments, when the reality is that they had been quite diligent in this respect and had come to conclusions that were hard to square with anything but the fact they were killing people.

Ecusta's experiments force us to enlarge our understanding of how the grand tobacco conspiracy came about. The Plaza Hotel meetings of December 14–15, 1953, are rightly regarded as the beginning of the industry's conspiracy to deny, deflect, or distract from the hazards of tobacco, with the immediate prompt for this meeting traced to Wynder, Graham and Croninger's demonstration that tobacco tars cause cancers when painted onto the shaved backs of white mice.[3] In fact, however, this run-up to conspiracy has a deeper and heretofore hidden history, in which the Ecusta experiments, the Runyon–NYU collaboration, and the joint action of the industry's "tobacco discussion group" were crucial to the recognition of the real dangers.

Indeed there is evidence that it was in trying to refute Wynder's experiments—and failing—that the industry came to realize that the cancer problem was not going to go away. Paul M. Hahn, president of the world's largest tobacco company, learned about the results of the Ecusta experiment only a week prior to inviting his fellow tobacco manufacturers to meet at the Plaza Hotel in New York, which suggests that the decision to launch the conspiracy was made not just in response to publicity surrounding Wynder et al.'s experiments—accompanied by a steep drop in tobacco stocks—but also in response to the industry's having demonstrated the cancer hazard in its own laboratories.

We begin with a history of efforts to induce cancers in experimental animals, including Angel H. Roffo's pioneering work, following which we turn to Claude Teague's unpublished "Survey of Cancer Research" (1953), the broadest review up to that time of the experimental induction of cancer using tobacco tars—and the document most feared by the lawyers defending the industry in court. We then examine the events surrounding the Ecusta experiment itself, looking also at how experimental carcinogenesis was ranked in the status hierarchy of medical rhetoric and reasoning. We finish with a discussion of how and when a "consensus" was established that cigarettes were killing people and some of the difficulties involved in disentangling honest and dishonest doubts.

9

Early Experimental Carcinogenesis

In my opinion, the harm from nicotine is greatly over-rated and I am saying this not because I am chief chemist of the American Tobacco Company but from strictly scientific facts.

A. L. CHESLEY, 1921

Ecusta scientists were not the first to conduct animal experiments with tobacco. As early as the 1820s German physicians had isolated a pure form of nicotine, showing the alkaloid to be a poison of the first order. A single drop on the tongue could kill a dog, several drops a horse. Tobacco throughout the nineteenth century was listed in the *U.S. Pharmacopoeia and National Formulary,* which characterized the distilled oil of tobacco *(oleum tabaci)* as containing the "highly poisonous" nicotine alkaloid.[1] Nicotine's pharmacologic properties later came under revisionist scrutiny, when reformers pushing for new laws to supervise food and drug safety wanted tobacco regulated as a drug. Tobacco was already becoming a powerful political force, however, and in 1905 James Buchanan ("Buck") Duke of the American Tobacco Company saw *tabacum* dropped from the official list of *U.S. Pharmacopoeia.*[2] Details are sketchy, but the deletion may well have been engineered to avoid having nicotine regulated as a drug. (Tobacco was still in the seventh revision of 1893, along with cinnamon, cannabis, and cubeb.) Tobacco was excluded from the Pure Food and Drug Act of 1906 (the Wiley Act, which established the FDA) and came instead under the rule of the Miscellaneous Tax Unit of the Bureau of Internal Revenue and later the Bureau of Alcohol, Tobacco, and Firearms, unregulated from a public health point of view.

Experimental oncology also began in the nineteenth century, when physicians started exploring whether a particular germ, chemical, or physical irritant could cause cancer in rats, mice, dogs, or even humans. Experiments were done to see whether salt, syphilis, or factory chemicals of various sorts cause cancer, or even whether tumors transplanted from one breast to another would continue to grow.[3]

Viruses were later explored, along with X-rays and radioactive substances and hundreds of different organic and inorganic chemicals.

Many of these early studies focused on exposure to toxics in the workplace. Coal tar was a culprit recognized early on, because the effects were so strong and often localized in a particular factory. Coal tar is derived from the condensed volatile distillates generated during the manufacture of *coke,* a pure form of carbon used in the making of steel. German chemists in the 1800s had discovered that coal tar extracts could be used to make colorful dyes and other useful chemicals, chemicals that, as was soon discovered, caused tumors of various sorts in exposed workers. In one horrific case in the United States, nineteen of twenty workers came down with bladder cancer after working with beta-naphthylamine, a potent carcinogen used in the manufacture of synthetic dyes.

Occupational cancers came to the attention of medical scientists, who sought to reproduce these in the laboratory. Katsusaburo Yamagiwa and Koichi Ichikawa produced coal tar cancers in laboratory animals in 1916,[4] and Ernest L. Kennaway in England in 1925 showed that coal soot and tars from heated acetylene and isoprene were carcinogenic. By the 1930s there was an enormous literature on experimental carcinogenesis. The Donner Foundation's 1935 *Index to Literature of Experimental Cancer Research* lists thirty thousand entries on the topic, with an entire section devoted to tobacco. Wilhelm Hueper, in his comprehensive *Occupational Tumors,* reviewed this literature, much of which also made its way into the monthly summaries of the *Zeitschrift für Krebsforschung, Cancer Research,* and a dozen-odd other specialized periodicals.[5]

CANCERS DES FUMEURS

The first known effort to induce a *tobacco* cancer in laboratory animals was by Anton Brosch in Vienna, who in 1900 rubbed "tobacco juice" onto guinea pigs, or perhaps onto only one (he doesn't say), causing a proliferation of epithelial tissues on an old scar. Brosch cited Hermann Tillmanns's 1880 characterization of tobacco, paraffin, petroleum tar, and soot as "well-known carcinogens," but his interest was more in crafting a more general theory of carcinogenesis—as in whether irritation, trauma, embryonic remnants, heredity, or infection should be considered the primary mechanism. Brosch's experiment is poorly described in his report, which treats the tobacco rubbing in only part of one paragraph in an article nearly 150 paragraphs long. Brosch in fact wrote less about his experiment than what I've devoted to it here.[6]

Tobacco by this time (circa 1900) was fairly well known as a cause of cancer of the lips, mouth, throat, and tongue—the French talked about *cancers des fumeurs,* "smokers' cancers"[7]—but smoking was not yet regarded as a significant threat *to the lungs.* The first suggestion of such a link seems to have been by Hermann Rottmann in his 1898 medical dissertation for the University of Würzburg, where we find it speculated that lung cancers might be caused by the inhalation of tobacco *dust*—not smoke. Isaac Adler in the United States in his 1912 text on lung cancer pathology hypothesized a tobacco–lung cancer link, but it was not until the 1920s and 1930s that statistical studies began to document the connection, following the perception of something new and sinister in that vital organ.

Statistical studies did not become important in establishing the lung cancer hazard until doctors in the richer parts of the world started noticing a dramatic rise in lung cancer. Quantifying this rate of increase with any precision was difficult, given misdiagnoses, incomplete registries, and confounding factors, but the epidemic was dramatic enough by the 1920s to attract the notice of physicians. Victor E. Mertens of Munich's University Surgical Clinic in 1930 surely jumped the gun when he reported that the increase of lung cancer was "conceded by everybody," but his statement does reflect a broad and growing recognition of the phenomenon. R. G. J. P. Huismann in Amsterdam—the German industry's point man on smoking and health—in 1940 characterized the increase as "certain." And more and more physicians were starting to suspect that smoking must have something to do with it.[8]

THE SCIENCE OF EPIDEMICS

A crucial piece of evidence for these early researchers came in the form of *epidemiology*—the science of epidemics—which had gained a boost from efforts to discover how living or working conditions might be making people sick. In its simplest form, epidemiology involved little more than comparing two groups to see whether people who, say, drank from a particular well were more or less likely to get cholera, or whether sailors who drank citrus on a ship were more or less likely to get scurvy. Early epidemiology involved a kind of detective work: John Snow in London in 1854, for example, plotted cholera deaths on a map and discovered that deaths clustered around a water pump on Broad Street. Recognizing fouled drinking water as the cause of the disease, he famously convinced the Board of Governors of St. James Parish to remove the handle from this pump and helped put an end to the epidemic. (Steven Johnson's *Ghost Map* is the best book on this.)

Early tobacco epidemiologists couldn't use maps—smoking is a mobile, multipoint-source pollutant—but they could look at whether people with lung cancer tended to share certain attributes or behaviors. Were they male or female? Did they tend to live in towns or on farms? Was there something about their work that might explain their malady or something they were eating or inhaling? The earliest studies of this sort were "case series," showing only that people with cancer were more likely to have been smokers. Studies along these lines were published in both Europe and America beginning in the 1920s,[9] as doctors started noticing that most of their lung cancer patients had been smokers. More sophisticated methods were eventually introduced, controlling for sex, age, occupation, and state of health. Controlling for age was especially important, given that cancer is typically a disease of the elderly—because time is required to accumulate the requisite mutations and cellular growth. A population with a high cancer rate might simply be one with a lot of old people, so it was crucial to ask, how common is cancer among people aged, say, fifty-one to fifty-five? And what can we say about *the habits* of people of a particular age that might explain why some get sick and others remain healthy?

A breakthrough came in the 1930s with the invention of experimental epidemiology, combining the realism of traditional diagnostics with the reproducibility of the laboratory experiment. The most important early study of this sort for tobacco was conducted in Germany, at Cologne's City Hospital, in 1939. Franz Hermann Müller, a young physician whom we know very little about, compared the smoking behavior of eighty-six lung cancer "cases" and an equal number of carefully matched "controls" and found a clear relationship between smoking and one's likelihood of contracting cancer. Lung cancer victims were far more likely to have been smokers, especially of cigarettes, which led Dr. Müller to conclude that tobacco was "an important cause" of lung cancer but also that the recent and dramatic increase in smoking was *"the single most important cause of the rising incidence of lung cancer."*[10]

Subsequent scholars improved on Müller's methods and came to similar conclusions. A sophisticated case-control study by Eberhard Schairer and Erich Schöniger at the University of Jena appeared in 1943, followed by larger and more carefully controlled studies in both Europe and America. The turning point for the United States and Britain was 1950, when five separate studies were published implicating smoking as a cause of lung cancer. Wynder and Graham's was the first, followed quickly thereafter by Doll and Hill's carefully reasoned (and mathematically adept) work. By the mid-1950s the floodgates were open, and the evidence was strong, consistent, and unambiguous. This new work was distinguished by large sample sizes, more careful attention to potential sources of bias, and efforts (notably in Doll and Hill's case) to quantify the probability of error. Epidemiologists were able to show that the correlation between smoking and risk of death and disease came neither from chance, nor bias, nor confounding; and this was strong enough by the 1950s—especially when combined with animal experimental evidence—to bring about the birth of a consensus. Epidemiology itself was transformed in the course of documenting the lung cancer hazard; there is an interesting sense in which modern experimental epidemiology was both the instrument by which the hazard was proven and the offspring of its proof.[11]

FALSE BUT REASSURING STEPS

It was not such an easy thing to get *mice* to contract cancer, however—especially in their lungs. And in the odd evidentiary hierarchy of the 1940s and 1950s it was experimental proofs that many people imagined would seal the case against cigarettes.

Mouse-painting experiments could be organized that would generate tumors, but when more "realistic" experiments were tried—mimicking more closely the human experience of smoking—the results were often inconclusive.

The most "successful" experiment of this sort—from the industry's point of view—was that conducted by Egon Lorenz, a biophysicist at the National Health Service, who in 1940 began working with the American Tobacco Company to test whether smoke forced into the lungs of mice could cause tumors. In late 1941 and early 1942 Lorenz, together with colleagues from the National Cancer Institute, forced a group of mice to breathe tobacco smoke to determine whether tumors could be produced by this means. Ninety-seven Strain A mice were exposed for several hours a day for up to a year, during which time about half a gram of tar was deposited in the lungs of each mouse. Another group of ninety-seven mice was left unexposed as a control. The team found that mice forced to inhale smoke were no more likely to develop lung tumors than the controls. This was great news for the industry, which quickly started using the "reassuring experiments of Dr. Lorenz" in its public correspondence. The companies also made sure the results got wide attention in the popular media. The failure of this one series of experiments was treated as a kind of golden event and would be used for decades thereafter to refute evidence of a cigarette–cancer link.[12]

Why did Lorenz's inhalation experiments fail? Pulmonary malignancies in humans often take twenty, thirty, or even forty or more years to gestate, which is much longer than the life span of your typical mouse. Tumor-sensitive mice were often used in such experiments—as they were in Lorenz's—but even here it was hard to control the dose, which in humans of course is self-controlled; people *try* to smoke. How much smoke, though, actually enters the lungs of experimental animals? This was never easy to say (Lorenz's mice were not really "smoking," but rather just running around in smoke-filled cages). Dosage was a crucial issue, however, since if too low the cancer detection threshold might not be reached, and if too high the animals would die. It also turns out that rodents have excellent defense mechanisms against dust and soot accumulating in their lungs, an evolutionary consequence of living close to the ground. Mice, for example, are equipped with nasal turbinates that effectively brush out dust and other foreign matter from their lungs, as was recognized by the early 1960s.[13]

Many early efforts to induce lung cancer in experimental animals failed on this account—though not all. Otto Mühlbock in Holland in 1955 reported experiments in which mice exposed to smoke *did* get lung tumors—prompting worries within the American industry that this would become "splendid material for our adversaries."[14] Mühlbock's work didn't make as much of a splash as it might because it was in Dutch; the experiment was also rather odd in that researchers administered the smoke simply by having a smoking human blow it into the mouse cages—which apparently was difficult to keep up day after day. None of this really mattered terribly much, as the hazard was already pretty well nailed down from the mouse-painting experiments and the epidemiology—and the finding of benzpyrene in tobacco smoke. Which brings us to the work of a little-known hero in the history of experimental carcinogenesis, an Argentine who ran the largest cancer institute in South America and produced shocking cancers on the ears of rabbits by painting them with tobacco tar.

Roffo's Foray and the Nazi Response

Tobacco causes cancer; of that there can be no doubt.
ANGEL H. ROFFO, 1936

Angel Honorio Roffo of Argentina (1882–1947) was the first to show *convincingly* that tars extracted from tobacco could cause tumors in experimental animals. As founding director of the Instituto de Medicina Experimental para el Estudio y Tratamiento del Cancer in Buenos Aires (established in 1922), Roffo was able to examine and treat a large population of cancer patients, from whom he had learned by the end of the 1920s that smoking was a cause of many kinds of cancer.[1] During the next decade and into the early 1940s he published a series of ambitious papers, blending clinical, experimental, and statistical reasoning with a strong sense that many of the world's most common cancers could be prevented. Roffo showed that cancers all along the "smoking street" (lips, tongue, throat, cheek, bronchial passages, etc.) must be caused by exposure to tars released in the course of smoking. He also stressed that a great deal of human suffering could be prevented by stopping smoking.

Roffo's work is interesting for a number of different reasons. For one thing, there is his defense of the use of animal experiments to investigate tobacco carcinogenesis— as if clinical observations had already proved the point. In 1931, writing in the *Zeitschrift für Krebsforschung* (much of his work is published in German), he noted that while there were cases in which tobacco was clearly to blame for certain malignancies (from clinical observations) it was nonetheless useful to re-create the phenomenon by animal experiments. Reasoning by analogy from the production of cancer using coal tars, he argued that cancer must be being caused by the complex, tarry, polycyclic aromatic hydrocarbons in smoke rather than the (chemically simpler) inorganic constituents or the nicotine alkaloid. To test this hypothesis, he separated tobacco smoke into three distinct distillation products, which he rubbed onto the ears of three groups of ten rabbits each. Roffo found that the tarry fractions produced cancers but that when nicotine alone was applied no cancers were produced, no matter how long he waited. The same was true (no effect) from the various inorganic components he had isolated from smoke—salts such as ammonium chloride, for example, or gases such as carbon monoxide and dioxide.[2] His graphic colored images of rabbit ears riddled with tobacco-tar tumors created a sensation (see Figure 23) and were often reprinted by industry critics—and mocked by the industry's defenders.

BRAVE IN BUENOS AIRES

Roffo ran many similar tests over the next ten years or so, using different methods of preparing tobacco smoke extracts, different chemical fractions of those extracts, and different species of test animals. He never seems to have doubted the role of the golden weed, and by the end of his career was able to claim, based on hundreds of his own published papers, that tobacco was the major cause of lung cancer, that tar rather than nicotine was the primary culprit, and that polycyclic aromatic hydrocarbons were the principal carcinogenic agents. Among these last-mentioned compounds was 1,2-benzpyrene, a five-ring aromatic hydrocarbon Roffo was the first to identify in tobacco smoke (on the basis of spectrographic signatures).[3] Roffo also concluded that blonde tobacco was more dangerous than black—by virtue of yielding higher quantities of tars—and that the most dangerous were Turkish, Egyptian, and Kentucky tobaccos. (This is an interesting mistake: the *tars* from dark tobaccos often contain more carcinogens, but blonde tobaccos, by virtue of being "milder," yield a more inhalable smoke and therefore end up causing more cancer.) Finally, and most important, he showed that cancers could be induced in experimental animals even by using nicotine-free tobacco, meaning again that it was the *tar* rather than the *nicotine* that was causing all this cancer. And tar was not a trivial component of tobacco smoke: Roffo calculated that smokers could inhale as much as four kilograms of tar in ten years of smoking.[4] That would be about a gallon of the black sticky stuff.

Roffo had access to a large pool of cancer patients at his institute in Buenos Aires and used this as an opportunity to explore cancer causation on a statistical basis. In 1934, for example, he described how 302 of his 500 skin cancer patients had presented with malignancies on the nose, the body part most directly exposed to the sun, which he used to infer that solar radiation must be to blame. He also directed a number of projects involving human experimentation—to determine the role of skin pigmentation in protecting against X-rays, for example. Sex differences had helped him incriminate tobacco: How else did one explain the fact that men were far more likely than women to contract cancers of the lips, tongue, gums, and cheeks, while cancers of the stomach were fairly evenly balanced by gender? Men and women eat pretty much the same food, but what besides tobacco could be causing such differences? Smoking was far more common among men, and Roffo drew the proper inference. This sex difference was particularly evident for cancers of the throat and larynx: fully 5 percent of Roffo's male patients' cancers struck the throat, for example, whereas among seven thousand women in his clinic with malignancies only three (about 0.04 percent) suffered from cancer at this site—and all three were smokers. A similar pattern was evident for cancers of the lung. This was convincing evidence for him, and the language he uses is interesting: he says the patterns were strong enough to have an "almost experimental value."[5]

Not everyone was convinced by Roffo's studies, however. Ernest Kennaway in England had pioneered animal experimental techniques for replicating occupational cancers (especially from petrochemicals), and his concern was that Roffo might have burned his tobacco at too high a temperature to be realistic. This same complaint appears in many subsequent accounts of tobacco health history: Sir Richard Doll, for example, in a 2001 article, stated that Roffo's experiments "should not have been cited as biological evidence of the plausibility of a causal relationship" since "the temperature at which Roffo burnt his tobacco was greater than the temperature at which tobacco is burnt in normal smoking."[6] (Doll's objection is not entirely fair, since Roffo obtained cancers using a variety of different types of tobacco tars, including fractions from tobacco burned at temperatures approximating those of real-world smoking—more on which in a moment.) Roffo's methods of detection also came under scrutiny. Spectrographic fluorescence he had used to identify a class of chemicals known as polycyclic aromatic hydrocarbons—large-ringed molecules that are often carcinogenic—and some critics thought this method too crude to reveal individual constituents.

Whatever flaws we today might identify in his work, from a purely historical point of view we have to acknowledge that Roffo was a force to be reckoned with—and was so judged by his contemporaries. Eberhard Schairer and Erich Schöniger in 1943 cited Roffo's experiments as evidence of the carcinogenicity of tobacco tar, as did Franz Hermann Müller in 1939 and Fritz Lickint in his magisterial *Tabak und Organismus* (Tobacco and the Organism). Roffo was the key prompt for Leonard Engel's widely read "Cigarettes Cause Cancer?" (in a 1946 issue of *Reader's Scope*) and was crucial for Edwin Grace's article in the *American Journal of Surgery* in 1943, where the Argentine's discovery of benzpyrene in cigarette smoke was foregrounded.[7] James Ewing in the fourth edition of his authoritative 1940 textbook, *Neoplastic Diseases,* devoted several admiring paragraphs to Roffo's work, as did Steinhaus and Grunderman in their 1942 brochure, *Tobacco and Health.* Roffo was also honored in his native land: today his name is on the foremost cancer institute of Argentina, the Instituto de Oncología Angel H. Roffo in Buenos Aires.

Roffo was also taken seriously by American tobacco manufacturers. A 1950 memo to the president of American Tobacco reviewing the "Alleged Causative Relation between Cigarette Smoking and Bronchiogenic Carcinoma" (by the company's research director, Hiram Hanmer) listed Roffo as "the chief protagonist of the theory that there is a causal relation between smoking and cancer of the respiratory organs." The same memo pointed to Edwin J. Grace's "echoing" of Roffo's opinion and conceded that cancer authorities had been dissenting from Roffo's view "until recently." Claude Teague of R. J. Reynolds in his 1953 "Survey of Cancer Research" cited nine separate studies by Roffo, noting also his isolation of "benzpyrene from a pyrolytic distillate of tobacco" and his observation that the compound was "highly carcinogenic in animal tests." A tobacco industry expert witness in 1959 referenced twenty articles by Roffo, and a thousand-plus-page bibliography compiled by Reynolds in the 1960s listed fifty-five Roffo articles. Tobacco industry attorneys would later prepare to defend themselves against charges they should have known about and warned of hazards prior even to the 1950s—principally from the work of Roffo. In 1990, for example, the firm of Jones, Day, Reavis and Pogue expressed its concern that "plaintiffs may focus particularly on the early work of Roffo and others to suggest that warnings should have been provided in the 1940s."[8]

Tobacco had in fact been keeping a close watch on Roffo from his first published work on this topic in the early 1930s. Indeed it is in their responding to him that we find some of the first industry engagements with cigarettes as a possible cancer hazard—at least at the level of public relations. In the 1930s and 1940s, for example, many people wrote to the tobacco companies, asking whether Roffo had reliably shown that cigarettes were causing cancer. And industry research authorities responded to many of these letters. On May 11, 1939, for example, American Tobacco's research director, Hiram R. Hanmer, replied to a scientist who had written to the company about Roffo: "We have been following Roffo's work for some time, and I feel that it is rather unfortunate that a statement such as his is widely disseminated." The "general acceptance" of statements such as Roffo's had kept the literature on tobacco "in a very beclouded condition," and Hanmer reassured his correspondent of "an abundance of evidence that the use of tobacco is not remotely associated with the incidence of cancer." He also hoped that "eventually all of the evidence relative to tobacco and health, both pro and con, will be presented to the public in an unbiased manner," relieving the industry of "much stigma."[9]

It is unfortunate that we don't yet have a good biography of Roffo. We need to know more about his earlier work in the 1920s and how scholars in his native Argentina viewed his research. We need to know more about how he first came to realize that tobacco was causing cancer and why he was more or less forgotten in the wake of Wynder et al.'s (more powerful) demonstration of experimental carcinogenesis. Was Argentina just too far away? Was the language gulf a problem? Did his German ties taint him? And what role did professional jealousies or corporate defamation play in his neglect?

Part of what has gone on has been a distancing of pre–World War II research from the scholarship of subsequent generations, perhaps to emphasize the novelty of the approaches taken in the 1950s—which often weren't so novel. Ernst Wynder, Evarts Graham, and Adele Croninger in their influential paper of 1953, for example, objected that previous scholars had carried out their experiments "for too brief a period of time or with too few animals to be regarded as significant." Examples cited by Wynder included German studies from 1911 and 1923, which had reported hair loss or cellular proliferation after only two or three weeks of exposure, respectively. Wynder et al. mentioned Roffo's experiments on rabbits only in passing, failing to note that some of these lasted up to three years, hardly a period "too brief . . . to be regarded as significant." Otto Schürch and Alfred Winterstein—distinguished European scholars—were also ignored, though some of their experiments had run for more than six hundred days. Wynder, Graham, and Croninger used more sophisticated controls and larger sample sizes, but they should not be seen as revolutionaries; theirs was more the culmination of a research tradition rather than the beginning of an entirely new one.[10]

CONSENSUS IN THE THIRD REICH?

One remarkable aspect of the Roffo story is his sympathetic reception in Nazi Germany. Germany under Hitler had the world's strongest anti-cancer campaign, buttressed by sophisticated medical methods and a political apparatus eager to identify and exterminate threats to the German body politic. Germans during the Third Reich were the first to show that asbestos was a cause of mesothelioma, that food dyes could cause cancer, and that smoking was a confirmed cause of lung tumors. German medical science at this time was the most advanced in the world—and the most murderous—but political ideology also played a role in the recognition of cancer hazards, insofar as Nazism encouraged the discovery and elimination of "threats" to the German *völkisch* body—real or imagined.

That is how the cancer question became politicized in Germany in the 1930s and 1940s. Medical evidence was already moving against tobacco, and Nazi medical authorities recognized the need to take action. Crucial here is that Nazism was an ideology of racial purity: the body was faced with myriad threats, real or imagined, from white bread and food dyes to X-rays and race mixing. Party officials worried that tobacco, too, was sapping the strength of the German people, weakening their resolve, creating an alien allegiance in a world where your body was supposed to belong to the Führer. Health was a moral obligation, disease a form of treason. Which again is why so much effort—including scientific effort—was put into the campaign against smoking.

Was there in Nazi Germany a scientific or public health consensus that tobacco posed real and substantial hazards? Publications from the era certainly leave us with this impression, though of course there were still doubters, just as there would be following the Anglo-American work of the 1950s. What is interesting about the German case is that the consensus was strongest at the highest levels of medico-political authority. The most powerful physician in Germany—Reich Health Führer Leonardo Conti—was convinced, as was Hans Reiter, president of Germany's Reich Health Office, and Karl Astel, president of the University of Jena and the man in charge of health affairs for the state of Thuringia. These were some of the highest-ranking health authorities in the Reich, which is consistent with the fact that Nazi ideology made it easier to believe that tobacco was killing people.

Hans Reiter, for example, as president of the Reichsgesundheitsamt, was the most powerful public health official in Germany. In his 1941 speech at the opening of the Institute for Tobacco Hazards Research at the University of Jena, Reiter asked, "Are tobacco harms only in the imagination of a few fanatics, or do we have sufficient well-tested evidence to recognize the harmful effects of smoking as proven?" Reiter pointed to nicotine and carbon monoxide as well-known poisons in tobacco smoke but stressed that smoking even of nicotine-free cigarettes would cause harm. (The industry had been pushing "nicotine-free" cigarettes in response to the anti-tobacco outcry, offering these as a "light" alternative to ordinary cigarettes. Low-alcohol "light beer"—Leichtbier—was also developed and sold at this time.) Reiter noted that smoking caused constriction of the arteries, leading to circulatory failure and gangrene of the extremities but also damage to the arteries supplying blood to the brain. He also cited scholarly work showing that angina pectoris is often caused by smoking, whence the French medical custom of talking about "tobacco angina" of the heart. Damage to the respiratory system was also common, resulting in chronic lung catarrh but also asthma and emphysema, diseases found disproportionately among "inhalers" in their forties and fifties. Memory loss, slowed reaction times, premature aging, wrinkled skin, gray hair, ulcers, blindness, and diabetes had all been linked to smoking, and different kinds of tobacco use caused different kinds of tumors. Cancers of the lip, for example, were found almost exclusively in pipe smokers, whereas chewing tobacco was a "definite cause" of cancers of the gum and cheek. Reiter also remarked on how, following "painstaking observations of individual cases," smoking had been linked to cancers of the human lung.[11]

Reiter recognized that people would very likely differ in their susceptibility to such ailments; he also emphasized that more research was needed to deepen our understanding, whence the need for institutes such as this new one at the University of Jena. The important historical fact, though, is that Germany's most powerful public health authority was already convinced—from mountains of evidence—that smoking was a threat to human health. Reiter cited the work of the American biostatistician Raymond Pearl, who in 1938 had shown that smokers even in their thirties and forties had mortality rates twice as high as nonsmokers. Reiter also cited studies showing that smokers raise the carbon monoxide in their blood from about half a percent to ten or even twenty times that level; he then stressed the threat to military performance—damage to heart muscle, for example—and diminished ability of pilots to withstand the rigors of high-altitude flight. Experiments on mice, fish, rabbits, and guinea pigs had shown corrosive effects of tobacco at the cellular level, and Reiter concluded that if animals such as these could be harmed, why shouldn't we assume this would also be true for humans?

Leonardo Conti's speech at this same 1941 Jena congress reveals an equally unambiguous recognition of tobacco's deadly power. Conti was not a marginal figure in this realm: as Reich Health Führer he was the most powerful physician in Germany, with broad police powers and the friendly ear of Hitler. Conti hailed the establishment of the Jena institute as a "fundamental change in how we go about public health," signaling a shift in focus from infectious diseases such as plague or pox to chronic diseases of the sort caused by threats to our air and water. Tobacco was chief among these threats, and "no reasonable person" could deny the evidence. Nonsmokers perceived this when exposed to smoke, and smokers realized it when trying to quit. Conti noted that while he, like Astel and Reiter, was "absolutely convinced" of this danger, it was easy to be misled by stories of smokers living to some ripe old age. And there was also this question: how could anyone prove with certainty that the surgeon who smokes twenty-five cigarettes a day and then collapses from heart failure died from smoking rather than from, say, stress or some genetic fault? Conti's answer: animal experiments had shown the power of the poisons in tobacco, leaving no doubt as to their power to damage the interior of the body. Tobacco was "far more dangerous" than drink, which wasn't necessarily even harmful if done in moderation. Alcohol and tobacco were different in this respect, since drinking could cause *acute* poisoning while smoking caused a more insidious *chronic* poisoning. Conti cited many of the same outcomes mentioned by Reiter—hardening of the arteries, for example—and came down hard on cancer: "There can no longer be any doubt that carcinoma of the larynx, cancer of the esophagus, and cancers of the air passageways all have been linked to the irritating effects of smoking. Statistical findings make this clear, and in a way that cannot be challenged. Heart disease has also been linked to smoking. These are certainties, and that is how matters stand today."[12] Conti emphasized that these "certainties" were not as widely known as they should be and that progress against tobacco had been hindered by its addictive power. Many smokers couldn't even sit through a meeting without suffering the pangs of withdrawal, making them not so different in this respect from opium addicts.

It should not be overlooked that Reiter's and Conti's remarks are summary assessments of a much larger body of empirical work. Lickint's monumental 1939 *Tabak und Organismus* cites more than seven thousand references in 1,200 pages, and works such as this were relied upon by German medical authorities when they made their summary assessments. I stress this fact because we often hear that it was first in Britain and the United States in the 1950s that smoking was shown to be a serious, and medically well established, threat to human health. That is simply false. It is true that the British and the Americans after the war provided stronger evidence, as well as new ways to measure and document the hazard; it is also true that for many people this was news, and news even today in historical retrospect (even for some Germans, interestingly, who still have a hard time grappling with events from this era). But it is not true that British and Americans were the first to establish the reality of tobacco hazards. The first medical consensus that tobacco poses a grave threat to human health comes in Germany in the early 1940s. That consensus was aided by Nazi sentiments and comes undone by the war, but that does not mean it never existed.

POLITICAL AMNESIA

Part of our difficulty appreciating this history—apart from the fact that few scholars have gone back to the original German texts—lies in our presumption of the cumulative nature of science. We like to think of scientific knowledge as growing steadily over time, with progress never sullied by regress and nothing ever lost from the storehouse of human wisdom. The history of science in this view is like a giant immortal brain with perfect recall, when the more apt comparison might be to a tree that sheds whole branches when they no longer reach into the light. Most of what has ever been known has been forgotten. Forgetting is often crucial for scientific progress, but not *everything* that is forgotten is for good reason—in science as in life. For Nazi-era research we have the added complication of a kind of guilt by association: the good has been thrown out with the bad, and to a certain extent for good reasons. The foul taint of Nazism pervading much of this work has made it difficult to honor, to reuse, or even to recall.

Another crucial fact is that many of the most prominent anti-tobacco scholars and activists did not survive the war. Franz H. Müller, author of the world's first case-control epidemiology of lung cancer, vanished during the war years, perhaps killed in combat. Leonardo Conti took his own life while awaiting trial for war crimes, and Gauleiter Fritz Sauckel, author of the proposal sent to Hitler to establish the world's first Institute for the Struggle against Tobacco Hazards, was hanged on October 16, 1946, following his conviction for having organized Germany's deadly system of forced labor. Hans Reiter survived the war but lost his position as Germany's leading public health authority and lived out the rest of his life in relative obscurity. (His name endures, though, in the form of "Reiter's syndrome," a kind of polyarthritis consisting of urethritis, arthritis, and conjunctivitis, which rheumatologists circa 2000 tried to rechristen when his Nazi past was exposed.)[13] And of course Hitler himself, the most vocal opponent of smoking to govern any twentieth-century nation, committed suicide in the final weeks of the war.

Karl Astel's case is one of the most revealing. Astel had been named to head the

Jena institute, rewarding his long support both for antitobacco science and German fascism. Astel was both an anti-Semite and a rabid antitobacco fanatic (and a high-ranking SS officer); and as president of the University of Jena he had imposed a ban on smoking at the school (effective May 1, 1941), where he gained a certain notoriety for snatching cigarettes from the lips of smoking students. In his speech at the founding of the new institute, Astel listed five reasons for opposing smoking: (1) tobacco damaged smokers' health, lowering the human life span; (2) it cost people money they should be spending on more useful pursuits—four billion Reichsmarks per year in 1941; (3) it took up prime agricultural lands that could be used to grow more useful crops like apricots or cherries; (4) it was an aesthetic abomination, fouling the ground with cigarette butts but also matches and empty cigarette packs (he proposed portable ashtrays, which the industry would not take seriously until half a century later); and (5) it was a failure of ethics, insofar as people did not consider how their actions affected others or the good of the whole. Smoking was also filthy and unpatriotic—and deadly. Astel knew that cigarettes were killing large numbers of people; indeed it was in his own institute that the world's most sophisticated epidemiological demonstration of the link to lung cancer was conducted.[14]

Astel was not unusual, though, in blending Nazi rhetoric and anti-tobacco science. Nazism was very much the language of the German anti-tobacco movement in the early 1940s. Smoking was a violation of National Socialist ethics, one's "duty to be healthy" and (thereby) to serve the nation and its Führer. Tobacco was selfish, unhealthy, and irresponsible; the industry was capitalist and some said Jewish; smoking was "a threat to culture" and, as the leading anti-tobacco journal put it, "the gymnastic apparatus of the weak-willed" (das Turngerät der Willenlosen). Language of this sort helped to legitimize the anti-tobacco movement and in this sense helped to carry the consensus. Crucial also was the fact that Hitler himself disliked the evil weed, characterizing it as "vengeance of the Red Man against the Whites, revenge for having been given hard liquor." The Führer claimed that Nazism might never have triumphed if he personally had not given up smoking (in 1919); he also came to regret having allowed his troops to smoke, fearing this had compromised their fighting power. Hitler supported the Jena institute; indeed it was his gift of 100,000 Reichsmarks from his Reich Chancellery that had established it in the first place. A telegram read to those at the opening celebrations pledged his aid in helping to free Germany from "one of man's most dangerous poisons."[15]

TOBACCO STRIKES BACK

Astel's was a highly moralizing rhetoric—tobacco use in his view contributed to criminality and "bordello culture"—but this again does not mean that he and others like him were not convinced of real, empirically established harms. There has been this odd tendency in tobacco historiography—encouraged by the industry to a certain extent—to see tobacco's early critics as *either* moralistic *or* evidence based, as if the two are somehow mutually exclusive. The fact is that many of the earliest anti-tobacco fanatics had good sound evidence for their passions.

German manufacturers, however, were just as eager to use Nazi rhetoric to *defend* cigarettes. Tobacco manufacturers were proud of the fact that tobacco had officially been declared "war important" and boosted cigarettes as crucial for the "victorious peace of our Fatherland." Tobacco was sold as patriotic, its critics branded suspect fanatics. This latter denigration was a common theme: German cigarette manufacturers launched barbs against "anti-tobacco fanatics" and *Muradisten,* a reference to Sultan Murad IV of the Ottoman Empire, said to have traveled through Turkey beheading anyone found violating his draconian ban on smoking. Tobacco's critics were also labeled "French" or otherwise foreign to the spirit of the Nazi regime. Tobacco manufacturers wrapped themselves in the Nazi flag, accusing their critics of being unpatriotic or worse—as in somehow linked to the Jews or gripped by a prohibitionist psychopathology.[16] (See Figure 24.)

German tobacco magnates also tried to capture a kind of scientific high ground by establishing journals, research bodies, and honorific academies dedicated to glorifying tobacco. An industry-friendly Institute for Tobacco Research in Forchheim had existed since the 1920s, along with two prominent tobacco trade journals, the *Deutsche Tabakzeitung* and *Süddeutsche Zeitung.* Nazi health fears prompted the creation in 1937 of a new journal devoted principally to defending the golden weed, *Der Tabak,* redubbed *Chronica Nicotiana* in 1940 with aspirations to be "the global journal of tobacco." An International Association for Scientific Tobacco Research was established in Bremen in 1938 to coordinate the industry's counterpunch, which included sponsorship of an international tobacco congress and an annual Prize for Progress in Tobacco Research. *Chronica Nicotiana* published a seemingly endless stream of articles testifying to the glorious history of tobacco, alongside cigarette news from the front and the predictable ridicule of "anti-tobacco fanatics." The whole point was to buttress the legitimacy of tobacco in German society by wrapping its makers in the authority of exact science, hoary tradition, economic indispensability, and international prestige. On this latter point: while *Chronica Nicotiana* was published mainly in German, articles also appeared in English, French, and Dutch, and sometimes even in Russian (after the Hitler-Stalin Pact of 1939). This helped the industry define itself as neutral and nonpartisan—which is perhaps also why the association gave itself (in 1940) the rather grandiose Latin title Academia Nicotiana Internationalis.[17]

Institutions of this sort allowed the industry to claim for itself expertise in all realms of tobacco. Paul Koenig, director of the Reich Institute for Tobacco Research in Forchheim, claimed that his was the "go-to" place for all tobacco matters, from seed to cigarette. In a 1940 speech reported in the *Deutsche Tabak-Zeitung,* Koenig boasted that "virtually all scientific disciplines" were represented at his institute, from agricultural economics and breeding technology to medicine, history, art, law, political science, and even theology (since smoking supposedly had its origins in spiritualism).[18] Cigarette manufacturers often claimed that "the tobacco question" should be left to the experts—as in 1940, when *Chronica Nicotiana* complained that "everyone seems to feel competent to judge the tobacco question," with those knowing the least making the most noise. This same article noted the industry's recent establishment of an Institute for Comparative Luxury Goods to study coffee, alcohol, tobacco, tea, chocolate, and other *Genussmittel* (luxuries of taste), with the goal clearly being to renormalize and glamorize nicotiana by linking it to other sensory delights.

The industry also played the economic scare card, emphasizing the dependence of the German economy and state on tobacco and tobacco taxes. Reich Economics Minister (and Reich Bank President) Walther Funk vouched for the industry, just as Conti vouched for its critics. In decades hence this would become a typical tension all across the globe: health ministers tend to oppose tobacco, while finance ministers can't seem to get enough of it. German industrialists stressed the vital role of tobacco in the army and the utility of nicotine as an insecticide. Hopes were even held out that the tobacco plant might prove one day to be a source of cooking oil and perfume. Not wanting to rock any political boats, the International Association for Scientific Tobacco Research put a bust of the Führer on prominent display in its Bremen offices.[19] And makers of German collectible "cigarette cards" attacked Britain as "the robber state" while boosting Hitler as Germany's savior. Here is the voice of the German industry as expressed in a popular tobacco card album from 1941:

> With every word and every command of the Führer, from every action of the German army, from the steadfastness of the German people, comes our determination to bring to a victorious end the war that England has forced upon us. That victory will mean the fall of British plutocracy and the end of England's exploitation of the world. It will result in the victory of the socialist idea and the establishment of a just order in Europe and the entire world.[20]

Clever rhetorical tricks were also used to tackle the health question. "Not proven" is the charge repeated time and again: when evidence was adduced that smoking injures the teeth or gums or heart or lungs, or that nicotine is addictive, *Chronica Nicotiana* would spring into action and claim "not proven"—and denied even that smoking produced tar. A distinction was also drawn between tobacco *use* and tobacco *abuse*, contrasting "moderate" (i.e., harmless) versus "excessive" indulgence. A parallel distinction was made between "low-quality" and "high-quality" tobacco: so whereas inferior grades might well be bad for you (so the German industry said), the high-quality stuff was unobjectionable. Not all harms were denied: German manufacturers took the interesting stance that *inhaling* tobacco smoke was not such a good idea, and one of the industry's leading defenders called it "crazy" to inhale the smoke of "twenty, thirty, or more cigarettes per day." Germans were not yet using a great deal of flue-cured tobacco, so there was not yet much of an incentive—or need—to promote inhalation. Athletes and pregnant women were also discouraged from smoking, as were people with medical conditions. But for the rest of us: relax and have a smoke![21]

The industry's critics saw this as ridiculous. For most of those writing in *Reine Luft* (Pure Air), the flagship organ of the German Anti-tobacco League—there was no such thing as "moderate" tobacco use: all use was abuse. Quality really didn't matter, since even the best tobacco would still cause heart disease and premature aging and a stinking gangrene of the extremities—and cancer.

The industry's position on cancer is best characterized as dismissive, with the evidence ridiculed as "political" or "literary" in nature. Anti-tobacco activists were playing "statistical games" and violating the calm that was supposed to sedate the true spirit of exact science. According to a 1941 article in Germany's leading tobacco trade weekly, cancer was merely a ploy devised by fanatics looking for new ways to instill fears:

> According to our anti-tobacco contemporaries all that is terrible, bad, and evil in this world stems from tobacco. Why should this not include diseases? The scratchy throat with morning cough . . . no longer interests our anti-tobacco contemporaries, even though this is probably the only harm proven to come from smoking. But a scratchy throat with cough cannot be used for any useful propaganda purpose; it's too innocuous. There must be something more frightful! Cancer was the answer arrived at after trying a couple of other diseases, like TB.

Roffo's work was singled out for criticism:

> Research of the director of Argentina's National Cancer Institute, Professor Roffo, figures big in the evidence that smoking can cause cancer. Professor Roffo is the leading figure in Argentina's anti-tobacco movement; he also edits a journal titled "Live 100 Years" and swims in the currents of French cultural propaganda, for which he was named a Chevalier of the Legion of Honor shortly before the war. Professor Roffo was able to produce cancer by painting the ears of a rabbit for several weeks with "tobacco tar," causing the formation of growths. The fact that smoke alone, without destructive distillation, produced no tar [sic—he may mean cancer] didn't bother him; nor did the fact that there is a big difference between smoking and painting with tar. Or that many rabbits vanished into the Happy Hunting Ground before developing cancer.[22]

This author goes on to suggest that anti-tobacco activists owed a debt of thanks to this rabbit for having so helped their cause, since not every kind of animal painted with tar developed cancer. The sarcastic suggestion is made that the rabbit should become the anti-tobacco movement's official mascot or heraldic animal *(Wappentier),* complete with a tumor on its ear.

NAZI TOBACCO'S HATCHET MAN

The flippant tone of such remarks is typical of the industry's response to the growing evidence of harms from smoking. Much of the time, though, they demonstrate either a poor or deliberately obtuse understanding of the methods and issues involved. When Raymond Pearl showed that smokers shorten their lives, for example, German industrialists asked how it could be that people living where lots of cigarettes were smoked tended to live longer than people in poorer parts of the world where fewer cigarettes were smoked.[23] The puzzle should have taken about five seconds to solve, since it is based on a simple flaw. People in richer parts of the world tend to live longer for many reasons—foremost among these being that they are far more likely to survive infancy, childhood diseases, and childbirth. Rich people had (and still have) better access to clean water, clean jobs, and quality health care. It also happens to be true—or at least used to be true—that the rich were more likely to smoke. People in wealthier parts of the world therefore live longer, despite also smoking more. Studies like Pearl's made it clear, though, that people in developed countries would live *even longer* if they didn't smoke. Apologists for the industry either failed to grasp, or refused to admit, such facts well into the 1990s.

In the 1930s and 1940s, however, the German tobacco industry seems to have had some difficulty finding a medical doctor willing to work with its so-called Chemical-Hygiene Division. A Dutch physician by the name of R. G. J. P. Huismann eventually agreed to serve as the industry's scientific hatchet man and in the early 1940s frequently reviewed scientific works for the German cigarette press. Huismann was in fact one of the Continent's first great denialist scholars. When evidence was published linking smoking and angina, Huismann dismissed the link as happenstance. When evidence of other hazards was advanced, Huismann said that the afflicted must suffer from an "excessive sensitivity." Huismann's job was made easier by the fact that some critics exaggerated tobacco harms, or found them in fantastic places. Claims that smoking caused impotence or poor performance on the job were easy targets (less so, though, in hindsight), as were efforts to link certain female maladies to exposure to tobacco dust in factories. Huismann in parallel fashion rejected claims that alcohol or exposure to X-rays could cause long-term chronic injuries.

Huismann also dismissed the tobacco–lung cancer link, albeit not without delving into the evidence. In a long, two-part article in the spring and summer 1943 issues of *Chronica Nicotiana,* he conceded the rise of lung cancers for Holland and other developed nations; he also recognized that since cancer was a disease of the elderly, any statistical data would have to be age adjusted—to eliminate bias. (An aged population would show higher death rates from cancer simply because there are more elderly in the population, when rates for, say, forty- or fifty-year-olds might not actually have increased.) Huismann was also keen to apply the theory of statistical error, to make sure that whatever differences might be found in cancer rates over time were statistically significant. Huismann granted that lung cancer *had in fact* increased dramatically in Europe and added that he himself as a medical student from 1917 to 1923 had never seen a single case of the disease—it had been so rare. He also reproduced a chart from a 1932 Ph.D. dissertation showing the changing percentage of lung cancers found at autopsy in various parts of Europe, year by year from 1902 to 1930. The chart showed that in *no* study prior to 1920 was lung cancer ever found in more than one percent of all bodies autopsied, whereas in no study *after* that time was lung cancer ever found in less than one percent of all autopsies. Lung cancer was clearly on the rise in Holland and in other parts of Europe; that much, again, was "proven."[24]

Huismann did not believe, however, that the case for tobacco causation was closed. He commented on how much city life had changed in recent decades—the increased pace of life and stress, for example, combined with exposure to automotive fumes and dusts from newly tarred roads. Smoking had been blamed for cancer since the eighteenth century, as he pointed out, but Huismann also insisted that "many questions remain open" and that the cigarette link remained unproved. And like many future denialists, he did no experiments of his own, or any original epidemiology, or any kind of chemical analysis of carcinogens. Nor does he seem to have published outside the "safe" orbit of the industry's trade organs. *Chronica Nicotiana* was full of such apologetics, including efforts to blame cancer on one's genetic constitution, or psychology, or some other alternate cause. Helmuth Aschenbrenner, editor of the journal, published numerous dismissals of this sort and even had the chutzpah to have his own testimonials reviewed in the journal—by himself! One such self-embrace was his "Cancer and the Psyche," a previously published article abstracted in the journal's April 1943 issue. Aschenbrenner here laid out his theory that cancer was a purely "psychogenic disease," with neurasthenics tending to suffer afflictions of the lungs and hysterics more likely to contract cancers of the digestive tract and sexual organs. Aschenbrenner went on to enjoy a postwar career defending German tobacco makers, psychoanalyzing anti-tobacco activists as paranoid psychopaths fearful of "the big fire," meaning nuclear war.[25] Huismann, by contrast, seems to have vanished into thin air—but not before establishing several of the key canonical arguments used by subsequent denialists.

CIGARETTES SURVIVE THE REICH

Reading journals like *Chronica Nicotiana* today, one is struck by the fact that many of the arguments fundamental to the denialist campaign launched in America in the 1950s were already being tested in Germany in the 1940s. Recognition is given to the broad suspicion of a cancer hazard, but the statistics are attacked, and "more research" is demanded. Refutations in the form of "puzzles" are offered: the fact that cancers of the larynx or tongue had not grown as fast as those of the lung, for example, or that women's lung cancer rates were not increasing so fast even though women had been smoking a lot, or that the period during which smoking had become popular had also seen a growth in overall life expectancy. The industry published evidence of therapeutic uses of nicotine—to treat Raynaud's disease, for example—and even philosophical work in which the entire concept of causality was denied. Nazi-era cigarette manufacturers were faced with a powerful, politicized, and medically sophisticated threat, and responded by establishing institutions, arguments, and authorities to neutralize that threat. Writers for the industry predicted the eventual demise of the anti-tobacco movement, expressing confidence that tobacco "will be around long after the present anti-tobacco movement has passed into its prohibitionist afterlife."[26]

German health activists saw through most of these stratagems, accusing the industry of using the pretense of science to dress up what, in fact, was a kind of surreptitious advertising and an exercise of raw economic power. The German Anti-tobacco League accused the International Association for Scientific Tobacco Research of being little more than a trade association, prompting the industry to sue the league for defamation, in 1937. A Hamburg court ruled against the industry, however, concluding that the association was more of a trade group than a scientific society.[27] The Anti-tobacco League relished this victory, reminding tobacco makers on more than one occasion that their pretense to "science" was really a form of fraud.

It is also crucial to keep in mind, however, the deep asymmetry of the industry and its critics at this time. Public health advocates had ideological support from the Nazi Party, but this was hardly a match for the brute economic power of the industry. Cigarette defenders had the financial clout of Germany's tobacco empire behind them, with virtually unlimited funds to finance conferences, journals, industry-friendly research, and denialist screeds. Anti-tobacco organizations, by contrast, had to rely almost exclusively on donations—including the RM100,000 from Hitler's Reichskanzlei—and suffered more when push came to shove in the final years of the war. And while cigarette manufacturers quickly regrouped after the demise of the Reich, anti-tobacco groups were in far worse shape—scattered and demoralized—and never did regain their publishing or political power. So while the Institute for Tobacco Research in Forchheim continued on as before the war—albeit henceforth as a "Federal" rather than a "Reich" institute—Jena's Institute for Tobacco Hazards Research, the world's first tobacco prevention research institute, collapsed with the death of Astel and its chief benefactors. And the defeat of Nazism more broadly.

At the end of the day, at least the day of Germany's imperial power, the financial clout of the industry triumphed over the scientific and ideological threat to Nazi-era Big Tobacco. The consensus that tobacco was a major cause of disease falls into a deep and prolonged slumber—in continental Europe at least, which loses its lead here as in many other areas of science. The center of gravity in the Great Tobacco Wars shifts to the United States and Britain, where parallel battles over science and industrial authority would be fought.

"Sold American"

Tobacco-Friendly Research
at the Medical College of Virginia

We need friends in unfriendly times.
We need friends wherever we can find them.
We need friends and strong support in state capitals.
We need friends to learn how to be human.

EXTRACTS FROM THE TOBACCO ARCHIVES RETURNED
BY SEARCHING "WE NEED FRIENDS"

On May 22, 2008, the *New York Times* published an exposé of a rather suspect relationship between Virginia Commonwealth University (VCU) in Richmond and its research sponsor, Philip Morris. The article reveals the university's having agreed to remarkably restrictive conditions in exchange for funding from the tobacco giant, which totaled $1.3 million in 2007. Virtually all patent rights had been given over to the company, along with whatever other intellectual property might come from the collaboration. The contract stipulated that Philip Morris alone would have the power to decide what results from the grant would be published; it also barred university administrators from talking to the press about the nature of the grant and required that anyone asked for such a comment notify the company that such a request had been made.[1]

What is remarkable about the *New York Times* story, though, is how little of the underlying history of this collaboration is actually exposed. Francis L. Macrina, VCU's vice president for research, is quoted defending the restrictive language of the grant as part of a "balancing act," but no mention is made of the fact that Macrina himself was appointed when his predecessor (Marsha Torr) lost her job for questioning the wisdom of such collaborations. No mention is made of the fact that VCU's president, Eugene P. Trani, sat on the board of one of the world's leading leaf tobacco merchants, the Universal Corporation, for which he received an annual fee of $40,000 plus stock options, plus another $2,000 for each of the board meetings he attended and $1,500 for committee meetings.[2] And no mention is made of the fact that Trani had helped bring a new $350 million research park to Richmond, the crown jewel of which is Biotech Nine, Altria's (i.e., Philip Morris's) 450,000-square-foot Center for Research and Technology devoted to the tobacco company's version of "the life sciences." The *Times* article asserted that Philip Morris historically "has not been a major contributor to the university," which is true but misleading given that there are few universities with closer ties to the industry. They just got the company wrong.

For nearly three quarters of a century, VCU has been the tobacco industry's most important academic ally and collaborator. Most of that relationship involved collaboration not with Philip Morris but rather with the American Tobacco Company. Indeed, as we shall see, as early as 1940 the company famous for its toasted Lucky Strikes was declaring the Richmond school "sold American," meaning bought for the cause of the world's largest manufacturer of cigarettes.

DEATH IN CELLOPHANE

The tobacco industry is notorious for its decades-long campaign to claim there was "no proof" that tobacco was a cause of death and injury. The campaign is widely thought to have begun in December of 1953, when plans were made to reassure consumers that if there was anything wrong with cigarettes the industry would be the first to know and quick to organize a fix. In a "Frank Statement" published in 448 newspapers on January 4, 1954, the nation's leading tobacco companies—all but Liggett & Myers—announced the formation of the Tobacco Industry Research Committee (TIRC) to explore potential tobacco hazards, promising also to aid and assist research into "all phases of tobacco use and health."

The "Frank Statement" does indeed mark a new level of audacity in the industry's campaign to defraud the American public, but how new was this defensive posture? Were American tobacco manufacturers honestly in the dark about hazards prior to this time, and if so, when did they discover them? When did the industry stop believing cigarettes were safe? And when did honest doubts turn duplicitous?

Tobacco companies are complex organizations with thousands of employees and highly diversified departments, each with their own subdivisions of labor. Who knew what and how early? are therefore questions that are not always easy to answer. Knowledge and ignorance can have complicated biogeographies, and we also have to reckon with the corporate equivalent of a kind of psychological *denial*: people don't always *want* to know what they could and perhaps should know, especially if the knowledge is going to be painful. Upton Sinclair in 1935 noted how difficult it was to get someone to understand something "when his salary depends upon his not understanding it."[3] Avoiding the truth is probably easier when that is what is expected of you on the job. Psychological and sociological complications of this sort can frustrate our search for answers to "who knew what and when" in the realm of tobacco hazards.

We cannot peer directly into other people's minds, but we can say what the documents tell us, which is that researchers at America's largest tobacco firms had begun wrestling with health harms long before the 1950s. I've mentioned the letters people wrote to the companies, often prompted by research by Roffo and others indicating a substantial cancer hazard, but there were also published reports, some of which hit close to home. A May 1, 1939, article in a popular science magazine reported Roffo's experiments with rabbits, showing how tars extracted from the tobacco of Virginia's Piedmont produced "quick and virulent cancer of the eye," and in November of 1940 the *Richmond News Leader* reported Roffo's experiments along with Alton Ochsner's characterization of smoking as "a cause of cancer of the lung." Popular anti-tobacco literature was also reappearing, having recovered somewhat from the repeal of Prohibition in the early 1930s. (Many anti-alcohol activists had also opposed tobacco use, whence the battle cry after the passage of the Volstead Act in 1919: "Nicotine next!") Charles L. Van Noppen's *Death in Cellophane* appeared in 1937, reporting evidence of smokers shortening their lives by "seven or more years" on average, with a total loss to the nation of "more than 100,000 deaths annually." Van Noppen also compiled anti-tobacco utterances such as that by Hudson Maxim, the American inventor of smokeless gunpowder, who once judged that with every breath, smoking boys "inhale imbecility and exhale manhood."[4]

Tobacco manufacturers kept a close watch on such jibes, responding only when there was an actual threat to sales. American industry authorities also kept abreast of European events, including the epidemiology and experimental work coming out of Hitler's Germany. Translations were sometimes done in-house, but commercial services were also employed. In the 1920s, for example, the Lorillard Company employed Berlin Translation Services to translate German tobacco patents, and other companies performed similar services for the industry in the 1930s. American industry researchers in the 1940s were familiar enough with European scholarship to cite long passages translated from the German. Many foreign patents from the 1930s can be found in translation in tobacco company archives; many of these describe new filter designs, new methods of denicotinization, and so forth.[5]

By 1940 the tide of incriminating science had risen high enough for the industry to realize it needed a more vigorous response. Roffo was at the height of his powers, Franz H. Müller's case-control epidemiological study had been abstracted in *JAMA*, and Raymond Pearl of Johns Hopkins had shown that smoking was associated with a definite "impairment of longevity"—about eight years per smoker. Alton Ochsner at Tulane had also reported (with Michael DeBakey) that an overwhelming fraction of his seventy-nine lung cancer patients had been smokers. Chemists in tobacco industry laboratories were chalking up an ever-lengthening list of nasty chemicals in smoke, including not just nicotine, carbon monoxide, ammonia, and phenols (well known since the nineteenth century) but now also lead, arsenic, hydrogen cyanide, and acrolein, a decomposition product of glycerol notorious for its use in World War I as a chemical weapon. The industry was active in identifying and quantifying many of these constituents, assisted by the American Tobacco Company's improved automatic cigarette smoking machine, modified from German predecessors, details of which were published in 1936.[6]

THE IMPORTANCE OF BIOLOGICAL RESEARCH

And so on February 3, 1941, in reaction to the bad news coming from both at home and abroad (including Müller's work in Germany but also Roffo's in Argentina), Edward S. Harlow, American Tobacco's assistant director of research, wrote a memo to his superior, Hiram R. Hanmer, outlining "The Importance of Biological Research." This is a fascinating document, reading as it does like an honest divulgence of opinions, albeit not very flattering to the industry. We can presume it was never meant to see the light of day, and we find in it no evidence of eavescasting. The context is one in which scholars were beginning to trace the lung cancer epidemic to tobacco use. The American Tobacco Company, the largest in the world at that time, was also expanding its research department, having recently opened a new building at 400 Petersburg Turnpike in Richmond, housing "35 young scientists" organized into seven divisions, including a Medical Division headed by Harvey B. Haag, professor of pharmacology at the Medical College of Virginia.[7] More on whom in a moment.

Harlow began his memo rather abruptly by noting, "It may be assumed that the medical profession is the group which it is most desired to reach and convince." Reach and convince of what? We are not told, but from the context we know he is talking about the safety of cigarettes. Doctors were easier to convince "if properly approached," he says, because they are "less skeptical than other scientific groups." Doctors are "jealous of their prestige and fearful of exploitation," however, and therefore difficult to reach. And not likely to be impressed with chemical research: "the only kind of research which may be expected to impress the medical profession is that obtained by the pharmacologist or the physiologist in a biological laboratory." Harlow then says that the Medical College of Virginia was already providing evidence that the "alleged serious effects of smoking on health" were "greatly exaggerated"; he seems to have been convinced that "impartial research" would show that smoking had only "a negligible effect on the health of normal individuals." This is then followed by a revealing qualification: "But this would never be suspected by reading the extensive medical literature on tobacco."[8]

Harlow here implies that "the extensive medical literature on tobacco" *was* already beginning to show that smoking *did* have a non-negligible impact on health, even for "normal individuals." His prior qualification is also significant, however, in that he implies that if tobacco does somehow injure your health, you must not be entirely normal. The memo concludes, "The tobacco industry is very much in need of some friendly research."[9]

Friendly research was supplied first and foremost by the Medical College of Virginia (MCV—and since 1968 known as the Virginia Commonwealth University), a small once-private medical school in downtown Richmond whose founding father—Augustus Werner—had left the University of Virginia to begin a new medical school "because he didn't like Jefferson's philosophy that Professors shouldn't corrupt their teaching by making money caring for patients."[10] In the mid-1930s, as serious reports about tobacco hazards began to multiply, the MCV became the industry's most trusted and enduring academic ally. For more than a half a century the MCV—only a short drive from American Tobacco's Research Laboratory on Petersburg Turnpike—would provide the company with expert advice, sympathetic research, and friendly public testimony on matters of tobacco and health. And the collaboration continues even today, albeit now with Philip Morris, successor to American as the nation's largest tobacco firm.

How, though, did this collaboration get started? What were the key tobacco health worries in the 1930s, and what kinds of "friendly research" were actually done?

SULFANILAMIDE AND POISON GAS

The American Tobacco Company began working with pharmacologists at the MCV in the mid-1930s, as part of the company's efforts to develop a response to two novel health worries: the questionable health impact of *diethylene glycol* (increasingly used as a humectant in cigarette manufacture) and questions over the presence of *lead* and *arsenic* in cigarette smoke. These were not the first-discovered poisons in tobacco—or the first public outcries about them—but they certainly were two of the deepest challenges to worry-free tobacco manufacturing in the 1930s.

Tobacco manufacturers had begun using diethylene glycol (DEG) in the early 1930s as a substitute for *glycerine,* a sweetish, oily, "sugar alcohol" commonly used as a moistening or texturizing agent in foods and in tobacco. Technically known as a "hygroscopic" (moisture-attracting) agent, glycerine was much admired for its ability to help keep foods moist and tobacco leaves pliable during rolling. Glycerine is still used today in many different kinds of foods—to soften and smoothen ice cream and candy bars, for example, and in certain kinds of mechanical lubricants.

Philip Morris was apparently the first to begin using DEG as a glycerine substitute, around 1930. Health was one reason for the switch: charges had been leveled since the First World War that glycerine when burned releases *acrolein,* also known as acrylic or ethylene aldehyde, a tear gas used as a chemical warfare agent by the French. DEG is not so unlike glycerine from a chemical point of view, but it did seem to produce a less irritating smoke when used to moisten cigarettes. It seemed like a healthier alternative, though it also came with baggage of its own. The compound had been widely used as an antifreeze, and people were known to have poisoned themselves by drinking the substance. A bigger challenge came in 1937, when more than a hundred people died from taking a DEG-adulterated medicine known as Elixir Sulfanilamide. Sulfa drugs had been used in powder form to treat streptococcus infections, and the fatal decision to add DEG was made by a Tennessee manufacturer wanting to market the drug in liquid form. The concoction was not tested prior to distribution, however, and even when people started dying—from convulsions and kidney failure—the manufacturer was slow to issue a warning.[11]

Outrage over the sulfanilamide scandal led to the passage of the 1938 Federal Food, Drug, and Cosmetic Act, but it also turned up the heat on tobacco manufacturers, who started having to answer questions about whether the DEG being added to cigarettes might be responsible for some of the harms being linked to smoking—including cancer. Philip Morris's research director asked *JAMA* editor Morris Fishbein about this and was reassured to hear that it would be "unwarranted" for cigarette manufacturers to abandon their use of DEG. Fishbein explained that the sulfanilamide deaths were from taking "a considerable amount of diethylene glycol internally over a long period of time," a situation "not at all similar" to what occurs when smoking cigarettes. Fishbein went out of his way to reassure the public, in a *JAMA* editorial, that while DEG was "an unstandardized, nonofficial product, not recommended or recognized for internal use," there was nonetheless "no evidence" that its use in cigarettes was harmful. Fishbein of course didn't disclose his financial relationship with Philip Morris, or the fact that pre-publication drafts of his editorial were submitted to the cigarette manufacturer for its perusal.[12]

Acrolein was also a focus at this time, since while DEG was supposed to be producing a less irritating smoke (than glycerine), some thought that acrolein levels were just as high or even higher with the new substitute. "Irritation" was still widely viewed as a generic cause of cancer (somewhat like "mutation" would later become), and one reason for looking for substitutes of this sort had been the hope that alternate tobacco formulas might prove less carcinogenic. Industry researchers may well have had cancer in mind when they pondered the value of eliminating "irritants" in tobacco smoke. Exposure to poison gas in World War I was one early theory for why doctors were seeing such a rapid rise in lung cancer, and finding acrolein in cigarettes caused more people to point a finger at smoking. American Tobacco by 1935 had measured acrolein in the smoke of nine popular brands, with values ranging from .02 to .1 milligrams per cigarette. Philip Morris had also measured acrolein in cigarette smoke.[13]

(Military urgency would soon become a far bigger concern than health: glycerine was needed for the manufacture of nitroglycerine, which is why the USDA met with tobacco makers early in World War II to look for glycerine substitutes. By 1942 "scores" of substitutes had been explored, with none proving acceptable apart from

DEG. Sugar was one hygroscopic substitute examined, but the industry already recognized by this time that too much sugar added to cigarettes would upset the acid-alkaline balance of the resulting smoke.)[14]

From the point of view of health, additional worries came from the fact that *lead* and *arsenic* were being found in tobacco. Lead arsenate was widely used as a pesticide prior to the organochlorine revolution of the 1940s, and broader fears of poisonings from lead paint, water pipes, and gasoline caused a headache for tobacco men worried about their public image. (Germans for a time feared that smokers were being poisoned by the leaded gasoline sometimes used in cigarette lighters.)[15] The combination with arsenic created a kind of double whammy, since arsenic was also coming to be known as a carcinogen—which again is one reason non-arsenic pesticides such as DDT were so quickly adopted by agriculturalists in the 1940s and 1950s. Lead and arsenic would remain big worries for tobacco men throughout this time, prompting some of our earliest examples of denialist science.

In 1935, for example, Hiram Hanmer at American Tobacco presented detailed calculations of how many cigarettes you would have to smoke to "ingest" the same level of lead and arsenic allowed by the FDA in apples. Arsenic was indeed in tobacco, Hanmer conceded, but the amounts were significantly less than what one found in seafoods such as lobster.[16] The argument was clever but entirely specious, ignoring the crucial fact that it is often far more dangerous to *inhale* a given chemical than to *ingest* it. A great deal of denialist rhetoric from the 1930s centers on this claim that, since chemical x, y, or z was safe to eat, it must be perfectly safe to smoke. The chemicals to which smokers were exposed were "trivial" because the dosages were below a significant threshold, or didn't remain long in the body, or were "diluted" by being spread over the vast surface of the lungs, and so forth.

One point worth noting is that the DEG and lead/arsenic scandals were both manageable in ways that subsequent health scares were not. DEG and lead, after all, were not *inherent* hazards in the tobacco plant: diethylene glycol was added to make the leaf more pliable, and lead arsenate came in as a contaminant from the pesticides applied by growers. A copper acetate/arsenite known as "Paris green" was commonly used on tobacco—and this was another source of arsenic in the product. DEG, lead, and arsenic were all major-league poisons, but none was essential to either smoking or the tobacco manufacturing process. The cancer worries of later years would be quite different, focusing on the inherent dangers of inhaling even "pristine" tobacco smoke of the very highest quality and purity.

A SPLENDID CONNECTION

The American Tobacco Company's liaison with the Medical College of Virginia began with an effort to tackle these mid-1930s "health scares." As early as 1936, J. H. Weatherby and R. C. Neale from the pharmacology department worked with Harvey Haag from the same department to produce a report for the company on the toxicity of propylene glycol, another proposed glycerine substitute. Professor Weatherby also worked with George Z. Williams from the school's pathology department to explore the toxicity of diethylene glycol. Professor R. J. Main studied the effects of smoking on heart rate and respiration, and Professor Howard B. Hucker examined the toxicity, metabolism, and excretion of nornicotine (a nicotine metabolite). E. C. L. Miller, the MCV's librarian, did literature searches for the company, earning $100 per month from this source until his retirement in November of 1953. The American Tobacco Company was happy to have this help—all funded by the tobacco giant—which Hanmer, as chief chemist, in 1937 characterized as a "splendid connection." MCV President William T. Sanger was equally grateful in 1941, when the tobacco giant doubled its grant to the college (from $5,000 to $10,000 per annum).[17] American Tobacco by this time was paying the entire salary of several of the college's faculty and staff, including Paul S. Larson, the MCV professor of pharmacology who, for the next three decades, would do much to help the cigarette industry flourish.

Harvey Bernhardt Haag (1900–1961) and Paul S. Larson (1907–88) for decades were American Tobacco's academic point men on matters of smoking and health. As successive heads of MCV's Department of Pharmacology, Haag and Larson were faithful collaborators, keeping tobacco abreast of the latest in cancer research while also producing medical literature reviews and attending medical conferences. Haag and Larson also testified for the industry before regulatory committees and helped organize "friendly" experiments and publicity.[18] The two men continued working for the industry after the TIRC was formed in 1954, and in 1961 they published, with Herbert Silvette, another MCV pharmacologist, a 932-page annotated bibliography on smoking and health—known to defense attorneys as "the Green Monster"—regurgitating the "not proved" mantra of the industry. Larson, Haag, and Silvette's *Tobacco: Experimental and Clinical Studies* can indeed be regarded as the bibliographic fundament of the industry's conspiracy. The book is one long parade of conflicting reports about the hazards of smoking, and in the long section on lung cancer, comprising seventy-eight pages of "he-said-she-said," we find the authors concluding that:

> One *one* fact—uncontroverted and incontrovertible—emerges from this dense smoke of interpretation and misinterpretation; guess and speculation; wishful thinking and equally wishful denial; rationalization; propaganda; special pleading; emotionalism; and every other fault of reasoning and expression we like to believe (in defiance of all Medical History) has no place in scientific discussion and conclusion.

That "one fact" was that smoking could not be *the* cause of primary cancer of the lung—since some non-smokers also contract the disease. As for the rest: "no-one can either confirm or deny that smoking is a contributory factor . . . and so the situation remains much as it was described by Boland in 1938; there is no evidence that carcinoma of the lung is produced by tobacco, any more than there is any evidence that it is not. . . . [T]here is no proof of causation." The authors compare the cancer question to that fruitless quarrel described by Jonathan Swift in *Gulliver's Travels,* where Lilliputians warred over whether eggs should be broken at the larger or the smaller end.

Small wonder, then, that for many years Larson and Haag were two of the most highly paid consultants working at this time for the tobacco industry. The reported total for Larson's remuneration from 1949 through 1966 was $72,000, and Haag's was even higher, $78,750 from 1944 through 1961, extraordinary sums for the time. The largest tobacco company in the world was happy to have these helpers: Harlow's "friendly research" memo of 1941 had rightly characterized the Medical College of Virginia as "sold American."[19]

Haag's relationship with the company had begun in 1935, when Hanmer enlisted him to help secure evidence "favorable to our advertising theme," which postulated less "irritation" to the throat and lungs from Lucky Strike cigarettes. American Tobacco had been claiming that "toasting" gave smokers greater "throat protection"; the process (i.e., the normal heat treatment involved in redrying after flue-curing) was supposed to eliminate certain "acrid" constituents of tobacco, but there was also a lot of talk (and print) about its value in "sterilizing" tobacco leaves. Medical themes were coming to feature in the industry's public relations, but the companies also needed real live medical men to polish their image. Harvey Haag was very much appreciated in this regard. American Tobacco's research director heaped praise on the man—for his medical qualifications of course (the company had never had a physician on its research staff) but also for not being "blind to commercial values": "Through him we will establish a connection with the Medical College and will have a fellow continuously working along lines in which we are chiefly interested." Hanmer's vision for such a collaboration was to "proceed with all haste to secure evidence favorable to our advertising" while also realizing that "we shall be dealing with a class of people at first very skeptical of our motives."[20] Meaning medical doctors.

Reassurance research was the order of the day. In 1943, for example, Haag and Larson presented a lecture at the Medical Society of Virginia, ostensibly to puzzle out why it was that for every ten parts of nicotine inhaled by a smoker, only one part was excreted in the urine. Haag and Larson didn't know what happened to the missing nicotine (they suspected a breakdown in the liver), but the point was really just how *fortunate* such a disappearance was, given how toxic nicotine can be in the body. Newspaper reports gave the lecture an almost comic spin, commenting on how "something in the human body takes the nick out of nicotine before it does the heavy smoker any discernible damage." No mention was made of the fact that the work had been sponsored by the world's largest tobacco manufacturer.[21]

The MCV–American Tobacco relationship intensified in the early 1940s, as the industry became increasingly worried about Roffo's work demonstrating health harms in the form of cancer. Throat scratch and morning cough were one thing, but cancer was something else, especially cancer produced with tobacco tars in a modern laboratory. Haag was particularly useful here, given his authoritative position as chair of MCV's Department of Pharmacology (1936–55) and later dean of the School of Medicine (1947–50). Haag was well known and, by some accounts, much loved for his loud and friendly way with students; he was apparently quite a showman, entering his classes with his signature cigar in hand while booming out, "Happy days are here again."[22] Students flocked to his lectures, and fêted him with an annual "Harvey Haag Day" in which everyone would dress up as the master with cigar and trademark bowtie and tweed.

("Happy Days Are Here Again" was a song popularized at the Democratic Party's 1932 presidential convention and became Franklin Roosevelt's campaign song for his successful bid for the presidency. The song was later sung to celebrate the end of Prohibition, which is one reason Haag found it so appealing. Haag had opposed the Eighteenth Amendment—also known as the Volstead Act—and anti-alcohol crusaders had actually burned a report coauthored by Haag in which a tolerance for moderate drinking was expressed. This seems to have left him leery of any effort to implicate tobacco in health harms and helps explain his visceral distrust of efforts to rein in the sale or consumption of cigarettes.)

And Haag remained quite useful to the American Tobacco Company. Throughout the 1940s he was trotted out as a kind of "anti-Roffo" whenever the company was asked about health. In July of 1946, for example, Hanmer received a letter from a certain John J. Trotter of Harlingen, Texas, who had been alarmed by a "hair-raising article" he had read in the August issue of *Reader's Scope*. The article, titled "Cigarettes Cause Cancer?" was by Leonard Engel, a popular medical writer who relied heavily on Roffo for his claim that tobacco "may be a cause of widespread, terrible forms of cancer." Trotter wrote that he had been smoking cigarettes for twenty years, and though he didn't want to live forever he would still "rather not die of cancer."[23]

American Tobacco took this letter very seriously. On August 2, 1946, John A. Crowe from the company's manufacturing department sent a memo to Hanmer enclosing a suggested reply, recording also his estimation of this as "a subject about which we cannot plead ignorance." Hanmer replied to Trotter three days later, explaining that his company was "quite familiar with the claims of Dr. Roffo," having carefully read his articles since they had begun appearing in the early 1930s. Hanmer found it noteworthy that Engel's article was based "almost entirely on Roffo's sweeping statements"; he also noted that the company had been researching the composition of tobacco smoke for fifteen to twenty-five years and that, though he and his colleagues were reluctant to intrude on medical matters, Roffo's procedures were "so patently unscientific" that their "fallacies" should be appreciated. Hanmer reaffirmed that tobacco smoke "does not contain any carcinogenic substances" and recommended to Mr. Trotter that he contact "Dr. H. B. Haag, Professor of Pharmacology at the Medical College of Virginia," for further information. Haag had already prepared an elaborate review and critique of the lung cancer allegation for the company, and Hanmer assured Trotter that Haag would be "glad to give you the benefit of his broad knowledge."[24]

The American Tobacco Company sent a similar response to C. Estelle Smith, a company employee or stockholder from Morristown, New Jersey, who on February 13, 1948, had written to the firm with similar concerns. Smith was worried about the strong claims made in Engel's essay, including Roffo's finding of benzpyrene in tobacco smoke. Alfred F. Bowden, American's assistant to the president, responded as follows: "You will be interested to know that your Company has been alert to both the scientific research and the 'claims' which have been made relative to the subject of tobacco and health. Through our own Research Department, consisting of more than forty research scientists, and a research grant which we established more than ten years ago at one of the leading medical colleges in the country, we have carefully followed the progress of research in this field." Bowden also mentioned that if she wanted further information, "may I suggest that you write Dr. H. B. Haag, Professor of Pharmacology, Medical College of Virginia." Haag had "an intimate knowledge of the literature" and had been engaged in "a critical study of the effects of smoking for many years." Bowden didn't mention that Haag had been on the company's payroll for all those years.[25]

MORE SATISFACTION

In these and other letters a number of the industry's most important public relations strategies are visible in embryo. The industry was beginning to characterize claims of cancer causation as "dangerous"; in a Christmas letter of 1946, for example, Hanmer wrote to the president of Herstein Laboratories in Manhattan that the Engel article had "dangerous implications," illustrating what may result "from the careless use of half-truths in the hands of fanatics." The bluster of reassurance was also developing: after all, how could "forty research scientists" be wrong? Hanmer in 1950 reassured another concerned writer that the library of the American Tobacco Company contained "more than 13,000 references to articles concerning tobacco which have been published in scientific journals throughout the world," with some four thousand of these dealing with the physiologic effects of tobacco. So why worry? Finally, if correspondents wanted "more satisfaction" they could address their questions to "Dr. H. B. Haag, Dean of Medicine, Medical College of Virginia."[26]

Half-truths and worse were also becoming more common in the industry's public pronouncements. Bowden, for example, in his above-mentioned letter, asserted with regard to Roffo that "we know of no one who has confirmed his findings," when the fact is that confirmations of the cigarette–cancer link were already becoming common—and commonly disputed—in the scientific literature. Franz Müller in Cologne had provided strong statistical evidence of the link, as had Schairer and Schöniger in Jena. Herbert L. Lombard and Carl R. Doering in 1928 at Harvard's School of Public Health had concluded that the 27 percent higher rate of cancer among smokers was "highly significant," suggesting that heavy smoking "has some relation to cancer in general." Raymond Pearl had concluded that smokers were dying from their habit, and Germany was full of scholars convinced of the tobacco–cancer link. None of these studies were mentioned by Bowden. Harris B. Parmele, Lorillard's director of research (since 1929), was more honest—at least in private—confessing in a 1946 memo to his Committee on Manufacture that there was "just enough evidence" to justify the presumption of a cigarette–lung cancer link. Parmele admitted this to his colleagues in the company but never to the public.[27]

Hanmer was also not entirely honest in his characterization of flaws in Roffo's work. The claim was that Roffo had not prepared his tars in a proper manner, using unrealistic smoking conditions. Roffo had not allowed his cigarettes to be (mechanically) "smoked" but rather had used a process known as *destructive distillation,* whereby you basically heat a chunk of tobacco in a flask until it burns and/or boils away, collecting the outgassing effluents in a condenser of some sort. This could have been a serious objection: if Roffo had indeed prepared his tars in an improper fashion, he could have been producing cancers with substances bearing little relation to what actually goes into a smoker's lungs.

American Tobacco's research chief was well aware, though, that destructive distillation *was* an important part of how smoke is generated in the normal course of smoking cigarettes. In 1936, in a memo summarizing the work of his research department in Richmond, Hanmer noted that the constituents of tobacco smoke were "intermediate between the gaseous products of complete combustion and the semi-solid and liquid products of destructive distillation." This makes sense when you think about how smoke reaches a smoker's lungs. Smokers light their cigarettes, proceeding then to draw the resulting pyrolyzed aerosols through the tobacco-filled rod into their mouths and lungs. The lit end burns at a fairly high temperature (over 700 degrees Celsius, as had been measured), but the smoke cools as it is pulled through the tobacco. As these hot gases are drawn toward the smoker's lips, some of the tobacco near the thermal peak is destroyed (boiled, really) just prior to being reached by the peak-temperature pyrolyzed gases. What actually goes into a smoker's lungs is therefore a warm steamy mix of tar, soot, nicotine, and thousands of more complex compounds produced through this dual process of combustion *and* destructive distillation. Hanmer was not really being fair (or honest) when he objected that Roffo "did not smoke tobacco; he destructively distilled it." Destructive distillation was in fact how American characterized what happened during the smoking process when presenting its analysis of cigarette constituents to the Federal Trade Commission, part of its defense of "toasting."[28]

American Tobacco's private, quiet defense against Roffo continued throughout the 1940s, with the MCV as the company's faithful and unflinching ally. Experimental cancer studies were part of this, including a series of tests in which rats were made to inhale tobacco smoke. One study coauthored by four scholars from the MCV's pharmacology department found sixteen "smoked" rats living slightly longer than a group of non-smoking controls and no lesions at necropsy. This was not sophisticated work: the sample sizes were small, no literature was cited, and the published paper was not even twenty-three lines.[29] Roffo was the presumptive target, but the quality of the science funded by the tobacco magnate was as night to Roffo's day.

The tobacco company's relations with the Medical College of Virginia went deeper than this, however. In 1941, for example, the MCV chemist Sidney S. Negus was hired to survey the nation's medical schools concerning their positions on Roffo and smoking and health more generally. Negus had come up with the idea for such a survey and proposed it to Hanmer, who gave it the go-ahead. Negus helped organize medical student tours of American Tobacco's research facilities (with Fred J. Wampler, the college's professor of preventive medicine) and in 1941, with the industry's blessing, assumed the influential post of directing "press relationships" for the American Association for the Advancement of Science (AAAS). In taking this position, Negus announced privately to his tobacco benefactors his plans to be "contacting intimately all the key science writers of the country"; he also hoped "ever so often to have fundamental tobacco research reported from your Laboratory given national play." Negus knew where his bread was buttered and promised his new employer a kind of power of censorship: "Obviously nothing will be done in this direction unless approved by you." Hanmer clearly valued Negus's survey and his AAAS work, characterizing these as part of the company's effort to create a "friendly atmosphere" for reporting on the papers of Haag and Larson. Negus continued to work as the AAAS's principal press liaison throughout the 1950s, during which time he also served as public information officer for the Federation of American Societies for Experimental Biology. As late as 1961 he was still contacting science writers to make sure they covered Hanmer and Haag's (deeply flawed) efforts to exonerate tobacco from the charge of causing lung cancer. Negus's work as an agent for the American Tobacco Company was rarely mentioned in press reports on his work.[30]

Professor Negus was an important figure for American Tobacco, but dozens of other members of the MCV's faculty ended up working for the industry giant. Haag in 1939 had been appointed to head the "Medical Division" of the company's research laboratory at its new location in Richmond, where he helped organize research for the firm, including Egon Lorenz's inhalation studies. Haag also helped introduce other MCV faculty to the company, many of whom ended up on its payroll. Larson was his most significant recruit (in 1941), but there were many others—Herbert McKennis, for example, who did nicotine metabolism work for the company from 1956 through the late 1970s and benefited from the largesse of the Tobacco Industry Research Committee (via Paul Larson as principal investigator). Haag and Larson also served as expert witnesses for the industry in court and at hearings organized by the Federal Trade Commission, and in at least one case briefed American Tobacco on witness tampering in tobacco litigation (the wife of a plaintiff's attorney seems to have contacted jurors to ask about their smoking habits). Haag and Larson were very much the eyes and ears of the cigarette industry in academia.[31]

THE ISOTOPE FARM

Another interesting aspect of the American Tobacco–MCV collaboration is the 1955 establishment of a C 14 labeling facility ("Isotope Farm" was Willard Libby's name for it) at the college to trace the movement of radioactive isotopes throughout the body. The industry by this time was scrambling to determine precisely what in tobacco smoke was causing all this cancer, and the hope was that radioisotope tracers might provide a clue. In 1954 the American Tobacco Company pledged $120,000 for the construction of a "Radiological Nutriculture Laboratory" on top of McGuire Hall Annex on the MCV campus, with the hope that by growing tobacco plants in an atmosphere of radio-labeled carbon dioxide one could find out how (and how fast) various constituents of smoke moved through the body. American Tobacco's Edward Harlow traveled to Argonne National Laboratory in August of 1955 to explore how the Atomic Energy Commission had set up its laboratory, the only other such greenhouse in the country. Larson and Haag were consulted at each stage of the project, including how to spin publicity, but American was always pulling the strings.[32]

MCV's Nutriculture Laboratory was not American Tobacco's first venture into nuclear studies. In 1949 the company had begun a five-year sponsorship of the University of Chicago's Institute of Radiobiology and Biophysics, creating radio-tagged isotopes for use in nicotine studies launched in 1951. By 1953 radioactive sodium 24, potassium 42, iodine 131, and arsenic 76 had all been used in tobacco tracer experiments. Three years later, in 1956, American Tobacco upped its nuclear ante by collaborating with several other firms to erect a five-megawatt nuclear reactor on a three-hundred-acre tract near Plainsboro, New Jersey, at a cost of $4 million. I don't think it's widely known that the world's largest tobacco company helped build a New Jersey nuclear reactor, but for more than a decade Industrial Reactor Laboratories, Inc., was used to prepare isotopes for clandestine tobacco research, including studies of polonium 210, one of the principal suspect carcinogens in cigarette smoke. Measurements completed in 1969—as part of the company's secret Project PTT-A-68-A—found that neither charcoal nor resin filters did much to remove the radioisotope from cigarette smoke.[33]

INNOCENCE BY ASSOCIATION

The aging Hiram Hanmer in 1964 looked back on his company's relationship with the Medical College of Virginia, asking, "What value are these grants and consultantships?" In his long letter to American Tobacco vice president Robert Heimann written shortly before his retirement, Hanmer noted that "Twenty years ago they were invaluable. In those days we needed a friendly climate where research in a little known field could be done. . . . We needed friends in court, and both Harvey [Haag] and Paul [Larson] went all out in testimony before the FTC." Hanmer was often skeptical of academics, but here he was clearly proud of his MCV helpers: Haag' and Larson were "old acquaintances," their positions on tobacco and health were "understood," and both men had "demonstrated loyalty."[34]

Hanmer's recollection is consistent with American Tobacco's earlier assessments of the value of MCV's help, especially via the Division of Collaborative Medical Research directed by Haag, whose ostensible purpose was to determine "the physiological effect of the usage of tobacco." An American Tobacco report from 1941 minced no words about the utility of Haag's division, housed inside the company's Research Laboratory in Richmond: "This work and the information gathered is certainly very valuable and without doubt disproves the common belief that smoking causes so many ill effects upon health."[35]

One interesting aspect of the American Tobacco–MCV collaboration is that the corporate research personnel were generally not allowed to publish with Haag and Larson, even when they had contributed substantially to the project in question. Hanmer in 1949 proposed to the company's vice president, Preston L. Fowler, this possibility of joint publication, but his letter of request has a large "NO" penciled in at the bottom, presumably by Fowler. Restrictions of this sort seem to have led to a certain disappointment or even jealousy in the ranks of tobacco research scientists, denied the glory of authorial immortality. Industry scientists are known to have asked their superiors for "a more liberal policy on publication." Haag and Larson were building up long résumés on the industry's dime, while people like Harlow were getting little or no publication credit. Industry scientists seem to have been caught between a desire to publish and the code of silence required by their employers. Larson et al. were allowed to talk about nicotine's value as a "tranquilizer"— but money also bought a lot of silence, which caused a certain amount of irritation in industry research circles.[36]

Fortunately from the industry's point of view, there were always plenty of scientists willing to take their money. One remarkable feature of this time (1940s and 1950s) is how easy it was for tobacco manufacturers to find academics willing to collaborate. Every company had its allies: American Tobacco had the Medical College of Virginia (Haag and Larson et al.) but also developed close relations with Duke University, the University of North Carolina, the University of Texas Medical School at Galveston, and New York University and Sloan-Kettering. Lorillard in 1946 contracted with Ohio State to have a cigarette smoking machine constructed and with NYU to study the skin temperature drop of Kent smokers. Liggett & Myers employed the Arthur D. Little Corporation to identify carcinogens in cigarette smoke. Reynolds in the 1940s established a Tobacco Research Laboratory at the Bowman Gray School of Medicine in Winston-Salem (part of Wake Forest), where research activities included measurements of nicotine in breast milk, the impact of nicotine on heart disease, and studies using radioactive tracers. And Philip Morris funded Columbia University pharmacologists Michael Mulinos and Frederick Flinn to claim that diethylene glycol made Philip Morris cigarettes "less irritating." This is only a tiny sampling from the universe of tobacco–academic collaborations, which would grow exponentially over subsequent decades.[37] (See chapter 23.)

Many of these early consultants/collaborators were highly paid. Morris Fishbein received $50,000 from Lorillard in 1954 for providing a number of services, including writing articles for the company, helping to organize research (at the Hektoen Institute, for example), and helping to place ads for Kent cigarettes and articles boosting Lorillard cigarettes in medical magazines. Fishbein was also handsomely paid to produce a book for the company "on the medical aspects of tobacco"; his completed manuscript was submitted to Blakiston Press in the summer of 1954, but the book never saw the light of day, probably because it drove a bit too close to the truth. He did help to have a number of articles published on the topic, including cigarette-friendly pieces in *Good Housekeeping* and *Reader's Digest,* but his readers were never told they were reading research contracted by the tobacco industry. Fishbein earlier (in the 1930s) had helped defend Philip Morris's use of diethylene glycol as a humectant, following the bad press from the sulfanilamide poisonings. Fishbein supported the advertising of cigarettes in *JAMA,* a practice not brought to an end until January 1954. Fishbein was in fact forced to resign as editor, in large part for his refusal to give up cigarette advertising in the journal. The man had already made many enemies, chiefly through his strong-armed opposition to any kind of socialized medicine.[38]

Outsourcing allowed the industry to respond to critics with a certain scientific authority. So when experiments showed that tars rubbed on the backs of experimental mice produced cancers, scholars could be found willing to object that the tars were not prepared using the most up-to-date equipment, or the sample sizes weren't large enough, or the smoke or tars used were "stale" rather than "fresh," and so forth. The industry also used outsourcing to acquire a kind of *innocence by association:* how could we be so bad if we are working with Harvard, Stanford, or the University of California? The industry could also hide, or release in a selective manner, the fact that it was footing the bill for such research, which gave it a certain discretionary power over what kind of science saw the light of day. Industry executives throughout the period of conspicuous conspiracy (1954–2000) frequently remarked on the value of hiding the corporate origins of "friendly research"—which paid off when people like Harvey Haag were treated as neutral experts by consumer organizations looking for the truth about tobacco.[39] Outsourcing allowed "independent scholars" to do the unpleasant work of exculpation: Lorillard's 1954 tally of outsourced research, for example, included payments to David N. Kendall, a consulting chemist in Plainfield, New Jersey, to support his work "attempting to prove the absence of harmful [asbestos] fibers in Kent smoke"; an Ernest F. Fullam of Schenectady was likewise being paid to "confirm the absence of any harmful fibers in Kent smoke."[40] Innocence in at least some such efforts was a foregone conclusion.

Strategies of this sort were in wide use by the 1950s. So when the American Tobacco Company provided $50,000 in research funds to Duke University in 1951, this was channeled through the Damon Runyon Fund to disguise its industry origins.[41] Duke was spared the taint of taking tobacco money, and whatever came of the research could be traced only to the Damon Runyon Fund.

A SALUBRIOUS SITUATION

MCV faculty continued to work for the industry throughout the 1950s, 1960s, and 1970s, and with new kinds of formal ties. In the 1950s, for example, the American Tobacco Company took the remarkable step of having a number of its researchers obtain university appointments at the college. Edward S. Harlow was appointed a research associate in pharmacology in 1952, as were P. M. Pederson and William K. Stephens Jr. Lovell J. Dewey, another company employee, was appointed a research associate in biochemistry. The initiative here seems to have come from American Tobacco, but the university was a full and willing partner. One typical pattern was for the MCV to make an academic appointment, whom American Tobacco would then hire onto its staff (or employ as a consultant). This cozy relationship meant that it was sometimes hard even to say where the company left off and the college began. William Stepka, for example, published articles listing himself as a "research plant physiologist for the American Tobacco Company and an assistant professor at the Medical College of Virginia."[42] The tobacco company shaped many of the research priorities of MCV's scientific staff, as the exchange of personnel between the two organizations came to be virtually seamless.[43] Biological work for American Tobacco's New Products Division was carried out almost entirely on the MCV campus, and scholars such as John L. Egle Jr. and Arthur W. Burke Jr.—both with joint appointments at both institutions—did research on aldehyde retention and carbon monoxide metabolism, springing from worries about cigarette-caused ciliastasis and cardiovascular impairment. Some of these joint appointees had limited academic credentials. Edward Harlow, American Tobacco's assistant director of research, had only a B.S. degree. Others, like Arthur W. Burke, "Coordinator of Biological Research" for American Tobacco at the MCV, had both an M.D. and a Ph.D. Ties of this sort kept the industry abreast of ongoing events of interest: when the patholo-gist Oscar Auerbach in 1970 lectured at the college on "Pulmonary Changes Fol-lowing Cigarette Smoking," a summary of his talk and discussions thereafter quickly made its way into American Tobacco's files.[44]

Over time, the American Tobacco Company increased its annual payouts to the college. The base-rate contribution (apart from special construction projects) rose from $5,000 per year in the 1940s to $20,000 per year in the 1950s and $27,000 in the 1960s, by which time the tobacco giant was financing many of the faculty and staff in MCV's Department of Pharmacology: Larson and Haag of course but also McKennis, Egle, Burke, and a number of others, not to mention American To-bacco's own employees working in one capacity or another at the college (Peder-son, Stephens, Dewey, etc.). Many others were working as consultants for the to-bacco giant. The arrangement was a cushy one: little effort seems to have been spent on *applying* for this money; the checks just kept rolling in, year after year, with the occasional extra sum to finance a new building or some special tobacco-tinged project. MCV's longtime president, William T. Sanger (1925–56), was deeply appreciative, as was his successor, R. Blackwell Smith Jr. (1956–68). President Smith in 1957 thanked Hanmer for his most recent $20,000 check: "I do not know of any relationship which has meant more to us across the years." Smith returned the fa-vor by reappointing senior American Tobacco research staff to his faculty year after year into the late 1960s while also allowing the company to assist with vetting new hires for the college. MCV faculty also participated in high-level legal discussions at American—on how best to keep the company in "a salubrious situation with re-spect to legal position on the matter of 'smoking and health.'" MCV faculty often helped the company with legal consultations and provided expertise in legal or reg-ulatory hearings. The most common contact involved consulting, as when William T. Ham from the biophysics department helped the company with radioactivity in cigarettes, or Kenneth S. Rogers from biochemistry ran gel chromatography sam-ples (to determine molecular weights) for the company. College personnel occa-sionally met with foreign manufacturers, as on March 10, 1967, when Gallaher's chief chemist traveled to the college with a crew from Britain's Tobacco Research Council to find out whether Larson knew of any "evidence that would establish nico-tine as detrimental to the health of smokers."[45]

MCV's tobacco ties were transformed somewhat after 1968, when the Medical College of Virginia became the Health Sciences Division of the newly formed Vir-ginia Commonwealth University. There is no further record of Harlow et al. con-tinuing as research associates—suggesting that higher-ups in the university must have realized it was odd, even in Richmond, to have senior tobacco executives as faculty in a medical school. Daniel T. Watts, dean of VCU's new School of Graduate Studies, asked American Tobacco to donate its former Research Laboratory to the university, confiding that even as "a newcomer to Richmond" he was nonetheless convinced of nicotine's eminence as "the most effective and safest mild [central nervous system] stimulant known to man." MCV's pharmacology department by this time was getting nearly $200,000 per year from the tobacco industry, including direct grants from American but also monies from the Council for Tobacco Research and the American Medical Association's Education and Research Foundation (AMA-ERF), a $10 million hush fund financed by cigarette manufacturers as part of a deal struck (in 1964) with the AMA to help stave off Medicare. (From the AMA, the industry got more than a decade of benign neglect.) Much of this was still "friendly research": when Marvin A. Friedman from the pharmacology department applied for funding from the Council for Tobacco Research in 1974, he proposed that the nitrogen dioxide component of sidestream cigarette smoke "will protect people from the carcinogenic effects of food contaminants and smoke components."[46]

Tobacco manufacturers cannot have been too happy, though, when Jesse L. Steinfeld was appointed professor of medicine and dean of the Medical College in 1976. As Surgeon General under Nixon (1969–73) Steinfeld had proposed a "nonsmokers' bill of rights," earning him the label of the industry's "Public enemy number one," but the man was hardly a radical. At a 1977 news conference he was upbeat about how people were smoking "primarily filter cigarettes now"; he also drew hope from falling tar and nicotine deliveries and from the fact that even though per capita consumption had not fallen much "the cigarettes that people are smoking are less hazardous."[47] (A big mistake, as we shall see.)

Steinfeld actually seems to have done little to stop the industry's collaboration with the college. One thing that did change, though, was the suite of companies providing the funding. American Tobacco had lost its place as the nation's leading manufacturer (already in the 1950s), and other companies had started courting the MCV. Philip Morris began financing research on campus, for example, including a series of experiments in which VCU students were used as subjects (electric shocks were administered to study smoking as a response to anxiety). "Smoker Psychology" had become of particular interest to the company, which also funded MCV work on the extent to which smokers adjust their smoking intensity to fit some accustomed level of nicotine intake—also known as "compensation" or "self-titration." Cary Suter from MCV's Department of Neurology worked with Philip Morris to set up a "psychophysiological research laboratory," and Paul Larson, Herbert McKennis, John A. Rosecrans, and a number of others continued to take CTR money. Brown & Williamson in 1983 provided the university with a $15,000 gift to fund John A. DeSimone's work on taste electrophysiology and chemosensory reception, and the Tobacco Institute shortly thereafter paid Professor S. James Kilpatrick from MCV's Department of Biostatistics to develop a database to help the industry chart progress in research on the health effects of secondhand smoke. Kilpatrick in 1988 also applied for and obtained grant monies from the industry's Center for Indoor Air Research to show, as the title of his proposal announced, that "The Association in the Hirayama Study between ETS and Lung Cancer Is Not Significant."[48] Hirayama's was the first major study to link secondhand smoke with lung cancer— the association found *was* significant—and the industry would invest massive efforts in trying to discredit him and his work.

MCV faculty also helped the companies with specific marketing projects. MCV scientists in the 1990s helped Philip Morris evaluate its smokeless Accord cigarette, for example, prompting news reports with glowing headlines like "Accord Device Cuts Nicotine, Eliminates Poison." MCV faculty also helped undermine public health advocacy: in 1990 James Kilpatrick from biostatistics, working also as a consultant for the Tobacco Institute, wrote to the editor of the *New York Times* criticizing Stanton Glantz and William Parmley's demonstration of thirty-five thousand U.S. cardiovascular deaths per annum from exposure to secondhand smoke.[49] Glantz by this time was commonly ridiculed by the industry, which even organized skits (to practice courtroom scenarios) in which health advocates were given thinly disguised names: Glantz was "Ata Glance" or "Stanton Glass, professional anti-smoker"; Alan Blum was "Alan Glum" representing "Doctors Ought to Kvetch" or "Doctors Opposed to People Exhaling Smoke" (DOPES); Richard Daynard was "Richard Blowhard" from the "Product Liability Education Alliance," and so forth.[50] VCU continues even today to have close research relationships with Philip Morris, covering topics as diverse as pharmacogenomics, bioinformatics, and behavioral genetics.[51]

SYMBIOSIS

It would be a mistake to characterize this interpenetration of tobacco and academia as merely a "conflict of interest"; the relationship has been far more symbiotic. We are really talking about a *confluence* of interests, and sometimes even a virtual *identity of interests*. The Medical College of Virginia was "sold American" by the early 1940s and remained one of the tobacco industry's staunchest allies for seven decades. The college's pharmacology department for most of these years functioned essentially as an outpost of the American Tobacco Company, providing expertise and apologies for the world's largest manufacturer of cigarettes. This collaboration was so deep, and so all-encompassing, that it is sometimes hard even to find a clear line dividing the work of the college from the business of defending cigarettes.

At the peak of this collaboration in the 1940s and 1950s, MCV published a newsletter, titled *Medicovan,* with a masthead promising: "To Preserve and Restore Health, to Seek the Cause and Cure of Diseases, to Educate Those Who Would Serve Humanity." Noble virtues that have long inspired the honest study and practice of medicine, but here in this dark chapter of history little more than smoke blowing in the wind.

12

A Most Feared Document

Claude E. Teague's 1953 "Survey of Cancer Research"

Certain scientists and medical authorities have claimed for many years that the use of tobacco contributes to cancer development in susceptible people. Just enough evidence has been presented to justify the possibility of such a presumption.

HARRIS PARMELE, DIRECTOR OF RESEARCH, LORILLARD TOBACCO, 1946

Most American tobacco trials in recent years have pivoted around two questions: How early did the tobacco industry know that its products were killing people? And how much did ordinary smokers know about the hazards of their habit?

The two questions are interestingly opposite in their legal implications, since the industry ideally wants us to believe that while popular knowledge of tobacco's hazards goes back centuries, scientific knowledge has emerged only rather recently. The distinction between popular and scientific knowledge has become a cornerstone of the industry's defense, with the point being that smokers must shoulder the blame for whatever maladies they have suffered. "Everyone knew" means that people only have themselves to blame (for smoking), while the "absence of proof" means that the companies acted responsibly in refusing to acknowledge hazards. Everyone knew, but no one had proof. Defense experts testify either to long-standing "common knowledge" or to a very late "state of the art." Historians have been brought in to testify to both prongs of this fork, which in many respects is an industry construct.

Cigarette makers have used other arguments in their defense, however. Prominent among these has been the claim that while statistical evidence is always suspect, experimental evidence is more solid. The conjoining argument is that the "case" against tobacco in the 1950s or even later was based on little more than *statistics* and that a higher standard of proof was needed. "Higher standard" usually meant experimental proof: you force animals to smoke, or rub tobacco tars into their skins, and see if they get cancer. The companies put forward this argument in the 1950s to dismiss evidence of hazards; they put forth similar arguments today to exculpate their actions in legal retrospect. Laboratory evidence, we are told, is the "gold standard" of causation, which is why the companies were right to question the epidemiology and prudent in their reluctance to acknowledge proof. The claim is sometimes even made that it would have been *irresponsible* to warn before all the evidence was in. Experiments also offered a certain plausible deniability, given that they are generally speaking *idealizations*. The argument could therefore always be made that any given demonstration was "unrealistic" by virtue of being on the wrong animal, at the wrong dose, via the wrong route of exposure, using the wrong substance. These were common industry refrains in the 1950s, 1960s, and 1970s and reappear even today in efforts to re-spin the history of tobacco science. The lawyers responsible for helping Claude Teague prepare for his 1990 deposition had something like this in mind when they stressed that his use of terms such as *carcinogen* be "put in context (species, dose, time, tissue)." Exculpation via contextualization, a common industry defense against embarrassing documents.[1]

Recognizing this premium on laboratory experimentation helps us understand the industry's strong reaction to Wynder, Graham, and Croninger's paper showing that tars extracted from tobacco smoke could induce cancers when painted on the skins of mice.[2] The article was published in the December 1953 issue of *Cancer Research* and became a key stimulus in the industry's decision to launch a public relations campaign to exonerate tobacco from the charge of causing cancer.

The story is actually more complicated, however, since there wasn't much new in Wynder et al.'s article that the companies didn't already know. Wynder had been presenting his results for more than a year with a certain measure of press coverage: an abstract of his experimental work was delivered in April of 1953 at the annual meeting of the American Association for Cancer Research,[3] for example, and preliminary results had been revealed even earlier—in November of 1952—in a paper he had presented at the National Academy of Sciences in Washington, D.C., titled "Cigarette Smoking and Cancer of the Lung." Wynder here announced that "in cases of cancer of the lung there is almost always a history of excessive cigarette smoking"—but also that he had recently obtained "direct evidence that tar obtained from cigarette smoke will produce cancer experimentally when painted on the skin of mice." Cigarette makers were paying close attention: shortly after his 1952 presentation, the American Tobacco Company received a copy of Wynder's paper from Dr. E. E. Clayton, a pathologist at the USDA's Tobacco Division, along with a "confidential copy" of a letter from Wynder to Cornelius Rhoads explaining Wynder's plans to publish his data.[4]

By the end of 1952, then, the world's largest tobacco company knew what was coming. How did they respond? The hiring of Hill & Knowlton and the formation of the TIRC and publication of the "Frank Statement" are well known—and we shall explore these, too, in a moment—but there are earlier reactions that warrant an accounting. The one I want to talk about first is a document prepared by a young R. J. Reynolds chemist, Claude E. Teague Jr., shortly after Wynder's November 1952 speech and a good nine months prior to his explosive publication in *Cancer Research*. Teague's "Survey of Cancer Research," dated February 2, 1953, is the most comprehensive summary of experimental tobacco cancer research prior to Wynder's; it was never published, however, and would surface only in legal proceedings in the 1990s, where it was introduced as evidence of the industry's early knowledge of the reality of tobacco hazards. And for good reason.

A GROWING SUSPICION

Claude Teague earned his Ph.D. in chemistry in 1950 from the University of North Carolina, where he graduated with a dissertation on heterocyclic fluorine/nitrogen compounds. Two years later, following a brief stint at American Viscose (then a rayon plant and now an EPA Superfund site), he landed a job as a bench chemist with Reynolds, where he was put to work synthesizing Turkish tobacco flavors. This was a time of growing concerns about harms from smoking, and Reynolds had been expanding its R&D capacity to deal with the new threat. As a 1990 industry document put it, the expansion transformed Reynolds's research headquarters from "what was essentially a flavoring laboratory to a full scale research organization." Industry officials were worried about the publicity being given to the growing flood of epidemiological studies, but they also knew that papers based on sophisticated experimental methods were in the works. Roy Norr in his widely read 1952 *Reader's Digest* provocation, "Cancer by the Carton," had cited Wynder and Graham's 1950 conclusion that smoking was "an important factor" in the induction of bronchiogenic carcinoma; publicity was also being given to Alton Ochsner's prediction of a "frightening" number of lung cancers in store for Americans in consequence of the rapid growth of tobacco use. It was in this context that Teague was asked to prepare a review of the cancer–cigarette question for the company.[5]

Teague's "Survey of Cancer Research" presents a state-of-the-art review of experimental tobacco/cancer research. The document is broad in scope, covering experiments from Anton Brosch's in 1900 through Angel H. Roffo's in the 1930s and 1940s. Teague's reason for writing was simple: "Because of the possible connection between tobacco smoking and cancer of the respiratory system it is well for manufacturers of tobacco products to be aware of past and present cancer research." And the picture he paints is not a pretty one.

> The recent rate of increase of cancer of the respiratory system rather closely parallels the recent introduction and rate of increase of cigarette consumption, and this, together with the fact that until very recently the vast majority of cigarette smokers have been men, has raised a very considerable question. There appears to be a growing sus-

picion, or even acceptance, among medical men and cancer researchers that the parallel increase in cigarette consumption and incidence of cancer of the respiratory system is more than coincidence.[6]

One of the novelties of Teague's survey was his detailed discussion of the carcinogenic compounds found in tars of various sorts. He reports at length on efforts by Geoffrey M. Badger, an Australian organic chemist at the University of Glasgow, to characterize how different chemical structures might be more or less likely to cause cancer. Badger thought that most of the most "active" (i.e., carcinogenic) polycyclic hydrocarbons seemed to be derivatives of phenanthrene; he also thought that the introduction of methyl groups into benzanthracene and benzphenanthrene and chrysene led to increased cancer activity, that alkyl groups other than methyl were progressively less active as the number of carbon atoms in the chain increased, and so forth. Teague pointed out that it was "reasonable to suppose that with increased data and study will come a more precise understanding" of how cancer-causing potencies change with changes in chemical structure.[7]

Teague reviewed a number of population studies conceding the reality of the increase in cancer of the lung, noting in addition that "many writers" (fourteen references are cited) had concluded that "smoking, and [in] particular cigarette smoking, may be a causative factor in the induction of cancer of the respiratory system." Wynder and Graham's famous 1950 paper is summarized, including their conclusion that "excessive and prolonged use of tobacco, especially cigarettes, seems to be an important factor in the induction of lung cancer." Teague faithfully recites their grim observations: the incidence of lung cancer was "considerably higher" among heavy smokers compared to the general hospital population; 94 percent of male patients with tumors in their lungs were cigarette smokers; lung cancer was rare in nonsmokers; the growing practice of inhalation was probably a factor in the increased incidence of the disease; there could be a time lag of ten years or more between cessation of smoking and first clinical symptoms; and several independent studies had confirmed these results with a uniformity indicating strength in the link. Teague also recorded his expectation that the American Cancer Society's ongoing multi-year prospective study (by E. Cuyler Hammond and Daniel Horn) would "firmly establish or disprove the relation between tobacco smoking and cancer of the respiratory system." And so it did: Hammond by October of 1954 was able to conclude that the case for smoking causing lung cancer had been proved "beyond a reasonable doubt."[8]

Teague then turned to animal tests, summarizing twenty-eight separate studies from 1900 through 1942. Many of these had appeared in publications "not readily available," requiring him to consult abstracts or secondary references. Teague notes certain deficiencies in this literature: some of the methods are poorly described, and some studies don't reveal the precise nature or source of the substances tested or what doses were used or how tumors were classified. He does, however, produce a table of the results, listing the type of tobacco extract used, how it was applied and for how long, and the kinds of cancers produced. His conclusion: the results of these tests, though not always definitive in any given study, "would seem to indicate the presence of carcinogens."[9]

Teague's "Survey of Cancer Research" is important in a number of different respects. It is one of the broadest reviews of tobacco–cancer research up to that time, covering research from twenty-two scientists in seven countries. His conclusion is also remarkable, coming as it does from the research department of a major tobacco company and echoing the language of Wynder and Graham: "The closely parallel increase in cigarette smoking has led to the suspicion that tobacco smoking is an important etiologic factor in the induction of primary cancer of the lung. Studies of clinical data tend to confirm the relationship between heavy and prolonged tobacco smoking and incidence of cancer of the lung." Teague also concluded that animal experiments had indicated the "probable presence of carcinogenic agents" in tobacco, though more work was needed to confirm this. He ended his review with a series of recommendations, among them that his survey be supplemented by "complete, detailed surveys of the individual topics covered above"; that the industry assemble files on pertinent literature; that "all tobacco additives, i.e. flavorants and humectants, used by this company be examined carefully with respect to their possible roles as carcinogens or carcinogen producing agents"; and that "management take cognizance of the problem and its implications to our industry, and that positive research action be planned and initiated without delay."[10]

BRILLIANT CAREER

Teague's unpublished "Survey of Cancer Research" displays a far deeper appreciation of the tobacco–cancer link than what the industry was admitting to the outside world. In April of 1954 the Tobacco Industry Research Committee published its first "white paper," titled *A Scientific Perspective on the Cigarette Controversy,* citing only William McNally's study from 1932 to claim that "only one tumor has been obtained in the course of subjecting a large number of mice to the action of tobacco tar, compared with the very high incidence of cancer in mice treated with coal tar." Tobacco was therefore "relatively unimportant in the causation of cancer." Apart from the "one tumor" found by McNally, none of the thirty-odd other studies reviewed by Teague are mentioned—not even the Wynder, Graham, and Croninger paper of December 1953 that had caused the industry so much grief.

(The TIRC's *Scientific Perspective,* I should note, was distributed widely: 176,800 copies were mailed to doctors, with another 15,000 going to members of the press and thousands more to deans of medical schools, radio and TV commentators, members of Congress, and other opinion makers. Press reports on the paper cited

"authorities from the Damon Runyon Fund" as "refusing to accept as a fact any relationship between smoking and lung cancer," with no mention of the fact that the
Fund was receiving massive support from the tobacco industry, as we shall see in
a moment.)[11]

Given its sophistication, the tobacco industry likes to trivialize Teague's "Survey." In one of his trial depositions from the late 1990s Teague claimed not even to
remember having prepared the document, recalling only that he had probably
turned it over to Murray Senkus, director of chemical research at Reynolds and his
immediate supervisor. The industry's official line has been that the survey was a
kind of private musing; the paper was just a "review of the literature" and emphat-
ically *not* a piece of original research.

Privately, though, the cigarette makers' lawyers have conceded that Teague's was
"the first comprehensive discussion of smoking and health to be prepared by an
RJRT scientist that was reviewed by at least some in upper management." Since the
review was prepared at the request of the company's director of research, Kenneth
H. Hoover, it would seem reasonable to assume that he, too, must have seen it.
Teague himself in an interview of May 3, 1985, recalled his paper also being seen
by John C. Whitaker, president and (later) chairman of the board of the company.
We also know that it "caused concern" for Henry Ramm, Reynolds's powerful general counsel. A brief by attorneys working for the company reveals that "an effort
was made by the Law Department to recall all copies." Ramm was later named chair
of the industry's powerful Policy Committee of Lawyers—also known as the Committee of Counsel or Legal Committee—a body responsible for "the high policy of
the industry on *all* smoking and health matters."[12]

And Teague himself went on to a brilliant career at Reynolds. From his original
position as research chemist, he rose to Director of Chemical Research (1959–69),
Assistant Director of Research (1970–77), and Director of Corporate Research (in
1978), before retiring in the late 1980s as Director of R&D Administration, with
responsibilities for "personnel, finance, facilities, security, report writing, planning,"
and even some agricultural research. Teague played a key role in deciphering the
chemical innovations that had led to Marlboro's success in the 1960s and 1970s—
the use of ammoniated tobacco sheet to freebase cigarette smoke, for example; he
also began Reynolds's practice of drafting long-range planning documents, pushing for the company to emulate Philip Morris in this regard. We also know something about his views regarding nicotine addiction and youth smoking. In lawyerly
circles Teague is notorious for his 1972 memo characterizing the tobacco industry
as a "specialized, highly ritualized and stylized segment of the pharmaceutical industry"; he is also known for his 1973 use of terms such as *pre-smokers* and *learners* while discussing how his company could recapture (from Marlboro) the youth
market. Teague knew that few smokers actually liked their habit and that most

wanted to quit; a 1982 memo has him declaring that "most of our customers would do without if they could," absent the disabling grip of addiction.[13]

Teague's 1953 "Survey" shows that a fair review of animal experimental evidence, intended purely for internal industry use, compiled prior even to Wynder et al.'s publication later that year, revealed strong evidence of a tobacco–cancer link. Tobacco industry officials would later deny much of what Teague had found—that tobacco contained carcinogens, that clinical studies had confirmed a causal link, and so forth. Reynolds scientists were actually proud of having found benzpyrene and nitrosamines in tobacco smoke (in 1954)—along with cholanthrene and several other polycyclic hydrocarbons—but were never allowed to publish or publicly discuss these findings. Teague himself as early as 1955 had proposed a method by which carcinogens could be eliminated from tobacco smoke, conceding "strong indications" that polynuclear hydrocarbons were "the active carcinogens." Topics such as these were always kept closely guarded within the companies. A 1971 memo from one of Reynolds's most powerful chemists noted that while company researchers were encouraged to publish on innocuous topics, papers on "polycyclic hydrocarbons, hydrogen cyanide, carbon monoxide and similar materials" were not to be submitted for publication. Alan Rodgman a decade previously had confessed that while Reynolds had done a great deal to document the existence of carcinogens in cigarette smoke, none of this had been published because it dealt with the taboo topic of "carcinogenic or cocarcinogenic compounds."[14]

AN HONEST DOUBTER?

A company man to the end, Teague always upheld the industry's line that there were "doubts" about the reality of tobacco hazards. But was he himself an honest doubter? One clue comes from an invention he conceived shortly after finishing work on his "Survey." On December 17, 1953, Teague filed a "Disclosure of Invention" with his superiors, announcing his idea for a new kind of filter tip, designed to darken artificially as a cigarette was smoked. Teague had noticed that people like to see their filters turn brown as they puff away, believing this to be "a criterion of filter efficiency." Teague therefore proposed adding chemicals to filter stuffings that would "undergo color change to a dark color, preferably brown," when exposed to smoke. Teague noted that while such a device would have "little or no effect on the actual efficiency of the filter," its advertising and sales advantages would be "obvious." Ten years later Philip Morris scientists were still claiming that "the illusion of filtration" was as important as "the fact of filtration."[15]

Illusions have always been vital for the sellers of cigarettes; this is a world where grim ends are masked by cowboys and romance and fresh mountain streams. The industry always needs to rescue its appearance, which is why such care has been taken to renarrate the tobacco past, to re-create an exculpatory history. Teague's "Survey of Cancer Research" has been subjected to a great deal of image management since its discovery in the 1990s. The document was first divulged in the discovery process for *Minnesota v. Philip Morris,* the 1997–98 case that forced millions of company documents into the open. And ever since, tobacco attorneys have had to try to explain away Teague's "Survey"—as a private musing, a review of no consequence, a one-off nothing we should not take seriously.

Teague himself was still alive when his "Survey" finally came to light, permitting lawyers for the plaintiffs to interrogate him about his text. And so for four days in July of 1997 he responded to questions about his life at Reynolds, including how and why he came to draft the document. In five hundred pages of testimony we find the seventy-two-year old Teague making claims that stretch the reader's credulity. Teague claimed not even to remember his "Survey," for example, when we know it was a key focus of his deposition preparation. The deposition reads as an exercise in professed incompetence: Teague says he drafted the document only because he had spare time on his hands; his department had moved into a new laboratory space with drainage problems, and the survey was just a make-work project to kill time. Teague calls his review unoriginal and inconsequential, and we are led to think of it as a kind of accidental scribble. Here is how he tries to make it go away, when probed by the plaintiff's attorney, Daniel A. O'Fallon:

Q: You did what you considered to be an acceptable job; right?

A: Exactly.

Q: And presumably what your supervisors considered to be an acceptable job as well; right? They advanced you to eventually become the assistant director of the research department—?

A: They maybe promoted me to my highest level of incompetency. Are you familiar with the Peter principle?

Q: In any event, you, as one of R. J. Reynolds' researchers with a Ph.D., concluded that, based on what you saw, the substances derived from tobacco had some degree of carcinogenic activity; right?

A: Well, I would—my degree was in chemistry. I have no training, zero, zip. I think I took one course in zoology in college and hated it. I'm not an expert, not even knowledgeable in biological things so me making an assessment of this stuff, you know, fairly presumptuous of me, but I was younger and I guess more brass in those days but—

Q: Did R. J. Reynolds have someone that was more qualified to do this survey?

A: I would assume surely they did.

Q: Did they have that person do such a study?

A: I wouldn't know if they had.

Q: Who was that person? Who would have been more qualified than you to do this?

A: I guess they could have gone almost anywhere and hired somebody to do a study like that.

Q: But the fact of the matter is: They didn't go somewhere, they came to you; right?

A: No. We went through—I don't know whether I went to them or they came to me. I don't think this was any big deal. It was something to occupy me while they were chiseling up and re-pouring the lab floor.

Q: You don't think that a study, a survey of the literature concerning whether or not cigarette smoking causes cancer was any big deal to R. J. Reynolds in 1953?

A: I don't know whether it was or not. I don't think it was to me.

Teague denies even having understood what he wrote when he wrote it.

Q: [citing from Teague's "Survey"]: "The closely parallel increase in cigarette smoking has led to the suspicion that tobacco smoking is an important etiological factor in the induction of primary cancer of the lung"; correct?

A: Uh-huh.

Q: Etiological factor means it causes the lung cancer; correct?

A: I was wondering what "etiological" meant. I just fished that out of somebody and I don't know what "etiology" means. What?

Q: Doesn't it mean a cause?

A: I don't know. I'm asking you. I don't know.

Q: I didn't write this document, sir. What did you mean when you wrote it?

A: I think I did a survey of stuff and if somebody had a nice conclusion, I just put it here. You know, I was not in any sense posing to be an expert to draw conclusions.

Q: Did you say that anywhere in this? Did you preface this all by saying I don't know what the hell I'm talking about?

A: No, but I wish I had.[16]

Teague's "Survey of Cancer Research" is one of the most feared documents ever faced by tobacco industry lawyers in court. They don't like it, because it shows what any right-minded judge of facts from the time should have known: cigarettes were killing people. When forced to confront this document, as they must in virtually every modern tobacco trial, the industry tries to diminish its significance and to isolate its author. They find it hard to get truth on their side, but sadly, and all too often, there are other ways to win in court.

13

"Silent Collaborators"

Clandestine Cancer Research Financed by Tobacco via the Damon Runyon Fund

Tobacco companies are like cockroaches; they spread disease and don't like the light.
STANTON GLANTZ, CIRCA 1996

Medical research was not a high priority for the tobacco industry prior to the 1950s. The publication of strong epidemiological studies in 1950 changed this, causing worries that people were going to stop smoking in consequence of fearing for their lives. All the major companies had been involved in health-related research, but the scope, scale, and urgency of such projects would dramatically increase in the 1950s. Teague's "Survey of Cancer Research" was part of this, as was American Tobacco's work with the Medical College of Virginia, but there were other projects that were even more ambitious, including some so secretive that some researchers didn't even realize they were working for Big Tobacco.

One of the most important involved a collaboration organized under the rubric of "Air Pollution Studies" conducted at New York University, the Sloan-Kettering Institute (SKI), and the Memorial Cancer Center of New York, with major funding from the American Tobacco Company and other cigarette manufacturers, channeled secretly through a foundation known as the Damon Runyon Fund. The collaboration is significant, in that it quickly became the nation's largest lung cancer research effort and the biggest to explore the possible role of tobacco. It is also significant because

a) the principal investigators—Anthony J. Lanza at NYU and Cornelius P. Rhoads at Sloan-Kettering—understood their goal as helping the tobacco industry clean up its act;

b) the tobacco industry hid its role in organizing the effort;

c) the industry—led by the American Tobacco Company—tried to control the research at every turn; and

d) despite efforts to control the research and its publication, the collaboration ended up helping to prove the tobacco–lung cancer link, though this was never publicly admitted.

Ernst Wynder was actually one of the beneficiaries, insofar as he was part of this collaboration in the period during which he was conducting his mouse-painting studies. This is one of the great untold ironies: Wynder's earthshaking research—which rattled tobacco stocks and drove a stake into the very heart of Big Tobacco—was partly funded by the world's largest tobacco manufacturer.

The collaboration is also notable in that it prefigures the kind of merger of research and public relations that would come into operation with the establishment of the Tobacco Industry Research Committee in 1954. The TIRC would be more thoroughly under the control of the industry, but that is largely the result of lessons learned from these earlier collaborations.

"AIR POLLUTION" RESEARCH

The Damon Runyon Memorial Fund for Cancer Research, Inc., was founded in 1947 as a nonprofit devoted to the fight against cancer. Its namesake was the prolific New York sportswriter and short-storyist famous for his "Broadway Stories," better known today as the Broadway hit *Guys and Dolls*. (The play opened in 1950 and ran for twelve hundred performances.) Runyon died of cancer of the throat in 1946, after a life of socializing with the likes of Al Capone, Jack Dempsey, and Babe Ruth. Following his death—quite likely from smoking; he had begun at age nine or ten and quit only when tumors in his throat made it too painful—a friend of his, Walter Winchell, a conservative gossip columnist and nationally syndicated radio announcer, took to the airwaves to call for contributions to combat cancer in Runyon's name. Buoyed by top-notch publicity and promises to keep "attacking the cancer cell from all sides," the campaign quickly gained the support of "Mr. and Mrs. America" but also of celebrities such as Milton Berle, Marlene Dietrich, Jimmy Durante, William Randolph Hearst, Joe DiMaggio, Bob Hope, and Ed Sullivan, all of whom served on the board of the Fund. By 1950 the charity had given out more than $3 million in ninety-three grants and eighty-eight fellowships to eighty-four institutions in thirty-seven states, making it one of the nation's leading supporters of cancer research. The American Cancer Society must have been green with envy.[1]

The idea for a tobacco industry collaboration (code named "Air Pollution" research) seems to have come from John H. Teeter, executive director of the Runyon Fund, who in September of 1950 sent letters to the presidents of American Tobacco, Philip Morris, R. J. Reynolds, and the other tobacco makers asking for their help to fund a broad program of cancer research.[2] Teeter enclosed clippings from the press about recent research linking tobacco and cancer, noting that it would be good to get the industry's "reaction." Hiram Hanmer at American was one of the first to react, arranging a meeting with Teeter in October of 1950. Hanmer thanked him for a clipping from a recent issue of the *Science News Letter* implicating arsenic in lung cancer causation.[3] Teeter then explained that the Runyon Fund had on file a request from NYU for a grant in the amount of $150,000 to support a long-term project on lung cancer—including $50,000 for "tooling up" and $50,000 per year for operations thereafter. Teeter realized this was an ambitious sum, given that the eleven projects currently funded by the National Cancer Institute (NCI), the American Cancer Society (ACS), and the Runyon Fund itself totaled only $96,768 altogether.[4] American Tobacco agreed to fund the collaboration—with minor contributions from the other manufacturers—provided certain conditions of confidentiality could be met. The Runyon-NYU-SKI collaboration would become the best-financed lung cancer research project in the world, albeit one with its ultimate source of funding hidden.

Hanmer had originally been looking for—and obtained—a parallel collaboration with Duke University. Duke had long-standing ties with Big Tobacco, dating from the establishment of Trinity College in 1892 with funds from Washington Duke, patriarch of the American Tobacco Company. In 1924 Washington's son, James Buchanan "Buck" Duke, had granted the college an endowment of $40 million in exchange for which it was renamed "Duke University," the world's only university still today named after a tobacco tycoon. (There are, however, scholarships, buildings, and even entire divisions within other institutions so named: the George Weissman School of Arts and Sciences at Baruch College, for example, honors a man who once, as vice president for marketing at Philip Morris, expressed his pride in having "our greatest strength in the 15–24 age group.")[5] American Tobacco developed close ties with several Duke scholars, including Paul M. Gross and Marcus E. Hobbs from the chemistry department, both of whom had earlier worked with Liggett to identify the chemical constituents of tobacco smoke.

Duke University officials in the 1950s were initially reluctant to accept Runyon funds, worrying about potential negative publicity from the tobacco taint (pro or con) and infringements on academic freedom. American Tobacco made it clear from the outset, however, that they did not want *any* of their Runyon-funneled funds publicized. Duke administrators were agreeable; indeed they themselves wanted to make "doubly sure" no publicity would come from any such collaboration. The fear seems to have been that the tobacco association might pop up on Walter Winchell's popular radio show. Winchell reported regularly on cancer research, and American Tobacco had to strike special deals with Teeter, Duke, and NYU to make sure these new collaborations would be kept under wraps. Teeter told Hanmer that the Runyon Fund was happy to provide however much or little publicity a donor wanted; he also agreed that the research could be limited to study of the "chemical and physical properties" of tobacco smoke, avoiding the third rail of smoking and health. Hanmer transmitted to his superiors his belief that limiting the project in this manner (and avoiding publicity) "would remove any fear of linking Duke University or the tobacco industry with cancer or any possible damaging effect of tobacco on health."[6] NYU, with feisty young Ernst Wynder on staff, would prove somewhat harder to control.

Even with "Air Pollution" as the nominal rubric of the collaboration, and even though the tobacco focus (and backing) was deliberately hidden, the cigarette sponsors were still not entirely pleased with the nomenclature used to characterize the collaboration. Hanmer told Teeter that American Tobacco "had been avoiding the use of the word 'pollution' because of its unsavory implications" and would prefer the phrase "air-borne materials." Teeter assured him that such hot-button words could be avoided—though project terminology did continue to slip around a bit. Lanza at NYU talked about "inhalation cancer," while Paul Gross at Duke liked the more neutral term *aerosols*. And Teeter in correspondence with Philip Morris talked about research into "airborne infection." Hanmer was pleased with the project's overall tenor, however, especially its sheltering of tobacco. Tobacco would be studied but only as "an extremely small" part of the whole, allowing the "spotlight" to be taken off tobacco. Hanmer confided to his superiors:

> I have gotten the impression that they [esp. Teeter] are trying to make this project as broad as possible and are almost as desirous as we are of getting the spotlight off tobacco, feeling that this is an extremely small phase of studies which involve traces of a great variety of metals, organic chemicals, automobile exhaust gases, and anything else which gets into the air in the form of fine particles or traces, mainly from industry plants throughout the country.[7]

Hanmer was happy to hear that Runyon was willing to keep the industry's role quiet (Teeter would "adapt himself to our convenience") but also seemed pleased that research at NYU and elsewhere (he mentions the Trudeau Foundation and Notre Dame) was "far removed from the clinical phase."

FALSE HOPES FOR A QUICK FIX

By 1952 the collaboration was under way. American Tobacco had given $100,000 to the Runyon Fund, Ecusta Paper had given $15,000, and the other tobacco companies had coughed up $10,000 or less. The first industry money came to Runyon in 1951, and by 1953 the American Tobacco Company had contributed three annual gifts of $50,000 each.

The two key scholars in the New York phase were Cornelius P. Rhoads, director of the Sloan-Kettering Institute, and Anthony J. Lanza, director of NYU's Institute for Industrial Medicine. Lanza already had a long record of assisting the world's

most powerful chemical, petroleum, lead, and asbestos companies with their cancer quandaries, with the point in each case being to minimize or deny such hazards. Teeter talked a lot about "cross-fertilization" between the industry's expertise
and academics supported by the Fund, but Lanza and Rhoads were also eager to
help tobacco solve its public relations predicament. Rhoads bragged to Hanmer
about how effectively Lanza had dealt with "the petroleum industry problem," and
the hope was clearly that NYU could do for tobacco what it had earlier done for
Big Oil and Big Chemicals: help restore confidence in the industry and its products. Rhoads also hoped—and apparently believed—that whatever in tobacco
smoke was causing all this cancer could be neutralized, removed, or filtered out,
rendering cigarettes safe.[8]

Rhoads's optimism is easy for us to belittle as 1950s naïveté, and it is true that
many scholars at this time had simplistic views of disease causation. Diseases were
often imagined as having single causes, and magic bullets were sought that would
either eliminate the causal agent or cure the disease once caused. Malaria had succumbed to quinine and scurvy to provisions of lime juice—so why not a miracle
cure for lung cancer? Penicillin was the most recent wonder drug, and time enough
had not yet passed for resistant strains of bacteria to spoil the euphoria. Chronic
disease was just beginning to surpass infection as the dominant disease pattern, but
diseases caused by long-term chronic exposures were still novelties for many
people. Hopes were therefore high that cancer, too, might fall to a magic bullet: an
Australian newspaper in 1954 announced that "Every Country is Looking for a
Single Chemical to Smash the Disease."

Also important to realize, though, is that tobacco industry researchers already
regarded the idea of a penicillin-like therapy for cancer or a cleansing of carcinogens from tobacco as naive. Hiram Hanmer in November 1953 ridiculed Rhoads's
"false hopes" for a quick fix: "He [Rhoads] knows nothing about tobacco technology, nor the difficulties that might be involved in 'neutralizing, removing, or filtering out' the mouse carcinogens said to be present in cigarette smoke." Hanmer
also noted that "the therapeutic chemical agent which he [Rhoads] hopes to find is
referred to somewhat derisively as 'Rhoads' cancer penicillin.'"[9] Cancer prevention
was part of neither man's mind-set—neither Lanza nor Rhoads; Hanmer is more
inscrutable. Rhoads also thought that medical technology was progressing so fast
that cancer would soon be cured anyway. So it didn't much matter whether you ever
found a way to prevent it.

TIGHT SECURITY

Collaborating in the American Tobacco–Runyon Fund "air pollution" project were
a number of scientists working under Rhoads and Lanza. Norton Nelson, director
of research at NYU's Institute of Industrial Medicine, was a member of the team,

as was William E. Smith, professor of medicine at NYU and an expert in the realm of carcinogenic bioassays. Others involved in the project conducted animal experiments of various sorts (tobacco tar painting, for example), identified tobacco constituents, or used radioactive tracers to study nicotine metabolism. The NYU organic chemist Alvin I. Kosak studied the chemical composition of tobacco smoke and Sid Laskin, a physicist with expertise in pharmacology and instrumentation, organized C 14 tracer projects to study nicotine metabolism. Kanematsu Sugiura and Ernst Wynder were involved in animal experiments, reporting to Nelson. It is one of those interesting ironies of history that Wynder's famous demonstration of the carcinogenicity of tobacco tars (with Graham and Croninger) was part of this larger, industry-financed project. No one seems to have noticed this link; Wynder's subsequent funding from Philip Morris (in the 1960s and 1970s, to the tune of several million dollars) has been well documented, but his earlier dependence on cigarette money has escaped notice. When Wynder published his influential mouse-painting experiments he was a resident in medicine at the Memorial Cancer Center "collaborating on the N.Y.U. investigations"; the tobacco source of the funds was so carefully hidden, however, that Wynder may not even have known the industry was funding his work.[10]

The secrecy surrounding this collaboration was always a matter of concern. On February 26, 1953, Hanmer reported to his superiors that Lanza "does not know that we are making a contribution" to the Damon Runyon Fund. Lanza was "very keen" to have an advisory committee appointed that would include representatives from the industry and told Hanmer et al. that since the industry would receive "much unfavorable publicity regardless of their attitude" it would be "to their advantage to declare themselves in support of scientific research directed toward the solution of this whole problem of smoking and cancer." Hanmer, however, was wary of publicity and didn't want his company joining any formal committees. Instead, he advised that his company participate as "silent collaborators."[11] Hanmer didn't (yet) see how his company could benefit from publicity of the sort Lanza was describing; the hope was still that the cancer problem could be quietly contained or controlled.

Tobacco executives at this time were of two minds about supporting cancer research. There was hope that the cancer problem could be solved by filters or additives or some other manipulation, but there was also fear that research might simply exacerbate the problem—by making the dangers more widely known or well established. Industry chiefs were therefore divided over the value of collaborating even with friendlies such as Rhoads and Lanza. A. Grant Clarke of Reynolds, architect of the "More Doctors Smoke Camels" campaign, and Robert N. DuPuis of Philip Morris were especially suspicious of the collaboration, whereas Harris Parmele of Lorillard and Hanmer of American Tobacco were generally supportive. Even Hanmer had his doubts, however, and often sent agents to keep tabs on the NYU work.[12]

Wynder's participation was always a sore spot for the industry. As early as 1950, in a letter to his president, Hanmer had characterized the young medical scholar as "somewhat more of a fanatic than a scientist." The American Tobacco Company would keep a close watch on Wynder over the next several years. Lanza, for example, after a November 5, 1953, meeting, reassured Hanmer, "I am not worried about Wynder. If we should shoot him tomorrow, another Wynder would bob up. I *am* worried about Graham. His is a big name in medicine. People listen to him, but he keeps shooting off his mouth."[13] Hanmer was increasingly bothered, though, by the fact that Rhoads seemed unwilling or unable to silence this young émigré upstart. (Wynder was born in Germany in 1922 and fled to New Jersey with his parents in 1938 to escape Nazi persecution.) Rhoads tried to argue that Wynder had "nothing to do with the tobacco research" supported by Sloan-Kettering (and therefore American Tobacco), but Hanmer pointed out that Wynder was listed as a participant in two of the five projects his company had been asked to support. Rhoads reassured Hanmer that Wynder had been "deliberately taken off tobacco work," but Hanmer countered that Wynder had lectured at an American Cancer Society meeting only two days previously and not on "circumcision, oral cancer and diet"— projects Rhoads said Wynder had been working on—but on tobacco and cancer. Rhoads confessed that while he could "control Wynder's work and his publications," the man was still free to speak wherever he wished.[14]

Wynder was in fact becoming the tobacco industry's number one enemy, a kind of *Roffo nouveau* and the target of a great deal of vituperative industry rhetoric. In one of his memos documenting the meetings of November 5, 1953, Hanmer claimed that Wynder had turned to tobacco only after failing as a surgeon; the young physician was "impetuous," immature, and "an out and out crusader." Hanmer also claimed to have reasons "to doubt his intellectual honesty." Evarts Graham, by contrast, was a distinguished surgeon who had received "all the honors the medical profession could bestow upon him." Alton Ochsner at Tulane was equally distinguished, and though "fanatical about smoking" was "probably intellectually honest because he refrained from condemning tobacco until he learned of the research being done by Wynder and Graham." So ruled Hanmer from his perch as research director of the world's largest tobacco corporation.[15]

PR was always paramount for the industry when it came to matters of smoking and health. The companies wanted friendly research, but they also wanted to make sure research could be packaged and publicized in ways that would help sell cigarettes. And in the years leading up to the conspiracy launched in December of 1953, the industry was not at all eager for the public to find out it was financing cancer research. (This represented a change from some of the braggadocio of earlier correspondence—and contrasts also with the approach taken after 1953, when the industry wanted everyone to know it was supporting research.) Runyon Fund officials were instructed on this need for secrecy and were happy to comply. The charity appreciated the industry's money and was happy to grant Hanmer's wish that "no publicity be permitted other than publication of results of research in accredited scientific journals." The net effect, though, was for this vital tobacco connection to go unnoticed in the popular press. When the *Wall Street Journal* cited Runyon Fund officials as prominent among those "refusing to accept as a fact any relationship between smoking and lung cancer," no mention was made of the fact that the world's largest tobacco company was bankrolling the Fund. Because this had been kept secret.[16]

IN A GOLDFISH BOWL

So prior even to the denialist campaign launched in the final weeks of 1953, tobacco companies were major funders of cancer research. They did so surreptitiously, channeling money through third parties that could be operated as puppets, without anyone knowing who was pulling the strings. Tobacco companies by this time were nervous about the attention being given to cancer: Hanmer complained about his company being "in a goldfish bowl," which was not where it wanted to be. The company wanted to be able to control discussions surrounding tobacco and cancer, but it also wanted to hide its role in orchestrating the effort. Hanmer was particularly worried about the NYU-SKI research getting out of hand: on December 1, 1952, he wrote to his superior, American Tobacco Vice President Preston L. Fowler, complaining that Teeter was "not controlling either the course of experiments or the publication of the results, even though Damon Runyon Memorial funds [i.e., American Tobacco funds] are being used for the purpose."[17]

Hanmer was also worried that NYU would produce "positive results"—meaning a demonstrated tobacco–cancer link—no matter what. At his November 5, 1953, meeting with Rhoads, Lanza, Nelson, and Teeter, Hanmer challenged Norton Nelson of SKI: "will you not increase the concentration of the so-called cigarette smoke tars or the frequency of application until cancers or their equivalent are produced on mice?" Nelson replied that this was indeed one goal, but Rhoads confessed that he did not expect "any direct relationship between mouse carcinogens and human carcinogens" to be established during his lifetime. Rhoads also affirmed, though, that "cigarette smoke does contain a mouse skin carcinogen—'That is a fact.'"[18]

The good news from Rhoads's point of view was that he and his men could probably do for tobacco what they had earlier done for the petrochemical industry, namely, identify the offending carcinogens, which the cigarette manufacturers could then "neutralize, remove, or filter out." Cigarettes would then "no longer be held responsible for contributing to lung cancer." Hanmer queried Rhoads on this: "I want to get this perfectly clear. As I understand it, you are saying that the mouse carcinogen in cigarette smoke should be removed and that, if it is removed, our problem will be solved, although nobody knows whether there is any relation between the mouse carcinogen and the carcinogen which is alleged to cause lung cancer in man." Rhoads at this point appeared a bit "nettled" and pointed out that tobacco manufacturers already recognized the need to remove carcinogens "because they are making filter tip cigarettes." Hanmer responded that the two largest cigarette companies were *not* in fact selling filters, and that the others were doing so not because they had conceded a hazard but rather simply to take advantage of publicity emanating from the medical profession. Filters were "purely a merchandising and sales promotion proposition."[19]

Hanmer was clearly annoyed by Rhoads's "That is a fact" assertion (on mouse carcinogens in smoke), noting that the "fact" in question was based on Wynder and Graham's unpublished two-year study reported at the April 1953 meeting of the American Association for Cancer Research. Hanmer was peeved: "The report has never been published in full, even in the Proceedings of the Society. The details are not known to us. This seems characteristic of Wynder's work and makes it doubly suspect." (Wynder had submitted his paper to *Cancer Research* in June 1953 but it did not appear until December, a month after Hanmer's rant.) Hanmer was also bothered by the fact that Wynder was getting positive results while others had gotten "negative or only occasional positive results." "Knowing Wynder," he declared, "we would expect prejudiced experimentation."[20]

MOUSE CARCINOGENS

Hanmer and his colleagues were hoping that whatever was wrong with cigarettes—and something clearly was—could be fixed. If there were carcinogens in the paper or the leaf or the pesticides, or in something having to do with the manufacturing, perhaps these could be eliminated or at least reduced to an acceptable level. Liggett & Myers's research chief in 1954 observed that Standard Oil had been able "to get around their difficulties with cancer by diluting or blending their oil in such a manner that they never had a concentration of the carcinogenic principle in excess of 6% in their oils." If carcinogens could be reduced in such a manner for petroleum, why not for tobacco?[21]

Tobacco industry researchers eventually decided they would have to accept the reality of "mouse carcinogens" in cigarette smoke, and the running together of these two terms—*mouse* and *carcinogen*—became a kind of dismissive mantra, with the implication that whatever was causing tumors in rodents might be perfectly safe for humans. Such would be the conspiracy's public face for decades hence, but internally the companies knew better. The whole point of the animal experiments financed through the Damon Runyon Fund was to shed light on whether smoking might be hazardous to humans. Researchers close to the project admitted this, noting that inferences about carcinogenic potency as revealed through such experiments "can be satisfactorily transferred from animals to man."[22]

The fact is that by 1953 the industry was already conducting other kinds of experiments—in secret—to explore not just *whether* but *what part* of cigarettes was causing cancer—as in whether it was the paper, or an added flavorant, or the burning tobacco leaf, or something else. That was the goal of a crucial series of experiments coordinated by American Tobacco with the Ecusta Paper Corporation, to which we now turn.

14

Ecusta's Experiments

Without Cigarette Paper there are no cigarettes.
HARRY H. STRAUS, PRESIDENT, ECUSTA PAPER
CORPORATION, MAY 1943

Tobacco manufacturers by the early 1950s were facing a new kind of quandary. The question was no longer whether but *why* smokers were so often dying from cancer. The tide was clearly shifting to cigarettes as the major cause—but what *precisely* was it about cigarettes that made them deadly? Arsenic was known to be in tobacco smoke, and Roffo had implicated benzpyrene, but there were lots of other candidates. By the 1950s compounds on the industry's list of suspects included arsenic, ethylene glycol (and its acrolein derivative), benzpyrene, chemicals released during the burning of cigarette paper and paper additives (including inks), tobacco flavorants of various sorts, gases released from safety matches and lighter fluids, a couple of different nicotine alkaloids, heat from the smoke itself, metals of various sorts (notably chromium or nickel), and radioactive isotopes that concentrate in tobacco leaf (potassium 40 was suspected in the 1950s, then polonium 210 in the 1960s). Paraffin was sometimes named, as were various aldehydes, phenols, and polycyclic aromatic hydrocarbons known to be in smoke.

It is also true, though, that a handful of scientific stragglers were still holding out for non-tobacco causes of the epidemic. Wilhelm Hueper at the NCI thought it was air pollution; Joseph Berkson from the Mayo Clinic blamed tuberculosis; and R. A. Fisher in Britain and Otmar Freiherr von Verschuer in Germany blamed the human genetic constitution.[1] Some diehards denied even the very *fact* of increase. Milton Rosenblatt, a New York physician and TIRC intimate, as late as 1964 denied that lung cancer rates had increased over time, characterizing evidence to this effect as an artifact of measurement: more people were being X-rayed, so more cancers were showing up.[2] There are lots of struggles over these questions in the months leading up to the Plaza Hotel conspiracy and the drafting of the "Frank Statement."

One little-known aspect of this run-up to conspiracy is a collaboration between American Tobacco and the Ecusta Paper Corporation to investigate whether tar from the smoke of tobacco *alone,* without the paper in other words, was capable of causing cancer. The collaboration began in 1952 and continued to a certain extent even after 1953,[3] by which time blame was squarely in the court of tobacco—rather than the paper or some other non-tobacco cause. Ecusta's involvement in cancer research grows out of the American Tobacco–NYU–SKI–MCV collaboration, from this effort to find out what part of the smoking process was causing cancer.

PAPER CHASE

This idea of *cigarette paper* causing cancer was nothing new in the 1950s. Henry Ford as early as 1916 had published a letter from Thomas A. Edison of lightbulb and phonograph fame, announcing that "the injurious agent in cigarettes comes principally from the burning paper wrapper." Edison was already known for his policy of employing "no person who smokes cigarettes"; here he asserted that the principal toxic substance in cigarettes was the acrid unsaturated aldehyde known as *acrolein.* Acrolein was already recognized as a powerful chemical irritant; the compound had been identified in cigarette smoke prior even to the twentieth century and gained further notoriety following its use as a chemical warfare agent in the First World War. So it wasn't such a big step for Edison and others to blame acrolein for cancers and other kinds of ailments thought to stem from "chronic irritation."[4]

Of course while Edison and Ford were crusading against the "little white slavers" it was not yet even suspected that cigarettes might cause *lung* cancer. Pipe smoking was often blamed for tumors of the lip or throat, but cigarettes were generally thought to be a "milder" form of smoke, with the danger lying only in their seductive appeal to the young and weak. Cigarettes were for dandies and sissies, and were widely regarded as a cheaper and less obnoxious form of tobacco use. And were not yet even a very common way to smoke. Americans smoked only 2.5 billion cigarettes in 1900—compared with the 330-odd billion smoked in 2011. Cigarettes wouldn't surpass cigars and pipes as the dominant form of smoking until the 1920s and 1930s.

The situation was different after 1950. Smoking was being confirmed as the principal cause of lung cancer, and cigarette paper was often cited as the reason why. Wynder had proposed testing paper tars for cancer activity in February of 1952, by which time the American Tobacco Company was also sending its trusted envoy— Dr. Harvey Haag—to speak with Sloan-Kettering and others about "the cigarette paper tar situation."[5] American Tobacco had also hired H. J. Rand & Associates to explore this paper tar problem, following the advice of Bruce F. Barton, an advertising executive with cigarette accounts who, in October of 1951, was worried that one of the company's competitors would beat American to the punch and produce the world's first "cancer proof" cigarette paper: "I shudder at the thought of some day reading in the papers that science has proved that it is cigarette paper, not the tobacco, that can be a contributing factor in cancer, and that one of our competitors has a paper that is cancer proof."[6]

H. James Rand, a Cleveland inventor (and grandson of the founder of Remington Rand Inc.), was hired to avoid this prospect. Rand was convinced that tobacco was innocent; tobacco was at most "an extremely weak carcinogenic material." He also believed that additives such as diethylene glycol or sulfurous fumes from matches posed little harm. Sulfur dioxide was indisputably an irritant, but the quantities inhaled by a smoker were not sufficiently large (.0023 grams per twenty matches) to be "a conceivable factor in carcinogenesis."[7]

Cigarette paper, by contrast, had been "notoriously ignored in efforts to isolate a carcinogen from cigarettes." Rand was a follower of the Hungarian novelist, chemist, and inventor Istvan Tamas, who had developed a synthetic cigarette paper (made from purified methyl cellulose) that was supposed to make cigarettes cancer-proof. To test this, or really rather to prove it—Rand clung obsessively to his idée fixe—Rand and his colleagues isolated tars from the smoke of cigarette paper and looked for the telltale signs of carcinogenic spectra. Spectrographic analysis showed fluorescence in the 400 to 440 mμ (millimicron, nanometer) wavelength range with peaks at 405 and 434 mμ, wavelengths "characteristic of carcinogenic substances" such as methyl-cholanthrene, dibenzanthracene, and benzpyrene, all powerful carcinogens. Rand claimed that fluorescence was a better indicator of carcinogenic potency even than mouse experiments, and concluded that "of all the substances connected with the smoking of cigarettes which might be investigated or have been investigated for carcinogenesis, only the paper tars exhibit the characteristic fluorescent spectrum [of a true carcinogen]." Cigarette paper tars had not been tested in experimental animals while tobacco tars had been "virtually exonerated of carcinogenic action by animal experimentation."[8]

All of this was news, and rather disturbing, to the world's largest maker of cigarette paper. On March 6, 1952, Hanmer had returned to Richmond and called Lawrence F. Dixon, vice president at Ecusta, to let him know about Rand's experiments. Dixon soon thereafter spoke with the vice president for R&D at Olin, Ecusta's parent company, bringing him up to speed. (Olin had bought the Ecusta Paper Corporation in 1949 and was licensed to produce cellophane, "one of the most important agents of protection and preservation" in the cigarette business.) Olin's president, John M. Olin, and Ecusta President John Haynes were also apprised of the situation, probably by Rand himself.[9]

This paper–cancer question was complicated by the fact that cigarette manufacturers were increasingly using the woody stems and ribs of the tobacco plant to make cigarettes, blurring the paper-tobacco boundary. Paper after all is most often made from wood, which from a chemical point of view is essentially cellulose. Processed tobacco also contains a great deal of cellulose—especially when made from stems and ribs, as was being done with the turn to reconstituted tobacco sheet. Tobacco manufacturers in the 1930s and 1940s had begun using stems and stalks in cigarette filler—mainly to squeeze more money out of every tobacco plant—and the question arose: could this new use of woody parts be what was causing all this cancer? And if woody stems burned pretty much like paper, maybe it didn't really matter whether it was the leaf or the paper that was responsible, since both were pretty much the same from a chemical point of view. Plausibility for such a dilemma was increased by the fact that lots of other things were being shown to cause cancer when burned and rubbed onto the skins of mice—including tars from the smoke of yeast, turpentine, sugar, rice polishings, and human skin.[10]

Ecusta in the meantime was continuing to provide other tobacco companies with experimental papers. American Tobacco had the closest ties to Ecusta, but other manufacturers had started working with the papermaker. Philip Morris had Ecusta running tests to identify the papers used in Camels and Cavaliers exported to France, for example, and Ecusta had helped test Philip Morris's Dunhill brand fashioned from chlorophyll-impregnated paper. Ecusta also supplied Lorillard with chlorophyll paper—for testing to oxidize acrolein and to "stop cigarette breath." There is no evidence Ecusta ever organized animal experiments for Philip Morris, though we do know that the two companies were communicating on the cancer question, judging from a letter of October 30, 1952, in which Ecusta expressed its hope that "the problems common to your organization and to ours will bring us closer together." The "problems" referred to here included the growing number of poisons identified in tobacco smoke, especially soot, arsenic, and aldehydes but also carbonyl compounds, benzpyrene, and the broad class of compounds known as polycyclic aromatic hydrocarbons (see the box on page 214).[11]

American Tobacco's primary interest throughout the Ecusta collaboration was to find out whether tobacco could be exculpated as a cause of cancer. One way this was pursued was to see whether tar extracts from the smoke of paper-free cigarettes were carcinogenic. To prepare for this, Ecusta's two leading researchers, Jim Rickards and Milton Schur, visited American Tobacco's Richmond laboratory on September 18, 1952, to confirm plans to produce a number of "experimental cigarettes." These were normal cigarettes in every other respect, apart from being wrapped not with paper but with an experimental (and "fantastically expensive") purified cellulose known as "Rand tape."[12] The goal seems to have been to determine whether cigarettes wrapped in something other than Ecusta paper could still cause cancer. Animal experiments were not yet under way, and these early tests seem to have been confined to chemical analyses of smoke using spectroscopy, chromatography, and other analytic techniques.

POISONS IN CIGARETTE SMOKE (SELECTED)

Compound	Inhaled per Cigarette		Inhaled per Annum (globally)
Carbon monoxide	19.0	mg	110,000,000 kg
Tar	10.0	mg	60,000,000 kg
Argon	5.0	mg	30,000,000 kg
Nicotine	1.5	mg	9,000,000 kg
Methane	1.5	mg	9,000,000 kg
Acetaldehyde	0.9	mg	6,300,000 kg
Acetic acid	0.8	mg	4,800,000 kg
Hydrogen cyanide	0.45	mg	2,700,000 kg
Formic acid	0.4	mg	2,400,000 kg
Isoprene	0.3	mg	1,800,000 kg
Nitrogen oxides	0.3	mg	1,800,000 kg
Phenols	0.24	mg	1,400,000 kg
Ethylene	0.2	mg	1,200,000 kg
Acrylonitrile	0.13	mg	780,000 kg
Glycerol	0.12	mg	720,000 kg
Acrolein	0.1	mg	600,000 kg
Ammonia	0.08	mg	480,000 kg
Formaldehyde	0.06	mg	360,000 kg
Benzene	0.03	mg	180,000 kg
Acetylene	0.03	mg	180,000 kg
Styrene	0.01	mg	60,000 kg
Tobacco-specific nitrosamines	0.0015	mg	9,000 kg
Anthracene	0.10	μg[a]	600 kg
Arsenic	0.08	μg	480 kg
Cadmium	0.05	μg	300 kg
Chrysene	0.05	μg	300 kg
Benzopyrene	0.03	μg	180 kg
Vinyl chloride	0.01	μg	60 kg
Radioactive polonium 210	0.04	picocuries	< 1 kg

Note: Per cigarette data are from the 1989 Surgeon General's Report, 81–87, with an average given when a range is specified. Global totals assume six trillion sticks smoked per annum.
[a] μg = micrograms.

A DAUNTING PROSPECT

Planning for Ecusta's animal experiments began in earnest in the winter and spring of 1953. Ecusta scientists drafted a set of instructions detailing how to prepare cigarette smoke condensate,[13] and set about designing their own set of animal experiments parallel to those of the NYU–Runyon Fund group.

This cannot have been a pleasant process for Ecusta, given what was at stake. Recall that while strong evidence was accumulating that cigarettes could cause cancer, it was not yet clear precisely *how*—whether it was from the paper, the heat, the arsenic, the polycyclics, or even fumes from safety matches or lighter fluid. Cigarette paper in these critical years (early 1950s) was a serious candidate, and Ecusta was the world's leading producer. Imagine their worry: what if it turned out that *they* and not, say, Reynolds or Lorillard or Liggett or Philip Morris, were responsible for tens of thousands of deaths every year from smoking? The prospect must have been quite daunting.

And we know they were worried. On January 14, 1953, Ecusta's Milton Schur met with Drs. Lanza and Nelson to find out how the NYU–SKI–American Tobacco "air pollution" (i.e., cigarette cancer) project was going—and asked if he could speak frankly. Schur cautioned that the two men didn't seem to understand that "what industry wanted most was to have them suppress irresponsible publications which might be damaging to industry." The whole question of cigarettes causing cancer was "in very much of a muddle."[14]

Equally muddled, or rather hanging in the balance, was whether the Ecusta Paper Corporation should be considered part of "the tobacco industry." Schur seems to have implied as much, and for good reason. The company produced both filters and papers for cigarettes and was actively involved in cigarette testing, including testing for safety. And when cigarette manufacturers launched their campaign to dispute and distract from the hazards in December of 1953, the papermaker was cordially invited to collaborate. Quite wisely they refused—albeit for reasons that don't seem to have left a paper trail. This refusal to join the industry's denialist conspiracy was probably the best business decision ever made by the company, allowing it essentially to vanish from the cigarette wars of subsequent decades. And ever since, cigarette paper makers have been pretty much invisible in the annals of tobacco history—even though people throughout the world inhale the smoke from about *300,000 metric tons* of cigarette paper every year. The papermakers are given a free pass, and whatever role paper may play in cancer causation disappears behind a cloud of smoke. Keep in mind that even if paper contributes only one part in a hundred to the total cigarette death toll, we are still talking about four thousand people killed every year in the United States alone. And more than ten times that globally.

POWERFUL FINDINGS:
THE SMOKE CONDENSATE TESTS

Ecusta remained at the center of the tobacco industry's cancer consternations in the spring of 1953. On April 7, for example, Schur sent Hanmer a copy of a press release on Wynder's mouse-painting paper, the published version of which would make such a splash eight months hence. Schur noted that Wynder's article was probably not yet in finished form and might well have a qualifying statement inserted "as a result of my request . . . to the effect that production of cancer in the skin of mice has not been proven to indicate that smoking has a tendency to produce lung cancer in man."[15] The chief scientist at the world's largest cigarette paper company was hoping he could control the conclusions reached in basic scientific research on the crucial issue of the day: whether cigarettes cause cancer.

In May of 1953 American Tobacco was working with Ecusta to establish how much acrolein was in cigarette smoke. Paper- and tobacco-wrapped cigarettes were compared, with the result that paper-wrapped cigarettes yielded significantly higher levels of this poison. A little over a month later Hanmer asked Schur if he could test Ecusta's new experimental filters, which were supposed to remove aldehydes from cigarette smoke.[16]

By this time, though, the Ecusta Paper Corporation was producing data showing that *regardless* of how they were wrapped, cigarettes yielded tars capable of causing cancer in experimental animals. In one crucial series of tests done in late May or early June, Ecusta researchers compared the tars from cigarettes wrapped in various kinds of paper against tars from paper alone. Tars from these different sources were painted on the shaved backs of mice, following which skin tissues were examined to see whether the tars had destroyed the sebaceous (sweat) glands. This was the "accelerated" bioassay developed by William E. Smith, the New York University pathologist also involved in the Runyon Fund–Sloan-Kettering collaboration. Ecusta summarized the results of these studies on June 9, 1953, in a remarkable chart (see Figure 25), showing that regardless of the kind of paper used to roll the cigarette—whether Minnesota or California flax or the purified cellulose known as Rand film or even burley leaf—in each case the "estimate of carcinogenicity" was positive (caused cancer, in other words). By contrast, tars from cigarette paper alone showed only a "mild" carcinogenicity. And a solvent control was negative—producing no cancer at all.

These were powerful findings, and apparently the first-ever industry experiments to show clear evidence of carcinogenic action from tobacco tars. Ecusta sent this chart to Lorillard's director of manufacturing, who forwarded it to the company's director of research, Harris Parmele, asking that the information be kept "very confidential" since Ecusta was making these tests "independent of other laboratories with which you are familiar"[17]—that is, the American Tobacco Company.

JULY AND AUGUST 1953: THE WHOLE SMOKE "IMPINGEMENT" EXPERIMENTS

It is hard to imagine today how frightening this all must have been. Cigarettes were being accused of causing cancer, and the industry's own experiments were confirming the charges. One response was to try to verify these results, using other meth-

ods. A letter of June 24, 1953, has Rickards thanking Hanmer for his "extremely interesting and fruitful" visit one week before, when a new series of whole smoke "impingement" experiments was first put into motion. The collaboration had already
resulted in infrared absorption curves for the combusted papers from Ecusta, and
the search was on for better ways to identify carcinogens in the resulting smoke—
and to see what kind of impact these would have on biological tissues. Larson and
Haag were requesting data, and while we don't have direct evidence that they or
even Hanmer had been given the "accelerated" test data from Ecusta's carcinogenicity chart, this is probably safe to assume. Rickards was also producing experimental filters for use in American Tobacco's experiments.[18] On July 1, 1953, Hanmer sent Schur five cartons of experimental cigarettes wrapped in different kinds
of paper; he also requested samples of the filters Ecusta was designing to help reduce some of the aldehydes in cigarette smoke.

Having already demonstrated carcinogenicity through mouse painting, the idea
was now to augment the realism of the animal tests—by using *whole smoke blown*
onto the shaved backs of mice rather than *smoke condensate painted* onto the shaved
backs of mice. Plans for these new experiments first show up in a letter of July 7,
1953, from Milton Schur to Hanmer. Rickards had met with Larson and Haag in
Hanmer's Richmond office on June 18 and now, two weeks later, the plan was to
launch these so-called smoke impingement tests. The idea was to confirm—or ideally, disconfirm—the "positive" results already obtained at Ecusta, along with the
mouse-painting experiments of Wynder et al. that, while not yet published, were
looming on the horizon.

Rickards played a key role in the research design, instructing Larson on the age,
sex, and strains of mice to be used. Schur and Rickards suggested to Larson the advantage of using only one sample of cigarettes, "one which has yielded positive results [i.e., cancers] by our solvent application method," until the project had established "the frequency and duration of direct impingement treatment which will yield
interpretable results." Once this "rational basis of procedures" had been established,
the group could then "run a whole series of samples by smoke impingement." Schur
also reported Larson's remarks about publication rights being reserved by the Medical College of Virginia; this is interesting, because it shows that the project was not
undertaken on the initiative of Ecusta but rather by the American Tobacco Company and its staff, including Larson and Haag. Schur allowed this question of publication to be "a matter which we leave entirely in your [i.e., American Tobacco's]
hands, knowing full well that you would not agree to any publication until the time
would be propitious."[19]

Rickards explained the design of the experiment in a July 8, 1953, letter to Larson at the MCV. Responsibility for designing, administering, and evaluating the experiments was to remain with Ecusta, but the animals were actually to be kept (and
exposed) at the MCV under the direction of Larson and Haag. Following the meth-

ods of William E. Smith, the mice were to be male and eight to ten weeks of age; exposures would begin on a Monday and take place three times daily, five days a week. The mice were to be shaved, exposed to blown smoke, and after an appropriate length of time sacrificed to obtain a section of exposed skin that would be clipped out, preserved in formaldehyde, and then shipped to Ecusta for analysis. The original plan called for six different cigarettes to be tested on six animals each; it was later decided to use only one cigarette type—the one already shown to be "positive" for causing cancer in the condensate experiments.[20]

On August 18, 1953, Schur wrote to Hanmer noting that the smoke impingement tests were about to begin. Results were already coming in from the condensate experiments, and Rickards was on a two-week stint in Hanmer's lab in Richmond, brushing up on infrared spectroscopy and fractionation column techniques (to identify smoke constituents). Schur and Rickards clearly knew they were on to something big: Rickards's visit to American Tobacco's lab had impressed on these men the gravity of the situation, judging from the uncharacteristically effusive tone of Schur's letter of thanks to Hanmer: "We consider sacred all the information Jim [Rickards] obtained during his work at your laboratory, and we will keep it strictly confidential even within the confines of our own laboratory."[21]

In this new set of experiments whole smoke—as opposed to extracted tobacco tars—was to be used to approximate what actually happens when smoke enters a smoker's lungs. The plan was to blow smoke onto the shaved backs of mice to see if cellular changes of a cancerous or precancerous sort could be detected. Smith's accelerated biological test would again be used to speed up the results; tissue samples would then be graded on a scale from 0 to 10, with 0 indicating no effect and 10 being complete destruction of the glands in question.[22]

The idea of using whole smoke to test biological reactions was an old one in the industry. The first mention in the internal documents dates from the mid-1930s, when American Tobacco scientists blew smoke into the eyes of rabbits to evaluate "the degree of irritation" caused by DEG-treated cigarettes. (Philip Morris used such tests, complete with graphic images of inflamed eyes, to advertise its cigarettes, though Harlow at one point confided that "a rabbit will scream if nicotine is introduced into the eye.") Philip Morris had substituted DEG for glycerine to keep tobacco leaves pliable during manufacturing, and the question for companies like American Tobacco was whether such a substitute was in fact less irritating. Harvey Haag from the MCV and A. M. Ambrose from Stanford were hired to test for toxicity and found that while no great danger seemed to arise from low concentrations, the smoke derived from DEG-treated cigarettes was actually harsher than that from glycerine: "the edema [swelling] seems to be definitely greater." Haag and Ambrose had published this in 1937, prompting internal grumbling from Philip Morris that Haag had failed to disclose his sponsorship by American Tobacco.[23]

Now, though, in the summer of 1953, whole smoke experiments would be used to measure the carcinogenicity of tobacco as against cigarette papers. Rickards on September 9, 1953, wrote to Harvey Haag at the MCV, providing him with reference samples of mouse skin tissues graded according to whether the sebaceous glands were "intact" (i.e., healthy), "altered," or "absent" (i.e., destroyed), along with an explanation of the grading system. And over the next two months, Ecusta and the MCV exchanged mouse skin samples in formaldehyde, evaluating the degree of destruction of tissue as an index of carcinogenic potency. Paul Larson sent one set of exposed samples to Schur on September 17, for example, and Schur responded on September 24, noting that the specimens would be examined within the next few days. Schur added that Hanmer, Rickards, Larson, and he himself were all looking forward to the results "with the greatest interest."[24]

BAD NEWS FOLLOWED BY WORSE

Bad news came from NYU on October 13, 1953, when Norton Nelson, director of research at the university's Institute for Industrial Medicine, delivered a devastating "progress report" for the past year on Runyon Fund grant 231, titled "Investigation of the Chemical Nature of Environmental Carcinogens." Recipients included the top research officers of the leading tobacco companies in the United States (Clarke from Reynolds, Cullman and DuPuis from Philip Morris, Hanmer from American, Parmele from Lorillard, Schur from Ecusta, and Tucker from Brown & Williamson), all of whom were instructed not to publish or circulate the report. The reason was evident from the very first sentence, which announced that "Tars collected from cigarette smoke have been shown to produce cancer on the skin of mice and rabbits."[25]

That was shocking enough, but equally alarming were the final results of Ecusta's whole smoke experiments, delivered to Larson at the MCV in a letter of November 6, 1953, marked "Confidential." Milton Schur, Ecusta's manager of research and development, reported that among the eight mice exposed to whole smoke "very strong" activity—meaning cancer or precancerous growths—had been found in five of the animals. "Mild" activity was found in one additional mouse and none in the other two. Rickards had obtained these results by telephone from "our pathologist" (apparently at Ecusta) and asked that all parties wait for the written report before exchanging views. Schur sent that written report to Larson on November 10, 1953, leaving no doubt about the strong biological activity of the tobacco tars tested. Ecusta had confirmed once again the industry's worst fears—that smoke from cigarettes can cause cancer.[26]

November and December of 1953 must have been something of a nightmare for U.S. tobacco manufacturers. Bad news was followed by worse, prompting ever more desperate attempts to either explain away the bad news or keep it under wraps. Larson, for example, was not satisfied that Ecusta's tests were adequate to establish carcinogenicity and challenged other aspects of the studies. Schur responded by pulling scientific rank, citing William E. Smith's view that "*any* product causing the destruction of the sebaceous glands under the conditions of accelerated tests would probably produce papillomata and eventual cancer under the conditions of the recognized standard test." Smith at this time was the chief proponent of the accelerated tests used in the Ecusta experiments; he was also a faculty member at NYU's Bellevue Medical Center and an important figure in the NYU collaboration—and one of those who would suffer professionally for recognizing the cancer-causing capacity of tobacco. Smith in fact would shortly thereafter be purged from the NYU faculty (by Lanza in 1956), a decision upheld despite protests to the chancellor.[27]

Ecusta was quite happy with these results, and for obvious reasons. Experimental tests had seemed to exonerate cigarette *paper* and put the entirety of blame for cancer on *tobacco*. In subsequent correspondence of the company it is taken for granted that "either 3 or 4 malignancies and a small number of benign growths" had been produced in the mice exposed to cigarette smoke, with no cancers and only a few benign growths on the unexposed controls—consistent with the chart shown earlier to Lorillard. And tars made from paper alone showed no more tumors than the tobacco-free solvent controls.[28]

Quite apart from exonerating paper, however, there is another reason Ecusta must have been pleased. Ecusta by this time was manufacturing not just *paper* for the industry, but *filters*. And not just for American Tobacco, but for the entire U.S. cigarette industry. We don't have documents showing filter makers cracking open the champagne, but it makes sense that a manufacturer of filters would stand to gain if people were to start demanding "safer" cigarettes. This may have been one reason Ecusta was willing to conduct such tests in the first place: the tobacco industry's lemons would become Ecusta's lemonade.

"BEYOND ANY DOUBT"

Ecusta's experiments were never made public. The results were never published, nor were they even mentioned by any of the corporate principals over the subsequent half century of conspired silence. Nor are they mentioned in any published histories of tobacco or cancer research. By the time the results were in, however—in November of 1953—the cancer cat was coming out of the bag, big time. Word was getting out that the tobacco companies were supporting cancer research, and journalists and editors wanted to know why.

Some of the tensions surrounding this issue were already revealed at a November 5, 1953, meeting of the NYU–American Tobacco–Sloan-Kettering "Air Pollution" group—with all the principals of the collaboration present, along with Hanmer from American Tobacco, Parmele from Lorillard, and Schur and Dixon from Ecusta. Never before in the United States had researchers come together in such strength to discuss tobacco and health. The conversation was clearly tense, and the focus was not so much on results as on crisis management. Lanza started out with a statement that he and his collaborators were "constantly being sought out" by journalists wanting to know "what they were doing, the purpose of their investigations and who was financing them." Hanmer summarized the event for his employers at American Tobacco:

> [Lanza] said that the situation was becoming embarrassing and a statement could not be much longer deferred. He anticipated that unless they themselves made a statement, someone would endeavor to publish an article without benefit of guidance from them. . . . Dr. Lanza felt that such publicity might be both inaccurate and more damaging to the cigarette industry than an authorized statement from the NYU group.[29]

Lanza then went back over the history of the collaboration, recalling that it was actually the industry that had first approached NYU—in 1951—perhaps via Schur from Ecusta or Parmele from Lorillard, he wasn't sure. Lanza and Rhoads had refused direct funding, suggesting instead that monies be channeled through the Damon Runyon Fund. Rhoads once again compared the tobacco situation to that of the chemical industry twenty-five years earlier, when beta-naphthylamine had been found causing bladder cancer in dye workers. The industry had responded with "very poor public relations"—but had eventually managed "to correct this condition." Rhoads was hoping that tobacco could be rescued by a similar campaign. The more immediate difficulty, though, as Rhoads communicated to his tobacco hosts, was that the situation was now so hot that some kind of press release was unavoidable. Rhoads had thus far managed to postpone meetings with reporters from *Fortune, Life,* and *Time* but "sooner or later" would have to talk with them. Hanmer wanted their research to continue "without any publicity," but Rhoads insisted this was no longer possible. The subject had become "a matter of widespread public interest."[30]

That turned out to be an understatement. On November 30, 1953, *Time* magazine ran a story announcing that tars from cigarette smoke had now been proven to cause cancer in mice "beyond any doubt." That was a quote from "famed surgeon A. Evarts Graham of St. Louis," but it was also the headline for the article, which cited Graham's revelation: "Dr. Ernest L. Wynder and I have reproduced cancer experimentally in mice by using merely the tars from tobacco smoke. This shows conclusively that there is something in cigarette smoke which can produce cancer. This is no longer merely a possibility. Our experiments have proved it beyond any doubt."[31] The industry by this time had decided it could no longer afford to keep silent, and in a press release of November 30, 1953, American Tobacco president Paul M. Hahn admitted his company's role in helping to finance "the Damon Runyon Memorial Cancer Fund, which supports New York University's Institute of Industrial Medicine, which is trying to find the cancer-causing factor in cigarette tar." *Time* reported Hahn's announcement, along with his claim that "no one has yet proved that lung cancer in any human being is directly traceable to tobacco." *Time* also noted, however, that "study after study" had established "a correlation between prolonged cigarette smoking and lung cancer."[32]

A final blow came on December 8, when Alton Ochsner, Ernst Wynder, and a number of other prominent medical scholars lectured at the Twenty-ninth Annual Greater New York Dental Meeting, announcing that medical men were now "extremely concerned about the possibility that the male population of the United States will be decimated by cancer of the lung in another fifty years if cigarette smoking increases as it has in the past." The *New York Times* minced no words in reporting on the event:

> Four Medical reports were presented here yesterday linking cigarette smoking and disease, particularly lung cancer, without qualification.
>
> The correlation between smoking and cancer was stated in unusually strong terms by leading medical specialists at the twenty-ninth annual Greater New York Dental Meeting.
>
> The meeting also marked one of the first occasions in which medical researchers, reporting before a professional group, have joined in insisting firmly that it is indeed smoking, and not some other environmental factor, that has caused the great increase in lung cancer among males noted in disease statistics of the last two decades.[33]

The combined effect of *Time*'s stories and the *New York Times* article, together with pent-up lingering rumors about the NYU–Sloan-Kettering–American Tobacco collaboration, caused an outgassing of panic on Wall Street, with tobacco stocks falling more sharply than at any time since the Great Depression. On December 9, 1953, American Tobacco's stock lost about 6 percent of its value; Reynolds's lost closer to 10 percent.[34] The cigarette trade was in danger of coming undone.

LUCKY TWIST

There are lots of different ways one could look at the cancer research funded by the tobacco industry in the early 1950s. One would be to regard these as essentially *intra-industry squabbles* over whether it was the paper, or the tobacco, or some additive or contaminant or method of processing that was causing all this cancer. This was not a debate that either side (paper or tobacco) wanted to air in public, which helps explain why the Ecusta experiments never saw the light of day.

One can also imagine, though, how differently things might have turned out if the experiments had exonerated tobacco. After all, this was still a period when experts could honestly doubt smoking's link to the lung cancer epidemic; the case was closing, but it was not yet entirely closed. If Wynder et al.'s work had been refuted, the world surely would have heard about it, and loudly. As history and the facts of the matter had it, however, the Ecusta tests turned up positive: tobacco smoke blown onto the bare backs of mice caused cancers, as did the painting of tobacco tars.

The lucky twist for Ecusta was not just that paper was (relatively speaking) exonerated, however. They were also fortunate to have decided—in December of 1953—not to accept the tobacco industry's invitation to participate in the prevarication project, despite "considerable pressure" from the rest of the industry.[35] The company seems never to have lied to the public (about cancer), which is probably why it has never been sued. Ecusta did, however, continue to supply millions of miles of paper to the industry, along with equipment and facilities for tobacco's various PR fronts. It also continued to research ways to make cigarettes "safer." On June 1, 1954, for example, Cowan Dengler, Inc., a New York advertising company, invited Ecusta to try its "new, improved paper," offered as a way to "reduce or eliminate the propensity toward lung cancer on the part of cigarette smokers which many medical authorities believe exists."[36] The Ecusta company itself never issued any kind of warning that the cigarettes they were helping make were causing cancer, even though they had helped to prove that fact in their laboratories.

Ecusta continued to work with the Tobacco Industry Research Committee and other industry research bodies—supplying the TIRC with tobacco tar distillates for use in industry-financed research, for example. The company also conducted research on the combustion properties of various kinds of paper and paper ingredients and as late as the 1980s was helping Philip Morris develop its adjustable "Dial-a-Taste" (or "Dial-a-Tar") gimmick, a cigarette that was supposed to give smokers a choice in how much tar to inhale (aka Project Data). Ecusta developed state-of-the-art automatic smoking machines for the industry and helped BAT develop "Reduced Visibility Sidestream" cigarette papers.[37]

And other agencies continued mouse experiments—at great cost, and to no good end. From 1974 to 1984, for example, industry-funded scientists forced ten thousand mice to inhale the smoke from 800,000 cigarettes, looking for—and finding no examples of—squamous cell lung cancer.[38] Such projects were oddly anachronistic: smoking had already been shown to cause cancer in humans, and post-1950s efforts to see how mice fared under such conditions are probably best characterized as pseudoscience married to animal cruelty. The industry kept hoping for ways to "spin" itself out of this grim charge of causing mass death, and while this worked for a time, history would eventually catch up with them.

Consensus, Hubris, and Duplicity

Cigarette smoking is a cause of lung cancer. And that's that and you can't talk your way out of it.

HARVEY GRAHAM, *SMOKING—THE FACTS*, PUBLISHED BY THE BRITISH
MEDICAL JOURNAL ASSOCIATION, 1957

We like to think of scientific knowledge as cumulative, that ideas once established as true cannot be undone. But the reality is that facts can come undone, there is forgetfulness, and not every good thing flourishes. That was part of the insight of Thomas Kuhn's great *Structure of Scientific Revolutions:* our views of the world change not so much by steady pilings-on of fact but rather by gestalt shifts in how we see the world. Science advances by leaping over the canyons of dried-up ideas, which also means that a certain kind of forgetting—or *unlearning*—is key to any scientific change. Old points of view must be abandoned, the strange becomes familiar, the familiar strange. Notions of what is true are transformed, along with what is real or even imagined as possible. Great science is supposed to be revolutionary.

Of course not every scientific advance, even if "proven," is accepted right away. Revolutions can encounter organized resistance, especially when powerful toes are being stepped on. The fact of smoking causing cancer is a stellar example: lots of science making this link had piled up by the 1950s, but the industry quickly learned that scholars could be found to dispute such facts—for a price.

So when can we really say that smoking was recognized as a cause of cancer? When did a consensus emerge?

A TILTED LANDSCAPE

The first thing to recall is that the landscape here is tilted; this is not a world of innocent inquiry, with researchers simply trying to discover the truth. We cannot even really talk about a world inside the industry and a world outside, because the industry has exerted such a powerful influence over academic research. We shall return to this when exploring scholarly collaborations; the industry's ability to tame and harness scientists is crucial for understanding how inquiries in this realm have unfolded historically.

Crucial also to keep in mind is that cancer of the lung is only one of several kinds of maladies caused by smoking and not even the first to be recognized historically. Pipe smoking was found to cause cancers of the lip and throat as early as the eighteenth century, when John Hill in England and Samuel Thomas von Soemmerring in Germany published medical papers on these topics. French physicians were talking about *cancers des fumeurs*—smokers' cancers—by the middle of the nineteenth century, and when President Ulysses S. Grant died from cancer of the throat in 1885 this was widely blamed on his fondness for cigars.

So it is *not* true that smoking was first recognized as a cancer hazard in the 1950s, as we sometimes hear from the industry's experts in court. Such a misconception is arrived at by focusing only on cancers of the lung and only on the science of Englishmen and Americans. Smoking was well known as a cause of tumors of the lip and throat in the nineteenth century, and even the lung cancer link was pretty well nailed down by Germans in the 1930s and 1940s. Lung cancer has become the signature mark of tobacco death partly for legal reasons: far more smokers die from heart disease, but it is easier to litigate on the basis of pulmonary tumors because over 90 percent of all such cancers are caused by smoking, whereas most heart disease is *not* caused by smoking (only about a third is—because there are so many other ways to injure your heart). Which also means that when lawyers want to try a tobacco case, they tend to choose plaintiffs with a lung disease rather than a heart malady.

That being said, there are still good reasons for highlighting lung cancer as the calling card of the cigarette epidemic. Chief among these is the fact that nine of ten people who contract the disease would never have developed it had they not been smoking or breathing other people's smoke. The fraction can be as high as 95 percent, depending on where you live and how much other filth there is in the air. In the early stages of a cigarette epidemic smoking will be only one among many causes of lung cancer—since the disease itself will still be rare. Mass smoking will eventually swamp all other causes, however. Lung malignancies are also notoriously difficult to treat, which means that even today, with the best access to modern medicine, most people who contract the disease will die from it. Lung cancer is not like tumors of the skin or even breast cancer; a diagnosis of pulmonary malignancy is usually a death sentence.

How, though, was the lung cancer hazard discovered? What kinds of evidence were adduced, and when can we say a consensus developed?

CONVERGING LINES OF EVIDENCE

The science of the mid-1950s actually involved a confluence of several distinct lines of inquiry, notably

- Animal experiments, showing that tobacco tar extracts could cause cancer;
- Epidemiology, including both retrospective and prospective studies of statistical patterns of human disease;
- Clinical pathology, meaning the microscopic study of cellular damage caused by exposure to cigarette smoke;
- Chemical analytics, meaning the isolation of known carcinogens in tobacco smoke;
- Presumptive arguments from the logic of medical inference, notably the fact that nothing better explained the rise of the lung cancer epidemic—and especially sex differences—than smoking.

Animal experiments.   Angel Roffo, as we have seen, was the pioneer here, showing that cancers could be induced by several different kinds of tobacco extracts on several different kinds of animals. Studies along these lines were replicated and deepened by the industry itself (in secret) and then by Wynder, Graham, and Croninger, whose 1953 publication became the most important prompt for the industry's campaign of denialist doubt mongering. The industry liked to trivialize animal experiments by talking as if laboratory mice had nothing to do with humans. Here a certain opportunism was at work: animal experiments were trumpeted when they failed to show a cancer link and ridiculed or disparaged when they confirmed the link. Or just kept quiet, as was done with the Ecusta experiments.

Tobacco epidemiology.   Lombard and Doering in Massachusetts produced the first significant study in 1928, showing that smokers were more likely than non-smokers to contract cancers of the lips, bladder, cheek, and tongue—and lung. Insurance agents had done even earlier work, but the focus on cancers of the lung was not strong until 1939, when Franz Hermann Müller at the University of Cologne showed that smokers were far more likely than non-smokers to contract cancers of the lung. Müller's paper is a retrospective case study, meaning that hospital patients with lung cancer were asked about their smoking habits, which were then compared with those of a similar group of patients who had not developed cancer. The result: lung cancer victims were far more likely to have been smokers. And though sample sizes would grow in subsequent years along with new methods to quantify statistical significance and to control for possible bias, the many studies that followed Müller's were not profoundly different in terms of design—or conclusions. In 1943, for example, Eberhard Schairer and Erich Schöniger at the University of Jena presented a more careful study with larger controls, showing again that people with lung cancer were far more likely to have been smokers. The Jena study was carried out at the university's Institute for Tobacco Hazards Research, a body established by funding from Hitler's Reich Chancellery. The research was rigorous, yielding results of greater statistical significance than those produced by Müller. Schairer and Schöniger didn't calculate that significance, but subsequent epidemiologists have shown that the odds of their results coming about by chance were less than one in ten million.[1]

The collapse of the Nazi regime and the stigma subsequently attached to German medicine meant that much of that country's pioneering cancer research was ignored. Müller and Schairer and Schöniger were occasionally cited, but credit for discovering the cigarette–cancer link was far more often granted to British and American researchers, notably Wynder and Graham in the United States and Doll and Hill in England. German research was seen as "tainted," albeit unfairly in this instance. A fairer assessment would be that the Germans discovered and produced solid evidence for the link in the 1930s and 1940s, after which the center of gravity of research shifted to the English-speaking world, where more nails were added to the coffin.

However one judges the early German work—and much of its neglect has simply to do with the failure of scholars to read the original German texts—one cannot deny that by the 1950s the river of evidence had become a flood, with the best work appearing in Britain and the United States.[2] Five separate epidemiological studies were published in 1950 alone. Wynder and Graham in their comparison of 684 cases and a comparable number of hospital controls showed that lung cancer victims were far more likely to have been smokers; prolonged use of tobacco seemed to be "an important factor in the induction of bronchiogenic carcinoma." Morton Levin and colleagues from the New York State Department of Health showed that people who smoked for twenty-five years doubled their chance of contracting lung cancer, with the data suggesting "a causal relation between cigaret and pipe smoking and cancer of the lung and lip." Clarence Mills and Marjorie Porter from the University of Cincinnati concluded that cigarette smoking bore "a highly significant relation to cancers of the respiratory tract," and Robert Schrek and his colleagues at the Tumor Research Unit of the Veteran Administration Hospital in Hines, Illinois, found "strong circumstantial evidence" of cigarette smoking as "an etiologic factor in cancer of the respiratory tract." Richard Doll and A. Bradford Hill in England provided even more convincing evidence of a "real association of carcinoma of the lung and smoking."[3]

Piling on, this German, British, and American retrospective work was soon joined by a relatively new kind of epidemiology known as "prospective" or "cohort" studies, in which large numbers of initially healthy people were followed over the years to see whether smokers were more or less likely to develop cancer. Prospective studies were designed to eliminate some of the potential sources of bias in earlier work, notably "recall bias." Müller's 1939 study, for example, had relied partly on relatives' reports of how many cigarettes their dearly departed had smoked. Skeptics had objected that people diagnosed with lung cancer (or their relatives) might be more likely to say they had smoked: an investigator might even prompt an answer along these lines from an unconscious hope to implicate cigarettes; or lung cancer sufferers might exaggerate how much they had smoked, perhaps from an overeagerness to blame some external cause. If people diagnosed with cancer were more likely to confess having smoked, or to exaggerate how much they had smoked, this would artificially inflate any estimate of the extent to which smoking had contributed to the disease.

Prospective studies eliminated this possible source of bias, since careful records were kept of participants' smoking habits *prior to* their developing cancer. Recall bias was eliminated, because records of smoking rates were being kept in real time. Smoking rates were also recorded by people with no stake in the outcome. The new studies gave the same results as the old: Doll and Hill in 1954 announced their confirmation of the retrospective evidence, concluding that smokers were *more than ten times as likely* as non-smokers to die from lung cancer. Risk also increased with amount smoked, as one might expect from a causal relationship. So whereas non-smokers died from lung cancer at the rate of about 7 per year per 100,000, the figure for light smokers was 57, for medium smokers 139, and for heavier smokers 227. And people who smoked more than thirty-five cigarettes per day were dying from lung cancer at a rate of 315 per 100,000, more than forty times that of non-smokers.[4] Similar results were found by E. Cuyler Hammond and Daniel Horn in the United States, working for the American Cancer Society.[5] The power of these studies was augmented by the large numbers involved: Doll and Hill's encompassed 40,000 British doctors, and Hammond and Horn's followed more than 180,000 American men. Few studies in the history of medicine had ever had such power, and doctors and non-doctors alike were impressed. Doll and Hill were both knighted for their efforts, and Hammond and Horn were broadly celebrated.

Clinical pathology.   Pathology is the science of the causes of disease, with the focus typically on the microscopic analysis of tissues. Clinical pathologists are expert in distinguishing normal from abnormal cells, as in whether a worrisome biopsied lump is cancer and, if so, what type. Pathologists use state-of-the art microscopes and cellular staining techniques to identify diseased tissues and by the 1930s had begun to realize that smoking could cause injury to the natural cleansing mechanisms of the human lung. A patent application from 1932 in the files of the American Tobacco Company noted that even "the merest traces of aldehydes completely paralyze" the cilia, the hair-like cellular projections responsible for cleaning the inside lining of the lungs. This same patent observed that "carbon monoxide destroys the unison of action, and ammonia increases the moisture film which weighs them down."[6] Aldehydes, carbon monoxide, and ammonia all were known to be in cigarette smoke by this time; American Tobacco was in fact getting so many letters suggesting ways to reduce carbon monoxide that it drafted a form letter detailing how to respond—as it would later do for inquiries concerning lead and arsenic.[7]

Pathologists in the 1950s set out to nail down this question of whether smoking could cause damage at the cellular level. One of the most remarkable studies was done by Anderson C. Hilding, an otolaryngologist at St. Luke's Hospital in Duluth, Minnesota, who confirmed that smokers were suffering from pulmonary *ciliastasis*—the deadening of the tiny hairs (cilia) lining the lung that are supposed to waft away whatever dust or soot might gain entrance into the lungs. In a healthy person the foreign matter is surrounded by a mucous blanket and slowly pushed up the trachea, ending up at the back of the throat where it can be safely swallowed or spat out. From a series of experiments using the lungs of humans recently deceased and freshly killed oxen, Hilding showed that cilia are immobilized at precisely those parts of the lung where smoke impinges most directly—at forking points in the bronchial tubes, for example—which also turns out to be where cancers are most likely to develop. Hilding was too cautious to say he had *proven* smoking causes lung cancer, but he did characterize his evidence as "suggestive" of such a link, especially considering that smoking created "islands" of deciliated tissue where tars could collect— and remain for months or even years—duplicating the conditions under which Wynder et al. had shown that skin painting could produce cancers in experimental animals.[8]

Oscar Auerbach, chief of laboratory services at the Veterans Administration Hospital in East Orange, New Jersey, about this same time showed that tissues taken from the lungs of 117 deceased smokers were far more likely to have cellular abnormalities—including enlarged nuclei, basal hyperplasia, and squamous metaplasia—than tissues taken from non-smokers. To prevent bias, the tissues were randomly coded to make sure the pathologists doing the classification wouldn't know which group they had come from. Auerbach found that smokers' lungs were damaged in direct proportion to how long they had smoked and that cellular aberrations were common even in smokers who had not yet developed cancer. He conducted this work over a number of years, but by June 1955 the national media had begun to cover his effort to find "direct biological evidence" and "a missing link" in the causal chain joining smoking with lung cancer. For Auerbach and his collaborators this new source of evidence was "fully consistent with the theory that cigarette smoking is an important factor" in the causation of bronchogenic carcinoma.[9] Important also was that a clear dose response was observed: the more people smoked, the more likely they were to develop abnormal cellular growths and patches of denuded cilia, paving the way for tars to accumulate in their lungs. Yet another nail was driven into this coffin when Hermann Druckrey, a distinguished German pharmacologist at the University of Freiburg, showed that the hazardous chemicals in cigarette smoke could penetrate into the interior of human epithelial cells. Ernst Wynder was particularly impressed, testifying for a congressional committee (investigating filters) that "the suspected agent has been found at the scene of the crime."[10]

Chemical analytics.   Angel Roffo was the first to find benzpyrene in tobacco smoke—which he identified by its fluorescent spectrum—but by the mid-1950s most of the tobacco industry's laboratories had confirmed not just benzpyrene, but a number of other polycyclics in tobacco smoke, joining the list of poisons previously identified. Arsenic, formaldehyde, and ammonia had long been known to exist in cigarette smoke, and acrolein had been found prior even to the 1920s, but the number of such agents expanded dramatically in the 1950s. Benzpyrene was verified in several different laboratories; Teague in his 1953 "Survey" reviewed Roffo's work along these lines from the 1930s, and Brown & Williamson by 1952 had also achieved "a partial isolation and identification of a carcinogenic hydrocarbon, benzopyrene," in cigarette smoke.[11] New analytic techniques developed after the war—notably chromatography, mass spectrometry, and methods using radioactive tracers—made it possible to find ever smaller quantities of chemicals in smoke, and Auerbach's and Hilding's work prompted efforts to identify ciliastats. The notion here was that even if they didn't directly cause cancer, chemicals harming the "mucociliary escalator" might still promote the disease by interfering with the lungs' natural cleaning mechanisms. Scientists in France and elsewhere by the end of the 1950s had identified several different ciliastats in cigarette smoke, notably phenols, aldehydes, and ketones.[12]

Techniques of this sort made it possible for tobacco company chemists to construct long (unpublished) lists of carcinogens in tobacco smoke. Arthur D. Little researchers working for Liggett in 1961, for example, concluded that cigarette smoke contained not just "poisonous" but also "cancer causing" and "cancer promoting" chemicals. Philip Morris's powerful chief of research that same year identified forty distinct carcinogens in cigarette smoke (see Figure 26). Industry lists such as these never saw the light of day, however, and for decades thereafter the companies would deny that any trustworthy source had ever established a link between smoking and cancer—which contrasts starkly with their concessions to one another in private. Alan Rodgman, Reynolds's powerful Senior Research Chemist, summarized the situation in a confidential 1962 report titled "The Smoking and Health Problem": "Obviously the amount of evidence accumulated to indict cigarette smoke as a health hazard is overwhelming. The evidence challenging such an indictment is scant." Rodgman held out hope for alternative causes but acknowledged that the Surgeon General was likely to indict cigarette smoke in the report then being prepared. And that the TIRC's own Paul Kotin had endorsed the 1957 assessment of the NIH/ACS Study Group on Smoking and Health that "the sum total of scientific evidence" had established "beyond reasonable doubt" that cigarettes were a causal factor in the ongoing epidemic of cancer of the lung.[13]

FACTS ON THE GROUND

Animal experiments, epidemiology, clinical pathology, and chemical analytics were all crucial for the cancer consensus of the 1950s. And researchers often appreciated these mutually reinforcing lines of evidence: Wynder cited Roffo and Doll and Hill; Doll and Hill cited Wynder and Graham; and so forth. And in Germany, methodological reinforcement of this sort was already a feature of the pre-war landscape. German scholars in the 1930s drew attention to the parallels between tobacco tar and coal tar, both of which had been shown to cause cancer in experimental animals. Smoking was recognized as tantamount to repeatedly "painting" the lungs with tobacco tars, with an impressive 100 grams of tar inhaled for every kilogram of tobacco smoked. Roffo had emphasized this comparison, calculating that a year of moderate smoking could bring nearly half a kilogram of tar into the lungs—enough to fill a small beaker. Roffo had also stressed that recognition of a tobacco–cancer link had sprung from the confluence of very different evidentiary traditions, ranging from clinical experience and epidemiology to chemical analytics and animal experimentation in the laboratory.[14]

Quite apart from the industry's obstinacy, however, it wasn't easy to recognize cigarettes as carcinogens until large numbers of people were smoking them. Lung cancer typically has a latency of thirty, forty, or even fifty or more years from first exposure to onset of symptoms, which is why the epidemic didn't appear until decades after the cigarette boom. Inhalation was also not such a common way of smoking until the popularization of low smoke-pH Virginia blend cigarettes in the early decades of the twentieth century. Cancer in this respect is different from the situation in, say, astronomy, where the objects of inquiry are uninfluenced by human actions. Cancer is *a historical phenomenon,* insofar as what actually causes the disease can change over time. Cancers of the lung are essentially twentieth-century phenomena, because inhalable cigarettes are essentially twentieth-century phenomena.[15]

Which brings us to yet another source for the lung cancer consensus, albeit one less tangible, more indirect. Ernst Wynder called it "presumptive" evidence, meaning basically that cigarettes were a plausible explanation; they were at the scene of the crime, and the explanation made more sense than the available alternatives. *Presumptive evidence* began building in the 1920s, when scholars started noticing the rise of lung cancers and looking around for explanations. Tobacco for a time was just one of many possible causes, along with poison gas from the First World War, asphalt dusts or vapors from newly tarred roads, urban air fouled from industrial pollution, and delayed effects (such as lung scarring) from the 1918–19 flu pandemic that killed tens of millions worldwide. Some scholars thought that cancers might grow from old scars or from exposure to tuberculosis or pneumonia; others imagined that the new fashion of eating tomatoes or using aluminum dishware might help explain the epidemic. All these theories (and many more) were in play in the 1930s and 1940s, though by the end of this period cigarettes had risen to the top of the explanatory pile.

One reason cigarettes rose to the top of this pile was that the evidence was never strong for the alternatives. German scholars in the 1930s had shown that smokers inhaled far higher levels of tar and soot than people driving close behind a car or a truck; there was also the fact that non-smokers living in the city seemed to be no more likely to contract cancer than non-smokers living in the clean-air countryside. Studies of air pollution showed that while acute effects could be significant—as with London's deadly "fogs" from the early 1950s—chronic cancer effects were not so clear. Negative evidence of this sort was as important as the positive: Jerome Cornfield et al. in an authoritative review of 1959 noted that while the epidemiology and animal experiments uniformly implicated cigarettes, there were "serious inconsistencies in reconciling the evidence with other hypotheses which have been advanced."[16]

KEY CONSENSUS STATEMENTS

This does not of course mean that all (honest) doubters disappeared. But it does mean that it becomes increasingly hard to deny the overwhelming mass of evidence—unless of course you are trapped in some intellectual backwater or ensnared by the industry's campaign of deception. Dissenters were progressively marginalized, and more often than not in the employ of the companies. Published expressions of this consensus are numerous in the 1950s and can be found in medical editorials, reviews, and textbooks; in annual reports of medical associations; and in "white papers" and resolutions issued by public health authorities. Key consensus statements include the following:

- In 1952 the International Union against Cancer, meeting at Louvain, Belgium, issued a resolution that "there is now evidence of an association between cigarette smoking and cancer of the lung, and that this association is in general proportional to the total consumption." The same organization two years later, meeting in São Paulo, resolved that "additional studies support the view adopted in the previous Symposium and point to the association mentioned (between smoking and lung cancer) as of causative nature."[17]
- In 1953, an editorial in the prestigious *New England Journal of Medicine* characterized Doll and Hill's recent epidemiology as yielding "evidence of an association between cigarette smoking and lung cancer so strong as to be considered proof within the everyday meaning of the word." Indeed "If similar data had incriminated a food contaminant that was not habit forming and was not supported by the advertising of a financial empire, there is little doubt that effective counter-measures would have followed quickly." This same journal in January of 1954 described the clinical statistical evidence linking smoking to lung cancer as "massive."[18]

- In November of 1953 a statistical panel set up by Britain's Chief Medical Officer in the Ministry of Health concluded that the statistical connection between
smoking and lung cancer was "real," with "a strong presumption, until some
positive evidence to the contrary is found, that the connection between smoking and lung cancer is causal." Geoffrey Todd, chief statistician at Imperial Tobacco and director of Britain's powerful Tobacco Research Council, was disappointed but "soon came to see that the Panel had reached the right conclusion."[19]
- On February 12, 1954, following a three-year investigation, Britain's Standing
Advisory Committee on Cancer and Radiotherapy announced that the relationship between smoking and lung cancer was "causal" and that "the risk increases
with the amount smoked, particularly of cigarettes." Iain Macleod, Britain's
minister of health, endorsed the findings of the committee in a speech before
the House of Commons, embracing its conclusion that the causal link between
smoking and lung cancer "must be regarded as established." The distinguished
Danish cancer statistician Johannes Clemmesen predicted "a steady rise in
bronchial cancer" as a result of addiction to "a Red Indian habit."[20]
- The American Cancer Society's National Board of Directors in October of 1954
announced "without dissent" that "the presently available evidence indicates an
association between smoking, particularly cigarette smoking, and lung cancer,
and to a lesser degree other forms of cancer." The Society in its *Annual Report*
characterized this association as "definite" and noted that there should be "no
question of the facts," namely, that a heavy smoker was "at least five times as
likely to develop lung cancer" as someone who had never smoked. Cornelius
Rhoads, research director at the Memorial Center for Cancer in Manhattan,
identified the "underlying medical question" as "settled," and the Sloan-Kettering
Institute for Cancer Research concluded that "The heavy inhaler clearly has a
much greater chance of acquiring lung cancer than does the non-smoker" and
that for anyone attempting to understand the cause of this epidemic, tobacco
smoke in the lungs "can no longer be ignored as a primary factor." The Public
Health Cancer Association that same year issued a resolution advising the public to stop smoking to prevent cancer.[21] And inventors filing patents for filters
started giving as a reason that cigarette smoke "has a tendency to produce
lung cancer."
- Cancer societies in Norway, Sweden, Finland, Denmark, and the Netherlands
over the next couple of years made similar statements, as did the Joint Tuberculosis Society of Great Britain and Canada's National Department of Health
and Welfare. On November 6, 1954, Dr. Horace Joules at a conference of Britain's Socialist Medical Association affirmed there was "no doubt whatever" that
the main cause of cancer of the lung was "excessive smoking of cigarettes."[22]
- Carl V. Weller, a distinguished pathologist at the University of Michigan, in
his 1955 *Causal Factors in Cancer of the Lung* wrote that though formerly a

skeptic, he now agreed "with many of the specialists in statistical analysis and in the epidemiology of cancer, that this association has been established."[23] Many other skeptics—Clarence W. Lieb and C. P. Rhoads, for instance—were "converted" by the evidence and started embracing the consensus.

· Charles S. Cameron, Medical and Scientific Director of the American Cancer Society and another former skeptic, in 1956 wrote, "If the degree of association which has been established between cancer of the lung and smoking were shown to exist between cancer of the lung, and say, eating spinach, no one would raise a hand against the proscription of spinach from the national diet."[24]

· The chair of Britain's Medical Research Council in 1956 characterized the smoking–lung cancer link as "incontrovertible" and noted that evidence from Britain and elsewhere had shown that lung cancer mortality was "20 times greater among heavy smokers than among non-smokers."[25]

· Britain's Medical Research Council in June of 1957 issued a statement concluding that "a major part" of the increase in lung cancer was associated with smoking, "particularly in the form of cigarettes," and that the relationship was "one of direct cause and effect." Britain's health minister endorsed the statement and reported to the House of Commons that "the most reasonable interpretation of the very great increase in deaths from lung cancer in males during the past twenty-five years is that a major part of it is caused by smoking tobacco."[26]

· Also in June of 1957 the Study Group of distinguished scholars from the National Cancer Institute, the American Cancer Society, the National Heart Institute, the American Heart Association, and several leading U.S. schools of medicine concluded after a year of intensive review that "the sum total of scientific evidence establishes beyond reasonable doubt that cigarette smoking is a causative factor in the rapidly increasing incidence of human epidermoid carcinoma of the lung." The report was endorsed by U.S. Surgeon General Leroy E. Burney, who pointed to "an increasing and consistent body of evidence that excessive cigarette smoking is one of the causative factors in lung cancer." The Surgeon General also concluded that "many independent studies" had confirmed "beyond reasonable doubt that there is a high degree of statistical association between lung cancer and heavy and prolonged cigarette smoking."[27]

· Also in 1957 the Netherlands Ministry of Social Affairs and Public Health published a statement recognizing the smoking–lung cancer link.[28]

· In 1958 Sweden's Medical Research Council reported to the king of Sweden, citing publications by the U.S. Study Group and Britain's Medical Research Council to conclude that substances inhaled with cigarette smoke "constitute, in all probability, an essential factor in the occurrence of certain types of lung cancer." The report also expressed the hope that smoke "could be made free from cancer-producing substances."[29]

· In 1960 the American Cancer Society Board of Directors reaffirmed as "beyond a reasonable doubt" that smoking is "the major cause of the unprecedented increase in lung cancer."[30] That same year a seven-nation panel of experts from the World Health Organization concluded that "the association between smoking and lung cancer has been demonstrated" and that "the available evidence indicates that cigarette smoking is a major causative factor." This was a conclusion based on "extensive research" about which there was "no serious doubt."[31]

- In 1961 the Council of the Canadian Medical Association meeting in Montreal released a statement characterizing cigarette smoking as the "principal causative factor" in the lung cancer epidemic. A review published by Norman Delarue characterized the link as "inescapable" and "beyond any reasonable doubt."[32]

- In 1962 Britain's Royal College of Physicians, after a two-year investigation, concluded that smoking was "an important cause of lung cancer" and that if the habit were to cease "the death rate from lung cancer would eventually fall to a fraction, perhaps to one fifth or even, among men, to one tenth of the present level."[33]

Even a few frustrated tobacco company attorneys were admitting this consensus—internally—as early as 1961. An American Tobacco Company lawyer penned a memo that year mocking the industry's public stance that "few" medical men acknowledged a danger:

> Regarding the "few" who ascribe a causal effect to smoking: these "few" would include the Surgeon General of the United States for the Public Health Service, the Commissioner of Health of New York State, the California State Department of Public Health, the Public Health Cancer Association, the Ministry of Health of England and Wales, the Study Group of the American Cancer Society, American Heart Association, National Cancer Institute and National Heart Institute, the Medical Research Council of Great Britain, the Netherlands Ministry of Social Affairs and Public Health, the State Medical Research Council of Sweden, the American Public Health Association, the National Tuberculosis Association and the Study Group of the World Health Organization, among others.[34]

This same lawyer would later admit that

> By the time of filing of the first suit [against the tobacco companies], *Lowe* in St. Louis in March 1954, the medical case against cigarettes was regarded as proved beyond question by the vast majority of the general public and the medical profession.[35]

THE 1964 SURGEON GENERAL'S REPORT

It therefore came as icing on the cake—or rather a kind of scientific anticlimax—when the U.S. Surgeon General concluded in January of 1964 that smoking was "causally related to lung cancer in men." That conclusion came as a result of thirteen months of careful examination of the scientific literature, assisted by 155 consultants and an energetic supporting staff, all trying to assess the state of scientific knowledge with regard to smoking and health. The document is significant by virtue of the methods used: scholars from several different disciplines were chosen to serve on the Advisory Committee responsible for drafting the document, and great care was taken to survey the entirety of literature available on the topic. Allan Brandt credits the report as the first example of what he calls "procedural science," meaning science deliberately organized in such a way as to guarantee a rock-solid armor against impeachment.[36]

The Surgeon General's report is nonetheless flawed in a number of interesting respects. For one thing, there is the odd fact that members of the Advisory Committee were required never to have taken a stand on the question of smoking and health. That is not how one might normally imagine the constitution of an expert body; imagine an expert report on, say, climate change or world hunger that required those drafting the report never to have published on the topic. This was an expert report of innocents: the experts were naive to a certain extent, more like a jury trying to reach a verdict than a scholarly body coming to novel conclusions of fact. The facts were pretty much already known to those closest to the evidence; the report produced what I prefer to call an *administrative* rather than a *scientific* consensus—as the science had been pretty much nailed down a decade earlier.

The report was also extraordinary in that the tobacco industry was granted power to veto anyone nominated to serve on the committee. As if polio had a vote in what kind of vaccine to develop. Recognizing this veto power, great care was taken not to allow on the committee anyone who was strongly anti-tobacco; about half the committee, in fact, were smokers. More sinister is the fact that two members had previously worked as consultants for the cigarette industry: Maurice H. Seevers, chair of the Department of Pharmacology at the University of Michigan, had consulted for American Tobacco; and Louis F. Fieser, a Harvard chemist and the inventor of napalm, had worked for both Liggett & Myers and Arthur D. Little (on benzpyrene in cigarette paper) since the early 1950s.

Fieser turned out to be relatively ineffectual, but Seevers ended up—as he had started—a crucial tobacco ally. It was his voice that convinced the committee to pronounce smoking "a habit" rather than "an addiction," despite significant evidence (and internal industry concessions) to the contrary. Twenty-five years would pass before this crucial oversight was corrected: the first U.S. Surgeon General's report to recognize tobacco as addictive did not appear until 1988.[37] For that delay we can thank not just Seevers but also decades of resistance from the industry, fearful of the legal consequences of any such admission. The industry's own internal correspondence makes this fear explicit, as in 1980, when lawyers from Shook, Hardy and Bacon characterized addiction as "the most potent weapon a prosecuting attorney can have in a lung cancer/cigarette case." Their reasoning was sound: "We can't defend continued smoking as 'free choice' if the person was 'addicted.' "[38] Which of course is why it was always crucial to keep this off the table. Seevers in 1964 managed this for the industry, paving the way for a quarter-century delay in official recognition of tobacco's addicting power.

Seevers was an important figure in the history of addiction obfuscation. His adamant refusal was based on his view that nicotine did not cause antisocial behavior and was not intoxicating. Richard Kluger puts it nicely in his *Ashes to Ashes:*

> To Seevers, addiction meant an overpowering desire to continue using a drug, a tendency or need to keep increasing the dose, a physical dependency, withdrawal symptoms that could be life-threatening, and the user's willingness "to obtain it by any means"—a none too thinly veiled reference to antisocial acts like robbery to pay for the habit. The alternative term, habituation—which was how Seevers characterized cigarette smoking—did not involve constantly escalating dosages, implied a psychological rather than physical dependency that could be rather more easily broken, and was not associated with antisocial acts.[39]

Kluger goes on to point out that the absence of the psychopathology we associate with "harder" drugs may have something to do with the fact that cigarettes have been "cheap, ubiquitous, and legal," which of course has not been true for heroin or opium. There was also the difficulty of grasping addiction on such a scale, given the ubiquity of smoking: was half the American adult population to be branded a bunch of addicts?

Nicolas Rasmussen of the University of New South Wales has shown that there is more to this story, however. Seevers in the 1930s had worked as a consultant for the pharmaceutical industry, spending quite some time defending amphetamines against the charge of being addictive. Seevers came up with the argument that amphetamines could not be addictive because they were *stimulants,* unlike debilitating intoxicants such as heroin or the opiates. Nicotine was a stimulant, which by his definition meant it could not be addictive. Nor could cocaine—or any other stimulant. Seevers was an influential member of the World Health Organization (WHO) committee that in 1957 ruled that cigarette smoking was a "habit" and not an addiction, and it was only in breaking with Seevers that the WHO recognized smoking as more than a habit—in 1964—too late for inclusion in the Surgeon General's report. Seevers also managed to have himself appointed head of the AMA's whitewash Committee for Research on Tobacco and Health, part of the Education and Research Foundation, which from 1964 through 1973 dispensed $10 million in tobacco industry money for research with little or no bearing on addiction or any other tobacco-related harm. Seevers supervised this "total fiasco" (as Kotin later characterized it) for more than a decade, cementing the joint embrace of Big Tobacco and Big Medicine that, even at the time, was regarded as "blackening" the AMA's public image. And all in exchange for the industry's support in quashing socialized medicine.[40]

It is therefore wrong to regard the Surgeon General's report as an "unimpeachable" assessment of the science of the time. It was biased by the contrived means by which it was constituted, by the exclusion of leading authorities, and by the infiltration of industry allies. It was biased by its cautious rhetoric of understatement and by its bizarre inclusion of marginal topics—the final distracting chapters on somato-types, for example, which waffle around in the mire of constitutional predispositions (thanks to Carl Seltzer, the industry's quasi-Harvard point man). A committee representing the best science of the time would have come to stronger conclusions, without so many of the qualifications that made their way into the final text.[41]

Also crucial is that the Surgeon General's Advisory Committee did not have access to the industry's internal work on smoking and health. The committee was never told about Teague's survey, or Ecusta's condensate and whole smoke experiments, or details of the Runyon Fund–NYU collaboration, or the long lists of smoke carcinogens compiled by Reynolds, Philip Morris, and the other companies. The committee wasn't privy to BAT's confessions from 1961 that smokers were "nicotine addicts," or to Brown & Williamson's 1963 confession that the company was "in the business of selling nicotine, an addictive drug." Nor were they told about the research underlying the 1962 brag by Sir Charles Ellis of BAT that his company possessed a knowledge of nicotine "far more extensive than exists in published scientific literature."[42]

A GRAVE CRISIS AVERTED

Of course it is still fair to regard the Surgeon General's report as a document of substantial *political* significance and a turning point in the broader public recognition of tobacco hazards. The report put the stamp of government approval on the reality of the cancer link—at least for men—and in some sense marked the beginning of the end for smoking in the United States. Per capita smoking rates began to fall from this point on—though we should also realize that this per capita drop was not very steep, and *total* U.S. consumption would continue to rise for nearly two decades, reaching a peak of about 630 billion cigarettes in the early 1980s. And even the political force of the Surgeon General's report was not what it could and should have been. Tobacco manufacturers were actually pleased with the response: smoking rates fell rather dramatically for a couple of months following the press conference announcing the report but had pretty much recovered by the end of the year. Less than a month after its appearance, Philip Morris Vice President George Weissman wrote to his CEO, Joseph F. Cullman III, expressing his relief that the public reaction had not been as severe as feared. Press reflections were "comparatively mild," and even the most serious opponents of the industry had not come up with "life or death" proposals for the industry; the "grave crisis" was averted.[43]

Tobacco industry profits would in fact continue to grow for decades. That is largely because the cartel wielded enormous political power in Washington and indeed throughout the Americas. Big Tobacco had friends at the highest levels of government, and resistance was widely recognized as treacherous. That is probably why President Lyndon Johnson never endorsed the Surgeon General's report, despite urgings from his cabinet to do so. Johnson of course had other things on his mind: President Kennedy had been assassinated less than two months previously, and the vice president had assumed the reins of power in some haste. Johnson was urged to embrace the report and to move against cigarettes by his undersecretary for health, the young Joseph Califano, but the president knew the Democrats were weak among whites in the tobacco-growing South, largely as a result of having championed the cause of racial desegregation. Johnson told Califano that taking on Big Tobacco could mean a loss for the Democrats in the next presidential election, a political risk he was not willing to take. [44] That's how powerful tobacco has been. More powerful arguably even than Big Oil, since Johnson felt no qualms about endorsing the reality of global warming ("This generation has altered the composition of the atmosphere on a global scale through . . . a steady increase in carbon dioxide from the burning of fossil fuels.")[45]

Though widely reported as news, the Surgeon General's report was actually something of an anticlimax for those on the frontiers of the relevant science. We also need to realize that the report never would have been written—there would have been no need—if the industry had not been so adamant in opposing the science. The U.S. government never would have felt compelled to organize such an odd and unprecedented inquiry. The scientific case against tobacco was largely closed by the mid-1950s, and the perceived need to test and certify this by a neutral board of inquiry—a kind of trial by scientific jurors—tells us more about the power of Big Tobacco than any purported precariousness of the science. Recall Charles Cameron's observation (from 1956) that if similar evidence had been found against spinach, it would have been barred from the national diet. Half a dozen food dyes were banned in the United States in the 1950s on far less evidence. The persistence of tobacco is a testament to the industry's political and economic clout, joined with an unparalleled mastery of the arts of denial, deception, and distraction. Plus of course the addictive power of the nicotine molecule.

INDUSTRY ADMISSIONS

For the Anglo-American scientific community, a consensus was established in the 1950s that smoking was a significant cause of lung cancer. We also have instances where tobacco manufacturers admitted as much, albeit only privately. Teague's "Survey of Cancer Research" and the animal experiments conducted by Ecusta and the NYU–Runyon Fund circle come to mind, but there are other examples. On March 25, 1954, for example, top researchers and executives from Liggett & Myers met with Arthur D. Little, Inc., to discuss plans for a series of experiments to verify Wynder et al.'s work with mice. Liggett had recently hired the firm to conduct a series of such tests, with the plan also being to test whether different brands might be carcinogenic in differing degrees. Toward the end of the meeting Frederick R. Darkis, Liggett's chief of research, commented to the group that "if we can eliminate or reduce the carcinogenic agent in smoke we will have made real progress." We have the minutes from this meeting,[46] and it seems that none of those in attendance challenged his premise, that there was in fact some cancer-causing agent in cigarette smoke. The question was clearly not *whether* but rather *how* such agents might be operating, with suspects including arsenic, polycyclics, phenols, sterol oxidation products, or even a virus carried over from the plant.

Another admission comes from 1952, when a U.S. company started marketing a stop-smoking aid under the brand name Nicotol, a dopamine releaser containing lobeline, an alkaloid derived from "Indian tobacco" *(Lobelia inflata).* Hanmer had been alerted to a two-page ad for the drug in the *Boston Sunday Advertiser* and noted in an evaluation for his company's advertising manager that the ad's identification of carbon monoxide, arsenic, and cyanide in tobacco smoke "could not be challenged." Hanmer also admitted that Raymond Pearl was probably right to have concluded that smokers die an early death: Pearl was "a distinguished scientist and his conclusions stand." Hanmer concluded that any attempt to quarrel with the ad would probably be regarded as quibbling, so no public comment was issued. "Perhaps the advertisers of Nicotol have an Achilles heel, but we haven't been able to find it."[47] Hanmer was clearly frustrated that the scientific tide was turning against his company, a frustration also expressed in a letter he wrote to President Hahn at American Tobacco on November 19, 1953, shortly before the launch of the formal conspiracy. Hanmer here described a conversation with the Stanford biochemist A. Clark Griffin about Wynder et al.'s soon-to-be-published mouse-painting experiments, noting Griffin's view "that if someone performed research which contradicted the studies and the conclusions of Wynder and Graham he would be able to publish it only at considerable risk to his reputation; that it would bring down the wrath of the medical profession on him and that if anyone had the courage to do so, he might lose his position, so great would be the pressure upon the institution and the department which he represented."[48] Of course there could be no "wrath" or "pressure" from the medical profession unless such views were strongly held. Hanmer and Griffin here reveal that Wynder et al. had sufficient authority to make tobacco–cancer deniers feel beleaguered, marginalized—which is yet another index of a consensus.

And European manufacturers were coming to similar conclusions. In France in summer 1958, John M. Moseley, Manager of Basic Materials Research at American Tobacco, recorded the "unavoidable conclusion" of Dr. Jean-Louis Cuzin of the French "Regie" (Tobacco Monopoly):

> Dr. Cuzin told me privately that they had reached the unavoidable conclusion, based on the results of animal experimentation and statistical studies, that there is a cause

and effect relationship between smoking and lung cancer and that he had been instructed by the French Regie to make an official statement to the effect at the London Cancer Meeting in July 1958. It is apparent that Dr. Cuzin has been greatly influenced by Dr. Ernest Wynder. I asked Dr. Cuzin what would be the next step by the French government concerning this matter and he did not know. He did not think that the French people could be dissuaded from smoking and said that they did not care.[49]

Moseley had earlier acknowledged the French monopoly's acceptance of "the anti-cigarette evidence as establishing a cause and effect connection between smoking and lung cancer"; Cuzin repeated this same conviction to Moseley three years later—in 1961—noting that it was "the official position of the French Regie that there is an association between cigarette smoking and lung cancer." Cuzin by this time had been charged by the French monopoly with producing a "safer" cigarette "with good taste"; he believed that by reducing benzpyrene it should be possible to make a cigarette "which is 30% safer," perhaps by reducing the width of cut of the tobacco to allow for a more complete combustion.[50] French investigators in Raymond Latarjet's laboratory in Paris were also investigating the use of palladium catalysts to burn up some of these polycyclic aromatic hydrocarbons, a trick later used by Liggett for its Project XA cigarette.

French tobacco makers in the 1950s had a more honest relationship with the scientific community than their British or American counterparts. It may have helped that the French industry was a state-run monopoly; crucial also, however, is that the French were not yet smoking nearly as many cigarettes as the English or the Americans. French smokers tended also to prefer black tobacco blends, which by virtue of being harsher—more alkaline—were less often inhaled and therefore less prone to cause lung cancer.[51] This help explains why less was made of the cigarette–cancer link in France than elsewhere: fewer French were smoking, not many of these were inhaling, and so fewer were dying from cancer. French male lung cancer mortality in the 1950s was only about one-third of that for males in the United Kingdom, a pattern nearly perfectly reversed over the course of the next four decades. For British males aged thirty-five to fifty-four, for example, lung cancer rates *fell* by more than a factor of three from 1960 to 2000, whereas comparable French rates over this same period *more than tripled*.[52] The difference stems from the fact that France and Britain have had very different smoking histories.

Recall that the British were smoking like chimneys in the 1930s and 1940s, yielding a hefty cancer harvest in the 1950s and 1960s. By contrast, the French were not such avid smokers in the prewar years, nor were they so much in the habit of inhaling, given their preference for harsh, high pH, black tobacco blends. Wartime occupation and postwar poverty caused shortages, and as late as the 1950s the French were smoking only about 600 cigarettes per person per year, compared with British levels four or five times this high (1,300 for women and 3,600 for men). This situation was reversed in the 1960s, 1970s, and 1980s, however, as British smoking rates fell (dramatically) while French rates rose. British lung cancer rates have been falling since the 1960s, whereas French rates didn't start to fall until the 1990s. Otherwise put: the French tobacco epidemic has unfolded very much like the British, albeit with a thirty- or forty-year delay.[53]

The important fact for the science historian, however, is that British industry researchers were as convinced as their French counterparts of the reality of tobacco hazards. John Moseley on his 1958 research tour visited Imperial Tobacco in Bristol, where he talked with Herbert R. Bentley, a chemist and number two man at one of the largest tobacco research laboratories in the world, with a staff of 125. Imperial at this time was supplying smoke condensates to T. D. Day at the University of Leeds for mouse-painting experiments but also to J. W. S. Blacklock at St. Bartholomew's Hospital in London for injection into rats' lungs and to Ilse Lasnitzki of Strangeways Laboratories in Cambridge for in vitro tissue culture of lung cells. Blacklock and Lasnitzki had already obtained tumors from smoke condensate, and all three of these scholars—along with Bentley himself—were convinced that cigarettes were causing cancer: "They think that the case has been proved," is how Moseley recorded it in his report to American Tobacco.[54] The question at Imperial was therefore not so much "whether" but rather "how" cigarettes caused cancer—with the hope being that the culprits could be isolated, identified, and removed.

As for identification, carcinogens known by the Imperial Tobacco Company to be in cigarette smoke as of 1958 included benzo- and dibenzopyrene, benz- and dibenzanthracene, beta-naphthol, butyric acid, and arsenic. The company had also had some success reducing benzpyrene via the addition of 5 percent ammonium sulfamate or one percent copper nitrate to the tobacco mix, tricks developed originally by H. J. Rand in Cleveland. These reduced the carcinogens in smoke by about half, but with extra copper nitrate this could be upped to about 80 percent. None of these made for a very tasty smoke, however, and the nitrate apparently also left a rather peculiar purple ash. Many other compounds had been tested but none with much success. Bentley was sorry to see Wynder's work holding up so well; he had hoped that the mouse-painting experiments would wither in the face of scrutiny. As of 1958 he was willing to concede—albeit only to his industry colleagues—that Wynder did have "good technique" and that his findings were "probably valid." British experimentalists had come to similar conclusions: Sir Ernest Kennaway, fêted for having proved the carcinogenic potency of coal tar dyes, in 1956 was "greatly impressed" by Wynder's work and blamed the failure of British efforts to replicate his experiments on improper technique, including their failure to use shaved mice. Professor Day at Leeds, working under contract from the Tobacco Manufacturers Standing Committee, was equally impressed—and by 1959 had managed to reproduce Wynder's experiments, a feat never revealed to the public.[55]

German manufacturers were more skeptical, owing perhaps to the stagnation of their science in the wake of the war and postwar poverty, perhaps also in reaction to the nazification of German science and the postwar survival of its denialist apparatus. A great deal of the country's manufacturing capacity had been destroyed during the war (or carted off to Russia), and in 1958 German smokers were smoking only ten cigarettes per day, compared with the thirty-six per day consumed by Americans. Dr. Franz Muth, head of research at Reemtsma's cigarette factory in Hamburg, found little reason to worry about cancer, given how few cigarettes were being smoked in Germany. Wynder had tried to draw attention to the cancer evidence during a May 6, 1958, trip to Munich but was disappointed: Wynder complained to his German colleagues about the American industry's suppression of two legal cases on behalf of widows of lung cancer victims and hoped for greater cooperation in the Fatherland. Reemtsma's lab had been unable to find benzpyrene in the smoke of German cigarettes, however, and Hermann Druckrey, working now for Reemtsma, was looking instead for carcinogens in some of the pesticides used on tobacco and in certain additives. (As director of the German Cancer Research Institute in Heidelberg, Druckrey was a powerful figure in German cancer research, despite some residual taint from his Nazi background.) Muth thought the Americans should coordinate their research with Heidelberg and with Reemtsma: "Everyone should work together to find out if and what is the cancer forming agent in smoke and then do away with it." Muth didn't like how TIRC research was being exploited in American advertising and informed Moseley of his view that "too much [was] being said about the amount of money being spent." Muth did perceive a danger to the industry from the cancer charge, however, and helped resurrect the denialist campaign in 1959 as chairman of the newly formed Scientific Research Station of the German Cigarette Industry. The German body maintained publicly that the cancer link was unproved and that assertions to the contrary threatened "investigation of the true causes of this disease." In a 1960 article written with Druckrey among others, Muth observed that tobacco smoke was only "weakly carcinogenic" by comparison with concentrated benzpyrene, though he did admit that the cancer-causing potential of smoke condensates could "hardly be subject to further doubt."[56]

John Moseley visited a dozen-odd research laboratories in as many countries, and there is probably no better assessment of European manufacturers' state of mind than his sixty-page report from 1958. Moseley recorded widespread criticism of U.S. advertising but also a "tacit agreement not to trade on, or refer to, the anti-cigarette charges beyond the simple use of the word 'filter.'" This so-called Gentlemen's Agreement helps explain the global silence of the industry on matters of smoking and health. European manufacturers by and large accepted the reality of the cancer link but would not admit this openly, given the delicacy of the American legal situation. As late as 1976, Sydney J. Green, BATCo's senior scientist for research and development, commented (privately) on how "legal considerations" dominated the British industry's position with regard to smoking and disease. Green again in 1980 observed that fear of litigation had led the industry to reject "any possibility of any causal relationship between smoking and disease"; he also characterized the level of scientific proof required by the industry as "impossible, perhaps ridiculous," and a "formula for inaction and delay." He also commented on the psychology of such denials, characterizing them as "usually the first reaction of the guilty."[57]

THE MATH OF MEGADEATH—AND THE INSURANCE INDUSTRY'S DISCOUNTS

One thing epidemiology allows you to do is to calculate how many people are actually dying from smoking. This is really only a matter of grade-school math, once you have fixed the rates at which people are dying. Some of the most interesting early work of this sort came from Richard Doll, who in 1955 produced a remarkable chart plotting cigarette consumption from 1930 against lung cancer death rates from 1950.[58] The comparison was only for men and only for eleven European nations, but the results were striking and consistent: countries with high per capita smoking rates also had high lung cancer mortality rates (see Figure 27). The relationship was clearly linear, meaning that the more a society smoked, the more people would die from lung cancer—and in a predictable fashion. Doll's chart actually lets you calculate the rate at which people will die on a per cigarette basis: so a country smoking 1,000 cigarettes per person will suffer a lung cancer death rate of about 300 per million twenty years later.

Which also means—though Doll doesn't seem to have drawn this conclusion—that one lung cancer death is produced for every three million cigarettes smoked. Obviously there will be variations according to how cigarettes are smoked in any given society, including how far down on the butt and how likely people are to inhale, but the relationship is remarkably consistent and can be used to predict lung cancer rates anywhere in the world. Basically you just look at how many cigarettes are being smoked in any given society and divide by three million, and that is how many lung cancer deaths you will have in that society some twenty years later. Divide by a million, and you get the number of smoking-caused deaths that will result.[59]

In 1955, for example, when the filter fad was just getting going, smokers in the United States smoked a total of 400 billion cigarettes. Twenty-five years later, in 1980, there were an estimated 320,000 deaths from smoking.[60] So 400 billion cigarettes caused about 320,000 deaths, or about .7 deaths per million cigarettes. By 1980, however, smokers in the United States were smoking about 600 billion cigarettes, and these caused about 440,000 deaths in 2005—which is still about .7 deaths per million cigarettes. This is an effective riposte to anyone who believes that cigarettes have become safer: they have not. Don't forget also that medical treatments have improved somewhat over time, which means that deaths from smoking would be *even higher* in the absence of such improvements. We'll see in a later chapter that cigarette makers also put less tobacco in today's cigarettes—to insinuate an impression of safety—which means that *gram per gram* cigarettes have actually become more deadly. The tobacco industry has, in effect, managed to squeeze more death out of a given quantity of leaf.

Estimates of the total death toll from smoking in the United States began to appear in the 1930s—recall Van Noppen's figure of 100,000 deaths per year—and by the 1950s and 1960s were fairly common. One group with an early interest in such matters was the life insurance business, which flourished by virtue of knowing what causes some people to live a century while others sicken and die young. Frederick L. Hoffman at Prudential Life Insurance had linked pipe smoking to mouth cancer in his 1915 *Mortality from Cancer Throughout the World* and by 1931 had become one of the first statisticians to explore the smoking link in detail. The question eventually arose whether discounts should be offered to people who didn't smoke: Harry Dingman, medical director at the Continental Assurance Company, in a 1946 treatise titled *Risk Appraisal* threw down this gauntlet: "Use of tobacco entails extra mortality. In assessment of risk, why ignore it?"[61]

Underwriters of course are a conservative lot and seem not to have offered non-smokers' discounts prior to the 1960s. Fortune National Life in Madison, Wisconsin, implemented such a policy in January of 1963, with Executive Life Insurance of Beverly Hills and Great American Reserve Insurance in Dallas announcing similar plans shortly thereafter. Senator Maurine Neuberger in her 1963 book, *Smoke-screen,* observed that the "contempt for statistical evidence" expressed by tobacco makers was not shared by actuaries, judging from the growing number of companies offering "a substantial discount on life insurance to applicants who have not smoked for 24 months prior to their application and who are willing to forswear smoking for the foreseeable future." Neuberger added that insurers were "hardly noted for reckless risk-taking."[62]

Insurance discounts for non-smokers proliferated after the 1964 Surgeon General's report—even in North Carolina, the heart of Camel country, where State Mutual Life Assurance had begun offering them within months of the press conference announcing the report.[63] State Mutual was in fact the first major firm to offer such policies nationwide and sold $5.8 million worth to abstainers in the first six weeks. Farmers Group by the 1970s was offering non-smoker discounts even for *auto* insurance—because smokers tend to have more traffic accidents. (Germans had recognized this since the 1930s, whence the Nazi-era campaign to prevent smoking-while-driving.) Tobacco makers recognized the threat and in 1975 accused Farmers of deceptive and misleading advertising—misleading because, as Tobacco Institute President Horace Kornegay insisted to yet another insurer offering such discounts, "smoking has never been scientifically proven to be the cause of any disease."[64]

Cigarette industry opposition strengthened in the late 1970s, as increasing numbers of insurers started offering non-smokers' discounts. One skirmish for which we have a paper trail took place in the summer and fall of 1979 when Allstate, one of the nation's largest insurers, unveiled a plan to discount life insurance premiums for people who had not smoked a cigarette within the past twelve months. Allstate had designed an ambitious campaign to kick off its "Healthy American Plan," which Philip Morris learned about from backdoor channels at Leo Burnett, the advertising agency handling both Philip Morris and Allstate accounts. (Burnett had surreptitiously forwarded advance copies of Allstate's ads to Philip Morris.) Philip Morris asked the Tobacco Institute to organize a response, which took the form of an effort to pressure advertisers and insurance regulators, assisted by tobacco allies in the U.S. Congress and state agriculture departments.[65] Philip Morris CEO Ross Millhiser contacted his counterpart at Allstate; the Tobacco Institute also informed Allstate that while it knew of no plans to organize a formal boycott, the insurer could certainly expect "other segments" of the industry to "cease patronizing" both Allstate and its corporate parent, Sears.[66]

One argument used by cigarette manufacturers was that discounts of this nature would hurt regional tobacco economies. More common, though, was the charge of "insurance discrimination." Peter B. Sparber & Associates of Washington, D.C., was hired to orchestrate a nationwide campaign to protest the "discriminatory nature of nonsmoker discounts," with the goal being to "identify and support existing critics of the insurance industry to achieve insurance reform that prohibits discrimination against smokers." The plan was to identify smokers with other groups that might be suffering discrimination, which is why someone at the Tobacco Institute scrawled this query on Sparber's recommendations: "Gays—are they victims of ins[urance] discrimination?"[67]

The tobacco industry by 1979 had managed to get North Carolina's Department of Agriculture and the Tobacco Growers Information Committee to warn of the specter of "insurance discrimination." Some states tried to bar insurance companies from offering discounts, while others—notably West Virginia and Massachusetts—launched efforts to *require* such discounts. Most bizarre of all, perhaps, was a 1981 Philip Morris plan to offer special life insurance to smokers of Merit cigarettes, the company's flagship "low tar" brand. Cartons were to come with special inserts announcing the offer—called "Merit Life-Savers"—with the insurance to be supplied through the National Benefit Life Insurance Company of New York. It is unclear how far beyond the proposal stage this scheme ever went; planning documents make it clear that all sides recognized certain risks of "liability exposure."[68]

We do know, though, that insurers defended their rights to offer discounts. In October of 1979, for example, State Mutual Life released a study showing significant differences in mortality between smokers and non-smokers, commenting that differences such as these were "too large to be ignored for individual insurance underwriting and pricing purposes." Surgeon General Julius B. Richmond endorsed the study, adding that non-smokers "live about eight years longer than smokers."[69]

Indeed by this time it was not at all unusual for insurance companies to offer non-smokers' discounts. The Tobacco Institute in 1979 compiled a list of seventy-six American companies offering discounts of this sort,[70] and by 1985 an estimated 80 percent of *all* U.S. insurers were offering non-smokers' discounts.[71] The remarkable fact is that even companies partnered with Big Tobacco offered the discounts. CNA and Franklin Life, for example, owned by the same mega-conglomerates that owned Lorillard and American Tobacco, offered such policies, prompting one economist to remark, "Not only do they kill you . . . they bet that you're going to die." Gordon Lindsay in his marvelous satire, *Make a Killing,* compares the situation to that of the veterinarian practicing also as a taxidermist: "Either way, you get your dog back."[72]

One reason discounts of this sort were not offered even earlier is that insurers often held substantial investments in tobacco stocks. George E. Moore, director of the Roswell Park Memorial Institute in Buffalo, New York, commented on this in the early 1960s, noting in a letter to the *British Medical Journal* that non-smokers were being "penalized by having to support the additional illnesses and deaths of their smoking brethren."[73] Moore pointed out that investments in tobacco stocks "deterred" such companies from "penalizing smokers with higher insurance rates"— and that the sums involved were often sizable. Tobacco industry observers summarized the situation as follows, based on Moore's investigations: "The 1961 edition of 'Corporate Holdings of Insurance Companies' records that one very large insurance company had 15,000 preferred shares of American Tobacco Company . . . the largest U.S. life insurance company held $8,800,000 of R. J. Reynolds bonds; and the largest individual holdings of Liggett & Myers was $28,000,000 in bonds held by [an insurance] company with total assets in excess of $10,000,000,000."[74] So it was hardly surprising that many insurers didn't want to rock this boat. Insurers were in the business to make a profit, and if that meant going easy on an enterprise in which they themselves had a stake, then this would have to be factored into their calculations.[75]

TO "DISCREDIT AND DISARM THE FOE"

One overarching goal of this book is to address the question, how and when did it become known that smoking was killing people? This is often what is at stake in lawsuits, where the industry is accused of negligence, or failure to warn, or conspiring to commit fraud, and so forth. The companies want us to believe there was no scientific "consensus" in the 1950s, or any real reason to warn about smoking until some time after the Surgeon General's report of 1964. The Surgeon General's report, however, is not the beginning but rather the *end* or *official certification* of a process—at least from the point of view of the science. We're talking about a *political* document that was very much responding to—and framed within the confines of—the tobacco industry's enormous political and economic power. By this I mean that the Surgeon General's report never would have come into existence had the industry not been so powerfully obstinate.

In saying that the scientific case against cigarettes was essentially closed by the mid-1950s, I am not saying there were not dissenters or laggards. The point is rather that scientific work after this time was essentially a mop-up operation, at least when it came to lung cancer.

One reason we know that deception was taking root by this time is that the industry started to become more concerned with appearances. I've mentioned Claude Teague's cosmetic brown-turning filter, but there are many other instances of deliberate deception, including scientific espionage and surreptitious infiltration of the scientific and popular press. In October of 1953, for example, Hiram Hanmer hired a malacologist (a scholar of mollusks) by the name of Stanley Truman Brooks to help refute the emerging tobacco–cancer consensus. Brooks was an expert on Pennsylvania land snails, having spent the better part of his career as curator of mollusks in the Carnegie Museum of Natural History (1928–46) before hiring on with American Tobacco. Brooks was supposed to gather information useful for the publication of "educational articles" on tobacco and lung cancer and for this purpose traveled to Washington, D.C., and Bethesda to meet with NCI officials (including Harold Stewart and his assistant, Howard Steffee);[76] he also visited Adele Croninger, Wynder's assistant in St. Louis and coauthor of the mouse skin-painting paper from December of 1953. The goal in hiring Brooks was to undermine Wynder, using whatever ammunition might come from the industry's allies in Britain.

Brooks had not even read Wynder et al's paper but nonetheless felt comfortable assuring Hanmer on December 24, 1953, "We have enough material to befuddle the Wynder combination . . . the remaining job is to discredit and disarm the foe." Brooks was particularly keen to find "evidence of fudging" in Wynder's study and proposed a rather devious method:

> If I could go to Wynder's laboratory as an interested zoologist who would like to work in the laboratory for a month or so in order to learn the technique, I think it could be done. It is "the mystery of the easy cancers!"

Brooks also volunteered to use his press contacts to discredit Wynder.

> The public is not interested in scientific reasoning. Therefore, the newspaper is the most important channel. What we need is a person like Ray Sprigle, Pulitzer Prize winner, who is on the *Post Gazette*. . . . He would be a good one for the exposé.

The *Pittsburgh Post Gazette* would be a good venue, he says, since it was

> away from New York, away from the tobacco industry and would be a very good (psychologically and strategically) primary vehicle. It is an AM paper so any exposé would go directly on the wire to all other papers and hit the street the same day throughout

the USA. The "man on the street" could not connect it with the Wall Street group—that is important. It is a Bloch paper and I have many friends there—including the Bloch brothers, Sprigle, etc.

If I could produce the evidence, Sprigle could certainly put it across—he is also a heavy smoker! I also think I could wrangle a job with the Wynder group. . . . There should be a constant stream of knowledge going out which could be a rebuttal(s) on each of these Wynder pronouncements. It would be done nicely, not viciously, and could be good propaganda for the tobacco industry.

To disguise the source, Brooks would send out the column under his own name and use his home address. "Magazine attacks" were also entertained, and Brooks offered that he had already begun drafting one of these:

It could go out for use by some known magazine writers or be published under a pseudonym. Name writers would be necessary for the top flight magazines—as we discussed. But are the slicks the place we want to hit? . . . I wouldn't lend my name (my real name) to an article in these but a lot of MDs do. These pulps pick up their stuff any place they can find it and perhaps they would take our propaganda (and that is a good word as its source indicates) if fed to them. I could send the columns under my name and perhaps articles under a pseudonym.[77]

Think about what we have here: a scholar is conspiring with the world's most powerful tobacco company to write articles defending cigarettes under false pretenses, to infiltrate a scholar's laboratory to conduct espionage, and to publish under a pseudonym in venues designed to conceal a financial source. Information was to be gathered with the goal of acquiring "ammunition" to combat anti-tobacco "propaganda"—and Brooks's is by no means the only example of such abuse. Hiram Hanmer often met with science writers to advise them on how to get the industry's point of view across, and Reynolds in the fall of 1953 informed American, Brown & Williamson, Lorillard, and Philip Morris of its plan to establish an ambitious "Bureau of Scientific Information" to confute Wynder et al.—with the Camel maker's role in orchestrating this "news service" deliberately disguised.[78] And the Tobacco Institute itself, founded in 1958 as a spin-off from the TIRC, was little more than a mouthpiece for the industry's "no proof of harm" propaganda.

"WOULDN'T IT BE WONDERFUL!"

The final months of 1953 were fateful for the tobacco industry. Facing the deepest crisis ever in its history, cigarette makers went on the attack, denying any solid evidence that cigarettes were causing disease. The first big salvo came on November 26, 1953, when the American Tobacco Company issued a press release in which President Paul Hahn blasted what he called the "loose talk" on lung cancer. The public was to be "reassured," since no one had yet proved that lung cancer was "directly traceable to tobacco or to its products in any form." Hahn claimed that "for every expert who blames tobacco for the increase in respiratory disease there are others who speak with at least equal authority, who say that there is no evidence to show that tobacco is the cause." He also addressed the question of experimental carcinogenesis:

> There are a few scientists who report that by using a high concentration of cigarette smoke—entirely different from the smoke which a person draws from a cigarette—and painting it on the skins of mice, they have produced skin cancers on the mice. On the other hand, there are many more scientists of high repute who have made similar experiments and have reported that no cancers were produced. Moreover all scientists agree that there is no known relation between skin cancers on mice and lung cancers in humans.[79]

Hahn's press release marks the beginning of a new and far-reaching campaign to thwart the consensus falling into place. Hahn's claim that "for every expert who blames tobacco" there were others who said there was "no evidence" was simply false—as was quickly pointed out to the company in private correspondence. On December 17, 1953, Dwight Macdonald from the *New Yorker* wrote a long letter to Hanmer, noting that there were at least forty-three published medical authorities affirming the hazard, compared with only fourteen known to have denied it (since 1948). Far from being in the minority, the affirmers actually outnumbered the deniers by a factor of about three to one. Macdonald listed the authorities on both sides—along with the dates of their publications—and advised Mr. Hahn to "correct his mistake," especially since the subject was "too serious a one to be fooled around with." Hahn, however, never made any such correction. And Hanmer delayed responding to Macdonald until January 4, when he explained that he saw no "useful purpose" in "debating the various shades of opinions of the authorities." Hanmer didn't challenge Macdonald's three to one figure, however.[80]

The tobacco barons by this time were really only interested in authorities who could be coached onto their side. And Hahn's press release flew in the face even of the *experimental* results the industry was receiving from the Ecusta company and elsewhere. Shortly after Hahn's press release, the head of one of the nation's leading tobacco research departments effused in a document now preserved in the Hill Archives at the Wisconsin Historical Society: "Boy! Wouldn't it be wonderful if *our* company was first to produce a cancer-free cigarette. What we could do to competition!" This same document, from December of 1953, preserves one of the earliest known industry admissions of addiction, with yet another research director confiding to Hill & Knowlton, "It's fortunate for us that cigarettes are a habit they can't break."[81]

We don't know for sure who uttered these words—their names are not given in the documents. We only know that they came from two of the four research directors interviewed by Hill & Knowlton to get the lowdown on what the industry knew as of December 1953. Most likely they were part of the group that had attended the meeting of November 5, 1953, which included Hiram Hanmer (American Tobacco), Robert N. DuPuis (Philip Morris), A. Grant Clarke (R. J. Reynolds), Harris B. Parmele (Lorillard), and Irwin W. Tucker (Brown & Williamson). As for the "Boy! . . . cancer-free" comment: given that DuPuis and Clarke were suspicious of the NYU collaboration and that Hanmer and Tucker were not given to such outbursts, it could well have been the more enthusiastic Parmele from Lorillard. Parmele we know to have read "with a great deal of interest" the 1946 article by Engel ("Cigarettes Cause Cancer?"), which asked: "Which manufacturer will then be the first to meet the challenge? Which will seek ways to eliminate carcinogenic agents from tobacco tar and first be able to say in full truth: 'in my brand there is no carcinogenic tar'?"[82]

Hahn's press release is also notable because it introduces language that would find its way into the "Frank Statement" of January 4, 1954, the magna carta of the American industry's conspiracy to deny any evidence of tobacco harms. The press release cites Hahn's words: "At one time or another within the past 350 years practically every known disease of the human body has been ascribed to the use of tobacco. One by one these charges have been abandoned for lack of evidence." This exact same "One by one . . . " sentence is repeated *verbatim* in the "Frank Statement,"[83] and several other passages bear striking resemblances, suggesting the strong hand of Hahn in drafting the statement. Some passages echo even earlier remarks by American Tobacco research director Hiram Hanmer. In October of 1953, for example, Hanmer had written to the American Cancer Society, boasting of his company's extensive research in the area of smoking and health. Hanmer here too claimed that "the long history of smoking shows that, at one time or another, practically every known disease of the human body has been attributed to tobacco." Hanmer then claimed further that "notwithstanding claims of suggested 'statistical correlation,' no proof has been advanced that tobacco smoking is the cause of malignant disease of the respiratory tract."[84] Both would become mantras of the industry in subsequent decades.

THE PSYCHOLOGY OF DENIAL

The psychology of denial can be complex, but it can also be quite simple. It must have been unpleasant for cigarette makers to acknowledge they were killing people, and we can imagine different strategies for coping. People must have reminded themselves they had a job to do, perhaps a family to feed; and some may have even viewed it as a kind of game. Some thinking executives may have believed some "higher cause" was being served—freedom or pleasure, perhaps, or their company's right to sell a legal product. It is not hard to concoct rationalizations: Yes, cigarettes are deadly, but they also offer comfort and solace to millions. Yes, there is risk, but what in this world is without? And if we don't make them, won't others just take our place? And what is so great about longevity, anyway? Should health really be ranked over all other virtues? What about the life well lived or made vibrant from a brush with death? Philip Morris president Ross Millhiser predicted the eventual disappearance of the desire "to die in good health," and libertarian "admitters" could always raise the greater specter (than cigarette death) of government intrusion. And no one was forcing anyone to smoke . . . [85]

Attitudes of the executives must also have been somewhat like those of smokers who, as was appreciated by the industry, had a series of rationalizations for their continued "stupid" behavior. Here is how one Brown & Williamson document from 1970 imagined a smoker thinking about his habit:

> I know the cigarette is bad and smoking is dangerous, but I don't want to think about it. I love smoking and I am going to continue smoking. But, please don't remind me (directly or indirectly) that I am illogical, irrational and stupid.[86]

Cigarette makers may well have thought much the same about making and selling cigarettes:

> I know that selling cigarettes is bad and dangerous, but I don't want to think about it. I love selling cigarettes and I am going to continue doing so. But, please don't remind me that I am a duplicitous, racketeering, social parasite responsible for millions of unnecessary deaths.

This latter, of course, is (my) pure speculation. What we do know is that astonishingly few people actually left the business, or rather few that have left any traces in the historical record. One we do know about is Robert Wald, a former legal counsel for Lorillard who, in 1971, quit the company when he stopped being able to justify it to his family. In an interview for the *Wall Street Journal* Wald confessed, "I haven't the slightest doubt that cigarets cause lung cancer. I had to come home every night and face my kids' saying, 'Daddy, why do you work for a cigaret company?' "[87] Wald's conscientious objection is strikingly rare, however, and the archives are silent on his case. The industry's internal policing seems to have been quite effective, just as retirement benefits were generous and penalties for the turncoat severe.

The simplest explanation may be the best: some people can be bought—not all, of course, but enough. And the money was so good that few of those once on the gravy train ever found the courage to jump off.

PART THREE

Conspiracy on a Grand Scale

All too often in the choice between the physical health of consumers and the financial well-being of business, concealment is chosen over disclosure, sales over safety, and money over morality. Who are these persons who knowingly and secretly decide to put the buying public at risk solely for the purpose of making profits and who believe that illness and death of consumers is an appropriate cost of their own prosperity?

JUDGE H. LEE SAROKIN, RULING IN *HAINES V. LIGGETT*, 1992

If you're worried about cigarettes—may we confuse you with some facts?

TOBACCO INSTITUTE ADVERTISEMENT, 1971

LYING IS, among other things, an art. There are many ways to deceive, however, and it generally works best when you can cast yourself as an authority—or better yet, harness the authority of others. The marketing genius of the tobacco industry was carefully developed in the 1930s, with the goal being to "engineer consent" through multiple methods of persuasion. One was to go for the gut; another was to capture the media; another was to make so many groups dependent on you that to question cigarettes was to undermine the economic well-being of the nation. Or at least to generate such a specter.

How, though, was *science* harnessed to exculpate cigarettes? How did this particular form of duplicity get going, and why was it so successful? The terrain here is different from what we sometimes imagine when we think of corrupt science. The key is not so much that the companies *suppressed* science (which they certainly did), nor even that they spent far more to promote cigarettes than to study their health effects—which is also true. The genius of the industry was rather in using even "good" science, narrowly defined, as a *distraction,* something to hold up to say, in effect: See how responsible we are? Look at how much research we are funding!

Most of the research funded by the industry, though, had little to do with smoking and health. That was the whole point, to throw cash at projects that would pose no threat to business as usual. And in this they succeeded. The industry becomes a substantial funder of basic biomedical research, albeit research whose principal raison d'être was to distract from the reality of tobacco hazards. In this, the industry's support even for "good" science was part of the largest and deadliest campaign of deception the world has ever known. And many of those who took this money became its unwitting pawns.

Our task here is to explore this support for science, recognizing the tobacco industry first and foremost *as a disease vector,* in the apt formulation of Eric LeGresley, a lawyer with the World Health Organization's Tobacco Free Initiative:

> The world's most widespread, serious infection is purposely spread by its vector: the tobacco industry. To reduce the 500 million deaths tobacco industry products are projected to cause amongst those presently alive, public health advocates must study the life patterns of the tobacco industry as earnestly as they would any other disease vector. The investigative tools, however, are different. Rather than a tiny insect, this vector has economic resources rivalling those of many of the world's largest governments. . . .
>
> With more than a billion smokers worldwide, tobacco is mankind's most widespread serious infection, and among its most contagious. The pathway has recently become known: Its spread is mapped out in mahogany-lined boardrooms; it breeds its resistance to countermeasures in political backrooms; and it seizes its victims in adolescent bedrooms.[1]

LeGresley goes on to point out that one difference between tobacco and, say, a mosquito transmitting malaria is that the cigarette men know they are being studied. That is why "third party" agents are so often used—to disguise the nature of the process of contagion. Which is also why, as LeGresley notes, the tobacco industry now "more often appears cloaked as something else." Science, as we shall see, has served this purpose rather well.

The Council for Tobacco Research

Distraction Research, Decoy Research, Filibuster Research

> Your questions were: "Have we tried to find carcinogenic substances in tobacco smoke?" And we have not because we do not believe that they are there.
> CLARENCE COOK LITTLE, SCIENTIFIC DIRECTOR, TIRC, TESTIFYING
> IN *LARTIGUE V. REYNOLDS*, 1960

The year 1953 marks a turning point of sorts in human health fortunes. Deceptive claims had been made in ads for years—that Camels wouldn't cut your wind or jangle your nerves, for example—but Wynder et al.'s experimental demonstration of cancer from cigarette tars in December of that year demanded a more dramatic response. Smoking was charged with causing cancer, and popular media were reporting on the facts. What was the industry to do?

Looking back, the companies should have admitted the problem and stopped selling cigarettes. And leading industry figures promised as much. Philip Morris Vice President George Weissman in March 1954 announced that his company would "stop business tomorrow" if "we had any thought or knowledge that in any way we were selling a product harmful to consumers." James C. Bowling, the public relations guru and Philip Morris VP, in a 1972 interview asserted, "If our product is harmful . . . we'll stop making it." Then again in 1997 the same company's CEO and chairman, Geoffrey Bible, was asked (under oath) what he would do with his company if cigarettes were ever established as a cause of cancer. Bible gave this answer: "I'd probably . . . shut it down instantly to get a better hold on things." The other manufacturers made similar assurances. Lorillard's president, Curtis Judge, is quoted in company documents: "if it were proven that cigarette smoking caused cancer, cigarettes should not be marketed," and Judge himself would "quit his employment." R. J. Reynolds president, Gerald H. Long, in a 1986 interview asserted that if he ever "saw or thought there were any evidence whatsoever that conclusively proved that, in some way, tobacco was harmful to people, and I believed it in my heart and my soul, then I would get out of the business." Such were the promises.[1]

One reason the companies never admitted proof, or even evidence of any gravity, may be that they found themselves too far along in their campaign of denial to backtrack without causing a corporate catastrophe. Like a giant Ponzi scheme, there wasn't any coherent exit strategy. How did they think it would end? The companies' own laboratories were confirming cancer hazards—so there was always the danger that this, too, might come to light. And the longer the conspiracy went on, the darker were the prospects for any kind of innocent exit. The industry was in a difficult spot.

THE "FRANK STATEMENT"

American Tobacco President Paul M. Hahn launched the formal conspiracy on December 10, 1953, by inviting the CEOs of the other leading manufacturers to meet to plan a response to this tightening noose. And so on December 14 and 15 at the Plaza Hotel in downtown Manhattan, with Hahn in charge and the other companies falling in line, a decision was made to have the PR firm Hill & Knowlton coordinate a campaign of reassurance, spreading the message that the industry was doing everything in its power to determine the truth and to fix whatever might be wrong with cigarettes. "More research" was the mantra—by which was meant "the jury is still out." Hill & Knowlton in a memo from Christmas Eve, 1953, reminded Hahn et al. that the matter was one of "extreme delicacy," with the first task at hand being "not to add fuel to the flames." The firm recommended a program of research and education, the goal of which would be "reassurance of the public through wider communication of facts." And not just any facts: the public had to realize there were "weighty scientific views which hold there is no proof that cigarette smoking is a cause of lung cancer."[2]

The first public salvo of this new operation was released on January 4, 1954, as a full-page "Frank Statement to Cigarette Smokers" in newspapers throughout the United States. (See Figure 28.) Wynder et al.'s tar painting was singled out for attack: the experiment was denigrated as not "conclusive," and readers were led to believe that the "theory" that smoking was in some way to blame for lung cancer was just that, a theory, and really there was "no proof" cigarettes were one of the causes. The statement claimed that the statistics invoked to make such a claim "could apply with equal force" to any other aspect of modern life and that though critics had long blamed tobacco for "practically every disease of the human body," those charges had been abandoned "one by one" for lack of evidence. The industry also claimed to hold its customers' health as "a basic responsibility, paramount to every other consideration in our business"; signatories therefore promised to cooperate "closely with those whose task it is to safeguard the public health" and to provide "aid and assistance to the research effort into all phases of tobacco use and health." And to bring this about, they announced the formation of a Tobacco Industry Research Committee (TIRC) to conduct research into "all phases of tobacco use and health."[3]

The "Frank Statement" may well be the most widely publicized—and expensive— single-page advertisement up to that point in human history. Four hundred forty-eight newspapers in 258 cities with an estimated circulation of 43,245,000 printed the ad, at a cost of more than $244,000. ("Negro newspapers" were not targeted, apart from the *Atlanta World.*) Costs went substantially higher when the companies ordered two hundred thousand additional reprints, plus further republication in the tobacco trade press. The National Association of Tobacco Distributors asked for another million copies to be handed out at retail outlets, pushing costs even higher.[4]

The "Frank Statement" itself was also news, however, and widely reported as such. Stories on the counterpunch appeared on television and radio, with additional commentaries in newspapers. The papers remarked on how the TIRC was to be governed by a Scientific Advisory Board, whose demeanor would be "calm and detached" in contrast to "some of the extremist attacks upon tobacco use." Comparisons to the recent fluoridation flap became fashionable, with at least one newspaper, the *Cincinnati Enquirer,* refusing to crusade "on either side" given the lingering taint from that scandal, where "groundless fears" had tipped the scales of public opinion. (Paranoid conservatives had warned of a communist plot to poison the nation's water supply—by adding fluoride to prevent tooth decay—prompting ridicule from progressives and mockery in films such as Stanley Kubrick's *Dr. Strangelove.*) This same paper recalled a time when tobacco had been linked with leprosy, a "fantastic and baseless rumor that spread across the country like a prairie fire." Some fun was also made of the fact that tobacco had once been blamed for tuberculosis—which from today's vantage point turns out not to have been so crazy. Smoking is a major cause of TB in modern India, for example, where more people are killed by this means even than by lung cancer.[5] All of this helped the industry, via the argument that since tobacco had once been falsely blamed for foolish fears it must be foolish now to blame *anything* on tobacco. The "one by one" rhetoric of the "Frank Statement" said as much—and many press reports followed the script laid out by the industry.

The plan to sponsor research via the TIRC was also widely reported, and with a great deal of sympathy. Telegrams to Hill & Knowlton were favorable by a margin of about two to one. This was not by chance, since the PR firm had contacted editors and writers from across the country to ensure favorable coverage. We know how hard Hill & Knowlton worked from the archival record left by the firm in the Wisconsin Historical Society in Madison: hundreds of magazines, newspapers, and radio shows carried news of the industry's launch of a research effort, and the response was generally favorable.[6]

But what did the TIRC actually do?

RED HERRING RESEARCH

For forty years, from the mid-1950s through the mid-1990s, the TIRC/CTR was the world's leading sponsor of (what appeared to be) tobacco and health research. It got its new name—Council for Tobacco Research—in March 1964; it had earlier changed from "Committee" to "Council" to avoid the political odor of the former term. Hundreds of thousands of dollars were spent in the 1950s, millions *per year* in the 1970s and 1980s, and tens of millions per year in the 1990s. The industry was always proud of the sums involved and made sure the public was duly impressed. In 1985, for example, the CTR announced that it had spent over $100 million up to that point, a figure that would grow to $204 million by 1993 and $282 million by 1997. By 1998, when the organization was finally dismantled under the terms of the Master Settlement Agreement, the CTR was awarding about $36 million per year in grants. Over forty-odd years more than $300 million was provided for "tobacco and health" research.[7] All of which was widely advertised, since the *fact* of having supported such research was crucial for the program to have any effect. The point was to be able to say, "We have funded such research," garnering laurels and legitimacy for the industry.

On paper, the ambition was to "explore and learn the causes of disease, including the role *if any* played by tobacco use."[8] The crucial fact about the TIRC/CTR, however, is that it rarely supported research that might reveal smoking as a cause of human harms. The primary focus was on the *mechanisms* of disease rather than on its preventable *causes*. The TIRC also didn't pay a lot of attention to tobacco and tended not to fund research that might cast cigarettes in a bad light. Its scientific director, Clarence Cook Little, in a confidential 1959 memo listed six areas for research by the group:

1. Heredity—how much does the biochemical nature of the individual depend upon its innate composition? Some individuals in the same environment develop the disease; others do not.
2. Infection—how much do bacteria and/or viruses, either present or previously experienced, influence cell or tissue changes? To what extent do they increase the risk of later disease?
3. Nutrition—how much do the various nutritive materials taken, absorbed, stored or excreted by the individual affect cell or tissue changes? Cholesterol is one substance now under extensive investigation, but vitamin deficiencies and other imbalances may be important.
4. Hormones—how much do the various glands of internal secretion affect cells or tissues . . . ? It is known that they have an important role in breast cancer, adrenal cancer, and that men have four to six times as much lung cancer as women.
5. Nervous strain or tension—how much do these factors influence the cells and tissues of various systems of the body other than the nervous system itself?

Ulcer is already recognized as a disease in which stress is important. Cardiovascular disease is also implicated.

6. Environmental factors—how much do physical or chemical components of
   the environment and introduced as foreign non-living agents affect the cells
   or tissues? In addition to tobacco, air pollutants, humidity and temperature are
   involved.[9]

Note that tobacco is mentioned only in the final paragraph and only within a clus-
ter of other environmental considerations, like "humidity and temperature." That
again was the policy and practice of the TIRC/CTR: smoking was slighted as a cause
of the lung cancer epidemic, while other causes—often treated as "confounding
factors"—were given far more attention. The goal was really to look in such a way
as not to find, and then to claim that despite the many millions spent on "smoking
and health" no proof of harms had ever been uncovered.

Tobacco industry observers outside the United States were well aware of this ruse
and commented on it privately. In 1958, for example, a team from British American Tobacco visited the United States as part of an effort to survey American views
on tobacco and health. In their long and revealing report, the BATCo team related
the opinion of Liggett & Myers that the TIRC and its Scientific Advisory Board had
done "little if anything constructive": "the constantly reiterated 'not proven' statements in the face of mounting contrary evidence has thoroughly discredited
T.I.R.C., and the S.A.B. [Scientific Advisory Board] of T.I.R.C. is supporting almost
without exception projects that are not related directly to smoking and lung cancer."[10] This was not so different from the American Cancer Society's assessment that
same year. In its *Bulletin of Cancer Progress,* the ACS accused tobacco manufacturers of conducting "a sideshow with smoke and mirrors." The whole point was
"to deny repeatedly," to "mislead," and "to convince the trusting, tobacco-consum-
ing public of the industry's eleemosynary, 'lasting interest in people's health.' "[11] The
great Alton Ochsner had hit this same nail on the head even earlier, ridiculing the
TIRC (in 1954) as "tapeworm research" designed "to postpone a day of reckoning
for the industry."[12]

"RESEARCH MUST GO ON AND ON"

Charged with bias and frustrated in their efforts to gain a solid reputation, the TIRC's
puppet masters soon realized more had to be done to separate the organization's
science and advocacy missions—or at least to create such an illusion. And so in 1958
the TIRC sprouted off a new body, the Tobacco Institute, with the more explicit mission of proselytizing for the cause. This didn't eliminate charges of bias or irrele-
vancy, but it did allow the companies to turn their more transparently propagan-
distic functions over to a distinct body, which thereafter operated openly as a trade
association. The Tobacco Institute (TI) became the industry's primary "go to" (or

"hear from") instrument on tobacco and health; it also made propaganda films, organized media friendlies, lobbied Congress and local legislators, conducted "educational campaigns," and published "white papers," pamphlets, press releases, and newsletters debunking or distracting from cigarette hazards. This gave C. C. Little at the TIRC a bit of breathing room: the plan had been to cultivate him as an expert witness for use in litigation, and the hope was that by separating the PR from the science, Little could be kept innocent "in his ivory tower."[13]

I've stressed the deliberate *irrelevance* of CTR-funded research to the question of whether smoking was causing harms—and admissions to this effect by cigarette industry observers in other parts of the world. American industry insiders conceded this as well. Brown & Williamson's chief counsel in 1963, for example, noted that the CTR was "conceived as a public relations gesture" and had functioned as such. Similar views were expressed in 1964, when higher-ups from Britain's tobacco establishment visited the United States and found once again that "CTR supports only fundamental research of little relevance to present day problems." Stronger language was used in 1973, when yet another BATCo delegation paid a visit, concluding in their thirty-eight-page report that the CTR had become "a backwater of little significance in the world of smoking and health." By this time even the American industry's lawyers had been confessing—albeit only privately—that "Most of the T.I.R.C. research has been diffuse and of a broad, basic nature not designed to specifically test the anti-cigarette theory."[14]

Of course it would have been simple enough to verify the hundreds and eventually thousands of studies demonstrating death and disease from smoking—if that is what the industry had really wanted. It would not have been hard to test, amplify, or improve upon these studies; the industry had lots of money, ample laboratory space, and many willing partners who could have helped. The companies for many years bragged about their state-of-the-art research facilities—which included comprehensive libraries, well-equipped labs, and sophisticated document retrieval and translation services; this was not an enterprise short on funds. The CTR's library was massive, containing an estimated 150,000 publications "readily available" and organized by author.[15]

But the companies never undertook any honest effort to evaluate this literature—at least not through channels that were supposed to see the light of day. Council for Tobacco Research monies went mostly to basic biology and biochemistry, leaving the big and really the only honest question unexamined: was smoking causing disease? The industry's vast PR machinery churned out its message—"not yet proven"—while never actually funding research that might have yielded such proof. Hundreds of press releases urged the need for "more research," with the claim sometimes even made that it was dangerous to jump to conclusions, given that the case was not yet closed. And that, of course, is how the industry wanted the health "question" kept:

forever open. As Imperial Tobacco once confided to the Tobacco Institute, "Research must go on and on."[16]

The Council for Tobacco Research is best thought of as an elaborate engine of distraction, a mechanism for blowing smoke. The whole point was to sponsor decoy research, whose hoped-for impact would be to draw attention away from cigarettes as a cause of harms (we can also think of this as "lightning rod research"). The goal was to be able to say the industry was "studying the problem," when it was actually doing everything it could to deny its existence. The CTR became a shield for the industry and a tool for its defense in court, where tobacco attorneys could say, "But look at how hard my client has been working on this problem!" Industry scientists confessed as much in private, as when Philip Morris Research Director Helmut Wakeham wrote to Joseph F. Cullman III, chairman of the company and head of the Tobacco Institute's powerful Executive Committee, arguing for a bit of internal honesty: "Let's face it. We are interested in evidence which we believe denies the allegation that cigaret smoking causes disease."[17]

One interesting twist is that the industry *did* occasionally fund animal research but not typically through the CTR and usually not past a point where it would get too close to any kind of embarrassing truth. We've seen how the Ecusta experiments revealed carcinogens in cigarette smoke, and we've seen how Claude Teague's "Survey of Cancer Research" conceded the same effects—both from 1953. Liggett & Myers beginning in 1954 funded mouse experiments through the Cambridge, Massachusetts, consulting firm of Arthur D. Little (ADL), which found evidence of cancer-causing chemicals but kept this pretty close to its chest. Liggett and ADL in 1963 produced a nine-volume review of these studies for the exclusive use of the Surgeon General's Advisory Committee but never publicized any of this research—nor the fact of smoking causing cancer—to the wider public. And even the Liggett/ADL report to the Surgeon General was "withheld from the general public at Liggett's insistence."[18] Liggett was certainly not the most powerful player in the conspiracy: the company refused to sign the "Frank Statement" of 1954, for example, and joined the CTR only for a five-year period, from 1964 through 1968. Liggett was, however, one of the founding members of the Tobacco Institute (from 1958) and adhered strictly to the broader industry's playbook, refusing to admit any kind of harm from smoking.

SUPPRESSION OF RESEARCH

Now, a lot of people when they think about tobacco industry abuse of research think in terms of *suppression,* and there are certainly some notorious examples. Among the more nefarious would be R. J. Reynolds's closure of its "Mouse House" at the company's headquarters in Winston-Salem, North Carolina, in March of 1970. The company had established a program to conduct in-house biological research, principally to understand the role of pulmonary surfactants in the genesis of emphysema. (Surfactants lubricate the air sacs of the lungs, keeping them from sticking together during exhalation. Several chemicals in cigarette smoke impair this natural lubrication.) When the researchers started getting results that could be embarrassing for the company, however, a decision was made to shut down the laboratory. Twenty-six Reynolds scientists lost their jobs overnight, in what has come to be known as the "Mouse House massacre." A former Reynolds scientist, Joseph E. Bumgarner, has recounted (under oath) how he and twenty-five other members of the company's biological research division were told to hand over their notebooks and leave the company. Strangely enough, a 1985 internal report for the company actually celebrated this research as "important," characterizing it as having come "close to showing what was thought to be the underlying pathobiology mechanism of emphysema."[19] None of this was ever disclosed to the public, however.

There are other instances in which research getting too close to the truth was nixed. Philip Morris in April of 1984, for example, closed its Nicotine Program, following worries that the research could expose the company to the charge of having demonstrated addiction. Victor J. DeNoble, an experimental psychologist, had been hired to develop nicotine analogs, ideally in the form of alkaloids without the cardiovascular negatives of nicotine. DeNoble also did work showing how nicotine and acetaldehyde when combined reinforced one another, producing a kind of dopamine euphoria synergy in the brain. All of this became dangerous, once it was realized that it could open up the company to the charge of having recognized the addictive power of nicotine. Shook, Hardy and Bacon lawyers in 1994 commented on this danger,[20] and Philip Morris's director of applied research, William Farone, later recalled how the research was halted "by order from New York City" (corporate headquarters) because it had produced "data which the company did not want to have in the records."[21] DeNoble was also forced to withdraw a paper he had submitted to *Psychopharmacology;* the company didn't want him revealing any information that would "not be favorable to the company in litigation." And to avoid further legal danger, on April 5, 1984, shortly before having to divulge documents for *Cipollone v. Liggett,* DeNoble was told (as Richard Kluger summarizes it) "to close down his laboratory, to kill the animals, to suspend all further investigation of possibly less toxic or harmful alternatives to nicotine, never to try to publish or discuss his work on addicting rats, and to find work elsewhere."[22]

There are also instances where the industry tried to hide its suppression efforts after the fact. Leonard Zahn, a PR agent working for the CTR, managed this for the industry in 1974, when it was feared that Freddy Homburger was going to present evidence that his funding had been cut after showing that inhaled tobacco smoke could cause cancer in the laryngeal tissues of Golden Syrian hamsters. As president and director of Bio-Research Consultants, Inc., in Cambridge, Massachusetts,

Homburger had been doing experiments along these lines since the 1960s and by 1973 had managed to confirm the work of Walter Dontenwill in Germany that inhalation could in fact produce tumors. The CTR was not happy with this result, however, and refused to renew his contract. Homburger had planned to talk about his work at a press conference scheduled for April 8, 1974, but Zahn managed to have this cancelled. Zahn was proud of his intervention, announcing to Henry Ramm and Willson T. (Tom) Hoyt at the CTR, "He [Homburger] was to have a news release with him and was to tell the press that the tobacco industry was attempting to suppress important scientific information about the harmful effects of smoking. He was going to point specifically at CTR. . . . I arranged later that evening for it to be cancelled." Zahn then tried to cover his tracks, ending his memo with one of the more poorly chosen lines in the history of corporate racketeering: "I doubt if you [Henry Ramm] or Tom [Hoyt] will want to retain this note."[23]

Suppression was never an easy or pleasant matter within the companies, staffed as they were by researchers trying to build up research résumés and networks of respect. Pressures not to publish—or rather to publish only along "approved" lines—raised an interesting problem of how to allocate credit for research performance. One solution arrived at took the form of industry-sponsored conferences, where company scientists could present papers to a limited circle of corporate friendlies. Foremost among these was the Tobacco Chemists' Research Conference, a series of annual meetings organized from 1949 to bring together researchers working in (or for) the industry. Papers from these meetings were often published in *Tobacco Science,* a journal established for this purpose in 1957. Most of these papers were on tobacco chemistry, always a strength of the companies. Indeed between 1949 and 1996 tobacco manufacturers spent "several tens of billions of dollars" in research along these lines, counting personnel, equipment, and supplies.[24] Research performance was also recognized through a series of prizes established to honor excellence in tobacco science. The Paris-based Cooperation Centre for Scientific Research Relative to Tobacco (CORESTA) awarded bronze and silver medals for this purpose, and Marlboro's makers in 1967 created the Philip Morris Award for Distinguished Achievement in Tobacco Science. Helmut Wakeham at Philip Morris was a prime mover in establishing this latter prize—and its very first recipient.

Tobacco Science provided a dedicated outlet for industry chemical work, but not every kind of topic was allowed to see the light of day. Papers on subjects that might compromise the industry's "intangible legal situation" were explicitly barred from publication; for Reynolds in the 1970s this included papers on "polycyclic hydrocarbons, hydrogen cyanide, carbon monoxide and similar materials." Philip Morris had similar rules: when William Dunn was exploring nicotine psychopharmacology in the 1970s, the policy was to "bury" any kind of results that made nicotine look too much like addictive alkaloids such as morphine.[25]

Research was sometimes even suppressed by its authors, for fear of giving exposure to a "controversial" topic. Lorillard chemist Alexander W. Spears in June of 1960, for example, submitted a paper on phenols in tobacco smoke for a Tobacco Chemists' Research Conference scheduled for October. Company lawyers feared airing the industry's knowledge of hazards in public, however, so Spears told the organizer he was pulling his paper: "it has been recently decided in the interest of the Company and the tobacco industry that a paper dealing with compounds which are controversial in the health aspects of smoking should not be presented." Spears withdrew his paper, and the conference organizer returned all copies of his abstract.[26]

There were other ways by which suppression took place. In 1956, for example, TIRC bigwigs objected when George E. Moore from Roswell Park Memorial Institute started talking about the reality of cancer hazards. Moore had given a talk in which he had mentioned this reality, along with his plans to conduct a series of animal tests using tobacco tars. The TIRC was alarmed to learn he had taken up with the "Hammond camp" (meaning scientists convinced of a hazard) and was planning to thank the TIRC for its support. The industry wanted none of this, and Willson T. Hoyt from Hill & Knowlton arranged for Moore to be instructed "not to mention the TIRC." The TIRC didn't want its grantees spouting off about cigarettes causing cancer and pressured them on this point—despite also admitting that censoring a scientist in such a manner was "ticklish."[27]

Similar suppressions occurred in other parts of the world. Walter Dontenwill's industry-funded Institute for Tobacco Research in Hamburg was closed down in 1975 when animal experiments there started implicating smoking in laryngeal cancer and heart disease,[28] and BAT's research at Southampton was always guarded when it came to matters with a certain legal gravity. Legal fears led Philip Morris to establish a sizable research facility at Cologne—INBIFO, the Institut für biologische Forschung—to conduct some of its more sensitive research safely distant from the long arm of American law.

In the United States there are instances in which the plug was pulled on CTR research when the investigator seemed to be getting too close to inconvenient truths. From 1971 through 1980, for example, Gary Friedman, an epidemiologist at Kaiser-Permanente in Oakland, California, had been handsomely supported by the CTR for his work exposing complications in some of the epidemiology linking smoking and heart disease. The CTR liked his skeptical bent, feeding as it did their hope that something—anything—other than smoking would explain the ills experienced by smokers. (CTR's governing lawyers in 1978 were still confiding that they "must find skeptical scientists.") Friedman obtained about $100,000 a year from this source, resulting in a number of papers coauthored with Harvard anthropologist Carl Seltzer, one of the most ardent of the industry's "no proof" ideologues. Friedman was not an ideologue, however, and in 1979 he made the fatal mistake of noting in one of his papers that "most scientists now agree that cigarette smoking is an important factor in causing death."[29] Friedman shortly thereafter had his funding faucet turned off, as was often the fate of "admitters" of this sort (honest scientists, one could say). That was the common practice of the CTR: scholars willing to play ball would be supported, but those who strayed too far from the party line were cut off or even punished.

"IS IT WISE TO SCARE THE PUBLIC?"

The TIRC/CTR was an odd body from the start, however. In certain superficial respects it operated like a legitimate research granting agency—the American Cancer Society, for example, or the National Cancer Institute. It had a scientific advisory board with distinguished scholars as members; it awarded grants on the basis of peer review (and lawyerly review) and printed annual reports containing abstracts of grantee publications. The ACS resemblance was not entirely accidental, since one of the goals in creating the tobacco body was to capture the aura and authority of the cancer body. The man eventually hired as scientific director, Clarence Cook Little, had previously headed the American Society for Cancer Control, which later gave rise to the ACS. The TIRC modeled itself on the ACS but more important saw itself as a competitor: the Cancer Society had begun publicizing the death toll from smoking, and the industry needed an authoritative counterforce.

The TIRC's public relations mission was never far from the surface. More than half its first-year budget (1954) went to Hill & Knowlton, the PR firm managing the science-as-distraction strategy (no money went to research at all in that first year). Its physical location should have raised eyebrows: the TIRC was headquartered on the fifty-third floor of the Empire State Building, one floor below the offices of Hill & Knowlton, which also provided its working staff. Thirty-five Hill & Knowlton staffers were employed full- or part-time for the TIRC in 1954, and there was always significant overlap in both personnel and operations of the two organizations. Hill & Knowlton helped the industry choose C. C. Little as scientific director and helped plan the kinds of topics to be treated—and avoided. Hill & Knowlton would also take over PR for the Tobacco Institute when it was founded in 1958 and remained tightly bound to the institute until the two parted ways in 1969.

The hiring of Clarence Cook Little to head the TIRC was a real coup for the industry. As a former president of both the University of Maine (1922–25) and the University of Michigan (1925–29), Little had proven himself an able administrator. He was a Harvard man from a wealthy Massachusetts family with a religious bent and a sense of corporate *oblige;* he often delivered Episcopalian sermons in Maine churches—and of course he smoked a pipe. He was also a geneticist of some note, and famous for developing pure strains of mice for use in medical research. In 1929 he had founded the Jackson Laboratory in Bar Harbor, Maine, where he bred rodents that were either reliably immune to, or highly susceptible to, cancer. His genetics (and eugenics) background proved useful in his tobacco reincarnation, allowing him to argue that cancer was a "constitutional" disease: chemicals of a certain sort might well cause cancer *but only in susceptible individuals*—a truism that allowed his benefactors to shift blame for tobacco maladies onto the idiosyncrasies of individual smokers. Little fixated on genetics while staunchly denying even the remotest shred of evidence implicating smoking. He also wanted people to worry more about psychological issues, like *fear*. Talk about a tobacco–cancer link was always "premature" but also fear-mongering, like "crying wolf when we know there isn't any wolf there as yet."[30]

Little here was simply following a script drafted prior even to his hiring on with Big Tobacco. In its *Scientific Perspective* white paper of 1954, issued as the industry's first propaganda blast after the "Frank Statement," the reader is cautioned: "Is it wise to scare the public and create widespread anxiety among millions of people on the flimsy evidence that has been presented?" Little was always worried more about fear than about smoke, testifying as late as 1967 that it was "too bad that the extensive propaganda [against cigarettes] has brought back fear into the minds of hundreds of thousands of Americans." Tobacco strategists often sounded such alarms: Brown & Williamson in 1969, for example, in secret planning documents for the company's Project Truth, expressed the company's Objective No. 5 as: "To prove that the cigarette has been brought to trial by lynch law, engineered and fostered by uninformed and irresponsible people and organisations in order to induce and incite fear." Industry spokespersons often raised this specter of tobacco being "lynched"—rhetoric deliberately crafted for use in Project Truth.[31]

Little was hired to direct the Tobacco Industry Research Committee in the summer of 1954, but he was not the first man offered the job. Harold L. Stewart, chief of pathology at the National Cancer Institute, had been made an offer and turned it down, as had Wilhelm Hueper and a number of others—E. Cuyler Hammond of the American Cancer Society and Hayden Nicholson of the University of Arkansas, for example, but also McKeen Cattell, chief of pharmacology at Cornell.[32] Hueper as head of the NCI's Environmental Cancer Section must have seemed an attractive candidate: the world's leading authority on occupational carcinogenesis thought that tobacco was being unfairly blamed as the cause-all of modern cancer and that other kinds of carcinogens were being let off the hook, notably asbestos and the many dangerous pollutants belched forth from the petrochemical industry. And he was partly right. It was easy for the Dows and DuPonts of the world to blame smoking or some other "personal factor" for whatever maladies their workers were contracting. Hueper was a kind of proto–Ralph Nader or Rachel Carson, keenly aware of the depth of corporate neglect and malfeasance. Much of his life had been spent documenting dangers to which workers were exposed, but he was no friend of Big Tobacco and scoffed at the idea of taking money to become their corporate poodle. He didn't think much about tobacco as a cancer cause—for decades he smoked a pipe and at one point credited 90 percent of all lung cancers to (non-tobacco) environmental and occupational causes, leaving only 10 percent for cigarettes—but he also had a strong moral compass and wasn't about to let himself be bought. So Hueper refused the industry's offer.[33]

Hanmer of the American Tobacco Company had made it clear that he wanted as director someone who was "safe for the industry," but as scholar after scholar balked he realized this was very much a "buyer's market." Despite the handsome salary, it was not so easy finding the right kind of person to shill for the industry. Distinction was one criterion, but the director also had to be willing to play according to the industry's rules. Paul Steiner of the University of Chicago, for example, was dropped from consideration when an industry confidant noted that he was "not reliable": "He will quit within a few months and go around saying that there is no question about it—cigarette smoking causes lung cancer."[34]

Desperate, the industry finally got lucky with its offer to Clarence Cook Little. At sixty-five the man was clearly past his prime, but that was presumably safe; the industry wanted a "yes-man," not someone wanting to shake things up. And Little himself could certainly survive on the pay: $20,000 per year, with many perks and fringe benefits. Little started work and proved very loyal. By 1960 he was praising his benefactors for having responded to the health scare in "a very fine and courageous way" (by establishing the TIRC); the industry was doing a "magnificent job."[35]

MICRO- VERSUS MACRO-BIAS

The question of whether the TIRC/CTR supported "good research" is often raised in litigation, and the industry always tries to argue that the organization performed admirably, consistent with the highest scientific standards.[36] And it is true that many CTR grantees were prestigious scholars from some of the country's leading academic institutions—places like Harvard, Stanford, Yale, and UCLA. Six CTR grantees went on to win Nobel Prizes, and thousands of CTR-financed papers were published in some of the world's leading scientific journals—6,400 papers by one count. So how could anyone say this was not good science?

The problem is not that the research was "bad" in some narrow technical sense; by and large it was not, judging by traditional performance indicators. No one has ever (fairly) accused CTR grantees of plagiarism or fraud or fabricating data; that is not where the bias lay. The bias stems rather from the fact that the CTR really wasn't designed to explore whether, how, or to what extent smoking caused illness. Experts hired by the industry to supervise the grant review process usually didn't know much about tobacco and were selected more with an eye to keeping the research "industry friendly." Grants were rarely given to anyone who knew much about tobacco and health, and CTR administrators were also by and large ignorant in this area.

Sheldon C. Sommers, M.D., is a case in point. Sommers was a member of the CTR's Scientific Advisory Board from 1967 through 1989 and held the office of "Research Director" from 1969 to 1972 and "Scientific Director" from 1981 through 1987. How much, though, did he know about tobacco? His curriculum vitae from 1991 lists 342 published articles, and whereas the word *hypertension* appears twenty-seven times and *cancer* seventy-three, the word *tobacco* doesn't appear even once. Nor does *cigarette* or *nicotine*.[37] Cigarette makers liked him not for any substantive contribution to identifying tobacco harms—which he did not make—but rather because he was willing to stand up in public and say that smoking was "not a cause" of human cancer. In 1985, testifying for the defense in *Galbraith v. Reynolds,* Sommers expressed himself as follows:

> Q: Doctor, do you have an opinion presently as to whether cigarette smoking is a cause of lung cancer?
>
> A: Yes.
>
> Q: What is your opinion?
>
> A: In the scientific sense, I believe it not a cause.
>
> Q: When you qualify your answer to say "in the scientific sense," what do you mean by such a qualification?
>
> A: Scientific evidence of a causative agent involves that it should be both necessary and sufficient to produce a condition.
>
> Q: What do you mean by "necessary" to produce a condition?
>
> A: The condition does not exist in its absence.[38]

Of course by such a definition there is not much in this world that causes anything. Drunk driving does not cause traffic accidents, because traffic accidents can be caused by fatigue or a slippery road. Playing with matches cannot cause fires, because fires can be caused by things other than matches. This is typical industry obfuscation, and it is why they loved (and hired) men like Sommers. The examining lawyer realized this and pursued the matter further.

> Q: Do you have an opinion as to whether cigarette smoking is a contributing factor to the development of lung cancer?
>
> A: Yes.
>
> Q: What is that opinion, Doctor?
>
> A: Epidemiologically, a relationship has been claimed.
>
> Q: I'm aware of that. What I'm asking for is your personal scientific opinion as to whether cigarette smoking is a contributing factor to the development of carcinoma of the lung? . . . I'm not asking what it's been claimed by others. I'm narrowing in now on your personal medical scientific opinion. Do you have one, as to whether cigarette smoking is a contributing factor to the development of bronchiogenic carcinoma?
>
> A: I have an opinion. It's actually bronchogenic.

Q: Bronchogenic. I'm sorry. What is your opinion, please?

A: My opinion is that it remains to be proved whether and in what way cigarette smoking is a contributory factor to lung cancer.[39]

Sommers was commonly called upon to make such weasely claims in court, including in overseas trials against the industry.[40] In trials such as these he grotesquely misrepresented the state of the science, but also its historical development.

As for the research supported by the CTR, the bias lay more in the kinds of research funded, the topics chosen. It is not so much micro- as *macro-bias*—a bias visible not in any one study but rather in the aggregate collective body of research. Additional bias lay in how support for research was used for purposes of public relations. The goal was distraction or red herring research, drawing attention away from tobacco as a cause of illness and onto the industry's munificent support for research. The industry wanted to be able to say it was funding research, and this fact alone was of PR value. It was therefore crucial for the CTR's annual reports to be widely distributed: the report for 1971, for example, was sent to 400 medical school libraries, 1,364 experts in allergies, 3,989 cardiologists, 3,291 pathologists, 6,577 radiologists, and so forth—21,496 recipients altogether.[41]

MECHANISMS VERSUS CAUSES

The CTR supported mainly basic research into human biology, and when specific diseases were addressed this was usually to investigate proximate disease *mechanisms* rather than ultimate disease *causes*. Topics explored included cellular and developmental biology, genetics, immunology, virology, and neuroscience, among others. Insofar as cancer was looked at, this was almost always in terms of biochemical mechanisms—so researchers would look at some biochemical pathway in tumorigenesis, or how certain genes were turned on or off during carcinogenesis. Nicotine was sometimes studied, but when addiction was a focus this was typically to stress differential genetic susceptibilities.[42] Studies were rarely conducted using the methods of epidemiology, apart from studies designed to find "confounding factors" and the like. Toxicology was rarely supported, and little was done to elucidate the nature or consequences of poisons in smoke. Ciliastasis was not much studied, nor experimental carcinogenesis, with any other purpose than to challenge previous work. The whole point was to whitewash tobacco, albeit not in such a way that would be apparent from looking at any one grant or any one grantee. Indeed it is probably safe to assume that few of the researchers taking such money had any idea they were part of a conspiracy. The goal was really to create the *illusion* of support for honest research, which could then be used to keep the public reassured. The goal was also, though, to cultivate and maintain a "stable of experts" ready and willing to serve in regulatory hearings or litigation. Public relations authorities from Hill & Knowlton, co-architects of the constructed ignorance strategy, articulated this defensive character of the TIRC in a 1962 review, noting that the organization had been an effective response to the 1954 "emergency," following the realization that smoking and health was a "public relations problem that must be solved for the self-preservation of the industry." The whole point had been to put out "brush fires"—meaning publicity of harms from smoking.[43]

Looking back over the history of the discovery of tobacco hazards, it is hard to name *any* that were uncovered through CTR research. CTR funding resulted in the publication of at least 6,400 scientific papers, but which of these can we credit for having advanced our knowledge of harms from smoking? Did CTR researchers help to confirm that smoking causes bladder cancer or spontaneous abortions? What about the dangers from chewing tobacco or secondhand smoke? What does the industry have to show for its three hundred million–odd dollars of research?

Not much. Little of what we know about health harms was unearthed by CTR scientists, which means that the Council failed in its mission as advertised. That is because its true purpose was not to find out how tobacco impacts health but rather *to give the appearance* of providing such support while simultaneously running a campaign to deny proven hazards. By this criterion, of course, the CTR was a success in its very failure. The whole point was to fail to find evidence of harms while misrepresenting the effort as honest. CTR staffers have admitted as much: Dorothea Cohen, who wrote research summaries for the CTR's annual reports for twenty-four years until her retirement in 1989, once characterized the organization as "just a lobbying thing. We were lobbying for cigarettes." Congressman Ron Wyden (D-Okla.) cited Cohen's words when questioning CTR Chairman James F. Glenn about the Council's conduct, prompting Glenn to dismiss his former colleague as having "mental problems."[44]

And what about those six CTR grantees who later went on to win the Nobel Prize? Cigarette makers love citing such scholars to defend themselves in court, but the fact is that little of the research supported by such grants had anything to do with smoking and health. A look at the grant applications submitted by these scholars—Baruj Benacerraf of Harvard (Nobel Laureate, 1980), Stanley Cohen of Vanderbilt (1986), Harold Varmus of UCSF (1998), Ferid Murad of Stanford (1998), Louis Ignarro of UCLA (1998), and Carol Greider of Johns Hopkins (2009)—reveals that only Murad mentions either tobacco, cigarettes, nicotine, or addiction. Ignarro mentioned cigarettes in a 1979 application that was *rejected*—and was only able to obtain CTR money after a re-submit in which all mention of cigarettes was deleted. No one can complain about the quality of the work of these scholars—it is fine basic research into genetics, immunology, virology, and the like—but Big Tobacco supported such work because it *posed no threat to the continued sale of cigarettes.* It was safe.[45]

THE "MOST PRECIOUS THING"

The Council for Tobacco Research was thus a sham and a fraud. The CTR's Scientific Advisory Board was made up of industry "yes men" (and one woman),[46] and all decisions of any consequence were made by the industry's powerful Committee of Counsel (i.e., lawyers). Also revealing is the rate at which grants were awarded: more than 40 percent of all applicants received funding. Legitimate granting agencies typically award a far lower proportion—NIH yields are now down to around 10 percent, for example. This was easy money and money the industry was able to advertise as "clean," since there was rarely any overt effort to manipulate the research being funded.

That is one remarkable aspect of this whole "distraction" research business: how easily the industry was able to use liberal rhetorics and values—such as freedom of inquiry and eternal questioning—to its advantage. "Open controversy" was a key pillar in the industry's conspiracy, and the CTR always professed its "openness" to alternate hypotheses when it came to disease causation. The industry played this card in ads, press releases, and testimony before the U.S. Congress and the Federal Trade Commission, stressing always this need to keep an "open mind" about whether cigarettes cause disease. Open-mindedness was also apparently a requirement for serving on the CTR's Scientific Advisory Board. Clarence Cook Little in 1960 made this clear while testifying for the defense in *Lartigue v. Reynolds*. Asked whether everyone on the CTR's board of directors was skeptical about the tobacco–cancer link, Little responded, "Yes. I would say that all of the committee has an open mind on this subject. Some of them say that they think that there is more probability of this than others, but we keep our independence as individuals. It is the most precious thing we have. It is what makes the committee strong . . . we are all in agreement."[47]

Conformity and independence are interestingly conflated in Little's statement, but his use of the word *precious* is apt, since the success of the CTR depended on the question of cigarette health harms remaining open. The companies played this card artfully, identifying "closure" as "closed-mindedness" and tantamount to antiscience. This was very clever rhetoric, and many scientists seem to have bought it. The industry cast itself as a defender and supporter of objective science while simultaneously tarring public health advocates as closed-minded zealots. Similar strategies have been used in other realms of health and environmental policy—in debates surrounding climate change or control of toxic exposures, for example, where calls for more research are often de facto calls for intransigence and inaction.[48]

For the tobacco industry, though, this new strategy meant that the manufacturers could ally themselves with science—or even prudence—while the antitobacco camp could be charged with trying to close down inquiry. Joined to this was a great deal of rhetoric about the dangers of coming to premature conclusions. Industry experts repeatedly claimed it would be dangerous to accept the cigarette theory, given the stultifying effect this would have on research. Thomas J. Moran, a Virginia pathologist, made this argument in 1964 testimony at hearings before the U.S. Congress, arguing that accepting the cancer–cigarette link was "dangerous" and would lead to "complacency concerning the etiology of this disease."[49]

"CANCER LINK IS BUNK"

A more radical version of this argument-cum-threat held that the cigarette theory itself was causing people to get sick. A Pennsylvania cardiologist by the name of Joseph B. Wolffe, for example, claimed that acceptance of the cigarette theory had "traumatized a great many people, particularly those who are impressionable." Such at least was the story told by Stanley Frank, a popular sports writer who cited Wolffe (misspelled as *Wolfe*) in a 1968 article for *True* magazine, an article later found to have been secretly commissioned by Hill & Knowlton. Frank was also found to have revised his article for publication in the *National Enquirer* ("Cigaret Cancer Link Is Bunk") under the pseudonym Charles Golden. The chicanery might never have been detected had the industry not gone to such lengths to promote the piece, which was reprinted for the Tobacco Institute and sent out to six hundred thousand physicians, scientists, educators, policy makers, and media interests throughout the country. Six hundred thousand copies (of an eight-page reprint) is difficult to fathom: picture a thousand two-drawer file cabinets stuffed to the gills, or a stack of 8 1/2 × 11 paper more than half a mile high. Recipients included 41,055 "biological scientists," governors of every U.S. state, all 100 senators and 432 members of the House of Representatives—and that was not even 10 percent of the recipients. This was no small operation, as was revealed when the *Wall Street Journal* and *Consumer Reports* exposed the scandal.[50]

Clarence Cook Little himself liked to caution that the cigarette hypothesis was "dangerous" and that constantly harping on it could be harmful to your health. Little's own views changed revealingly over time, following his employment by the tobacco industry. In 1944 in a booklet titled *Cancer: A Study for Laymen* published by the American Cancer Society, Little had stated that it was surely "unwise to fill the lungs repeatedly with the suspension of fine particles of tobacco products of which smoke consists."[51] In 1960, however, when asked whether he still thought this unwise he replied, "No, as a general answer."[52] Key for Little was a kind of constitutional cop-out: so while some people might be "irritated" by tobacco smoke, the majority escaped with no apparent harm. Or at least no reliable evidence of harm. Which for him meant it was wrong to say that smoking "caused" cancer.

Indeed for Little, every living smoker was proof that cigarettes don't cause cancer. Here is how he put it when testifying for the defense in *Green v. American Tobacco,* one of the first tobacco trials:

> Q: Doctor, do you know of any one specific statistical study that shows that there is no relationship between smoking and lung cancer, any original study?
>
> A: That's a hard question to answer, in a way. . . . I would say that wasn't a question of statistics. It is just a question of fact, that the living people who smoke prove that there is no relationship in their case between cancer and smoking, because they haven't got cancer.[53]

Assuming he was telling the truth, which may be overly generous, we can only conclude that Little had an extraordinarily narrow and mechanical conception of causation, one that would never have passed muster in elementary physics or chemistry, let alone medicine. As with Sommers, there is this notion that if *B* doesn't *necessarily* and *invariably* follow from *A,* then we cannot say that *A causes B.* Little's failings in the realm of logic stagger the imagination, but tobacco was able to get away with it. Deep pockets, polished rhetoric, and lawyerly finesse all helped keep this festering logic zombie alive, long past its rightful time of interment.

Of course the irony is that throughout this time, the industry was constantly accusing health authorities of bias, blinding passions, unbridled enthusiasm. This is odd on the face of it but perhaps not hard to imagine how it came about. The companies must have tired of being accused of bias and decided they could flip this back against the anti-tobacco folks. A great deal of effort went into insinuating that while tobacco-financed researchers were striving for objectivity, groups like the ACS and NCI were mired in self-aggrandizing zealotry and prejudice. The industry's consorts became quite adept at exposing how an experiment or study might be flawed, incomplete, or inconveniently interpreted. Cancer researchers were accused of extrapolating from animals to humans and of improperly preparing tobacco condensates. Epidemiologists were charged with using outdated or improper statistical techniques or flawed mathematical models. Extrapolation of experimental results from skin to lungs was questioned ("skin tests we think are irrelevant to the lung problem"), as were generalizations about the nature of cigarette smoke. Bias became a major focus, along with research into the sociology of knowledge, the material culture of print, the sociology of citation, even the rhetorical force of different kind of fonts. Why is so little known about experiments *not* causing cancer? Because "negative results are rarely published."[54] Scholars in the pocket of the industry became expert at countering the argument that the industry failed to warn or lied to the public or failed to keep its promises. Scholars were handsomely paid to discredit some inconvenient scholar, argument, or document. To read the industry's critiques is to feast on a cactus of deconstruction, with a thousand tiny spines—one could say pinpricks—all hoping for an entry.

SPECIAL PROJECTS

The Council for Tobacco Research was ordered disbanded by Judge H. Lee Sarokin of New Jersey in the early 1990s, though it was not until 1998 that the body was finally interred as part of the Master Settlement Agreement. The Tobacco Institute was also dissolved at this time, along with the Center for Indoor Air Research— which had basically done for secondhand smoke what the CTR had done for the mainstream variety. Judge Sarokin had been uncompromising in his ruling, declaring the industry's conspiracy "vast in scope, devious in purpose and devastating in its results"[55]—which caused him to be removed from the case. The industry's conduct has been so horrific that a simple expression of the truth can be easily misread as prejudice.

Sarokin's judgment has been upheld by subsequent history, however. Most of the lawsuits filed against the industry since the decision in *Cipollone v. Liggett* (1992) have introduced evidence of the CTR's role in the denialist conspiracy. And court rulings have recognized its sham nature. In *United States v. Philip Morris,* Federal Judge Gladys Kessler, after sifting through millions of pages of documents, concluded that the TIRC/CTR was "a sophisticated public relations vehicle based on the premise of conducting independent scientific research—to deny the harms of smoking and reassure the public." Research was used to distract from hazards, to cultivate witnesses, and to perform "guided research" for company lawyers.

The most notorious were the so-called Special Projects—typically projects that had been turned down by the CTR's Scientific Advisory Board, or were not expected to qualify for such funding, or were simply hatchet jobs commissioned by the lawyers to deconstruct inconvenient science. The Special Projects helped provide a platform for the industry's obfuscatory propaganda, but they also allowed the industry to ask questions they didn't want anyone to know they were asking. The bagmen were often accomplished scholars, many of whom were later recruited for use as witnesses in litigation or to trumpet industry-friendly "science."

Special Project (SP) 109, for example, begun in 1965, involved a "collection of cases of emphysema among nonsmokers and among young people." SP-12 investigated the possibility "of additional statistical studies, such as those made by Perrone and Poche, which showed no association between smoking and lung cancer." Yet another Special Project involved the study of lung cancer among non-smoking Amish, Mennonites, and Mormons to show that non-smokers can contract the disease. Dozens of such projects had been launched by the mid-1960s,[56] all shielded from ordinary scrutiny, peer review, or disclosure—and often dealing with "hot topics" the industry didn't want to see publicized. SP-30, for example, was designed to check the accuracy of Radford and Hunt's demonstration of radioactive polonium in tobacco smoke and included a series of experiments to establish dose-response relations in exposed dogs. SP-31 and SP-32 were organized to examine levels of free radicals and nitrosamines in cigarette smoke.

Many of these were deliberate hatchet jobs. The statistician George L. Saiger from Columbia University received CTR Special Project funds "to seek to reduce the correlation of smoking and disease by introduction of additional variables"; he also was paid $10,873 in 1966 to testify before Congress, denying the cigarette–cancer link. The goal of SP-100, authorized in December 1965, was to assemble a panel of experts to repudiate the statistics relied on by the Surgeon General in his recent report; panelists included Saiger but also Leo Katz, K. Alexander Brownlee, and Theodor D. Sterling, all of whom were expected to show that the conclusions in the Surgeon General's report were "not justified." Ingram Olkin, chairman of Stanford's Department of Statistics, received $12,000 to do a similar job (SP-82) on the Framingham Heart Study, a long-term epidemiological study (organized by the National Heart Institute) best known today for nailing down the smoking–heart disease link. Lorillard's chief of research okayed Olkin's contract, commenting that he was to be funded using "considerations other than practical scientific merit." Many of these Special Projects were essentially lawyerly assignments, with the biases—or foregone conclusions—expressed in their titles. SP-103, for example, was titled "Specific Refutation of Misleading Statements Regarding Cigarette Smoking Commonly Appearing in Anti-smoking Propaganda." Another Special Project involved an "Epidemiologic Study to Find Pockets of High Lung Cancer Incidence without Relation to Smoking Habits." Yet another fostered clinical studies to show that "duration and amount of smoking have no relation to the age of peak incidence of lung cancer." Project SP-26 was similarly designed "to expose the inadequacy of the Harris inhalation index" for carbon monoxide, part of an effort to demonstrate flaws in unfriendly measurement methods.[57]

Between 1966 and 1990 more than $18,000,000 was allocated for CTR Special Projects, with most of the money coming from Reynolds ($6+ million), Philip Morris ($5.8 million), and Brown & Williamson ($2.6 million). Lorillard, Liggett, and American Tobacco contributed lesser sums, proportionate to their cigarette sales. Former CTR vice president Harmon C. McAllister has testified that more than 130 separate Special Projects were administered through the CTR, each of which had its own principal investigator, typically a professor in a medical school or science department.[58] This included scholars from leading universities, people like Alvan R. Feinstein from Yale, Richard J. Hickey from the Wharton School of Business, Carl Seltzer from Harvard, and Victor Buhler, president of the 4,500-strong College of American Pathologists. At least thirty such Special Projects operatives testified before the U.S. Congress or in some other legal capacity, often without revealing their financial ties to the industry.

Victor Buhler in 1969, for example, testified before the House Committee on

Interstate and Foreign Commerce (investigating tobacco ads on television): "The cause of cancer in humans, including the cause of cancer of the lung is unknown. No amount of speculation, no amount of suspicion, no amount of repetition of now familiar findings and no amount of emotion can alter this fact. The cause of cancer of the lung is not known."[59] Arthur Furst, director of the Institute of Chemical Biology at the University of San Francisco, testified before this same committee that "much more must be known" about cancer before concluding that smoking was one of its causes. Furst was adamant in his skepticism: "I am not convinced that the placing of tars on the skin of mice shows anything. . . . I am concerned that the publication of premature conclusions has helped to create an impression that the answers have already been found."[60]

The industry also trotted out experts to oppose limiting the televised broadcast of tobacco ads. Eugene E. Levitt from Indiana University's School of Medicine testified there was "no scientific basis" for inferring that television commercials influence the smoking behavior of young people, while K. Alexander Brownlee, a Fellow of the Royal Statistical Society in London, testified that the U.S. Public Health Service had "failed to prove that cigarette smoking is the cause of lung cancer." John P. Wyatt, chairman of pathology at the University of Manitoba, testified there was not yet a "scientific basis" for tying smoking to emphysema; and Duane Carr, a surgeon at the University of Tennessee, testified that government health authorities had let "emotionalism and zeal" infect their pursuit of scientific truth—and that the cause of lung cancer remained "unknown."[61]

Nowhere did either Buhler or Furst reveal they had taken Special Projects funds. That was hardly by accident or oversight: the industry often used "third party" scientists to do its dirty work and tried whenever possible to disguise the financial arrangements. And the sums involved were often substantial.

Theodor D. Sterling, for example, a professor of applied mathematics at Washington University in St. Louis, testified before this same House committee, opining that the conclusions drawn by the Surgeon General about smoking and cancer were "probably invalid." In the 1960s and early 1970s Sterling received about $4 million to conduct research for the industry, mainly on indoor air pollution but also to develop statistical methods useful for challenging the smoking–cancer link. As late as the 1990s Sterling was ridiculing calculations of hundreds of thousands of U.S. deaths from smoking as "exaggerated propaganda" bordering on "the ludicrous"; he also accused health authorities of "resorting to misinformation to encourage people to stop smoking." Sterling was one of the Special Projects operatives exposed by Stanton Glantz and colleagues in their 1995 Cigarette Papers, though Sterling earned substantially more even than was realized in this early exposé. From documents subsequently released, we learn that the man probably received close to $10 million over a thirty-year career with Big Tobacco.[62]

By such means the industry was able to clog congressional hearings, to distort popular understanding, and to delay or weaken legislation designed to regulate smoking. Targeted funding gave a podium and megaphones to dissenters, warping the honest give-and-take of untainted inquiry. Tobacco charlatans gained a voice before the U.S. Congress and were often able even to insinuate themselves into peer-reviewed medical literature.

In 1968, for example, the biophysical chemist Richard J. Hickey from the University of Pennsylvania's Wharton School of Business was offered Special Projects funding (grant 56-B) to prepare a statement for Congress. Hickey had been turned down for normal CTR funding, but for the next several years he received millions of dollars from special industry accounts, primarily to use multivariate statistical methods to claim that air pollution was more important than smoking as a cause of lung cancer. Hickey published denialist articles in prestigious journals such as *Lancet,* without identifying himself as a Special Projects agent. A U.S. federal court later concluded that Hickey's work was funded because of his willingness to act "as a witness in litigation or before congressional hearings on behalf of the Enterprise."[63]

Special Projects were also organized to refute studies judged painful or embarrassing for cigarette makers. Efforts were initiated in the 1960s to undermine Hammond and Horn's epidemiology, and in the 1980s Domingo M. Aviado, a pharmacologist at the University of Pennsylvania, received Special Projects money to run a series of secret dog inhalation studies, designed ostensibly to succeed by failing. Inhalation experiments had been popular with the industry since the 1940s, largely because it turns out to be quite hard to give mice, rabbits, or even dogs lung cancer simply by exposing them to tobacco smoke. Lung cancers typically take twenty or thirty years to develop in humans, and small animals usually don't live long enough to get the disease. Aviado had earlier worked for Allied Chemical and in 1974 published an article in *Executive Health* titled "The Case against Tobacco Is Not Closed: Why Smoking May Not Be 'Dangerous to Your Health'!" The tobacco crowd found him a willing co-conspirator and hired him to help cast doubt on the hazards of both mainstream and secondhand smoke in publications such as the *New England Journal of Medicine.* By 1982 Aviado was getting more than $114,000 per year for research on twenty different projects for the industry, including "psychosocial aspects of burns" (from cigarettes), lung cancer in Greek and Japanese women (criticizing Hirayama and Trichopoulos), a critique of the FTC's 1981 "Staff Report" (which had found millions of Americans still poorly informed on tobacco hazards), and surveys of South American and Philippine views on smoking. Aviado also spearheaded an effort to develop a new computerized coding system for some fifty thousand publications on smoking and health, employing methods "dictated by priorities of interest expressed by Shook, Hardy and Bacon," the industry's long-standing legal defenders. Aviado testified before the U.S. Congress on behalf of cigarette makers and reassured Australian smokers that cigarettes pose "no health hazard to normal non-smokers." Many of his Shook Hardy assignments were of an activist nature, as when he testified before a New Jersey Assembly public hearing "questioning the health reasons" of a proposed law barring smoking in public places. Aviado seems to have been quite eager to do the industry's bidding, and one wonders what kind of work he might have refused.[64]

Special Project grantees sometimes investigated non-tobacco hazards. Professor Thomas F. Mancuso at the University of Pittsburgh received a Special Projects grant in 1972 to research air pollution, with the hope that he would counter, Hueper-like, the "cigarette hypothesis." Industry lawyers were pleased with his emphasis on occupational causes and saw him as a way to rebuke the view that "90% or more of lung cancer" was caused by cigarettes.[65] Richard J. Hickey was similarly paid to endorse R. A. Fisher's "genotype hypothesis," the idea that people smoke because they have a certain genetic yearning to do so, which happens also to be linked to a propensity to contract cancer. This was the so-called itch in the lung hypothesis: people smoke because they already have an "itch" (i.e., cancer) that needs to be "scratched" (by smoking). An equally plausible theory would be that people who accept such far-fetched notions must have a gene that allows their credulity to be stretched.

FEINSTEIN'S FOLLY

Alvan R. Feinstein, an influential epidemiologist at Yale University's School of Medicine, was one of the very first scholars to receive Special Projects funding. His SP-2 grant from 1966 involved publication of a report on health statistics expected to produce "helpful data"—data that would aid in the industry's ongoing effort to discredit the recent Surgeon General's report. Feinstein worked for cigarette manufacturers for more than three decades, earning many hundreds of thousands of dollars in the process. Big Tobacco appreciated his work on "detection bias" and praised him for allowing the industry to maintain (as late as 1988) that "lung cancer may not be directly linked to smoking."[66] Tobacco lawyers at Jacob, Medinger & Finnegan offered the following rationale for financing the man:

> Dr. Feinstein has long thought that one reason for the reported association between cigarette smoking and lung cancer, as well as the apparent rise in the incidence of lung cancer, is "detection bias." It is Dr. Feinstein's view that cigarette smoking may contribute more to the diagnosis of lung cancer than it does to the disease itself because smokers are given more rigorous physical examination and, therefore, a greater number of lung cancers are diagnosed in smokers than in non-smokers. In the early 1970's Dr. Feinstein did a research project to test his theory. He concluded that detection of lung cancer during life is greater in smokers and that the more a patient smoked the greater the likelihood that a particular diagnostic technique would be used.[67]

Feinstein helped the industry exculpate tobacco, by uncovering ever more sophisticated ways by which epidemiology might be flawed. His extensive work on bias helped him become one of the pioneers of what we now know as "evidence-based medicine"; indeed the *British Medical Journal* recently praised his role in "defining the principles of quantitative clinical reasoning." No mention was made, however, of how his push for ever higher bars of epidemiologic proof played right into the hands of his cigarette industry paymasters.[68]

Feinstein's complicity is significant, because his was such a powerful voice in the field of clinical epidemiology. As editor of one of the field's most important journals and author of several widely read textbooks, he used his position of authority to publish tobacco-friendly articles and letters, including refutations of the secondhand smoke threat. Former students and colleagues remember him as a "contrarian"—he was also a lifelong smoker of Camel cigarettes—but he clearly knew where his bread was buttered. Feinstein once compared the tobacco industry's hiring of consultants to the right of the accused to an attorney; he also likened the treatment of tobacco-friendly scholars (such as himself) to Galileo's persecution by the Catholic Church. And only a maverick, or so he thought, could go against "the current fervor of anti-smoking evangelism." In 1992, in thinly veiled autobiography, he published an article lambasting the "current atmosphere" in which a consultant's "stature, credibility, and integrity become instantly impugned and tarnished by the depravity of associating with the tobacco 'bad guy.'" Nowhere did he mention, though, that he himself was a long-standing tobacco industry consultant—one of the "bad guys"—and a recipient of secret Special Projects money.[69]

Cigarette makers for their part knew that some of Feinstein's colleagues were skeptical of his pro-cigarette slant; indeed some of the money he received from the CTR was deliberately awarded to counter the suspicion that his tobacco-friendly work had earned him in certain quarters. Feinstein's work on *colon* cancer was supported, for example, to neutralize some of this suspicion. The industry's evaluation of his 1988 request for funding noted that his "studying this tumor, which has not hitherto been associated with tobacco, will lessen some of the preconceived prejudices about the results of his research on lung cancer."[70]

It is unclear even today, though, how many of Feinstein's former colleagues and students knew (and know) about his work for the tobacco industry. One wonders which of his Yale colleagues knew about this in 1974, when he founded the Robert Wood Johnson Clinical Scholars Program, or in 1988 when he founded the *Journal of Clinical Epidemiology,* or in 1991 when he was named Sterling Professor of Medicine, the university's highest academic honor. Or in 2005, when a prize was established in his name, the Alvan R. Feinstein Award for outstanding clinical skills, honoring this long-standing collaborator with Big Tobacco. Harder still is to say how much of an impact tobacco funding has had on the rise of evidence-based medicine. Feinstein's was a career based on skepticism, and many of the statistical techniques he helped develop have been useful in challenging the reality of other kinds of medical and environmental hazards. Big Tobacco has clearly left an odious stain on scholarship, though we may never be able to say precisely how deep it has gone or how far it has spread.

THE COMPLICITY OF LAWYERS

Tobacco monies were sometimes provided just to keep a scholar in the industry's favor, or even to compensate them for embarrassment stemming from their work for the industry. A. Bennett Jensen, a Georgetown University pathologist, received Special Projects funding in 1988, for example, causing him problems with his university. Lawyers from Shook, Hardy and Bacon proposed therefore to pay him $40,000 "not for specific research" but rather "solely in order to maintain a good relationship with him and secure his continued help in making contact with other scientists." The money was to come from an expert witness slush fund administered by the firm, with the goal being just (as Shook Hardy attorney William Allinder put it) "to keep him happy." The tobacco lawyers admitted there was "no immediate value to his research"; Jensen had value as a potential witness, however, and keeping him happy was envisioned as helping the industry acquire "legislative witnesses." Special Projects by this time (1992) had been moved out of the CTR to become the direct responsibility of Shook, Hardy and Bacon, raising this question (in the minds of the industry's lawyers) of whether the joint industry funds administered in this manner "were used to purchase favorable judicial or legislative testimony, thereby perpetrating a fraud on the public."[71]

This last-mentioned musing highlights a little-probed aspect of the modern world's tobacco wars: the deep complicity of *lawyers* in the industry's long-standing campaign of deception. It is surprising how little outrage there has been about this aspect of the conspiracy. Are lawyers held to no ethical standards? How should we judge their conduct throughout this enterprise? And what are we teaching our young law students about professional ethics and social responsibility? Judge Kessler grasped part of this nettle on page 3 of her 1,652-page "Amended Final Opinion," ruling for the government in *United States v. Philip Morris*, finding the industry in violation of federal racketeering laws:

> Finally, a word must be said about the role of lawyers in this fifty-year history of deceiving smokers, potential smokers, and the American public about the hazards of smoking and second hand smoke, and the addictiveness of nicotine. At every stage, lawyers played an absolutely central role in the creation and perpetuation of the Enterprise and the implementation of its fraudulent schemes. They devised and coordinated both national and international strategy; they directed scientists as to what research they should and should not undertake; they vetted scientific research papers and reports as well as public relations materials to ensure that the interests of the Enterprise would be protected; they identified "friendly" scientific witnesses, subsidized them with grants from the [Council] for Tobacco Research and the Center for Indoor

Air Research, paid them enormous fees, and often hid the relationship between those witnesses and the industry; and they devised and carried out document destruction policies and took shelter behind baseless assertions of the attorney client privilege.

What a sad and disquieting chapter in the history of an honorable and often courageous profession.[72]

I am no lawyer, but if participation in such a conspiracy qualifies one for inclusion among the defendants in a lawsuit, then I cannot fathom why law firms such as Shook, Hardy and Bacon or Covington & Burling have not been brought before the bar of justice. Law firms were deeply complicit in the campaign to hide the hazards of smoking and played a crucial role in helping to maintain the business legitimacy of cigarettes.

Indeed, this complicity of lawyers goes to one of the most enduring deceptions of the conspiracy, this notion that the companies have turned over a new leaf and are now acting as "responsible corporate citizens." Nothing could be further from the truth—as anyone will know who has ever attended a tobacco trial, where the CTR and other arms of the conspiracy are held up as examples of the industry's honesty and beneficence. In later chapters we will see how the cigarette itself remains fraudulent in certain vital respects—and defective, which means that unnecessary killing is ongoing and will continue for however long cigarettes are sold.

MARCH BIRTHS AND BALD MEN

The tobacco industry's Special Projects have acquired a certain notoriety, but other kinds of manipulation probably had a more lasting overall effect. One commonly used trick was to cherry-pick extracts from scientific literature sympathetic to the industry and then to publish and distribute those extracts to a broad audience. This began already in 1954 with the release of the TIRC's first *Scientific Perspective* white paper and would continue throughout the formal conspiracy.

One remarkable example is the *Tobacco and Health Report,* a newsletter published by the Tobacco Institute from 1957 through 1969 to publicize "material which rebuts and discredits" the health charges against tobacco. According to a 1962 Hill & Knowlton document, 536,000 copies were sent free of charge four times a year to doctors, dentists, science writers, editors, and publishers throughout the United States. The point was to draw attention to doubts raised about the "cigarette theory" by abstracting, reprinting, and disseminating research by cigarette-friendly skeptics. The topics covered are extraordinary—and from the comfort of historical distance even comical. Lung cancer is said to be caused by mites from the feathers of birds and the month into which one is born. A report on lung cancer being "rare in bald men" is followed by one on the role of stress, pesticides, or industrial pollution. Here is a sampling of titles from the months surrounding the release of the 1964 Surgeon General's report:[73]

"28 Reasons for Doubting Cigarette–Cancer Link"   (Jul.–Aug. 1963)
"No One Yet Knows the Answers"   (Jul.–Aug. 1963)
"Rare Fungus Infection Mimics Lung Cancer"   (Nov.–Dec. 1963)
"March Birth, Lung Cancer Linked"   (Nov.–Dec. 1963)
"Viral Infections Blamed in Bronchitis Outbreaks"   (Mar.–Apr. 1964)
"Nicotine Effect Is Like Exercise"   (Mar.–Apr. 1964)
"Lung Cancer Rare in Bald Men"   (Mar.–Apr. 1964)
"English Surgeon Links Urbanization to Lung Cancer"   (Winter 1964–65)

As silly as these may sound today, a physician casually perusing the *Tobacco and Health Report* in the 1950s or 1960s might well have been led to consider cigarettes only a trivial cause of lung cancer. Indeed, relying on this publication alone, one would scarcely have reason to believe tobacco was causing *any* disease whatsoever. A Hill & Knowlton memo from 1968 listed the following "Criteria for Selection" for articles:

> First, the reports should be on new research, if possible. It need not always deal with some aspect of tobacco; for example, a report indicating some factor or factors other than smoking may be involved in one of the diseases with which smoking has been associated. Other examples:
>
> - a report in which the statistics of a smoking-associated disease are questioned.
> - one in which death certificates or classifications of such a disease are questioned.
> - one showing that many lung cancers may be metastatic from some other organ.
> - one indicating that a virus may cause human cancer, whether or not that cancer is associated with smoking.
> - one on research with animals, indicating that some other factor be involved with carcinogenesis or ciliostasis *[sic]*.[74]

The goal, in short, was to cast doubt on cigarettes as a cause of disease. Hill & Knowlton made this explicit: "The most important type of story" (for *Tobacco and Health*) was "that which casts doubt on the cause and effect theory of disease and smoking." And we know from correspondence preserved in the archives that some doctors at least liked the publication. An Illinois Public Health official wrote, praising "the willingness of industry to fight for truth in science"; others wrote to request reprints, or to subscribe, or to find out where they could apply for CTR funds.[75]

Quite a different impression would have come from the industry's own *Current Digest*, a newsletter distributed to "a controlled list" of industry friendlies by Hill & Knowlton via the TIRC/CTR. This was a more honest organ than the *Tobacco and Health Report*, summarizing tobacco and health research in the form of short abstracts. *Current Digest* was produced from 1956 into the mid-1990s, though it was always an in-house organ for executives' eyes only—and always kept confidential.

Though formally issued through the TIRC, the *Digest* was "almost entirely a Hill & Knowlton production."[76]

The *Current Digest* is important because it shows that the industry did make an effort to keep up with the science on tobacco and health. Hill & Knowlton also compiled a catalog of the relevant papers published up to 1955, classifying these according to whether they were "favorable" or "unfavorable" to the industry. Hill & Knowlton graded hundreds of scientific papers according to whether they were useful (A), neutral (B), or negative (C) for the industry's PR effort; a section titled "Tobacco Products Linked to Cancer," for example, included twenty-two articles in the "C" category, meaning that a cancer link had been established. Economists from the University of York have analyzed such evaluations along with the literature abstracted in the *Current Digest,* showing that the industry was actually fairly honest (to itself) when it came to assessing whether literature was favorable or unfavorable on the cancer question. What is striking, though, is how this internal assessment contrasts with the industry's public pronouncements. The TIRC/CTR issued annual reports beginning in 1956, claiming in each instance that the case against tobacco had not been proved. The industry was two-faced on this issue, keeping honest tabs internally on the evidence while pressing the "not yet proven" thesis onto the general public.[77]

To summarize: What is significant is the contrast between the industry's public and private stance. Publicly, and loudly, the industry was always denying evidence of hazards, typically by claiming this to be an "open question." Privately, however, the CTR was collecting medical reports on tobacco and summarizing them for internal industry consumption. We also know that the scholars receiving funds from the CTR had very different views about causation from those trumpeted via CTR or Tobacco Institute literature. Michael Cummings of the Roswell Park Cancer Institute in Buffalo, New York, has shown that the overwhelming majority of CTR grantees by 1990 *agreed* with the public health consensus—contrary to the industry's public stance. Cummings wrote to more than a hundred former CTR grantees and found that among the seventy-seven who responded only one was a smoker—and over 90 percent agreed that most deaths from lung cancer were caused by smoking. All but one agreed that smoking was addictive, and most also agreed that secondhand smoke endangered nonsmokers. Cigarette makers had not yet admitted any kind of harm from smoking, but their own CTR grantees were clearly already convinced.[78]

OPARIL'S EXCULPATION

Clarence Cook Little died in 1971 at the age of eighty-three from a heart attack. Most obituaries ignored or trivialized his tobacco work, and some even praised him—as if in grotesque mockery of the facts—as "one of America's foremost cancer researchers." The *New York Times* mentioned his work for the companies but also parroted their line that evidence of health harms from smoking was based "largely on statistical grounds." The *Times* also characterized Little's denials of tobacco–disease links as his "hobbyhorse," as if this were some kind of pet theory or idle indulgence.[79]

The fact is that for the last sixteen years of his life Little was little more than a puppet for Big Tobacco. His public pronouncements were carefully staged, his veneer of objectivity carefully protected. One reason for the establishment of the Tobacco Institute as distinct from the TIRC in 1958 was to sequester Little from explicit trade association activity, allowing him to be "immunized" for use in litigation; Little's sequestration, though, was simply a ploy to maintain this illusion of independence. The TI and the CTR were supposed to have different missions, but they were actually part of one integrated whole. Revealingly, with the formation of the TI in 1958 the TIRC's budget declined by exactly the amount allocated to the TI.

The Council for Tobacco Research was shuttered in 1998 as part of the Master Settlement Agreement reached between cigarette manufacturers and the attorneys general of forty-six states. By this time, however, the body was already moribund. The CTR had stopped accepting grant proposals on June 20, 1997, with the last grant going to Judith A. Shizuru, a physician at Stanford's School of Medicine, for work on a project titled "Bone Marrow Stem Cell Transplants for the Treatment of Autoimmune Disease." The Council did not disappear but by the terms of the MSA was no longer allowed to offer grants. Staffing was stripped down to a skeleton crew of four, having as their sole purpose to respond to litigation. James F. Glenn, president and CEO of the expiring body, in 1998 wrote to Stanford's Judith F. Swain, the first and only woman ever to serve on the Scientific Advisory Board, lamenting how the CTR had been "stripped of its benevolent and productive enterprise." Swain herself refused to attend the last few meetings of the SAB, having been surprised to learn in recent months that "the Council may not have been totally independent of the tobacco industry." Swain therefore thought it "best that I resign from any involvement with the Council."[80]

Equally naive, though, would be to imagine the industry so easily giving up this ghost. The CTR has in fact had a remarkable afterlife, principally in litigation. Even after its closure and dismemberment, the CTR lives on as a kind of legal zombie, touted by the industry as a legitimate research organ and as evidence of the cartel's stellar social responsibility. Scholars are actually paid to research the history of the CTR as part of an effort to polish its reputation in court, where CTR research is upheld as "good science."

Such has been the argument of Suzanne Oparil, M.D., a former president of the American Heart Association (1994–95) and ever since a paid expert witness for the defense in numerous tobacco trials. Oparil is typically brought in to say that the CTR was a legitimate scientific organization, turning a blind eye to the record of lawyer involvement in the selection of CTR projects. Indeed she denies that a primary purpose of this organ was to give credence to the denialist project. She herself received substantial funding from the CTR—about half a million dollars from 1989 through 1995—and was on a first name basis with its research director.[81] Her testimony shows how easy it is for scholars to get drawn into the industry's denialist orbit; it also shows, though, how much of its courtroom defense has relied on a continuance of the denialist project.

In June of 1997, for example, Oparil testified for the defense in *Broin v. Philip Morris,* a class action suit brought on behalf of flight attendants suffering from exposure to in-flight secondhand smoke. Under oath, Oparil claimed that the CTR was "a legitimate valuable scientific research organization" supporting "cutting edge" work of "excellent quality." Oparil's opinion was based on little more than a reading of CTR annual reports and a few representative papers, though she also claimed to have become an expert on the CTR—Sarah Palinesque—simply by accepting funding from this organ.[82] Her utility as a witness, however, stemmed from her willingness to keep to the industry's legal script. Asked whether she thought that smoking caused cancer, Oparil characterized this as "a complex question" given that smoking was not a *sufficient* condition for contracting the disease. Smokers were at a higher *risk* of developing certain kinds of cancer, Oparil said, but she refused to admit causality or that smoking was addictive. She also testified to having smoked "at parties, or occasionally one or two cigarettes after dinner," and that she didn't mind sitting in the smoking sections of restaurants or planes.[83] She was also forced to admit that she herself had never done any research "that supports the proposition that someone is more likely to get diseased because they smoke cigarettes."

Oparil continued testifying for the industry for several years thereafter, keeping pretty much to this same legal script. In *Engle v. Reynolds* she defended the right of sponsors "to discourage or prevent publication" and denied that tobacco manufacturers had tried to cast doubt on the cigarette–cancer link. She also denied that a causal link had been established between smoking and disease:

Q: Does cigarette smoking cause any disease?
A: By the strict definition of causality, no.

She admitted an "association" and various "risks" but would not come out and say, yes, smoking kills:

Q: You do know within a reasonable degree of medical certainty that cigarette smoking kills hundreds of thousands of people each year, don't you?
A: That statement is a statement made based on epidemiologic studies and based on the multiplication of an assessment of the increase in risks due to—which is attributed to the use of cigarettes.
Q: And you find those epidemiologic studies very convincing, don't you?
A: I—first—I—it's difficult to respond specifically to that question. Because the

specific studies that are used to make these statements and establish these statistical risks are studies that are not directly known to me. These are old data. How accurate they are is really not clear to me. How good the methods were to establish these levels of risks are also not known to me. I am not an epidemiologist.[84]

One might imagine a former president of the American Heart Association catching flak for collaborating so intimately with cigarette makers; the AHA, after all, has taken strong stands against smoking since the 1950s and by the 1990s had only harsh words for the industry. Judging from her long list of honors and awards, however, it appears that Oparil's colleagues may not know about this side of her career. Oparil was awarded the Founders Medal of the Southern Society for Clinical Investigation and the President's Achievement Award from the University of Alabama in 1995, the year she was also named one of the nation's "Top 20 Women Health Leaders" by the *Medical Herald*. In 2002 Oparil won the AHA's coveted Lifetime Achievement Award, presented annually to an individual "who has had a lifetime of outstanding achievements in the field of hypertension and has served as a role model through service, research and teaching." Did the AHA's prize committee know about Oparil's defense of the tobacco industry in court? Would that have mattered? What about the American Society of Hypertension, which elevated Oparil to the office of president in 2006, following a power struggle amid revelations that the Society had taken large sums of money from drug manufacturers trying to broaden the class of patients eligible for drug therapy? Is Oparil's view that "smoking does not cause hypertension" consistent with the state of the art as recognized by the Society? Does the Society for Hypertension condone the expression of such views in a court of law?[85]

The American Heart Association's official website highlights its struggle with the tobacco cartel in the mid-1990s, remarking: "Despite strong opposition from the tobacco industry, the American Heart Association continued to be an advocate for the American public."[86] The irony is that the highest-ranking officer of the AHA during these same years was not only taking money from the industry's fraudulent research arm (the CTR), but would also (subsequently) work for the industry as an expert witness in court, denying addiction and causal links and helping to buttress the central fraud of the conspiracy. People who wonder about the continued ability of the industry to defend itself against charges of fraud and conspiracy need look no further than the willingness of such experts to service the industry in this manner. All for a price, of course.

17

Agnotology in Action

Doubt is our product.
BROWN & WILLIAMSON, 1969

Deception has long been the tobacco industry's bread and butter. And though we probably cannot trace the strategy of manufacturing doubt to any one evil genius, the strategy does have a history, and key players and principals. High on my list for influentials would be Paul M. Hahn, president of the American Tobacco Company and chief architect of the 1953 Plaza Hotel meetings where the denialist campaign was set in motion. Edward A. Darr, president of Reynolds, seems to have helped craft the "no real proof" strategy, and Hill & Knowlton certainly helped polish this turnip. The idea was simple: the industry would fight science with science, exploiting Gibson's law that "for every Ph.D. there is an equal and opposite Ph.D." The court of public opinion was more than a metaphor: the entire public sphere was turned into a spectacular arena of deception, with tobacco on trial and two sides to every story and cigarettes presumed innocent until proven guilty—with the bar for proof set so high that no one could ever get over it.

From the archives we have a number of "smoking gun" memos and notes in which this doubt-mongering strategy is made explicit. The most infamous, perhaps, is the text of a speech attached to a memo dated August 21, 1969, from John W. Burgard, vice president of marketing for Brown & Williamson, to R. A. Pittman, senior brand marketing supervisor (and later director of advertising), and C. I. McCarty, who later served as the company's president and CEO. Here in this attached speech, titled "Smoking and Health Proposal," are these notorious lines:

> Doubt is our product since it is the best means of competing with the body of fact that exists in the mind of the general public. It is also the means of establishing that there is a controversy. If we are successful in establishing a controversy at the public level, then there is an opportunity to put across the real facts about smoking and health.[1]

Burgard's memo and the attached speech were squirreled away among seven tons of documents produced by the company in response to a 1979 subpoena from the Federal Trade Commission, part of a U.S. government inquiry into the industry's marketing practices. The company had hoped to overwhelm the FTC by the sheer volume of its response, but the strategy—known to lawyers as "dumping" or "papering"—backfired as page after page was read by diligent FTC staffers. (The entire treasure trove of documents would eventually find its way onto the Internet, which still was tiny on the horizon when the "dumping" began). Burgard's memo was cited in a classified version of the FTC's 1981 "Staff Report," which recognized the doubt-mongering as cynical and a sham: "By emphasizing and playing up areas where there is a genuine scientific controversy about the particular effects of smoking, Brown & Williamson proposed to cast doubt on the validity of the much larger body of uncontroverted medical evidence."[2] The memo was soon thereafter leaked to the press: the Sunday *Herald Leader* of Lexington, Kentucky, was the first to publish it—on July 5, 1981—but the Associated Press quickly picked up the story, which found its way into hundreds of newspapers across the country.

STRATEGIES FOR CREATING DOUBT

There are other instances where the tobacco industry makes explicit this goal of creating doubt, and not just in the United States. In 1984 in Britain, for example, Keith Richardson of BAT described the strategy to fight "the case against smoking" in an internal memo: "The Royal College of Physicians claims that 90% of all lung cancer deaths can be attributed to smoking. There can be no doubt that this is widely believed to be true and that lung cancer is the most emotive single issue. If we can cast doubt on the relationship between smoking and lung cancer then we have cast doubts on the entire case against smoking."[3] Similar confessions from other parts of the world could surely be unearthed, if governments or attorneys had the power to obtain the documents.

What kinds of strategies have been used to manufacture doubt? One of the more common has been simply to assemble and reproduce statements by authorities willing to deny the hazard. Dozens of such compilations were produced beginning in 1954, shortly after the counter-blast of the "Frank Statement." Most had titles like *A Scientific Perspective on the Cigarette Controversy* or *How Eminent Men of Medicine and Science Challenged the Smoking-and-Health Theory during Recent Hearings in the U.S. Congress.*[4] That, though, has been just one of many methods to promote ignorance. Expressed as imperatives, others would include the following:

1. Publicize statements from scholars skeptical of the hazard.[5] Fund the research of these scholars to entice them to testify in court or in regulatory hearings.
2. Publicize examples of people living to a ripe old age despite decades of smoking.[6]

3. Raise questions about "anomalies" that seem paradoxical: why, if smoking causes cancer, do some countries with high rates of smoking have low rates of cancer? Why don't laboratory animals exposed to whole fresh smoke develop lung cancer? And so forth.

4. Redefine terms. Deny there is "tar" in cigarettes and insist on using words like *biological activity* or *hyperplasia* rather than *cancer* or *pre-cancer*. Deny, deconstruct, or trivialize addiction, turning it into a matter of semantics— or "weak will" or free choice.

5. Wrap yourself in the authority of science. Contrast the "rush to judgment" approach of anti-tobacco "fanatics" with the cautious "wait and see" attitude of the industry. Insist on laboratory proof when faced with statistical evidence, and on human studies when faced with laboratory evidence. Claim also that the manufacturers know more about tobacco than anyone else, so they should be trusted.

6. State that the evidence linking tobacco and disease is merely "statistical" and then deride statistics as an improper method for reasoning about causality. Finance your own epidemiology and publish this in engineering journals if medical journals won't take it. Then hire experts to say such studies are "difficult to refute" and make sure such remarks get coverage in the popular press.[7]

7. Put a positive spin on uncomfortable facts. Yes, some mice develop tumors after exposure to cigarette tar, but don't forget that many of these mice *do not* develop tumors.[8] Just like most smokers never develop lung cancer. And yes, the surface area of the human lung is the size of a tennis court, but think of this as a strength and not a weakness: think how *dilute* the smoke must be to have to cover such a large area! Think of the body not as weak in the face of carcinogenic onslaughts but strong in its capacity to resist such onslaughts.

8. Construct graphs and charts in such a way as to make it look like cancer trends are chaotic ("graphic agnotology"; see Figure 29).

9. Hire journalists to write industry-sympathetic articles in the popular press and pressure media organs to ignore or suppress reports unfavorable to the industry. Threaten to withhold advertising from magazines that give too much attention to tobacco–disease links.

10. Undermine the authority of health organizations such as the American Cancer Society, the Surgeon General, the American Heart Association, or the National Cancer Institute. Denigrate these as "advocacy" or "government" organizations aligned with an anti-tobacco "cause" or "movement" (with an "agenda," etc.). Imply that such organizations are irremediably biased or one-sided.

11. Hire historians to rewrite history from an industry point of view and then use such scholars as experts in court. Hire lawyers who can convince juries that the industry was never dishonest and operated a responsible business.

12. Proclaim the smoking and health controversy to be "nothing new," the "same old same old," and so forth. Plan for ways to make the public tire of hearing about "accusations" against tobacco by deriding them as "old news," "centuries old," overly familiar, "notorious," and so forth.[9]
13. Keep people smoking by reassuring them that the industry is doing everything it can to make cigarettes as safe as possible and claim the high moral ground of corporate or environmental responsibility.
14. Always keep thinking of new ways to defend the industry.

Strategies of this sort are explicit in the industry's internal documents. Burgard's memo from 1969 and BAT's 1984 "cast doubt" confession are two of the more outrageous, but there are numerous others. The Tobacco Institute also occasionally let the cat out of the bag—when they thought no one would be listening. In 1972 TI Vice President Fred Panzer issued a memo talking about the "brilliantly conceived strategy" of "creating doubt about the health charge without actually denying it." British tobacco researchers in the 1980s commented on how Philip Morris was piloting a "global strategy" to deny secondhand smoke hazards, spending vast sums of money "to keep the controversy alive."[10]

In most instances the claim was simply that there was not yet sufficient evidence to "convict" cigarettes of causing any real harms; the question of causation was supposed to remain "open." In 1969, when the *New York Times* announced it would no longer publish cigarette ads without a health caution, the American Tobacco Company published a series of full-page ads in newspapers and magazines across the United States carrying the headline "Why We're Dropping the New York Times":

> Sure there are statistics associating lung cancer and cigarettes. There are statistics associating lung cancer with divorce, and even with lack of sleep. But no scientist has produced clinical or biological proof that cigarettes cause the diseases they are accused of causing. After fifteen years of trying, nobody has induced lung cancer in animals with cigarette smoke.
>
> We believe the anticigarette theory is a bum rap. . . . [11]

Hundreds of similar examples could be cited.

INTERNAL AGNOTOLOGY

Now, one point rarely appreciated is that the industry's propaganda was directed not just *outward* to the smoking public but also *inward* to the cigarette makers' own employees and commercial partners. Reynolds's president, E. A. Darr, took the denialist message to his stockholders on July 8, 1954, assuring them that "no real proof has been presented that there is a relationship between cigarettes and cancer." American Tobacco presented this same message to its shareholders, reporting Hanmer and Haag's purported "direct evidence refuting anti-cigarette charges." The companies' annual reports often rolled out the "not yet proven" mantra, as did the many newsletters printed for company employees and and their families (including re-tirees). Liggett's *Annual Report* from 1965, for example, reassured stockholders that "the U.S. Surgeon General's Report published last year was not conclusive" and that "a great deal more research is urgently needed." Lorillard's president three years later was expressly advised (by his research chief) not to bring up possible health harms when talking with shareholders.[12]

In some instances company newsletters invited employees to "test" themselves on the "tobacco/health issue" by answering mini-quizzes like

The cause of lung cancer is:

    a. cigarette smoking
    b. air pollution
    c. unknown

Non-Smokers who contract lung cancer get the disease:

    a. earlier than smokers
    b. later than smokers
    c. at about the same age.[13]

Or consider this extract from Philip Morris's *Call News,* a newspaper distributed to all corporate employees:

Philip Morris agrees with industry critics that cigarette smoking should be studied. We disagree, however, with those who feel that all the answers are in. We maintain that no causal relationship between smoking and health has been proved.

One thing seems abundantly clear to us: Without further research we will never know the true answers. Further, assuming a causal connection between smoking and illness, when one has not been established, takes attention away from the other im-portant subjects for study.[14]

Notice here again this intimation of a *danger* in concluding that smoking causes harm—by distracting from "other important subjects for study."

The fact is that virtually *all* the industry's classic denialist tactics were also di-rected at the companies' own employees. Copies of the Tobacco Institute's *Tobacco and Health Report* were sent to corporate staff, for example, to keep them plied with the latest information on how "New Statistics Contradict Anti-Cigarette Theory" and the like. Similar messages were sent to tobacco farmers and the many thousands of retailers, wholesalers, and warehousers responsible for keeping the wheels of the tobacco engine turning. Company lawyers were brought in to lecture to assemblies of tobacco farmers, salesmen, or retailers on tobacco and health, and speeches along these lines were read into the *Congressional Record.*[15] It seems as if no audience was off limits—including factory workers on the floors of tobacco plants.

R. J. Reynolds, in particular, devoted a great deal of effort to keep its employees properly aligned. A 1982 document lists the following means by which the company planned to "increase employee support of RJRT and management's positions on key tobacco issues":

A. *Smoking and Health*—Public Relations is responsible for all employee communication necessary to conduct this corporation-wide campaign to increase employee knowledge of company and industry positions on key tobacco issues.

 1. Minimum of two stories on tobacco issues will be prepared for each issue of *Caravan* [a Reynolds employee newsletter]
 2. *RJR World* [another corporate newsletter] will be supplied with a minimum of one story per month.
 3. A minimum of three brochures on tobacco issues will be prepared and distributed through RJRT break areas each quarter.
 4. A minimum of three posters on tobacco issues will be prepared and placed on all RJRT bulletin boards each quarter.
 5. Minimum of two mailings to homes of RJRT employees and retirees will be conducted to distribute significant booklets or other materials on tobacco issues.
 6. An information packet with appropriate RJRT and tobacco industry materials on tobacco issues will be put together for use in various ways. Packet will initially be tested for use in Whitaker Park tour area [in Winston-Salem] for visitors.[16] [Etc.]

Newsletters intended purely for corporate eyes—and there are dozens—carried denialist propaganda, reminding readers that even the American Medical Association agreed that questions about smoking and health "remain unanswered." R. J. Reynolds's *Tobacco International Communiqué* published elaborate refutations of the lung cancer link, reassuring employees that there was "no demonstrated relationship between smoking and any disease." The same company's *Management Bulletin* went even further, twisting reports to make it seem as if moderate smoking might even *prevent* cancer. As one early report put it: "A pack a day keeps lung cancer away."[17]

SPAM SANDWICHES AT REYNOLDS
AND JOKES FROM PHILIP MORRIS

One motivation for internal policing came from surveys showing that employees at Reynolds were paying too much attention to public media, including news reports. In 1979, for example, an "Employee Attitude Survey" found that most of the information available to employees was "anti-smoking in nature." The company responded by establishing a Communication Program on Smoking and Health, the goal of which was to deliver "pro-tobacco information to employees" through company newsletters such as *Caravan, Longbow,* and *RJR World.*[18] Smoking and health propaganda was typically sandwiched in between more benign stories of birthdays or promotions; this sandwich method was to play a role in the company's new corporate-wide "action program": "Our basis approach on all corporate-wide communications will be to introduce at least two other issues in our communications before presenting any significant information on the smoking and health issue. Then we will 'balance' information on smoking and health with material on a variety of other issues."[19] (Surveys were sometimes used to influence voting behavior: in Los Alamos County, New Mexico, for example, residents in one Reynolds-commissioned poll were asked whether they agreed with the view of "some people" that "if the law prohibiting smoking is passed, it will cause arguments and conflicts between people, possibly even violence." Local residents protested, recognizing such questions as surreptitious "campaigning against the ordinance.")[20]

Smoking and health was also one of the topics covered in the training manuals issued by Reynolds for its new sales personnel. The 1996 edition of Reynolds's two-volume, 549-page manual included a module on smoking and health designed to instruct Reynolds sales reps on "how to respond correctly when faced with questions." Employees were also instructed on how to talk to the press, with emphasis on the line that while smoking was "a risk factor for certain diseases" it was "not a proven cause." A 1996 *Issues Guide* prepared for this purpose warned of the human judgment involved in interpreting any statistical study, adding that animals forced to inhale "fresh, whole cigarette smoke" had never developed cancer, heart disease, or emphysema. And that estimates of hundreds of thousands of deaths from smoking in the United States and millions globally were "without exception" based on "complicated mathematical models" using "unproven" assumptions. And that the smoke constituents most often blamed for cancer were also found in auto exhaust and in broiled and grilled foods.[21]

Philip Morris printed similar guidelines, detailing how "the controversy" should be spun. Employees were instructed on how to respond to questions on hot button topics, with the bottom line always that there are "outstanding scientists who do not accept as proven a causal relationship between smoking and disease." Public demeanor was part of the program: spokespersons were to appear calm and confident with "nothing to hide"; "you will undoubtedly know more than the other person about the issues." Humorous quotes were also to be handy, like Fletcher Knebel's "Smoking is one of the leading causes of statistics" and C. A. d'Alonzo's "Sleep is to be avoided, since most heart attacks occur then."[22] Cancer denial was the most obvious and urgent imperative, but spokespersons were also to know that smoking has "little or no effect on birth weight" and that smoking is "a practice, a custom—not an 'addiction.'" Such manuals tell us a great deal about how the companies wanted us—and their employees—to think about cigarettes, with "guideline" chapters explaining how to talk about cancer, addiction, public smoking, social costs, advertising, and warning labels. Here is typical advice from one such manual:

Avoid flat assertions that "smoking is not dangerous." Our belief is that smoking has not been established or proven to cause disease. We do not claim to have all the answers and do not believe that the anti-cigarette crusaders have them either.

Analogies between cigarettes and alcohol are dangerous, since it is accepted that alcohol is detrimental to health in many cases, and causes a wide range of social problems. Consider animal fats, sugar or coffee.[23]

A higher level of indoctrination came from the industry's College of Tobacco Knowledge, an annual series of training seminars organized by the Tobacco Institute in the 1970s and 1980s to teach global tobacco elites how to communicate the party line on smoking and health. The college attracted tobacco-industry apologists from all over the world, helping the global industry maintain a unified legal-PR front on "the tobacco controversy."[24] Fifteen such seminars had been offered by 1987, training hundreds of legal and communications personnel from tobacco firms around the world. BAT's Christopher Proctor (no relation) organized similar programs in the 1990s under the rubric of "issues training"; in 1993 and 1994 alone Proctor conducted issues and/or witness training in Zimbabwe, Singapore, New Zealand, Costa Rica, Bali, and Shook Hardy's own Kansas City, assisting also with media briefings in a number of other locales.[25]

SELF-CENSORSHIP WITH CIGNA

A striking example of internal indoctrination involved covert censorship of the *medical information* to which tobacco employees were exposed. Philip Morris in the 1990s was worried about its workers learning the truth, so it asked its insurance providers to eliminate certain passages from the health information sent to employees. This self-censorship is remarkable enough, but perhaps even more astonishing is that a reputable insurance company was willing to collaborate in such brazen censorship, albeit for a price.

The background here is that Philip Morris, like many other large corporations, provides its employees with health insurance, vacations, pensions, and treatment for certain kinds of drug abuse. The company's health insurance provider in the 1990s was CIGNA, one of the oldest insurers in the United States. CIGNA had begun insuring marine voyagers in the nineteenth century and was the first American insurer operating in China. And like most other health insurers it provided information to its clients—in this instance thousands of Philip Morris employees—on how to keep fit, how to treat a sick child, and so forth. What is hard to believe, however, is that CIGNA also allowed Philip Morris to limit what its workers were told about the health effects of smoking.

Between 1996 and 1998, and perhaps at other times, CIGNA collaborated in an effort to censor the health information Philip Morris employees were receiving via the quarterly *Well-Being* newsletter sent to everyone on the Philip Morris payroll. And not just to Philip Morris the tobacco manufacturer but also to subsidiaries such as Miller Brewing and Kraft General Foods, makers of Velveeta cheese and Oreo cookies. In a recent analysis for the *American Journal of Public Health,* Monique E. Muggli and Richard D. Hurt of the Mayo Clinic in Minnesota show how Philip Morris benefits personnel would review prepublication drafts of the newsletter, deleting passages they found offensive or sometimes even barring the entire issue from being sent out. Passages deemed objectionable included remarks about cigarette smoke triggering asthma and an article advising people with high blood pressure to quit smoking.

The spring 1996 issue of *Well-Being,* for example, was released only after removal of an ad for a series of Time-Life videos narrated by Surgeon General C. Everett Koop. The summer 1996 issue was not sent to Philip Morris employees at all, because (as company censors put it) "several articles contained anti-smoking references." The winter 1996 issue was not sent out because the director of employee benefits at Philip Morris didn't want to pay $3,000 to replace an article containing this advice for asthma sufferers: "Do not allow smoking in your home or in any other environment that you can control." The summer 1997 issue was not published because it contained "objectionable" references to secondhand smoke. Philip Morris censors clipped out smoking references from at least two issues in 1998, including a passage on the importance of avoiding secondhand smoke when a child has an inner ear infection. After censorship, parents with a child suffering from an inner ear infection were told only to have the child blow his or her nose, to sleep with a pillow, and to keep good hand-washing habits. With no mention of avoiding secondhand smoke.[26]

Philip Morris clearly wanted its employees not to know the truth about smoking and went to great lengths to keep them in the dark. Even when it meant risking the health of their children.

A similar callousness was extended to stockholders. In 1996, at the annual meeting of RJR Nabisco shareholders in Winston-Salem, Reynolds chairman Charles M. Harper responded as follows to a question from shareholder Anne M. Donley about whether he thought it was right for children to be exposed to secondhand smoke:

> *The Chairman:* I will not restrict anybody's right to smoke. If the children don't like to be in a smoky room, and I wouldn't like to be, they'll leave. I don't know if you've got any grandchildren; I do. And if there is smoke around that's uncomfortable, they'll leave.
>
> *Ms. Donley:* An infant cannot leave a room.
>
> *The Chairman:* Well—okay. At some point they begin to crawl, okay? And then they begin to walk, and so on. Anyway, I guess that's enough said. Thank you very much.[27]

IGNORANCE AS ETIQUETTE

Corporate higher-ups do often seem to have wanted to know the truth, and we've seen how they kept up with current science while simultaneously fostering ignorance among their own employees.[28] And of course the scientific literature summarized for upper management told a very different story from the industry's public "no proof" bluster. It is also important to appreciate, however, how "bad news" circulated—or failed to circulate—in such an environment.

Inside the companies, knowledge of cancer hazards seems to have been impolite knowledge, a kind of dirty little secret you weren't supposed to talk about, at least not in ways that would stray too far from the party line. Corporate etiquette made it hard to talk about cancer without a denialist slant. To accept the reality of harms was like an expression of disloyalty, a traitorous act. Cancer concessions were de facto threats to corporate security, which is perhaps one reason we often find denials expressed in the language of "caution" or even "safety." The industry portrayed itself as being "cautious" in calling for more research or better proof. One can even imagine ignorance becoming honest in such an environment, through a kind of self-imposed blindness. It was, after all, often "safer" for the companies not to know, and the conditions needed to safeguard this ignorance were carefully engineered. According to Helmut Wakeham, the most powerful researcher at the world's most powerful tobacco company, it was the view of Philip Morris lawyers that "you couldn't be criticized for not knowing something." Self-imposed ignorance was a calculated legal strategy, a means (as William Dunn put it) of defending the industry against claims on behalf of "heirs and deceased smokers: 'We within the industry are ignorant of any relationship between smoking and disease.'"[29]

Evidence of this process of securing internal ignorance can be found in job descriptions for new hires at the various companies. Jobs that required a certain PR expertise, for example, often asked an applicant to recognize "the controversy." In 1993 applicants for the position of "Scientific Advisor" at BAT were expected to be aware that health authorities "continue to attack tobacco companies world-wide and publicise papers alleging the ill-effects of smoking." Applicants were also supposed to be able to assist in "explaining the BAT position on smoking issues to internal or external audiences."[30] The industry recognized the value of keeping itself in the dark about certain matters, consistent with Wakeham's view that you cannot be faulted for what you don't know.

Blame for creating ignorance in this realm cannot be restricted to the manufacturers, however. The industry has had many friends: in academia, agriculture, government, sports, law, journalism, and virtually every other part of society. Tobacco farmers tend not to be included as part of "the industry," but they have certainly participated in doubt-mongering. The Tobacco Growers' Information Committee published a newsletter beginning in 1958 containing much of this same denialist rhetoric. Growers' associations and wholesalers were also members of the Tobacco Institute, contributing funds and embracing its know-nothing, "no proof" posture.

Tobacco trade unions are not innocent in this respect. In the United States the Tobacco Workers International Union was established in 1895 and in 1978 joined with bakery and confectionery workers to form the Bakery, Confectionery, Tobacco Workers, and Grain Millers International Union. (Oddly enough, the BCTGM's webpage presenting "Union Companies and Products" has a long list of things made by the rank and file with no mention of any tobacco product.) When I checked in 2008 the union's website listed two locals from tobacco manufacturing plants, one in Greensboro and another in Richmond. The Richmond link wasn't working, but the Greensboro website directed me to a speech by the president of BCTGM Local 317-T, a Lorillard worker by the name of Randy W. Fulk, who rants about the "mind boggling" statistics thrown up against the tobacco industry. Fulk says that Lorillard has never encouraged anyone to smoke and compares smoking to driving a car with a speedometer that goes up to 160 miles per hour (caveat emptor, in other words). Government estimates of 400,000 Americans killed annually by tobacco he characterizes as "propaganda" and invokes the Bible to remind us that "we will all die of something." He also claims that the costs of smoking have been "ludicrously exaggerated," citing Kip Viscusi's macabre view that smoking actually *saves* society money by lowering health care costs. (Viscusi is a Harvard economist who has testified for the industry in court.) As examples, Fulk mentions "financial gains that arise from lower nursing-home costs" and "foregone retirement pensions and Social Security claims." (Because smokers die earlier, he means to say.)[31] It is sad to see a shop floor steward so buffaloed by his bosses, but perhaps that is what we have to expect from someone whose union requires him to defend his coworkers' jobs, whatever harms those might be causing to the larger community.

JOURNALISTS DROP THE BALL

Some historical ignorance of cigarette harms must be traced to the timidity of the mainstream media, stemming from their financial dependence on cigarette advertising. George Seldes was already lamenting this in the 1940s, but the strength of this dependency grew in subsequent decades as advertising budgets soared into the hundreds and eventually thousands of millions of dollars. Elizabeth Whelan of the American Council on Science and Health in the 1980s showed that women's magazines receiving ad revenue from the industry were woefully reluctant to publish anything critical of smoking or the tobacco cartel; Gloria Steinem, founding editor of *Ms. Magazine,* once called this situation "a kind of prison." Whelan more recently has shown that in 1998 and 2000 tobacco ads in American women's magazines outnumbered anti-smoking messages by more than ten to one. In terms of number of pages published, cigarette ads overwhelmed anti-smoking articles by a whopping thirty to one. Readers of *Mother Jones* in 2009 or *Wired* in 2010 or *Ebony* in 2011 may be surprised to find such magazines still publishing full-page color tobacco ads—as if American Spirit cigarettes (manufactured by Reynolds) were any less tainted than your ordinary redneck Camels or Marlboros.[32]

For many years, tobacco companies were able to use even highbrow organs like the *New York Times* to push their "we need more research" message.[33] In the mid-1980s the *Times* allowed Reynolds to publish a series of ads disputing the science linking smoking to heart disease. America's "newspaper of record" continued to print cigarette ads until 1999, when it finally bit the bullet and quit. In the 1970s and 1980s the paper was repeatedly urged to refuse tobacco advertising but balked, claiming that this would set a "dangerous precedent." When the paper finally made the right move and the sky did not fall, there was no more talk of any "dangerous precedent." What is perhaps most remarkable, though, is that for many years the *Times* actually paid to place its *own* ads in the tobacco trade press—to drum up advertising business. One such ad, placed in the *U.S. Tobacco and Candy Journal*, offered that "Lifestyles are made, not born."[34] In other words: please advertise in the *New York Times* if you want to get more people to smoke your product!

Indirect ads for the industry still appear from time to time in the *Times*. On May 4, 2009, for example, the Washington Legal Foundation published an op-ed in the paper attacking trial lawyers as part of an unregulated, greedy, "parasitic," "multi-billion-dollar" business that "restrains U.S. economic recovery." Morton Mintz in a commentary for the *Nieman Watchdog* pointed out that the Washington Legal Foundation has close ties to the cigarette industry, which uses such groups as fronts to get friendly opinions into the mainstream media. Journalistic penetration has also been achieved through what Simon Chapman of the University of Sydney calls "corporate schmoozing." In 2008 Pfizer and Philip Morris sponsored a training program for journalists in Brazil, with the endorsement and support of that country's largest newspaper, the *Folha de São Paulo*.[35] Training sessions of this sort allow corporate logos to appear in newspaper ads and give the sponsor a certain journalistic street cred.

But journalists have also been coaxed into working more directly for the companies. Stanley Frank's ventriloquizing for the industry in *True* magazine is one outrageous example, but there are many others. In 1977, for example, the New York writer Ruth Rosenbaum published an article in *New Times* magazine attacking the American Cancer Society and the National Cancer Institute for their (not altogether unfounded) mollycoddling of industrial polluters. Rosenbaum blasted the "cancer establishment" as a "self-perpetuating bureaucracy," 40 percent of whose funding went to "barely reviewed" contract research, a mechanism inviting "abuse and poor quality work." The article made it sound as if Big Medicine had been unwilling to take on Big Business, resulting in a self-interested suppression of alternative therapies. Rosenbaum accused the ACS's Committee on Unproven Methods of being "a network of vigilantes prepared to pounce on anyone who promotes a cancer therapy that runs against their substantial prejudices and profits."[36] Readers came away with an impression of the ACS as a bunch of self-satisfied defenders of medical orthodoxy, and indeed some people were fooled into regarding her article as a courageous exposé. Carl Jensen's left-leaning Project Censored, for example, honored and reprinted Rosenbaum's article in its annotated chronicle of "20 Years of Censored News in the U.S."[37]

Rosenbaum was fêted as a lefty maverick, but a search of the tobacco industry's archives reveals a more sinister story. Rosenbaum wrote her article with the help of Hill & Knowlton, the industry's public relations firm; she was also a personal friend of Fred Panzer at the Tobacco Institute and he, too, helped her with it. None of this was known to Jensen when he celebrated Rosenbaum's review for his Project Censored—nor, apparently, the fact that her articles had earned her invitations to work for the industry in litigation. Jensen et al. relied on Rosenbaum when they claimed that "the most serious problem with cancer research in this country has been the lack of attention given to banning carcinogenic chemicals." Tobacco is not mentioned among these chemicals, and the real story missed by Project Censored is that the attack on the American Cancer Society they naively endorse was crafted with the assistance of the Tobacco Institute and Big Tobacco's PR staffers.[38]

TOBACCO AS CHOCOLATE, APPLESAUCE, AND FREEDOM

Our focus has been on the creation of ignorance, but it is also important to realize that the industry does not want the minds of smokers and potential smokers to be empty: the goal is not an *absence* of knowledge but rather the insinuation of a specific body of knowledge, or belief and feeling, that will further the continued legal sale of cigarettes. The companies want us to believe we need more research, that it is dangerous to jump to conclusions or to shut off debate. They want us to think that smoking is safe, or at least safer than it used to be, or safe enough to be an "acceptable risk." They want us to think that it's not so hard to quit, that addiction is really only a matter of semantics, that smoking is an "adult choice," that Winston tastes good like a cigarette should.

The use of trivializing analogies is one way this is achieved. Tobacco is likened to coffee, chocolate, brandy, or some other naughty yet legitimate pleasure. Nicotine addiction is also trivialized by comparing it to far less noxious "habits"—like jogging or watching TV. Tobacco Institute VP Brennan Dawson in 1994 compared smokers to "news junkies" and "chocoholics," observing that nicotine was "also found in things as scary as potatoes."[39] Sharon Boyse at British American Tobacco was equally dismissive: "It has been suggested that smoking must be addictive because it contains nicotine. So do many common vegetables, including tomatoes, aubergines and potato skins. Are vegetable eaters also drug users?—physically dependent on their ratatouille, perhaps, in the same way that heroin addicts are dependent on their heroin?"[40] Cigarette apologists have commonly defended smoking by such means, likening it to applesauce, chewing gum, or Twinkies. A search of the industry's archives for "no worse than" returns hundreds of documents, with cigarettes described as no worse than alcohol, chocolates, caffeine, coffee or dessert, fatty hamburgers, milk, or sitting next to people with stinky perfume or bad breath. Academics have been hired to generate such comparisons: Theodore H. Blau, a Tampa, Florida, psychologist, in 1982 testimony before the U.S. Congress compared smoking to attachments to "tennis, jogging, candy, rock music, Coca-cola, members of the opposite sex and hamburgers."[41] Blau's remarks were cited in a Tobacco Institute press release, with no mention of his being on the take from the industry's Special Account No. 4—administered through the law firm of Jacob & Medinger. And no mention of his being a member of the "Tobacco Institute Team."

(The applesauce comparison is most vividly displayed in Peter Taylor's marvelous 1976 interview with Helmut Wakeham at Philip Morris, preserved for posterity in *Death in the West,* the film Philip Morris tried to suppress. Wakeham is asked whether he believes that smoking causes cancer and responds that *anything* can be bad for you if consumed in excess—even applesauce. Asked whether he thinks people are dying from eating applesauce, he responds that if not, then only because "they're not eating that much." He also dismisses the suggestion that doctors are an appropriate source for health advice.)[42]

The companies want us to believe they are responsible corporate citizens. They want us to think they have high moral standards, and they want us to know they support anti-litter campaigns and sustainable agriculture. The overarching goal, of course, is to generate good feelings for manufacturers and the tobacco habit. So cigarettes are to be thought of as more like chocolates and fine liqueurs and not so much like crack cocaine or carcinogenic smokestacks. Dangerous perhaps in excess but fine in moderation, a kind of edgy adventure like sky diving or some other extreme sport. And above all an *adult choice,* if not the last bastion of freedom.

Which is also why so much consternation has come from the fact that cigarettes kill not only smokers but also lots and lots of *non-smokers:* fifty thousand per year in the United States alone and perhaps ten times that globally. Hirayama and Trichopoulos published rock-solid indictments of secondhand smoke as a cancer hazard in 1981, and the U.S. Surgeon General and National Academy of Sciences by 1986 had concluded that the danger was real.[43] Which means that smoking as experienced by most people is less a free choice than a toxic intrusion, a pollution of personal space. Secondhand smoke turns out to cause far more deaths than oil spills or air pollution or even nuclear accidents like Chernobyl or natural disasters like earthquakes or tsunamis. Or all of the world's modern wars. The specter of death from "involuntary smoke" also gave tobacco a new political dimension, poking a big hole in the story of smoking as a free choice. And so required—at least from the industry's point of view—new ways to manipulate knowledge, belief, and desire.

Secondhand smoke was a serious challenge. Industry executives predicted a "devastating effect on sales," with people stopping smoking not just at work, but at parties and on planes and in countless other social spaces. Here was the "anti's silver bullet." As John Rupp from the law firm of Covington & Burling put it, secondhand smoke had put the industry "in deep shit."[44]

Cigarette manufacturers knew they needed an aggressive response, and the first was simply to extend the denialist campaign that had been used against the mainstream hazard. Secondhand smoke denial was, in a sense, the industry's intelligent design to an older generation's young-earth creationism. Scientists were hired to testify that "environmental tobacco smoke" (ETS) was a trivial or nonexistent hazard and that more research was needed prior to decisive action. Cigarette-friendly conferences were sponsored, along with research and political agitation. Front groups and third parties were organized to spread this message, including the ETS Consultants Program, the Associates for Research in Indoor Air (ARIA), the Center for Indoor Air Research (CIAR), and an umbrella group called Indoor Air International, created in 1989 to challenge nascent moves to restrict indoor smoking, especially in California.[45] A barrage of industry-funded advertisements helped create a climate of broad public confusion surrounding the topic. The denials were well funded and of global reach; Japan Tobacco's website in November 2010, for example, in the section on "Smoking and Health," part of a larger treatment of "Corporate Responsibility," comments: "We do not believe that the claim that ETS is a cause of lung cancer, heart disease and chronic pulmonary diseases in non-smokers has been convincingly demonstrated or that a reliable causal link between ETS exposure and chronic diseases has been established."[46]

Here again the work of analogies has been crucial. The industry has spent a lot of time trying to get us to think of "environmental" smoke (ETS) as more of an *annoyance* (or nuisance) than a real cause of harms. ETS is more like a baby crying on an airplane or a person with strong body odor or cloying perfume. The point, in other words, is not just to insinuate ignorance, but to guide us away from dangerous thoughts and onto thoughts safe for the industry. The interest has been to create not distrust in the abstract but rather distrust of certain bodies of knowledge—of unfriendly statistics, orthodox medicine, the Surgeon General or the EPA or "the government" more generally. Many different instruments have been used for this purpose, from ridicule in political cartoons to the sale of American flags and copies of the Bill of Rights. The hope has been to associate smoking with free speech, free trade, patriotism, and the unfettered pursuit of happiness.

Which is also why so much money was shoveled to the American Civil Liberties Union (ACLU), a freedom-loving organization famous for defending rights to march or to speak or, as it turned out, to smoke. Philip Morris in the late 1980s and early 1990s gave the ACLU over half a million dollars, with Reynolds chipping in several hundred thousand more. The money was funneled into the ACLU's Task Force on Civil Liberties in the Workplace, which fought for the right of smokers to smoke on the job while doing little or nothing for non-smokers. A writer by the name of John Fahs discovered the intrigue while working for the ACLU in the early 1990s and published some of the canceled checks in his 1996 book, *Cigarette Confidential*. Morton Mintz then covered the story for the *Progressive*, telling how he himself had been asked to donate to the organization, advertised in beg-letters as supported "*exclusively* by caring, concerned people like you"—with no mention of Big Tobacco's apparent quid pro quo. The ACLU had fought for the freedom of smokers to smoke—leaving the rest of us to suffer exposure to secondhand smoke without any aid from "our nation's guardian of liberty." Even Melvin Wulf, the ACLU's legal director from 1962 to 1977, was appalled to hear of the ACLU's taking tobacco money, commenting that its basic integrity had been "corrupted by the attraction of easy money from an industry whose ethical values are themselves notoriously corrupt and which is responsible for the death annually of 350,000 to 400,000 persons in the U.S. alone."[47]

CREATING DESIRE

It is not enough to think about the industry as creating or destroying knowledge, or even as creating and controlling desire. At the end of the day they really only care about enticing *behavior*, meaning the shelling out of cold hard cash for cigarettes. All else is secondary. Ignorance versus knowledge has only been an issue insofar as these can be twisted to help keep selling cigarettes. So the mind is targeted but also the gut, the emotions. Smoking is happy friends at the beach, an off-road race, a keep-me-thin therapy, or sexual liberation or adult cool. Smoking is what you do to relax or to unwind or to attract the opposite sex, or to overcome stress or seal a deal. All of which has been the job of advertising—image making—which trades in seductive semiotics and fantasies far from the real mortal ends of smoking. We are encouraged to think of cigarettes as more like coffee or chocolate or a very fine brandy—and not like choking phlegm and a ghostly shadow life in the hospital with tubes up your nose. Smoking is not supposed to be like lead paint or toxic waste or the white-knuckled grip of addiction but rather like hope and peace and choice and the very satisfaction of life itself.

Measuring Ignorance

The Impact of Industry Disinformation on Popular Knowledge of Tobacco Hazards

After smoking Camel cigarettes for twenty-four (24) years, my lungs are as clean as a whistle.
SYLVIA SINDELAR TO REYNOLDS, APRIL 28, 1958

Take old George Burns for example; he's been smoking for (probably) 60 years now, and is probably healthier than average for a man of his age. You might say that old George is living proof that tobacco smoke is not harmful to health.
M. WHITE TO REYNOLDS, OCTOBER 30, 1985

We've seen some of the techniques used by the smoke folk to manufacture and disseminate ignorance. How, though, do we measure the success of such efforts? After all, maybe the companies are right when they say that smokers have always known that tobacco is bad for you, that knowledge of hazards is "common" or nearly universal. If that is true, then perhaps the companies are innocent, or guilty only of puffery: if everyone is fully informed when they begin smoking, why should anyone be upset when disease sets in? The manufacturers may well have lied in denying harms, but is it really fraud if no one believes you? What can we say about the extent to which people have or have not known about the hazards of smoking?

Agnometrics may be a new word, but it is a well-developed field of inquiry. Since the 1950s, in fact, polling agencies such as Roper and Gallup have been paid substantial sums to explore what people know *and don't know* about specific topics, including the dangers of smoking. Polls can be used to test the industry's claim that such harms have long been "common knowledge," but there are other sources for gauging popular understanding. There is the testimony of smokers themselves, as revealed in letters written to the companies and telephone logs preserved in corporate archives. We also have the industry's own assessments of the extent to which people appreciate the dangers.

Here I want to explore these different ways of measuring ignorance, recognizing that there are difficulties in how we define some of the crucial terms. How do we gauge what is common or uncommon knowledge? The tobacco industry in staking its claim for "universal awareness" likes to confuse knowledge and awareness, ignoring the crucial difference between *knowing* that cigarettes are dangerous and simply *having heard* this to be the case. The error is so blatant that one marvels at its bravado: it would be hard, after all, to find someone who hasn't "heard" that cigarettes may be hazardous—and the warning is right on the pack. But there are obvious differences between awareness and belief. Many of us will have *heard* that some people *think* there are alien spacecraft being held at Area 51 in southern Nevada—but does that mean we actually believe it?

The industry seeks to perpetuate a similar confusion in its effort to prove that the dangers of smoking have long been common knowledge. A body of knowledge is common, they say, if large numbers of people have heard about it or have heard someone putting it forward as true—which is convenient in the cigarette context. Cigarettes in the United States have had cautions on the packs since 1966 and warnings since 1970; most smokers have seen such labels or at least are "aware" of them, so surely anyone with even half a brain must have been fairly forewarned. (The industry started making this argument when warnings were first proposed: people didn't need a warning since they already knew.) Common knowledge is also supposed to be evident from the broad dissemination of writings by health authorities, including discussions in textbooks or news media to which anyone but an ostrich or a hermit must have been "exposed."

But is this really evidence of public understanding? What, in fact, do people believe about the nature of harms from cigarettes? How seriously do they take such threats, and how have such views changed over time? These are questions that cannot be answered simply by looking at, say, high school textbooks or articles in magazines and newspapers, as the industry wants us to believe. If convictions could be measured simply by exposure to authoritative texts, then teachers would have no need to assign grades; we could just grade the textbooks. The industry's claim is sort of like saying that everyone in the 1930s must have been a communist, because communist literature was widely disseminated. Exposure is not a measure of belief; what people *know about* a topic and what *has been written* (by others) are two very different things—which the companies want us to conflate. They would rather we not distinguish between "having heard that" cigarettes may kill you and believing this to be true. But surely people may have *heard* that tobacco may be harmful without actually *believing* this is the case.

In court, the tobacco industry's "common knowledge" experts go to great lengths to confuse knowledge and awareness. Called to testify on what was known about the risks of smoking at some point in time, these experts produce countless exam-

ples of what people *might have been* exposed to—typically newspaper and magazine articles and the like—inferring from this that smokers must have known what
they were doing. Media reporting on such topics is taken as evidence of "common
knowledge": so if newspapers reported on, say, smoking as a cause of Buerger's disease or bladder cancer, then ordinary people must have understood such dangers.
They were properly forewarned.

Surveys of actual attitudes and opinions tell quite a different story, however. They
make it clear that knowledge of smoking's hazards has varied widely over time and
space but also by age, class, and sex—and (especially) by whether or not one smokes.
It turns out that *smokers* are significantly less likely to recognize hazards than *non-
smokers* and less likely to see themselves as vulnerable. Many smokers find it hard
to apply whatever knowledge they have to their own situation; they often feel that
they personally don't smoke enough to pose a real danger, or that their brands are
not the really bad ones. Many people who smoke only a few cigarettes per day do
not even regard themselves as smokers. And a surprising number do not think there
is anything wrong with moderate smoking. The answers people give in such surveys depend very much on how the questions are asked: virtually everyone will agree
that smoking *might* cause lung cancer, for example, while far fewer will realize it as
the *major cause* or that the evidence constitutes irrefutable proof.

There are several different ways to get at this changing history of ignorance. Here
we explore three different sources: *public opinion polls,* including qualitative assessments based on interviews; *consumer letters* and *logs of phone calls* to and from the
industry; and *statements by the industry itself* about the nature or extent of popular knowledge. Sources such as these shed light on what people have or have not
known, and in a more reliable way than looking only at the media to which people
have been "exposed." Exposure does not guarantee belief, any more than propaganda
guarantees patriotism. We have to look at what people actually believe, as revealed
by surveys, interviews, and testimonials in people's own words.

So first the polls.

HAVE YOU HEARD? DO YOU KNOW?

In the United States polling agencies have been interested in what people know and
don't know about tobacco since the 1940s. The first Gallup poll to address this question dates from 1949, when 52 percent of American smokers were found to agree
that cigarettes were "harmful," though the question was vague and didn't distinguish
different kinds of harm—as in cancer versus cough. And no effort was made to gauge
strength of conviction or degree of concern.

More sophisticated polling techniques were developed in the 1950s. In 1958, for
example, a Gallup poll reported that "among cigaret smokers, the sentiment still is

that cigaret smoking is not one of the causes of lung cancer." George Gallup found that when asked, "do you think that smoking is or is not one of the causes of cancer of the lung?" smokers answered as follows:

Yes, is a cause	33 percent
No, is not	43 percent
Undecided	24 percent

The report also showed that smokers of filter-tipped cigarettes were more likely to believe in cancer causation (38 percent vs. 28 percent). And that nearly three quarters of the smokers of *unfiltered* cigarettes said "no" or were undecided.[1]

Polling agencies hired by tobacco manufacturers came up with similar results. Elmo Roper and Associates at Williams College in 1958, for example, was hired by Philip Morris to conduct a study of smokers' attitudes for the company. Five thousand smokers from all across the country were asked several dozen questions about the dangers of cigarettes and how these compared with other kinds of hazards. While most of these people had *heard* that smoking had been linked to cancer—were aware of a controversy—nearly 70 percent agreed that "as long as you are careful not to smoke too much, cigarettes won't do you any real harm." And unprompted recall of cancer was quite low. When asked to complete the sentence, "The trouble with cigarettes is that they . . . ," only one percent volunteered "could cause cancer." And only 3 percent offered that cigarettes could be "harmful to your lungs, wind, breath." A "Highlights" section of the report concluded that while cigarettes were regarded as "bad for you to a greater extent than the other products we asked about" (air pollution, climbing out of a bathtub, etc.) there was "surprisingly little concern" about cigarettes. What little concern there was seemed "largely directed at the avoidance of throat irritation and the consequent search for mildness" in the form of filters. The survey found "fertile ground for promoting cigarettes as a good friend—a friend that relieves tension, permits one to relax, and is comforting when alone or idle." The good news (for the industry) was that while fear of cancer was "certainly present," smokers seemed to be "more preoccupied with the fact that cigarettes make them cough and cause sore throats."[2]

Polls can of course be misleading, especially when a clear distinction is not drawn between "awareness" and "belief." A 1954 Gallup poll, for example, revealed that 90 percent of those surveyed had "heard or read about" the connection between smoking and lung cancer, and this is often cited by the industry's polling experts in court. But when this same survey asked whether people *believed* what they had read— that cigarettes could cause cancer—less than half of those polled answered "yes." And smokers were even less convinced. A 1965 Louis Harris poll found that when 1,250 Americans were asked whether smoking was a "major" or a "minor" cause of lung cancer, only 20 percent of the heavy smokers said "major cause." Twenty-four percent said "minor" cause of the disease, and 56 percent answered "can't yet tell."

Surveys conducted in 1966 for the U.S. Public Health Service found only 46 percent of the adult population answering "yes" when asked, "Is there any way at all to
prevent a person from getting lung cancer?" Only 21 percent said "yes" in response
to the same question about emphysema and chronic bronchitis.[3]

Surveys have sometimes looked at the extent to which people are *worried about*
what they've heard. A 1956 series of interviews conducted by Lorillard Tobacco found
that most smokers had been unaffected by the recent cancer publicity and that since
many smokers' friends and physicians still smoked there was little pressure to change
habits. Here, as in all such studies, smokers were found to be less knowledgeable and
less worried than non-smokers.[4] That makes sense, given that many non-smokers
are former users who have quit, fearing for their lives. The ranks of smokers get de-
pleted of people savvy in such matters, pushing their average knowledge downward.

We should also not be surprised that people with different educational backgrounds have learned about health harms at different rates. Prior to the 1964 Surgeon General's report even doctors were slow to accept the reality of tobacco mortality. The scientific consensus of major health harms emerges in the 1950s, but a
1960 poll conducted for the American Cancer Society by Chicago's National Opinion Research Center found that *only a third* of all physicians in the United States
were convinced that smoking was "a major cause" of lung cancer. Doctors were
asked, "Is cigaret smoking a major cause of lung cancer?" Only 33 percent said
"definitely," with another 31 percent saying "probably." Thirteen percent said "probably not," 9 percent said "definitely not," and 14 percent expressed no opinion. This
same poll revealed an astonishing 43 percent of all American physicians still smoking cigarettes on a regular basis, with occasional users accounting for another 5 percent. Of the 52 percent who didn't smoke, more than three quarters were former
smokers who had quit when the cancer connection started generating publicity.[5]

SMOKERS WANT AND EXPECT TO QUIT

There are many graphic examples of ignorance in this realm—even among physicians. Dr. Kenneth M. Colby in his 1951 *Primer for Psychotherapists* asked and answered, "Should the therapist smoke during the interview? Why not?" Morris Fishbein, the former *JAMA* editor, in 1954 boasted to Lorillard's chief of research, "I
offer on my desk nothing but Kents." Some doctors scoffed at the 1964 Surgeon General's report: as recently as 1984 one Virginia physician recalled it as "the opinion
of a bunch of eggheads" and "just another attempt by the d__ yankees to destroy
the tobacco industry." The industry's pollsters found results similar to those of the
American Cancer Society: a 1959 poll of American doctors conducted for Hill &
Knowlton and the TIRC found only 14 percent of physicians willing to say that the
cigarette–cancer link had been "conclusively proven"—with nearly as many (about
10 percent) admitting to having *advised* their patients to smoke.[6]

Lung cancer of course is only one of smoking's many maladies, each of which has its own distinctive ignorance microclimate. A 1966 report on Philip Morris's secret Project 6900 concluded that while medical authorities had recognized a heart disease threat from cigarettes, the general public was still "not fully aware of the relationship." A 1970 survey conducted by Roper for the Tobacco Institute showed that most Americans considered smoking "only one of many causes" of smokers being sicker—with only 24 percent recognizing it as "the major cause." Most Americans by this time regarded cigarettes as "bad for you" in the abstract, but fully a third thought that only heavy smoking (defined as 1.5 packs or more per day) was dangerous.[7] That is massive ignorance. If there were 60 million smokers in the United States in 1970, this means that 20 million American smokers believed that only heavy smoking was dangerous.

This same Roper poll also looked at quitting expectations. Fifty-nine percent of those surveyed had tried to quit at some point, and among those who had managed to quit only 12 percent said they had been advised to do so by a doctor. Few, though, said they had *no* intention of quitting. One of the most striking findings was that two-thirds of those interviewed said they *didn't even enjoy cigarettes* but rather smoked them just from habit. Only 32 percent said they enjoyed "most things about smoking." Enjoyment was even rarer for smokers of menthols (26 percent) and filtered cigarettes (28 percent). Answers differed significantly by brand: 42 percent of all Benson & Hedges smokers said they enjoyed smoking, for example, as compared with only 29 percent of Marlboro smokers. Not even a quarter of all Kent smokers enjoyed their habit and only one in five smokers of Kools.

Does this mean that the makers of Marlboro, Kent, and Kool were doing something that made people smoke while also making them not like it? Or just that people who didn't much care for cigarettes smoked Kools, Marlboros, and Kents? Several companies by this time were beginning to juice up their cigarettes, making them more potent by means of ammonia chemistry (see below on "crack nicotine"); Kent cigarettes also seem to have appealed more to what the industry called "guilty" smokers, people who disliked smoking but thought that low-delivery cigarettes would be less likely to cause them harm. A surprisingly large fraction of Kent smokers (over 20 percent) said there was "nothing good about smoking." Light smokers were less likely than heavy smokers to enjoy smoking, and women were less likely than men. Only about one in three female smokers said they enjoyed the habit. African Americans were less likely to enjoy smoking than whites, and for the entire sample enjoyment was so rare that when people *did* like smoking they were called "enjoyers" and considered "rather unique."[8]

This is an insufficiently recognized but crucial fact: *most smokers dislike smoking and don't like the fact they smoke*—which has become increasingly true over time. A 2007 Gallup poll found an astonishing 81 percent of smokers in the United States saying they would like to quit, with a comparable percentage considering them-selves addicted. These pollsters concluded, "Current smokers widely agree on two things—they are addicted to cigarettes and they would like to quit."[9] It could well be that the very survival of the industry depends on the perpetuation of this myth, that people who smoke do so because they "like" it. The reality is that few smokers like the fact they smoke.

RANKING HAZARDS

Surveys conducted in the 1960s and 1970s reveal an increase in public apprecia-tion of hazards, though opinions did not change as fast as one might imagine. A 1964 poll conducted just prior to the release of the Surgeon General's report found only 25 percent of smokers believing that smoking was "a major cause" of lung can-cer. An industry survey later pointed out that the Surgeon General's report caused this to jump to 46 percent, a substantially higher figure but not yet even a major-ity. Doubters also remained dominant in Britain, where a 1964 survey of five thou-sand people found 60 percent skeptical of any connection between smoking and cancer. Twenty years later, in 1984, another British poll found about half of all adults disbelieving that smokers were more likely to suffer from heart disease. And only one in four realized that smoking fewer than twenty cigarettes per day conferred an increased risk of lung cancer.[10]

Interpreting such surveys, we should keep in mind that the answers people give will depend on how the questions are asked. Virtually everyone will answer "yes" when asked, "Have you *heard* that smoking *may cause* cancer?" But fewer will give the same answer when asked, "Are you *convinced* that smoking is *the leading cause* of lung cancer?" Asking about *proof* will also reduce the number answering in the affirmative. In 1967 a telephone poll conducted by C. E. Hooper for the Tobacco Institute found that when 1,996 people were asked whether the U.S. government had "proof" that smoking causes serious health problems, only 48 percent of heavy smokers answered "yes." One goal of this poll was to find out whom people were willing to blame for ill effects from smoking, with the remarkable result that over 90 percent of those polled agreed that "the smoker has himself to blame." Only about 10 percent said that cigarette manufacturers should shoulder any of the blame. Wide variance was found by age and level of education, however, and in ways we today might find surprising. Very few young people (only 8 percent) were willing to say that cigarette manufacturers should be blamed, whereas people aged fifty-five and older were far more likely to attribute fault in this manner (21 percent)—perhaps because they were more familiar with the grip of addiction. Nearly 30 percent of those with only an elementary school education blamed the manufacturers, com-pared with only 7 percent of those with a college degree. For reasons that are not entirely clear to me, educated people were far less willing to hold the industry responsible for health harms from smoking.[11] It would be interesting to see if this has changed in the intervening years.

Understanding this reluctance to blame the industry may help explain why juries have so often sided with defendants in tobacco litigation. For many years it was virtually impossible to win a lawsuit against the industry. A 1964 Florida jury, for example, refused to award damages to the family of Edwin M. Green, who in 1958 had died from lung cancer after several decades of smoking. The jurors, many of whom were smokers, found cigarettes to be "reasonably safe and wholesome for human consumption."[12] A later judgment found that while Mr. Green's cancer may well have been caused by his smoking of Lucky Strikes, the American Tobacco Company could not have known that smokers were increasing their risk (at least not as of 1956 when his cancer was diagnosed). Of course neither the jury nor the judge nor the attorneys bringing the case had access to the incriminating documents we have today.

Polling has also revealed unrealistic expectations of how easy (or hard) it is to quit. The U.S. Department of Health, Education, and Welfare (HEW) in a series of polls conducted in 1968 and 1970 showed that teenagers had unrealistic expectations of whether they would ever take up smoking and how easy it would be to quit. Close to 90 percent of those interviewed (smokers and non-smokers alike) didn't think they would be smoking five years hence, when the reality was that about 35 percent would be. Personal expectations diverged radically from statistical facts, and what these and other surveys show is that young smokers have been poorly informed about their capacity to quit. The HEW researchers also concluded that the high fraction of those answering "yes" when asked whether smoking is harmful was misleading, given that "there seems to be a feeling among young people who smoke that cigarette smoking is detrimental to health at some time in the far distant future, perhaps at middle age, but that they can smoke for a few years while they are young and quit later as they approach the age when cigarettes might hurt them."[13] Young smokers seem to regard the dangers of smoking as distant but also as transient— like a bullet they may dodge if they are lucky and don't indulge too much. Otherwise put: they don't appreciate the *cumulative nature* of the threat, which is different from, say, driving too fast on the highway. Driving's dangers are not cumulative: the risk resets to zero each time you make it home. With smoking, however, each cigarette does its own little bit of damage, which is never fully undone. This incremental nature of the risk makes it easy to imagine that "just one more" can do no harm, especially if one thinks that the body somehow cleanses itself between each cigarette. In reality the lungs are an excellent filter, which is why smoking changes them from a healthy pink into a speckled necrotic black.

This same study reported that the number of American teens using cigarettes was growing at a rapid pace: from three million in 1968 to four million only two years later—with significant geographic and cultural variations. Teenagers in the east were more likely to smoke than teenagers in the west, but smoking was also more common in cities than on farms and in blue-collar than in white-collar homes. And in homes with only one live-in parent. Children in homes where *both* parents smoked were twice as likely to smoke as those from homes where neither parent indulged. Sibling smoking was an even stronger predictor: girls with an older brother or sister smoking, for example, were more than four times as likely to smoke as girls with smoke-free older siblings. A curious fact about the 1960s, though, is that most Americans still trusted the industry to tell the truth. A 1966 U.S. Public Health Service survey found *well over half* of all smokers agreeing that people would not be convinced smoking was harmful until "the tobacco industry itself" made this admission. This same survey found over 60 percent of all smokers agreeing that the cancer link was "not yet proved" because it was "only based on statistics."[14]

The turning point for when a *majority* of smokers in the United States realized that cigarettes are a *major* cause of death does not come until the 1970s and 1980s, though most people still ranked smoking lower on the scale of hazards than the reality as recognized by medical authorities. A 1972 Roper poll found only one in three smokers realizing that a pack a day made "a great deal of difference" in how long a person lived. Remarkable also is that *not even one in ten* ranked smoking among the two or three things they considered most threatening to health—with far more worrying about water pollution, food additives, and the safety of prescription medicines. Most were aware that smoking was "bad for you," but few took this very seriously. That may be one reason smoking and cancer was so often the butt of comedic humor: it just wasn't taken very seriously. We don't find a lot of people making jokes about polio or malaria, because these were recognized as being rather horrific. Today, though, we no longer hear so many jokes about smokers' cancers—perhaps because people finally realize that the diseases caused by tobacco are pretty serious.

Roper conducted another poll for the Tobacco Institute in 1982—their eighth such survey—and found smoking still "low on the list of things people are concerned about." Asked whether smoking a pack a day made "a great deal of difference in longevity," for example, only about half of those polled answered "yes." (Living under "a lot of tension and stress" was more often listed as something that was likely to curtail one's life, interestingly.) Many people were also poorly informed about secondhand smoke, with only about two-thirds believing it was "probably hazardous to be around people who smoke." Non-smokers ranked secondhand smoke lower on their list of concerns than drivers who don't dim their headlights, parents who fail to control an unruly child, and sitting near someone in a restaurant who hasn't used deodorant. Smoking was also ranked *second to the last* in a list of fourteen potential hazards considered appropriate for governmental intervention, behind crime, chemical waste, narcotics, nuclear radiation, air and water pollution, food additives, and a number of others. The survey concluded that both smoking and secondhand smoke "have always ranked low" on the list of things people worry about.[15]

Louis Harris and Associates did a similar poll in 1983, comparing the views of ordinary American smokers to those of 103 health professionals. Deans of medical schools and schools of public health and other scholars were asked to rank a list of twenty-four steps people could take to improve their health, from most to least effective. As readers of this book will appreciate, "quitting smoking" was ranked number one by the overwhelming majority of medical scholars. When the same task was assigned to a group of randomly sampled adults, however, quitting smoking was ranked in tenth place, below "taking steps to control stress" and "getting enough vitamins and minerals" and "having smoke detectors in the home."[16]

This business of how much people know (or don't know) has also been addressed by regulators trying to find out whether the public has been adequately informed. In 1981, as part of an inquiry into whether warning labels should be strengthened, the Federal Trade Commission completed a five-year study of popular attitudes toward smoking. More than a dozen carefully designed polls were consulted, including surveys by Gallup, Roper, and Yankelovich, along with polls contracted privately by the Tobacco Institute. The conclusion of this detailed synthesis, summarized in a 330-page report to the U.S. Congress, was that despite more than a decade of warnings "a great many Americans" still did not know much about the health risks of smoking. Thirty percent were unaware of the relationship between smoking and heart disease, for example, and nearly half of all women didn't know that smoking during pregnancy increased the risk of stillbirth and miscarriage. Twenty percent didn't even know that smoking could cause cancer. The situation had improved somewhat by 1989, when Surgeon General Koop cited studies showing that about 15 percent of adults in the United States still held smoking *not* to be a major cause of death or injury.[17] Fifteen percent may not sound like much, but that was still around 30 million Americans.

Global data are not so abundant, but we do have some interesting figures from Britain. In March 1999 a MORI poll conducted for Britain's Action on Smoking and Health showed that 88 percent of British smokers didn't know that smoking could cause impotence. The British Medical Association used this to push for new warning labels on U.K. and E.U. cigarettes reading, "Smoking causes male sexual impotence." Scholars have also shown that many Canadians don't realize that "light" cigarettes are no less deadly than regulars. In 2008 researchers from the University of Waterloo looked at how people thought of cigarettes labeled "light," "mild," "smooth," and "silver" and found that cigarettes with such labels were consistently judged as having a lower health risk than regular "full flavor" brands.[18]

Chinese surveys reveal similar gaps. In 1996 a study of Chinese smokers found 61 percent agreeing that tobacco did them "little or no harm." And in 2009 Yang

Gonghuan from China's Center for Disease Control and Prevention reported that 67 percent of Chinese did not know that secondhand smoke could cause lung cancer. Many Chinese smokers seem to believe that foreign cigarettes are more dangerous than domestics and that herbal brands are significantly safer. In a country where nearly half of all physicians still smoke, we should probably not be surprised that accurate medical information is not widespread.[19]

CHARTING ITS POWER TO CREATE DOUBT

Even today it is probably fair to say that the full range of harms from smoking is not well known. Public understanding of tobacco has never been sophisticated, and few people even today know there is cyanide in cigarette smoke—or insect excrement or radioactive isotopes or "impact boosters" and "ameliorants" of various sorts. Tar and nicotine are often misunderstood, as when people write to the companies asking why tobacco cannot be "de-tarred" just as coffee is decaffeinated. Few seem to know even the rudiments of cigarette design.[20] There is a diversity even of *expert* opinion when it comes to questions like whether smoking causes breast cancer— so it is hardly surprising to find nonexperts in the dark. The more salient fact, though, is that decades of industry propaganda have left their mark.

Indeed, we have some instances in which the industry set out to *quantify* the impact of its propaganda, measuring the ignorance thereby created. In the late 1960s, for example, Brown & Williamson conducted before-and-after tests of an advertising message crafted to weaken public acceptance of smoking–disease links. Separate groups of smokers and non-smokers were asked, Do you regard the smoking–health relationship as "proven," "maybe proven," or "not proven"? The goal was to see whether an editorial attached to a Kool cigarette ad could weaken the confidence people had that smoking was a proven cause of disease. As hoped, the fraction of those answering "proven" *dropped by more than 10 percent* after being shown the denialist ad. Smokers were more easily persuaded than non-smokers, with the "proven cause" fraction dropping from 73 to only 60 percent. Those already in the "not proven" camp were little affected, but the fraction answering "maybe proven" *doubled* following exposure to the denialist message, from 7 to 15 percent among non-smokers and from 14 to 28 percent among smokers.[21] This was clearly the opportunity the industry was looking for, these fence sitters vulnerable to the denialist message. Cigarette companies after all don't need to convince *everyone;* all they need is enough converts to keep the enterprise going—meaning cigarette sales—via whatever slivers of doubt can be insinuated.

We have other, equally blatant, examples of the industry charting its power to create doubt. In the summer of 1973, for example, Tobacco Institute VP Anne Duffin wrote to her superior, William Kloepfer, informing him that test showings of the Institute's propaganda film, *Smoking & Health: The Need to Know,* had generated "large and statistically significant shifts in attitudes favorable to the Tobacco Industry." A survey commissioned by the Institute showed that watching the film had reduced by 17.8 percent the number of people agreeing that "Cigarette smoking cause[s] lung cancer." Duffin reported that the film had also caused more people to agree that "the Surgeon General could be wrong about the dangers of smoking cigarettes" and that "reports have overemphasized the dangers of smoking." These successful results encouraged additional showings, and by October 1973 the film had been viewed by "37,000 in community audiences . . . including 18,000 men, 9,600 women, 5,400 boys and 3,200 girls." Four years later the film's distributor, the Modern Talking Picture Service, reported that the movie had been shown to 318,724 people, including 38,851 boys and 27,429 girls. And that was just for one of several industry-distributed films. An equally misleading propaganda piece, titled *The Answers We Seek,* had been shown to 324,512 viewers by 1982, including tens of thousands of children.[22]

TESTIMONIALS OF SMOKERS:
THE CONSUMER LETTERS

Public opinion polls show that millions of Americans still do not appreciate many of the dangers of tobacco use.[23] That is perhaps not surprising in a nation where huge swaths of the population don't know that humans share a common ancestor with apes, or cling to the preposterous notion that Iraq—or the CIA or Israel—conspired to blow up the Twin Towers of the World Trade Center or that Barack Obama is a secret Muslim. H. L. Mencken once observed that no one ever went broke underestimating the intelligence of the American public; of course the real issue is not lack of intelligence but rather the lingering effects from one of history's most powerful disinformation campaigns. What can we say about knowledge, beyond what we've already learned from polls?

The letters written to the tobacco companies are useful in this regard, since here we have the unfiltered testimony of consumers, or at least of those going to the trouble of writing and mailing a letter. Tens of thousands of letters by people from all walks of life are preserved in the industry's archives, most of which are to or from R. J. Reynolds, maker of Camel, Salem, and Winston cigarettes. People wrote to offer suggestions or to lodge a complaint, or even to ask for help with medical bills or to find out where they might buy their favorite brand of smoke. Still others wrote to brag about their health, despite having smoked for thirty, forty, or even fifty years. Much can be learned from such letters, as from the phone and email logs kept by the companies recording comments or complaints.[24]

One thing we learn is that people have had lots of ideas about how the industry should be running its business. "Suggestion" letters are preserved going back to the 1930s; people wrote to propose cigarettes that would make colored smoke or new ideas for tobacco substitutes or filters. Financial and marketing advice was offered, along with advice on how to win a legal case.

Many of these letters recommend ways to make cigarettes safer—by adding certain chemicals or modifying some aspect of cigarette design. In 1954, for example, two women from Pine Bluff, Arkansas, wrote to Reynolds suggesting that the company incorporate penicillin into its cigarettes, to help people ward off colds in the winter. Other correspondents suggested packing cigarettes with the filter end up, so workers with dirty hands could nab a fag using only their lips. Still others proposed ways to fight anti-tobacco "hysteria" or "zealots," or offered themselves as guinea pigs to test claims useful to the industry—that smoking cures allergies, for example. Smokers volunteered to serve as witnesses in litigation and asked for advice on how one might sue for discrimination. A Vanderbilt engineer wrote to propose stuffing wildflower seeds into the filter ends of cigarettes, so that butts tossed from cars would end up germinating flowers, adding "beauty to our roadside berms."[25]

We also learn that many people have been profoundly ignorant about cigarettes. One commonly encountered view is that simply having survived smoking is proof it is safe. In 1985, for example, a Pocatello, Idaho, woman wrote to say she'd been smoking for sixty years and found it "neither addictive, habit forming or fattening." A fifty-year Camel smoker from Granite Falls, Minnesota, reported that same year, "This idea of smoking being bad for one's health to me is a lot of malarky. . . . I don't think smoking is bad at all." A Newcastle, Wyoming, man wrote of his view that "drunk driving kills more people than smoking ever did," and a man from Quebec wrote to emphasize "how many lives have probably been saved, and most likely prolonged due to smoking when under stress . . . most likely many more than lost due to lung disease!" (Reality check: in 2005, according to the U.S. Department of Transportation, 16,885 Americans died from alcohol-related traffic accidents, compared with 440,000 deaths from smoking.) Smokers characterized the cancer claim as bogus, bunkum, balderdash, and baloney—and often jumped from this to complain about people suing the companies. A woman in Casco, Maine, ruminated (in 1985):

> I think the case of the woman suing for her husband's death is full of baloney. I know people who have died of Lung Cancer that never smoked.
>   Also no way can they pin point this is caused by cigarettes. When I put my white lawn umbrella on the lawn in the summer and it is black in the fall—like soot—I am sure it is not caused by cigarette smoke. In fact I don't believe the lung association can prove anything either. With so many other things in the air, where you work etc! I love to smoke—why don't people mind their own business. . . . This country is getting just like Russia. No rights!

Reynolds was more than happy to agree, responding that "medical science" had not shown that "any element in cigarettes, tobacco, or tobacco smoke causes human disease." The true causes of human disease were to be determined "by scientific research, not by statistics."[26]

Many of these letters follow a kind of testimonial format: smokers claim to have indulged for years without adverse effects, and the industry is urged to defend itself against charges from medical authorities or anti-tobacco fanatics. The cancer evidence is often simply dismissed, as in 1970, when an Oklahoma City woman wrote to inform Reynolds of her view that "all the hooy about cancer is all a big nothing as far as I am concerned." A Hartford, Connecticut, man in 1984 characterized the cancer consensus as a bunch of "hysterical propaganda, shoddy science, and bully tactics." Many such letters are clearly from people with little formal education, but some are from professionals with advanced degrees. The director of the "National Institute of Inventors" wrote to say he had proof that "Smoking does not create cancer"—and offered to share his secret for $5 million. A retired mathematician formerly employed by the National Institutes of Health wrote that the war on tobacco had been "a scam—the danger of smoking is vastly exaggerated." And many "alternate causes" are proposed for the lung cancer epidemic. Another man from Hartford wrote to express his view that "cancer is caused by your emotions, not cigarettes." A retired navy man from Brooklyn protested all this talk about cancer as "a lot of bunk . . . you don't get cancer from cigarettes, you get it from treated foods." Some of these skeptics linked the fingering of tobacco to other unwarranted ideas, as when a Rialto, California, man compared the cigarette theory to Darwin's theory of evolution. Public health authorities were trying to "brainwash the country": "That smoking causes cancer is a theory just like Darwin's theory of evolution. It's someone's idea of how things might be, but is by no means proven fact."[27]

Ignorance of this sort is not surprising, given how hard the industry worked to spread its denialist message. In 1958, for example, a Bloomington, Illinois, man wrote to Reynolds asking about a rumor he had heard that Salem, "among a few other brands, is conducive to lung cancer." William S. Koenig from the company's public relations department wrote back to reassure him that despite all the "confusing publicity," the reality was that cancer claims were based "almost completely on statistics" and disputed by "doctors and scientists of high professional standing." A similar exchange took place in 1959, when a Boston woman wrote to ask why the companies didn't "refute some of these allegations about cancer." She was convinced that "a great many doctors do not believe it" and that many people contract lung cancer "who never smoked." Reynolds wrote back, assuring her that many distinguished medical scientists had "failed to verify the charges of a causal relationship" between cigarettes and lung cancer. Indeed the ongoing rise in cigarette consumption had led the company to believe that "a vast number of consumers are of the same opinion as you are."[28]

Many other kinds of letters were sent to the companies. Parents complained about free cigarettes being sent to their kids (some as young as twenty months) and protested infomercials disputing a hazard from secondhand smoke. Physicians wrote to express their support for the companies, with some confiding in their belief that moderate smoking was fine and problems arose only from overindulgence.[29] People wrote to ask about tobacco ingredients, or to protest finding foreign matter in their cigarette. (From Honolulu: "This letter is a complaint letter. I can't smoked this cigarettes. Because worm in cigarettes so dirty and gross! Reexamine this cigarettes. Please send new cigarettes to me.")[30] And while most of these letters sympathized with the industry, many are more open-ended, asking whether cigarettes really were as bad as people were saying. To which the industry invariably responded with its denialist routine.

COLD HARD FACTS

The volume of such letters increased dramatically in the 1950s, and by the 1960s R. J. Reynolds alone had more than a dozen people working in its public relations department responding full-time, with the rhetoric in each case quite tightly scripted. To a woman in Grapeview, Washington, Reynolds wrote, "notwithstanding all the theories bandied about, actually the real cause of cancer in human beings is still unknown." And to a man in Cottage Grove, Oregon: "the truth is that in spite of what the Surgeon General's Committee had to say on January 11, the cause of cancer in human beings is still unknown." T. A. Porter from Reynolds's Department of Public Relations was a frequent author of such letters, which often included his calming balm, "The fact still remains that the cause of cancer in human beings is unknown. Research must go on to determine the real cause."[31]

Reynolds employed skilled writers to draft such letters, and though each had his or her own distinctive style, the common thread was reassurance. Thomas Dixon concluded one such letter by emphasizing "the plain fact" that "notwithstanding all the theories bandied about, actually the real cause of cancer in human beings is still unknown. Condemnation by association has never managed to get very far with the American people." William S. Koenig from the same office characterized the 1964 Surgeon General's report as having "nothing new in it, nothing that had not been heard before. The fact still remains that the cause of cancer in human beings is unknown. Research must go on and is still going on to determine the real cause." Thousands of letters offered this same basic message. Here is a version sent to a man in Secaucus, New Jersey, reaffirming that "the case" against tobacco had "by no means been proven":

> In spite of all the excitement stirred up, the cold hard fact is that no one knows the cause of cancer in human beings.

And another, sent to a woman in the Ideal Trailer Park in Ontario, California:

> Now with regard to the present controversy relating to smoking and health, one inescapable fact stands out. No one yet knows the real cause of cancer in human beings. The Surgeon General of the United States in releasing his committee's report himself indicated that there was a great deal yet to be known and rejected out of hand the suggestion that no further research was needed.

And to a man in Punxsutawney, Pennsylvania:

> I earnestly hope you have not lost sight of the fact that after all no one knows the real cause of cancer in human beings. This statement can be made with positiveness, notwithstanding all the statistical fireworks with which the anti-tobacco forces have tried to dazzle and befuse the American public. All of us know that cancer was an affliction of the human race long before tobacco was introduced by the Indians to European explorers in the Seventeenth Century.[32]

Reassurances of this sort continued into the 1970s, 1980s, and 1990s. Tim K. Cahill in 1973, for example, wrote to assure a biology teacher from Drake University there was "no conclusive evidence that the ingredients in tobacco are causative of any disease." To a teacher in Wellesley, Massachusetts, Cahill characterized recent work on tobacco as full of "a great deal of misinformation" and "faulty statistical interpretations." Cahill et al. were especially fond of saying that the "cold fact" or "cold hard fact" was that "no one knows the real cause" of cancer; and from 1964 through the 1970s there are more than a hundred letters to the public using this morbid turn of phrase.[33] Reynolds's PR department generated a seemingly endless stream of such letters, always with this same basic message: "cold hard facts," which in reality were cold-hearted lies.

COMBING THE ARCHIVES

One thing we learn from this correspondence is that many ordinary smokers trusted the industry and distrusted "the government," the Surgeon General, and doctors generally. The industry's archives are full of letters from people ridiculing medical authority, deriding all the cancer talk as "nonsense," "hooey," "hoopla," "hysteria," "bunk," "balderdash," or "brainwashing." Many of these letters warn about infringements on smokers' liberty, as when a South Carolina man in 1991 cautioned that caffeine could be "the next to go": "You could be arrested for having a second cup of coffee and be hauled off to jail in your housecoat, with curlers still in your hair."[34]

How widespread, though, were such sentiments? It turns out there is a fairly simple way to find out.

What is wonderful about the seventy million pages of documents now online at http://legacy.library.ucsf.edu is that they are full-text searchable by optical character recognition—which means you can search a term, or string of terms, and obtain (theoretically) every document in which that term or string appears. Google's search engine works on essentially the same principle: you enter a phrase, and Google will find and display that phrase wherever it appears. The same can now be done with the tobacco archives. The archives can be combed for hot button expressions such as "cold hard fact" or "please destroy" or "no conclusive proof," and every document containing such a phrase will be displayed—theoretically. I say "theoretically" because the system is not perfect: documents that are handwritten, for example, don't generally show up, and not every odd font can be read, or old fuzzy carbon copies or texts that are smudged or otherwise illegible. But the system is fairly robust, and the possibilities virtually endless. The novelty (and utility) is ultimately in the form of *search speed:* rhetorical diamonds can be sifted from archival dunes, and searches that might well have taken five hundred years if done manually can now be done in a matter of seconds. Scholars are going to have to think much more about search theory, about new ways to comb and navigate through massive online digital archives.

So how can this be applied to the consumer letters? One thing we can do is search the archives for terms like *propaganda* or *brainwash* to see how or how often people writing to the industry used them. We can then ask, when people used such terms, were they using them against the tobacco industry or against public health authorities? Whom did these people trust or distrust?

A search of "dt:consumer letter propaganda," for example, returns 140 documents, each of which is a consumer letter (dt: means "document type") written either to or from the industry containing at least one use of the word *propaganda.* Typical is this 1989 letter from an eighty-year-old Camel smoker in Pine Beach, New Jersey:

> It is obviously impossible for government propagandists to state that smoking shortens life since only God . . . and certainly not the government . . . knows how long each of us will live and therefore cannot reasonably predict how many years will ultimately be lost to smoking. . . .
>
> Contrary to those who *state,* as if it were a scientific fact, that smoking causes illness and shortens life, it has enabled me to live healthily into my eighties because stress is the root of most illness. . . .
>
> I expect you to defend your customers, not bow to governmental blackmail and propaganda intended to fill Treasury's coffers.[35]

Not everyone who used the term *propaganda* was referring to the government, however. Some people denounced the industry's propaganda, as illustrated in this 1991 letter from "a concerned parent" in Vincennes, Indiana:

> Gentlemen,
>
> I am disappointed that a company can send propaganda to a boy that is only 17 years of age. Will you please stop sending CRAP through the mail to him. He is not legally even able to buy your products.[36]

So the question is, when the term *propaganda* is used in such letters, how often is it used to characterize actions or opinions of the industry versus actions or opinions of the public health community?

For those letters that have been preserved, it turns out that people have been more likely to apply the label "propaganda" to public health authorities than to the tobacco industry. Among the 140 letters using the term, 7 are from the industry (all of which talk about public health propaganda) and 8 others are duplicates. Among the remaining 125 letters, 70 are pro-industry, meaning that the reference is to public health or governmental propaganda. And only 51 are anti-tobacco, complaining about the industry's propaganda—typically promotional materials or denialist advertising. So people writing to the industry were more likely to worry about medical than about tobacco industry propaganda.

Similar results are obtained when one searches for uses of the term *brainwash* and related cognates (*brainwashed, brainwashing,* etc.). A search of "dt:consumer letter brainwash*" yields 53 letters, more than three quarters of which reveal consumers placing their trust in the industry. Here is a typical letter from a Hillsboro, Texas, citizen worried about "brainwashing":

> I am appalled and angry at the misleading and erroneous information which is bombarding and brainwashing the public by the news media with so-called health hazzards [sic] as determined by "doctors."
>
> The facts are that people are living longer even to 100 years and over. These are the people who were born at home with a mid-wife or other family member, smoked, dipped and chewed tobacco and in their earlier years knew nothing of "doctors" and their toxic drugs and medicine. . . . It is absurd that anyone would attribute any problem to only one cause when every day the very air we breath [sic] is contaminated with toxic fumes from factories, carbon monoxide from cars, buses, trucks, etc., dangerous chemicals in drinking water and toxic chemicals used by "doctors" in lab tests. . . . I can easily see where it would be to the advantage of "doctors" to brainwash the public through whatever means, into believing that all Americans problems are caused by cigarettes.[37]

Or consider this 1968 letter from a woman in Bel Air, Maryland:

> Gentlemen,
>
> Operation Brainwash has got me scared. . . . I have an excellent doctor who has vanquished my depressive state . . . and who assures me that a pack a day and twenty or thirty cups of coffee will do me no harm. He is far more competent in internal medicine than the Public Health Service, which has strained "statistics" in its cigarette attack. I'd be much interested in knowing how much lung cancer has increased incidence as a result of their subtle scare psychology.[38]

Reading this entire set of "brainwash" letters, what we find is that correspondents have been more likely to trust the industry than the public health commu-

nity. Some people clearly *believed* the companies when they offered their reassurances. Of course we don't really know how representative such people were of the
general population; it could well be that industry supporters were more likely than
their opponents to write, for example. We don't find a pro-industry bias among
correspondents in general, however, since those who wrote to the industry about
advertisements were critical of the industry by a ratio of about two to one.[39] Notable also is the fact that people who wrote to the companies were more likely to
say they were "addicted" than "not addicted."[40] All we can really say is that a significant fraction of the American public seems to have taken the industry at its word,
or at least felt that "doctors" and "the government" were no more trustworthy than
the manufacturers.

Of course there are other kinds of letters that don't mention health at all. A number of teenage girls seem to have fallen for the dark-haired mustachioed Winston
Man, for example, and wrote to request copies of his poster for their personal use.
Girls wrote on behalf of their (female) teachers, and mothers asked for such posters
for their daughters (to put up in their bedrooms). Anyone who doubts that such
ads appealed to teenagers should consider letters such as the following, sent to
Reynolds in 1976 from a girl in Wayne, New Jersey.

> Dear Winston-Salem Co.,
>   During the last few months, I have greatly admired your Winston Box billboard.
> It is the one with the man with dark hair and moustache.
>   I was wondering if you could possibly send me a copy. I would be glad to pay
> a reasonable price for it. Please let me know if this could be worked out.
>   By the way, I have been smoking Winston cigarettes for nearly 3 years. And that's
> a lot considering I am only 15 years old.[41]

We also find letters of protest, many of which are heartwrenching. The companies often sent out promotional offers, and though some effort was made to weed
out the dead or underaged the volume was such—millions of mailings—that mistakes were sometimes made. In June of 1990, for example, a disgruntled parent wrote
to Reynolds:

> I would appreciate it if you would stop sending my son your unhealthy literature
> to try and sell him cigarettes.
>   Please take him off your filthy mailing list. He is only fifteen years old and we as
> parents resent your corporation trying to brainwash our youth for your own greedy
> purposes.[42]

Sharon Marvin of Mesquite, Texas, responded to a 1999 offer mailed to her home:

> Please remove [my husband] from your mailing list—
> I buried my daddy because of cigarettes. I'm not going to bury my husband
> because of them.[43]

Not everyone, though, was so polite or so well spoken. Many people returned promotional items, as did Jana Clyne of Clive, Iowa, accompanied by a note saying that the recipient "has been DEAD for 31 months" as a result of smoking. Clyne scrawled "DEAD" in large capital letters all over the offer-insert and returned it to the company.[44] Others expressed anger in a form so harsh I cannot even print it here. The word "filthy" often appears in such letters, as in, "How dare you name a filthy cigarette after a noble Indian tribe and my home state?" (The reference is to Reynolds's Dakota brand.) Or: "Our only daughter died because of your filthy to-bacco products." Absent or invisible, of course, are the thoughts of those too dis-heartened or angry to write to the companies—or the laments of those already dead.

THE "SIMPLE AND UNFORTUNATE FACT"

Viewed in the aggregate, we can also find certain patterns in the letters written by the companies. In 1986, for example, Miriam G. Adams, manager of consumer cor-respondence at R. J. Reynolds, responded as follows to a certain Annette Rodrigues from Cupertino, California, who had asked for information on smoking.

> Despite all the research going on, the simple and unfortunate fact is that scien-tists do not know the cause or causes of the chronic diseases reported to be asso-ciated with smoking. The answers to the many unanswered smoking and health questions—and the fundamental causes of the diseases often statistically associated with smoking—we believe can only be determined through much more scientific research. Our company intends, therefore, to continue to support such research in a continuing search for answers.[45]

This exact same paragraph appears in *hundreds* of Reynolds letters to the public: a search for the phrase "unfortunate fact" returns 660 separate documents, almost all of which are letters from the company denying evidence of harms from smok-ing. Indeed the archives preserve the original form letter instructing the firm's PR agents to use this terminology when answering questions about smoking and health. A stamp on this document indicates that this phraseology was to be used for in-quiries concerning "S & H" (smoking and health) in correspondence "Primarily for Children."[46]

Reynolds prepared hundreds of different form letters for such purposes. Form letters were drafted for children, for "high school & below," for people inquiring about teen smoking or cancer or secondhand smoke or warning labels or tar and nicotine yields—and so forth. Letters of this sort were usually handled by public relations departments, but higher-level executives sometimes got involved. In 1977 William D. Hobbs, Reynolds's chairman and CEO, reassured one angry woman from Richmond, California, that "no element as found in cigarette smoke has ever been shown to be the cause of any disease." Hobbs assured her that "the questions of smoking and health are indeed still open" and that "the answers will be found through careful research, not anti-smoking propaganda."[47]

Not every letter, though, was judged deserving of a reply. Angry letters were often simply ignored. In 1996 an exasperated woman from Charlotte, North Carolina, wrote to Reynolds about her son:

> I have a 16 year-old son who is addicted to cigarettes—he is very open about it and wants to quit, but the addiction is so strong that thus far, he has been unable to stop. My husband and I are both non-smokers—my father died of a smoking related cancer at the age of 57. I also lost an aunt and a cousin to lung cancer—both were heavy smokers. My son knows all of this, but he is as addicted to nicotine as were my three now-deceased relatives. I find it totally ludicrous that you continue to deny the addictive power of nicotine, and I am outraged that my young son is now hooked to such a deadly product. He has no trouble buying cigarettes, even though he is under-age. I want you to tell me what I can do—I am angry yet I feel totally powerless to help my son, short of sending him at great expense to a drug rehabilitation center. You tell me why 3,000 teenagers a day start smoking, and why they cannot stop until, like my father, they are dead and buried way before their time.[48]

The policy seems to have been not to reply to such letters, which were numerous. In 1996, for example, a man from Metuchen, New Jersey, wrote to protest the company's call for people to speak out against tobacco regulation, accusing Reynolds of being "nothing but organized thugs and criminals." The company did not bother to answer. Nor was any answer given to Meghan E. Colasanti of Denver, who in 1990 wrote to ask, "Do you guys find it pleasing to kill people?" Colasanti's letter, preserved in Reynolds's files, is stamped "Pub. Concerns—Unfav. NO RESPONSE" and filed as part of a large collection of "unfavorable" correspondence, including missives comparing smoking to slavery or asking questions like, "Why are you still killing people with your lousy cigarettes? You should be in jail for attempted murder."[49]

Opinion polls and letters sent to tobacco manufacturers reveal many smokers poorly informed about cancer, heart disease, and other cigarette-linked maladies. Addiction also falls into this class, though many smokers do develop an intimate grasp of this excruciating fact, as a result of trying and failing to quit. Most smokers want to quit and eventually do try; smokers can even become "experts" in a sense, experiencing addiction in ways quite foreign to non-smokers or to thirteen- or fourteen-year-olds just starting to smoke. The sixty-year-old repeat quitter is understandably different from the novice in this respect. Letters documenting this desperate "awareness" have been preserved, as when a woman from Lakewood, Colorado, sent Reynolds a 1994 letter she had published in *Time* magazine:

> Your report [i.e., *Time*'s] on scientific experiments involving nicotine . . . quotes a researcher as saying, "There's an overwhelming body of evidence that it does produce an addiction in humans." No kidding! There is also an "overwhelming

body of evidence" when my rear end hangs out of our fireplace as I rummage through six-month-old butts trying to find one long enough to light up again. This is after I "quit" for the 173rd time in three years. And I consider myself to be somewhat dignified! There's your proof of addiction. No kidding![50]

Smokers prior to this time, however, don't seem to have liked using the term *addiction* to describe their relationship to cigarettes. A 1982 Roper poll conducted for the Tobacco Institute found 52 percent of smokers considering smoking "a habit," while only 25 percent considered it "an addiction." An additional 19 percent volunteered that it was "both"—a habit and an addiction. Roper's conclusion: "smokers consider smoking to be only a habit (52%) rather than an addiction (44%)."[51]

Of course when smokers try to quit, most learn fairly quickly how difficult that can be. Quit attempts increased following the 1964 Surgeon General's report, which is when millions of smokers discovered the strength of their addiction. Thousands of consumer letters in the industry's archives incorporate the word *addiction,* and by the 1980s the writers of such letters—judging from those that have been preserved—were more likely than not to recognize they are addicted. People do seem to differ in how easily or deeply they become addicted, but for most smokers we cannot really say that smoking, as the industry wants us to believe, is a "free choice." Smokers may well "choose" to smoke when they are first trying cigarettes at the age of thirteen or fourteen, but the reasons people start are quite different from why they continue. New smokers are not yet addicted and haven't yet learned how hard it is to quit. The industry has known about this for decades, and more recent studies provide confirmation.

In 2001, for example, the Annenberg Public Policy Center of the University of Pennsylvania published a sophisticated study—based on four thousand interviews—showing that young people underestimate how hard it can be to quit. Ninety-five percent of the adult smokers interviewed reported cravings stronger than they had expected, and few were happy they had ever begun smoking. Over 80 percent expressed regret at having ever started. The survey also found that young smokers had profoundly unrealistic expectations for how long they would be smoking: only 5 percent expected to be smoking five years down the road, when in reality most would still be smoking.[52]

This was old news for the companies, of course, who had long realized that most smokers—even young smokers—want to quit. Imperial Tobacco's Project 16 had come to this conclusion in 1977, based on their study of English-speaking kids in Canada, where it was found that teenagers once hooked "cannot quit any easier than adults" and that most likely "few will."[53] Cigarette makers realized that while smokers *start* smoking for one set of reasons (advertising, peer pressure, etc.), they *continue* for very different reasons—with the most important being physiological addiction. Trying to quit gives you basically a crash course in what it means—what it *feels like*—to try to loosen this addictive grip. The letters written to the industry, and especially those from after the 1970s, make it clear that most longtime smokers are painfully familiar with the realities of addiction. But this is a lesson most often learned after trying to quit and failing, by which time for most it is already too late—or at least too late without a painful struggle.

STATISTICAL JIGGERY POKERY

For decades the mainstay of the industry's legal position has been that the public has long been "well informed" about the hazards of tobacco. Defense attorneys want us to believe that people make an informed choice when they decide to take up smoking or fail to quit—and therefore have only themselves to blame for whatever illnesses they contract. Smoking by this logic is a calculated risk, a "risky decision," as one well-paid expert likes to put it.[54]

We have already seen from opinion polls and customer correspondence, however, that lots of people have what charitably might be called "gaps" in their knowledge. That is also the assessment of polling professionals, appalled by the tobacco industry's misuse of polls in litigation. In 1999 Lydia Saad and Steve O'Brien of the Gallup Organization commented on how

> Time and again, the tobacco companies have successfully convinced juries that the connection between smoking and diseases such as lung cancer has been common knowledge in the American culture for at least a century and, therefore, plaintiffs are responsible for the results of their voluntary decision to smoke. . . .
>
> [A] review of historical Gallup surveys suggests that there was, in fact, a high degree of public doubt and confusion about the dangers of smoking in the 1950s and 60s. There may have been widespread awareness of the controversy over smoking, but public *belief* that smoking was linked to lung cancer trailed far behind this general awareness of the controversy.
>
> The legal question at the core of these cases is whether average Americans (or average teenagers) understood the risks they were taking when they began smoking thirty or forty years ago. Looking at Gallup data in the public domain, it is difficult to conclude that they did.[55]

This poor state of understanding is hardly surprising, given how hard the industry has worked to obscure such hazards. The basic script never varied much, despite some variance in the rhetoric used to belittle or ridicule the evidence. I've listed below some of the terms used by the industry to denigrate the science implicating tobacco in health harms; such terms were used in correspondence with the public but also in Tobacco Institute brochures, press releases and "white papers" and the like:[56]

"Astounding," "unwarranted, absurd"   (1945)
"colored by prejudice"   (1945)
"crude experimentation," "mere opinion"   (1945)
"half-truths in the hands of fanatics"   (1946)
"at best, only suggestive"   (1955)
"nothing new"   (1957)
"opinions of some statisticians"   (1957)
"oversimplified thesis"   (1957)
"biased and unproved charges"   (1959)
"scare stories"   (1959)
"time-worn and much-criticized statistical charges"   (1959)
"extreme and unwarranted conclusions"   (1959)
"the tobacco guilt theory"   (1960)
"modern Carry Nations in science"   (1962)
"foggy thinking"   (1962)
"the easy answer to a complex problem"   (1962)
"largely a rehash of the same old data"   (1962)
"easy answers that may turn out to be misleading or false"   (1962)
"fanciful theories"   (1964)
"wild guesses"   (1964)
"propaganda blast"   (1964)
"theories bandied about"   (1964)
"guesswork . . . statistical volleyball"   (1965)
"statistical fireworks"   (1965)
"utterly without factual support"   (1965)
"slanted publicity . . . exaggerations and misstatements
    of fact . . . fantastic figure of 300,000 premature deaths
    annually . . . so-called 'new evidence' against smoking"   (1967)
"guilt by association"   (1968)
"'guesses,' assumptions, and suspicions"   (1968)
"this game of statistical volleyball . . . worse than meaningless"   (1969)
"claptrap"   (1969)
"contrived semantics"   (1969)
"a bum rap . . . half-baked"   (1969)
"speculation," "suspicion," and "repetition"   (1969)
"statistical allegations . . . products of surveys and
    computer tapes"   (1969)
"ridiculous statements"   (1970)
"colossal blunder"   (1970)
"one of the great scientific hoaxes of our time"   (1970)
"claims of the anti-cigarette forces"   (1971)

"repeated assertion without conclusive proof"	(circa 1971)
"a disservice to the public"	(circa 1971)
"a great deal of misinformation . . . faulty statistical interpretations"	(1972)
"press-conference science"	(1972)
"conventional wisdom"	(1974)
"the health furor"	(1975)
"speculations, and conclusions based on speculations"	(1978)
"weak conjectures based on questionable assumptions"	(1979)
"an amalgam of unproved charges, exaggerated conclusions and largely one-sided interpretations of statistical data"	(1979)
"media events, propaganda barrages, self-righteous zeal, or cabinet-level fiat"	(1979)
"half the story"	(1981)
"dogmatic conclusions . . . inconsistent statistics"	(1982)
"Orwellian 'Official Science,'" "Scientific Malpractice"	(1984)
"irresponsible and scare tactics"	(1988)
"unfounded and sometimes ludicrous"	(1991)
"the current fervor of anti-tobacco evangelism"	(1992)
"flawed . . . real travesty"	(1992)
"outrageous claims"	(1995)
"bogus statistics"	(1995)
"biased rehash of old news"	(1995)
"statistical jiggery pokery"	(1995)

Such attacks were widely distributed. Addison Yeaman, vice president and general counsel of Brown & Williamson, managed to have one especially vituperative tirade printed in the *Congressional Record* (December 4, 1967), launched with a quote from North Carolina governor Dan Moore characterizing the recent U.S. Surgeon General's report as "unwarranted harassment and unnecessary confusion created by headline seekers using biased information." Yeaman then mocked Surgeon General William Stewart as basically a scientific fraud, warning that the nation's top medical cop either had "lost the quality of objectivity" or was "misinterpreting the information available to him." Yeaman went on to denounce the "vicious attack" on the industry organized by

a formidable coalition of government agencies, legislators, fund-raising organizations, propagandists, and do-gooders—all engaged in a crusade against tobacco . . . disregarding and even stifling the truth . . . doing slight [sic] of hand manipulations with statistics . . . weaving a tangled web of propaganda and deceit . . . blind to all but their own position . . . outright statistical nonsense . . . devoid of ascertained facts . . . a shabby piece of propaganda . . . bamboozled . . . arrogance of bureaucracy . . . the dangers of demagoguery and arbitrary government actions [etc.].[57]

Yeaman's bottom line: "no one—and I mean *no one*—knows whether cigarette smoking causes any human disease."

Yeaman's vitriol in the *Congressional Record* was prefaced by an equally dismissive rant by Samuel Ervin, the U.S. senator from North Carolina best remembered today for his feisty role in the Watergate hearings. Ervin attacked Senator Robert F. Kennedy's reproach of the industry and had seventeen denialist screeds read into the record. In Ervin's view the arguments advanced in favor of the causal hypothesis contained "little more than old platitudes, new hyperbole, and blatant nonsequiturs," all based on statistics either "erroneous, irrelevant, or statistically meaningless." Ervin ridiculed the idea of requiring a health warning as an "absurdity" and declared that Americans had "a right to know that there is no proof that smoking causes lung cancer and heart disease." Indeed it was "far easier to show statistically that smoking cigarettes prolongs life." The senator mostly followed the Tobacco Institute's playbook—he had obviously been well briefed—but also felt it worth noting that the *Encyclopedia Britannica* (he doesn't say what edition) defined cancer as "an autonomous new growth of tissues of an unknown basic cause."[58] As if archaic definitions could resolve matters of fact.

Ervin may have been just plain ignorant in this realm; lots of people were, after all, and the senator may have been thinking only of the financial well-being of tobacco farmers in his native North Carolina. Such was still his view in 1972, when he objected to a proposal for federal limits on tar and nicotine from cigarettes as requiring "a police state far beyond that envisioned by Hitler."[59] It is unclear whether his opinion changed after being diagnosed with emphysema, following a lifetime of smoking.

ASSUMPTION OF RISK

One thing we can say is that the industry's assessment of popular understanding has been opportunistic. In the 1950s and 1960s, for example, it was common to hear them say that *no one* took such hazards seriously. By the mid-1960s, however, we start to hear that *everyone* was "aware of the issue," a theory first advanced as part of a tactic to forestall warnings and to protect against lawsuits. Congressional hearings on whether to require a warning label of some sort began shortly after the 1964 Surgeon General's report, and the industry responded by claiming that people were already aware of the "alleged health harms" caused by smoking—and therefore didn't need to be warned. The strategy was outlined at a secret meeting in May of 1964, where the industry's powerful Committee of Counsel decided to finance a survey to help buttress the point: "At our meeting in Washington on May 7, 1964, a decision was reached to proceed, on a preliminary basis, with a public opinion survey which we hoped would establish that there is a very high level of public awareness concerning the health issue involving cigarette smoking. It was contemplated that the results of this survey would be used as a basis for testimony at a Congressional hearing."[60] The survey had actually been proposed by two scholars of marketing and communications—Gary Steiner from the University of Chicago and David Berlo from Michigan State—who suggested to the committee that a public opinion survey might help to provide "strong support" for the industry's position that warnings were unnecessary. As recorded by an attorney working for Arnold, Fortas & Porter, the goal would be to try to establish six "basic propositions":

1. That there is greater public awareness of the charges against smoking than there is of numerous other important public issues;
2. That a very high percentage of the American public believes there are risks to health involved in habitual smoking of cigarettes;
3. That the risk to health is overestimated (accepting as a basis for comparison the statistics in the Surgeon General's report and the Royal College report);
4. That there is substantially greater public awareness of the possible risks of cigarette smoking than there is of such other health issues as the cholestorol [sic] question, drinking and obesity;
5. That persons who do not know of the health issues probably would not be reached by warnings in any event;
6. That advertising does not have as much to do with the social acceptability of smoking as do numerous other personal and psychological factors.[61]

Projects of this sort were always carefully lawyered, and in this instance the Committee of Counsel sequestered polling results to make sure "unfavorable data" would never see the light of day. All interviews, analyses, and statistical results were to be forwarded to the committee; the goal was to reduce the danger of a successful subpoena and to make sure inconvenient findings "could be destroyed and there would be no record in any office of the nature of the returns."[62]

Similar arguments—about the universality of awareness—would be revived in the 1980s, to counter calls to strengthen warnings but also to buttress the industry's "common knowledge" defense in court. Typical is the testimony of Reynolds CEO Edward A. Horrigan on March 16, 1982, at congressional hearings on the adequacy of warnings:

The evidence shows that over 90 percent of the American public is aware of the claim that smoking is harmful. . . . This awareness level is virtually, if not totally, unprecedented in comparison to the awareness of the major issues facing this nation. The facts demonstrate that the Federal Cigarette Labeling Act is working, that the public has been made aware of the claimed health hazards of smoking, and that people are in a position to make a free and informed choice of whether or not to smoke.[63]

Opposition to warnings and legal defense were the two main reasons industry lawyers emphasized "universal awareness." Indeed, this was precisely how the industry kept winning all its lawsuits: the argument was that people had long known about the hazards, or at least had known enough to make a free and informed choice.

The oddity, of course, is that the companies themselves throughout this time were refusing to admit such hazards, a disjoint finessed by radically separating expert from popular knowledge. Expertise demanded caution and "more research"; popular knowledge—spun as "awareness"—was supposed to be universal. And so by the 1990s the industry's public stance on smoking and health had crystallized into "We believe the general public has long been aware of the contention that smoking may be injurious to health"[64]—but we ourselves, the experts, don't believe there is any proven harm from smoking. Such confessions were always carefully worded, since the intent was not to admit that smoking *was* injurious but rather only that some people had made this "contention."

One last legal fact is relevant here. Historians of the law often point to the importance of a 1963–64 treatise known as the "Second Restatement of Torts," edited by William Prosser and his colleagues at the American Law Institute and a bible of sorts for American liability doctrine. Prosser et al. here state, in a famous passage in Section 402A, that whereas a manufacturer might be held liable for selling "bad whiskey" (containing, say, a poisonous contaminant), a maker of "good whiskey" cannot. And the same is claimed for tobacco. A maker of "bad tobacco" might be held liable, but makers of the good stuff cannot. The theory again was that people were supposed to *know* that whiskey or tobacco can cause harm and that a product to be *defective* would have to be *unreasonably* dangerous:

> The article sold must be dangerous to an extent beyond that which would be contemplated by the ordinary consumer who purchases it, with the ordinary knowledge common to the community as to its characteristics. Good whiskey is not unreasonably dangerous merely because it will make some people drunk, and is especially dangerous to alcoholics; but bad whiskey, containing a dangerous amount of fusel oil, is unreasonably dangerous. Good tobacco is not unreasonably dangerous merely because the effects of smoking may be harmful; but tobacco containing something like marijuana may be unreasonably dangerous.[65]

What is remarkable, however—and not discovered until recently—is that the *Restatement (Second) of Torts* (as it is also known) is partly a tobacco artifact. It turns out that lawyers working for Big Tobacco—including H. Thomas Austern from Covington & Burling, chairman of the Tobacco Institute's Committee on Legal Affairs—were deeply involved in drafting this document, notably the tobacco-friendly Section 402A, the founding text of strict liability. Elizabeth Laposata discovered the intrigue in documents preserved in the archives of the American Law Institute, where she found a record of tobacco industry attorneys trying to influence early drafts of the *Restatement,* including the crucial passage about what can be considered "unreasonably dangerous." Similar efforts were undertaken to influence the *Third Restatement,* issued in 1997. We should perhaps not be surprised that Tobacco tried to have its voice heard in such a crucial legal arena; what is surprising is how successful that effort has been. If American law exempts "good tobacco" from liability, that is partly because Tobacco helped draft the law.[66]

A FREE AND INFORMED CHOICE?

In court, the claim that the dangers of smoking have long been "common knowledge" is deployed to suggest that smokers make a free and informed choice when they light up. In private, however, the industry has been perfectly willing to admit there is much that people don't understand about cigarettes. Tar and nicotine numbers for many years were printed on packs, but few smokers knew the levels for their preferred brands or (more important) the deception behind such numbers. And few today know about the many poisonous *gases* in cigarette smoke—such as carbon monoxide and hydrogen cyanide. "Gas" became an area of intense industry research in the 1960s, with the goal of reducing some of the more noxious ciliastats. Several companies thought about educating smokers on this topic but quickly realized this could backfire, stirring up fears of yet another tobacco menace. Smokers didn't seem to know or care about "gas," so why raise the issue? Gas turned out to be one of those many areas where the companies decided to "let sleeping dogs lie." American Tobacco had already decided this for carbon monoxide in the 1930s, and forty four years later Brown & Williamson was still satisfied that "The subject of 'harmful' gases in cigarette smoke is an issue of which the general public is presently unaware."[67] And thankfully, from their point of view.

Radioactivity was treated in a similar manner. Harvard scholars had found radioactive polonium 210 isotopes in cigarette smoke in 1964, and the industry quickly verified this fact, as we shall see in Chapter 26. Despite having several different techniques to remove this isotope from cigarettes, however, the companies never took such steps and never warned consumers. Public ignorance was clearly the industry's bliss—and Philip Morris made a conscious decision not to wake this "sleeping giant."[68] Here, too, the industry preferred its customers ignorant.

There are other examples where the industry knew many people were in the dark about specific aspects of smoking. Philip Morris research chief Helmut Wakeham in a 1979 memo noted that people take up smoking long before they become aware of its addictive grip, and Brown & Williamson about this same time remarked that "Very few consumers are aware of the effects of nicotine, i.e., its addictive nature and that nicotine is a poison." The U.S. Federal Trade Commission in 1999 expressed its concern that millions of Americans were wrongly interpreting the tar levels marked on cigarette packs, imagining that a "5 mg" cigarette would deliver only one-third the tar of a "15 mg" cigarette. The companies have long known that smokers who switch to low-tar brands often end up smoking these more intensively, but smokers have been poorly informed on this point.[69]

We should also keep in mind that there are many different kinds of tobacco use, each of which has its own ignorance micro-environment. Water pipes have recently become quite popular on college campuses, for example, and many students smoke "hookah" without even realizing this is tobacco—and no less hazardous. Most hookah smokers believe water pipes are less harmful and less addictive than cigarettes and that quitting will not be difficult.[70] The industry appreciates such naïveté, and depends on it to a certain extent. New tobacco fads often have health effects that might not become manifest until twenty or thirty years down the road—which means that a nimble industry can profit by changing fashions from time to time. Think of people shifting from pipes or cigars to cigarettes, thence to long-stemmed holders, king-sized, filters, menthols, "hi-fis," slims, hookah, oral snuff, snus or "e-cigarettes," and so forth, apparently ad infinitum. *Plus ça change . . .*

Of course the industry itself is part of the public, and their long-standing refusal to admit any evidence of harms has always created certain difficulties in the realm of logic. How could knowledge of hazards be "common," for example, if the manufacturer wouldn't even admit it? This is perhaps the biggest contradiction in the industry's "common knowledge" defense: if everyone always knew, why were manufacturers so adamant in denying proof? The industry for many years denied the reality of harms but also any knowledge of harms even among its own research staff. Milton E. Harrington, Liggett's former president and CEO (1964–72), in 1985 responded to questions along these lines by insisting that "Nobody in the company thought smoking was harmful."[71]

The example of Sam Ervin shows that politicians have also been ignorant in this realm—which is hardly surprising. Politicians have often ignored tobacco hazards, perhaps for fear of offending a powerful source of jobs and potential donations. U.S. presidents have been required by Congress to issue an annual proclamation on cancer control ever since 1938, for example, recognizing April as "Cancer Control Month," and the remarkable fact is that neither smoking nor tobacco was even *mentioned* in any such proclamation until 1977, when President Jimmy Carter stated that the fight against cancer depended on the willingness of Americans "to alter their eating, drinking, and smoking habits and to seek early and appropriate medical care." (Carter in 1978 irritated health officials in his own cabinet when he claimed that cigarette manufacturers were striving to make smoking "even more safe than it is today"—implying it was already safe.) Smoking was not mentioned in any of the next four presidential Cancer Control Month proclamations, and Ronald Reagan did not issue a strong statement until 1984, when he announced that avoiding smoking was the "single most important step which can be taken" to decrease one's risk of cancer. Smoking has figured in most subsequent presidential statements but not in Bill Clinton's from 1998 or 1999 or in George W. Bush's from 2004. President Obama—himself a smoker until 2010—in his 2009 proclamation noted only that smoking "accounts for thousands of cancer deaths every year" and that quitting "can greatly reduce the risk of cancer."[72]

Pundits and presidential contenders have sometimes denied even the reality of harms. Senator Robert Dole of Kansas, while campaigning for the presidency in 1994, denied the addictiveness of smoking, comparing it to drinking milk. The conservative syndicated columnist James J. Kilpatrick as recently as 1985 was still publishing widely read articles with titles like "We Still Don't Know if Cigarettes Really Do Cause Cancer." And Rush Limbaugh—the notorious disinfotainer—gained further notoriety for this 1994 pontification: "It has not been proven that nicotine is addictive, the same with cigarettes causing emphysema."[73]

PHONE AND EMAIL LOGS

I should mention one final way to assess public understanding, using the records kept of phone calls and emails to the various companies. The companies sometimes kept logs of such calls, and these, too, reveal the persistence of ignorance even in the face of long-established medical wisdom.

The background here is that like many other large corporations, tobacco manufacturers often receive thousands of calls per day from consumers. In 1997, for example, R. J. Reynolds received 260,000 calls to its consumer relations department, plus an additional 400,000 calls via its outside telemarketing contractors.[74] Philip Morris fields an even larger volume, which can increase dramatically during periods of special promotions. At the turn of the millennium the company was receiving three to four million consumer-initiated calls per year, most of which were responses to promotions.[75]

Calls are handled in a number of different ways, according to what the company hopes to gain from such communications. In the late 1980s, for example, Philip Morris launched a "Bill of Rights" campaign essentially to identify smoking as a form of free speech. Toll-free numbers were created for people to call to obtain a free copy of the Bill of Rights, and by 1990 the company had received over three million requests for the document. An even bigger response followed the company's 1993–94 Marlboro Adventure Team promotion, during which smokers were invited to call 1–800 MARLBORO to obtain free brand-linked merchandise after accumulating "Marlboro Miles" (for smoking that brand). The response was one of the largest in the history of telemarketing, generating 900,000 calls in the first forty-five minutes and 2.5 million during the first four hours. Nearly 10 million smokers participated in the frenzy, which Philip Morris marketers characterized as "the largest promotion in consumer products history." Some 4 million orders were placed and 11 million items shipped.[76]

Telemarketing on such a scale requires complex and coordinated management. In 1993, for example, just to receive calls and process orders for its Marlboro Adventure Team promotion, Philip Morris established a new 450,000-square-foot "fulfillment facility" in Lafayette, Indiana, staffed by 350 employees, and a new Customer Service Telemarketing Facility in Kankakee, Illinois, with a staff of 25 to handle phone orders. Philip Morris in the year 2000 expanded its call-receiving capabilities, implementing natural-language speech recognition, standby promotional and apology mail packages, and a "new attitude" tailoring personal service to the individual smoker. Callers were given a personalized consumer ID and PIN to allow personal logins, and email and fax programs were installed to reach consumers more quickly. For a time the industry hoped to replace its telephonic contacts with fax, email, and web-based interactions, though phone calls apparently still remain important, with texting and interactive web 2.0 advertising close on their heels.[77]

Philip Morris is not the only tobacco company to engage outside firms for such purposes. R. J. Reynolds in 1997, for example, contracted with the Young American Corporation (YAC) in Young America, Minnesota, to handle its promotions fulfillment at a cost of $11 million. YAC responded to over 400,000 phone calls to the company that year, handling also certain aspects of computer security. YAC was the largest fulfillment vendor in the country at the time, with 250 separate packaged goods accounts. Three of YAC's facilities in 1997 had operators constantly standing by, with up to 350 staffers taking calls for the Camel maker. Brown & Williamson's operations were on a smaller scale, but in the 1990s the company contracted with the Cognos Corporation to handle its telemarketing and data processing, including help with assembling logs of calls to the company.

Though tobacco companies may receive millions of calls and emails in any given year, only a tiny fraction are recorded and preserved in the online archives. Phone logs are generally low on the industry's priorities for retention, which is why they don't usually survive for very long. Phone and mail logs are typically held for only a year prior to destruction,[78] and those few that have survived are probably just the result of either bureaucratic accident or the chance timing of a subpoena. I stumbled onto one such log while searching for references to one of my books: a caller had recommended my *Nazi War on Cancer* and two of my other publications to Brown & Williamson's PR department, a recommendation buried in a set of logged calls to the company from 1999 treating "Smoking and Health."[79]

Brown & Williamson's phone log from 1999 summarizes 129 recent calls to the company in which "smoking and health" was the principal focus. We usually have only a sentence or two summary for each, but callers reveal a wide range of views on cigarettes and their makers, from fawning sycophancy to derisive contempt (see Figure 30).[80] Accidents involving cigarettes are reported by a number of callers, as are various kinds of contaminants in tobacco. A father called because his ten-month-old daughter had swallowed some filters, for example, and a Japanese man called because he had found a "glass fiber-like substance" in his cigarette and was "anxious and worried about its harmfulness." Some callers were looking for health information: one wanted to know if the company had data about harms based on cigarettes smoked per day; another asked whether smoking was addictive. Several were clearly irate: one said that the company "lied to our customers" about addiction; another effused, "You are killing people with KOOL cigarettes. I hope you are happy."[81]

Many of these callers reveal substantial ignorance. One had heard that whereas filtered cigarettes cause cancer, nonfilters cause emphysema. Another expressed his view that it was not cigarettes but rather cigarette *lighters* that cause cancer. Another asserted that "petroleum products cause more health problems than cigts." And another had heard Rush Limbaugh on the radio and endorsed his view that "smoking is not addictive." One was upset that people "blame every disease on cigarettes," and another revealed his own personal cure for lung cancer—caused, as he imagined, by a virus.

As in the written correspondence, many of these callers reported being in good health despite having smoked for many years. This is a common refrain in the consumer letters: a search for expressions such as "forty years" and "fifty years" returns hundreds of documents, most of which are people bragging about having smoked for decades without apparent harm. George Burns, the cigar-smoking comedian who lived to the ripe old age of one hundred, is mentioned dozens of times in such letters. A search for "George Burns" returns ninety-seven documents, most of which are either contractual negotiations for the actor's appearance in industry-sponsored shows (such as *Hollywood Palace*) or letters from ordinary smokers extolling his longevity.

One interesting aspect of Brown & Williamson's phone log is that only six of the 129 callers were clearly angry with the company. One accused the company of having "lied about cigt addiction," another "ranted and raved" about how smoking "kills people," adding "You guys are worse than Hitler." A much larger number, however, were apparently unconvinced of smoking's hazards. The sample size is not enormous, but in these 129 calls touching on "Smoking and Health" callers were more likely to say smoking *did not* cause disease than to say that it did. Email logs tell a similar story: a 121-page Reynolds log kept by CEO Andrew Schindler snapshots more than 1,400 emails from the year 2000, with correspondents (still) offering that cancer is caused "by your emotions, not cigarettes," or that people exposed to high levels of radon "are prevented from lung cancer." A Tyler, Texas, man in 1997 took the trouble to fax a letter to Charles A. Blixt, Reynolds's general counsel, assuring him that "Microscopic Mites Cause Cancer Not Tobacco."[82]

Perusing such correspondence, we learn that the techniques used by the industry to respond to inquiries have changed dramatically over time. In 1958, for example, the Tobacco Institute acquired its first electric typewriters—two sixteen-inch Royals—at a cost of about $470 each. The IBM machines acquired in 1962 were even more expensive ($535) and typically the costliest equipment in such an office. Typewriters with storable memory meant that letters could be generated by changing only the address and salutation, and in 1967 use of the IBM Magnetic Tape Selectric was credited with allowing Reynolds's public relations department to operate with eleven fewer people processing correspondence. Form letters were in wide use by this time, as were computers by the 1970s and email by the 1990s. Automation of correspondence allowed the industry to ramp up volume and to save on costs while preventing potentially dangerous deviations from the syndicate's PR and legal lines.[83]

New clerical technologies (and media) are often easier to use and cheaper, but they can also be used to target more consumers—in this instance smokers—more directly. Highly focused communications also render marketing and promotions essentially invisible to the non-smoking world. People who don't smoke are often shocked to learn that the tobacco industry still spends about $13 billion annually on marketing and promotion just in the United States—mostly via discounts and direct mail—since much of this is unseen by non-smokers. This is precisely how the industry wants it: a fungus always grows best in the dark.

MORBID DISINFORMATION

Public opinion polls, consumer letters, and internal industry assessments make it clear that the hazards of smoking were anything but "common knowledge" in the 1950s and 1960s—or even later in many respects. Smokers in particular seem to have had a hard time grasping the breadth of the threat, which encompasses not just lung cancer and heart disease but also emphysema, chronic bronchitis, cancers of the lip, mouth, and tongue, blackening gangrene of the feet, injuries to the developing fetus, and myriad other maladies. Not to mention corruption of academia and the legal profession.

Much of that difficulty can be traced to the industry's coordinated campaign of reassurance. The hucksterism of the 1930s and 1940s was followed by the "Frank Statement" of 1954 and the barrage of distracting research, misleading ads, manipulation of governmental and professional organizations, and false marketing of filters, "lights," and low-tars. The companies said they would find and fix whatever might be wrong with cigarettes and on occasion even promised they would "stop business tomorrow" if genuine evidence of harms was ever uncovered. Such promises were never kept; indeed, the industry abandoned this responsibility while also doing everything it could to prevent the public from learning the truth.

Tobacco use has now spread into other parts of the world, propelled by many of the same strategies perfected in the United States. The golden weed already kills about six million people every year, and that number will grow before it begins to decline. Smoking rates are the ultimate proof of "common knowledge," and while total consumption peaked in the United States in the early 1980s there are many places where cigarette use is still on the rise. And even in health-conscious California we still have about eight hundred cigarettes smoked per person per year, a figure not much lower than the global average. Each of these cigarettes is a measure of the industry's morbid campaign of disinformation, combined with the lasting grip of addiction. Ignorance is the seed, death the harvest.

It would be wrong, though, to place too much emphasis on knowledge or its absence. The "consumer sovereignty" so often sanctified by economists places all responsibility for tobacco death—or quitting—on consumer choice, giving the industry a free pass. We tend to forget that cigarette makers also have choices, that they are the ones keeping nicotine in tobacco, fomenting addiction, robbing smokers of their ability to make a free choice. So "full disclosure" is not enough; we should not be satisfied with a highly addicted, even if highly informed, citizenry. And we don't have to grant unlimited freedom to manufacturers. The manufacture or sale of cigarettes is not an inalienable right or the sine qua non of freedom; the opposite is actually closer to the mark.

Filter Flimflam

The air you breathe through a Kent cigarette is several times cleaner than the air you normally breathe in an average American city.

HARRIS B. PARMELE, DIRECTOR OF RESEARCH, LORILLARD TOBACCO, 1954

The filters currently available are a hoax.

ALTON OCHSNER, PROFESSOR OF SURGERY, TULANE UNIVERSITY, 1954

Overwhelming evidence had accumulated by the mid-1950s that cigarettes were behind the explosive growth of lung cancer. Evidence was also strong that something in the *tars* in cigarette smoke was to blame. Fritz Lickint in Germany as early as 1935 had concluded that nicotine was "probably innocent" of carcinogenic potency and that benzpyrene was the more likely guilty party, basing much of his argument on Roffo's work.[1] Two decades later several *dozen* dangerous chemicals had been identified in tobacco smoke—and not just carbon monoxide, ammonia, and polycyclic aromatic hydrocarbons of various sorts (including benzpyrene) but also carcinogens such as arsenic, chromium, nickel, and nitrosamines. Richard Doll in a 1955 review identified arsenic, 3,4-benzpyrene, radioactive potassium, and a fistful of tobacco-pyrolysis products as cigarette carcinogens,[2] and industry scientists would greatly lengthen this list in the 1960s and 1970s.

Tobacco manufacturers often conceded the existence of carcinogens in tobacco smoke—albeit only privately. A December 24, 1952, report by Brown & Williamson's technical research department mentioned having isolated and identified several cancer-causing chemicals in smoke, including "a carcinogenic hydrocarbon, benzopyrene." (This same document recommended that a "correspondence" be initiated with Angel Roffo "by an independent laboratory not connected with Brown and Williamson"—which would have been difficult, as the man had been dead for six years.) Claude Teague in his 1953 "Survey of Cancer Research" acknowledged the presence of carcinogens in smoke, as did his chemist colleague, Alan Rodgman, in several of his reports for Reynolds. And Philip Morris scientists were not very far behind. In 1961 Helmut Wakeham presented a twenty-three-page report to the company's R&D Committee listing forty distinct carcinogens in cigarette smoke, admitting this was only a "partial list." (See again Figure 26.) The report also pointed to a dozen additional "tumor-promoting" agents, including phenols, liquid paraffin hydrocarbons, benzene, ethanolamine, and various organic acid esters. Company officials appear to have been proud of the fact that, among the more than four hundred compounds found in cigarette smoke by that time, Philip Morris had identified about fifty. Wakeham proposed a seven- to ten-year program to reduce "the general level of carcinogenic substances in smoke," with the goal of generating "a medically acceptable cigarette." The task would not be an easy one, he stressed; it would require time, money, and "unfaltering determination."[3]

None of these facts or plans was ever made public. Indeed it would have been hard for the companies to acknowledge any kind of effort to remove carcinogens from smoke, given their adamant refusal to admit their existence. There always was this awkward gap in tobacco logic: if the tar in cigarette smoke was really nothing to worry about, then why such a fuss about brand X being "lower in tar" than brand Y? The companies never liked talking about cancer facts—as such. And outsiders were never told about the steps taken by Wakeham and others to measure the carcinogenicity of specific compounds in smoke. We know about these efforts only because U.S. courts forced the disclosure of internal documents—aided by a handful of courageous whistle-blowers.

What the archives also reveal, though, is the industry struggling to figure out how one might eliminate—mainly by filtration—carcinogens and other poisons from tobacco. Efforts of this sort go back centuries, depending on what you count as a "filter." Water pipes have been popular since the earliest days of smoking, with part of the draw being this desire to purify the smoke by bubbling it through water. (It doesn't work: smoke from water pipes is just as deadly.) Hookahs and narghiles are inventions of the Orient, though similar effects were obtained by the long-stemmed pipes of Europe, with the point in each case being to *cool* the smoke—a reasonable goal for those who believed that *heat* might be to blame for its irritating or carcinogenic properties. Filters became a topic of interest in the second half of the nineteenth century, especially with the rise of manufactured cigarettes and nascent caterings to health-conscious smokers. Cork, paper, wool, cotton, and a number of other materials were tried, along with diverse physical and chemical means and blending tricks, most often with the goal of protecting smokers from some of the poisons known to be in smoke.

MANIPULATING NICOTINE

The first known efforts to develop low-nicotine tobaccos were by Karl A. Mündner (1835–91) of Brandenburg, a German tobacco manufacturer and colleague of Otto

Unverdorben, the first to identify nicotine in pipe residues. Mündner developed a low-nicotine "health cigar" using selective breeding techniques and new chemical extraction methods; his son Richard went on to develop filter-tipped cigars, using filters made from wool and cork. Paul Koenig, director of Germany's Reich Institute for Tobacco Research in Forchheim, in 1940 characterized Mündner as "the first to combat nicotine through his discovery of a method to de-nicotinize tobacco," offering this as evidence of the moral responsibility of the German tobacco industry then under attack from Nazi health authorities.[4]

Manipulation of the chemical properties of tobacco had also begun in the nineteenth century. High-nicotine tobacco plants were cultivated to obtain the alkaloid for use as a pesticide, and by the 1890s techniques were available to lower or remove entirely the offending/entrancing substance. Germany's Reich Institute for Tobacco Research pioneered much of this research, exploring how to augment or remove nicotine from tobacco through novel breeding techniques, grafting, and chemical treatments. By the 1930s German manufacturers were able to produce tobacco containing "however much nicotine was wished." And by 1940 fully 5 percent of the entire German tobacco harvest was "nicotine-free."[5]

American tobacco manufacturers kept a close watch on this European work and knew from their own experience that tobacco plants could be grown containing higher or lower levels of nicotine. They also knew that the alkaloid was easily removed from the finished leaf simply by soaking in ammonia or even in water. Alkaloids are typically water-soluble, which is why it's so easy to make a cup of coffee or tea, both of which contain the caffeine alkaloid. The American Tobacco Company noticed Forchheim's efforts to produce nicotine-free tobacco: a 1930 "Press Memorandum" in the company's archives acknowledges the German work, remarking on how the nicotine content of tobacco plants "can be diminished or increased by natural means" while still retaining traditional taste and aroma. Treatment with chlorine and proper culture and fertilization could increase the nicotine to as high as 12 percent, and close planting and a prescribed watering regimen could cause it to be "almost entirely" eliminated.[6] Countless inventors spent time designing new ways to manipulate the alkaloid in the finished leaf. An 1882 patent obtained by Richard Kissling in Bremen, for example, described "a novel process of denicotinizing tobacco" involving treatment of the leaf with calcium chloride, followed by steam treatment to drive off the nicotine. Dozens of such patents were awarded in the second half of the nineteenth century. Entering "nicotine" in the Google Patents search engine turns up hundreds of other claims filed with the U.S. Patent Office, many of which describe ways to adjust—or to eliminate—the nicotine in tobacco. All of which should be kept in mind when pondering whether the industry has ever "manipulated" the nicotine in cigarettes: they have been doing so for more than a century.[7]

HOPE AND HYPE—AND ASBESTOS

Filters have long been one of the primary ways cigarette makers tried to make cigarettes "safer"—with no great dishonesty originally attached to the practice. Cigarette holders, after all, were thought to have some virtue either in cooling the
smoke or in forcing it to travel through a series of barriers, causing it to lose some
of its noxious power. In the 1930s and 1940s filters were typically made from paper, wool or cotton, though it was fairly quickly realized that pretty much any
porous or fibrous material would work just as well—or as poorly—as anything else.
Denicotea's filters were made from silica gel crystals, and the American Tobacco
Company tried a porous clay porcelain. Germans developed a large number of filter materials and filed for patents in both Europe and the United States.[8]

The first American filter cigarette of any commercial significance was Brown &
Williamson's Viceroy, rolled out in May of 1936 with a $300,000 advertising fan-
fare. Slogans claimed a "safer smoke for any throat," and sales reached 400 million
sticks in the first six months. This wasn't too bad for a newbie, but nothing was taken
from the really big brands selling in the tens of billions per annum. Filtered cigarettes remained pretty much a novelty throughout the 1940s, and some brands
(Philip Morris, for example) even bragged about offering "unfiltered" smoking pleasure. Viceroy's sales tapered off and reached a nadir in 1946, having captured only
about a tenth of one percent of the American market. Lucky Strike that year sold
more than a hundred *billion* sticks, whereas the nation's leading filter sold only a
couple hundred *million*.

Those ratios would change dramatically in the 1950s, as the companies reori-
ented advertising and production to address the so-called health scare. Viceroy by
1956 would be churning out more than 23 billion cigarettes but couldn't even keep
ahead of the number two filter, Lorillard's upstart Kent. (Leading the pack was
Reynolds's much-hyped Winston, which sold a whopping 40 billion in 1954, its first
year on the market.) By 1958 Lorillard's flagship brand, Kent, had outstripped Brown
& Williamson's Viceroy, and all of the other companies were scrambling to out-gim-
mick each other in what quickly became a filter flood.

I've highlighted the duplicity campaign launched with the 1954 "Frank Statement,"
but filters were a fraud built into the cigarette itself. (Think about it: if filters are so
great, why don't we ever find them on cigars?) The whole point was to convince a
worried public—with little or no evidence to back it up—that baffles and barriers
of various sorts in a "filter tip" would somehow reduce the deadly tars in smoke.
The hope, and implicit hype, was that carcinogens might be trapped and filtered
out. Hundreds of different filter gizmos were patented for cigarettes in the 1930s,
1940s, and 1950s, which makes one wonder about the patent approval process. The
most popular were based on cellulose acetate for the fibrous "tow," or "filtering," ma-

terial, but filters were also made from crepe paper, wool, cork, cotton, and plastic foams and fibers of various sorts to which silica gel, activated charcoal, and numerous other substances had been added. Physical barriers were tried, along with microfibers such as nylon, rayon, dacron, polyester, fiberglass, and crocidolite asbestos.

Yes, *asbestos*. This deadly mineral fiber was the secret ingredient in Kent's Micronite™ filter, rolled and sold to millions of Americans from 1952 through 1956. An estimated 15 billion cigarettes were smoked through Kent's Micronite "blue asbestos" filter—by as many as four million smokers—and the company knew quite early on that bits of the mineral fiber could escape from the filter end of the cigarette.[9] Lorillard's competitors even sounded the alarm, albeit not very loudly: Liggett & Myers in 1953 advertisements hinted that use of a "mineral" filter was unsafe, prompting John H. Heller of Yale—a distinguished medical physicist—to write to the company asking what exactly was meant by this "non-mineral" boast. Liggett responded by noting that the use of minerals such as asbestos or glass in a filter "exposed the smoker to the possible danger of drawing mineral dust out of the filter into his lungs," leading possibly to "diseases of the pneumoconiosis type such as silicosis, asbestosis, etc."[10]

And as if that weren't bad enough, hundreds and perhaps thousands of workers were exposed while making the stuff for Lorillard. Asbestos dust levels were so high in the factories making these filters that many workers fell ill and died from lung cancer or mesothelioma. These were veritable death factories, wherein a higher proportion of employees died than in any other known asbestos plant.[11] When the Lorillard company finally stopped attaching asbestos filters to its cigarettes in 1956 the switch was made quietly, without alerting anyone to the change (or the danger). And cigarette stocks were not pulled from the shelves. Retailers just kept selling them until they were gone. Those few packs that escaped unsmoked are now collector's items, fetching hundreds of dollars on auction sites like eBay. And researchers take them apart to study what smoking them must have been like. The industry has been conducting such studies since the 1950s—which may well be why Lorillard's head of research, Alexander Spears III, died of mesothelioma, a disease found almost exclusively among people exposed to asbestos. Spears died from this lung-corrupting malady in 2001, seven years after testifying before Congress that smoking posed no known health risks.

Lorillard scientists knew that asbestos might pose a health hazard but seem not to have worried too much about particles entering smokers' lungs. On November 13, 1951, Lorillard's Harris B. Parmele wrote to his executive vice president, Robert M. Ganger, assuring him that asbestos was not fraying into the smoke of Kent cigarettes, based on measurements of the force required to smoke such cigarettes. One worry was that people might suck extra hard on a very tight filter, especially since smokers were already known to pull harder on filtered cigarettes "in an attempt to compensate (!) for the large proportion of smoke removed by the filter."[12]

We shall return in a later chapter to this question of *compensation,* which turns out to be the main reason "low-tar" cigarettes aren't any safer. Here I should also note, though, that Lorillard considered using its Micronite filter material to make surgical masks, with the goal of celebrating these in advertisements for the cigarette. The plan was to announce the masks only after making sure that asbestos would not make its way into the lungs of surgeons.[13] No such precautions were taken with Kent cigarettes, which were not thoroughly tested for fiber release until after they were being sold to the public.

"CLEANER THAN THE AIR YOU NORMALLY BREATHE"

Smokers flocked to filters in the 1950s, believing these to provide some genuine margin of safety. Lorillard's Kent (asbestos) cigarette, for example, skyrocketed from essentially zero sales in 1952 to more than 8 percent of the American market within six years. Colorful and sciency names were often given to such gimmicks, names like *millicell* and *selectrate* and *alpha cellulose.* Cigarettes were sold with "dual," "chambered," "granulated," and "deep weave" filters; others boasted filters with elaborate (or at least fancy-sounding) "gas traps" or "safety zones" of one sort or another. New Vision cigarettes had "tri-phase filters," Brown & Williamson's Belair came with a "recessed" filter, and Philip Morris sold "fluted" filters. Old Gold's patented "spin filter" was said to "spin" and "cool" the smoke; Parliament had a "star filter"; Reynolds had a "Multijet" filter; the Canadians had a "percolator" filter— and so forth. Smokers bought these contraptions believing harmful chemicals were being removed, and the industry did nothing to disabuse them of the illusion. Quite the contrary.

In the midst of this filter fest, grandiose claims were advanced on their behalf. Lark's charcoal filters were compared to water purification devices and to air filtration systems used in hospitals, spacecraft, and atomic submarines. L&M's alpha cellulose filter was a "miracle product" and "just what the doctor ordered"; it was also "entirely pure and harmless to health." Winston's filter was not just "pure" but also "snow-white"; Viceroy offered "Double-Barreled Health Protection" through its "Health Guard" Estron filter tip. Tareyton's activated charcoal filter promised a taste "worth fighting for"; Kent's Micronite filter incorporated the same material used to remove "airborne radioactive materials" from atomic energy plants (i.e., crocidolite asbestos). Brown & Williamson introduced an "all-tobacco filter" for its Kentucky Kings (in 1960) to "fill the gap between regular cigarettes and brands with artificial filters."[14]

This last-mentioned claim is interesting, since cigarette manufacturers already knew that tobacco itself was as good—or as poor—a filter as anything else. In 1935, in a report evaluating cellulose acetate as a filter material, American Tobacco researchers had concluded that the nicotine content of smoke from cigarettes with cellulose filters was "practically the same as that of ordinary cigarets." Special filtering devices, in other words, worked no better than the filtering action of tobacco itself. Similar observations are found repeatedly in the industry's archives, where filters are often characterized as "gimmicks." In 1946, for example, another American Tobacco report commented on how use of a filter tip on a cigarette was "actually of no benefit as far as filtration is concerned." In fact, so this report concluded, "tobacco is a better filtering agent." That is why smokers were often advised to smoke cigarettes only partway down, since the unsmoked half would trap many of the poisons from the first half. Because tobacco itself was "an excellent filter."[15]

Which also helps to explain why the American Tobacco Company, the world's largest tobacco manufacturer, with the world's most sophisticated laboratories, refused to move big-time into filters until 1963. (The company as a result suffered a dramatic loss of market share, from which it never really recovered.) Those companies that *did* produce filters did so mainly because they knew people would buy them, thinking they were "safer." But filters provided only an illusion of security. The era of explicit medical claims was over, but the advertised implication was still that atomic age technology would bring you medical peace of mind through advances in filter science. Liggett & Myers in 1963 compared its newly introduced "gas trap" filter (incorporating charcoal, aka the "Keith filter") to methods used to purify the air "in atomic submarines and space capsules, where men must breathe the same air over and over for days on end." The suggestion was sometimes even made that filters could make smoking *safer even than breathing ordinary air*: Harris B. Parmele at Lorillard, for example, worked hard to show that "the air you breathe through a Kent cigarette is several times cleaner than the air you normally breathe in an average American city."[16]

Ever clever, the industry farmed out part of this job of generating hype to the public. Brown & Williamson in 1955, for example, sponsored a $50,000 contest for college students, who were invited to submit names for a new and yet-unnamed Viceroy filter. Thousands of entries were received from universities all across the United States. Ten brand-new Ford Thunderbirds and an equal number of RCA Victor color televisions were awarded, along with 40 Columbia "360" K Hi Fi sets as second prizes. The contest generated the desired attention: eighty-nine college newspapers covered the event, yielding 712 column inches of publicity, plus extensive radio and TV coverage.[17] College students were prime marketing targets at this point, with ads often splashed throughout university newspapers and magazines.

Companies also praised the virtues of filters in other realms of life. In 1971 the American Tobacco Company offered smokers the opportunity to buy a cheap, Tareyton brand *water* filter as part of its "struggle for cleaner, better-tasting water." Smokers had only to send in $5 plus two wrappers from their Tareytons. Tareyton cigarettes, like the best water filters, were offered as exploiting the filtering action of activated charcoal, a "black magical material" first proven of use "in the gas masks of World War I." Better still, this same magical material was used "to protect air in spacecraft, atomic submarines, hospitals and auditoriums." Housewives were also advised to discover what soft drink manufacturers had known for years, namely, that "proper filtration makes a distinct difference in palatability—not only in a glass of water itself but in such water-based products as coffee, tea, frozen juices, shellfish, gelatins and vegetables."[18] Tareyton got lots of free publicity by this means—since many newspapers reported on the water filter as a way to fight pollution.

Cigarette companies sometimes made their own filters, but the process was more often contracted out to chemical manufacturers. Hoechst Celanese made cellulose acetate filters beginning shortly after the Second World War and quickly became one of the leading fabricators, the other being Tennessee Eastman, a division of Eastman Kodak. Cellulose acetate by 1950 had become the industry standard (often sold under the Kodak trade name "Estron"), with U.S. production growing from 3 million tons in 1953 to 22 million tons only two years later.[19] Filters must have been quite a sizable chunk of Kodak's business, though no one seems to have researched what the company thought about its aid to the cigarette business. (Kodak didn't participate in the conspiracy and therefore hasn't fallen prey to tobacco lawsuits—which also means we don't have access to internal documents.) Outsourcing continued into subsequent decades: American Filtrona of Richmond, Virginia, made "Fluted" plastic filters for Philip Morris in the 1970s but also the "low denier tow" (the actual filter material) for B&W's Capri cigarettes in the 1980s. The fibers most commonly used were the same as those used for the tips of marking pens and highlighters, albeit not so tightly packed.

The companies liked using fibers as filter materials, since they were easy to produce and allowed manufacturers to introduce additives of various sorts. The fibers could also be packed arbitrarily tight (or loose), allowing the manufacturer to block as much or as little of the smoke as desired. Packed too tight, however, a filter would not allow a smoker to obtain "satisfaction," which is why many early filters were loosened over the course of the 1950s. The industry developed elaborate techniques by which to measure filtration "strength," including a kind of barometer that basically told how hard you had to suck to obtain a requisite level of "taste" and "satisfaction"—tar and nicotine, in other words. Manipulating fiber packing densities allowed cigarette makers to control the rate at which smoke would enter the mouth and lungs for a given strength of suction ("pressure drop").

Health, of course, was the promised virtue of all cigarette filters. And as the "health scare" unfolded, smokers moved en masse to suck up (and on) the new gimmicks. So whereas in 1950 less than one percent of all cigarettes smoked in the United States had a filter, by the end of the decade their share had streaked past 50 percent. The craze was hastened by clever ads but also by free publicity in the form of media endorsements. *Reader's Digest* in 1953 reported on studies by the AMA showing that Kent's Micronite filter removed more tar and nicotine than other leading brands; the same magazine in 1957 identified Kents as having "filter tips that really filter."[20] Boosted by such free (and misleading) advertising, sales of Lorillard's flagship brand took off like a rocket. From only 495 million sticks in 1952, sales rose to over 3 billion in 1953, 14 billion in 1957, and 36 billion in 1958. Sales grew from 300 million per month to 3 *billion* per month in only ninety days, following the popular magazine's endorsement. *Reader's Digest* gets lots of credit for sounding the alarm on tobacco harms, but in this instance billions of asbestos-laced cigarettes were smoked as a result of the magazine's ill-informed endorsement.[21]

No one at *Reader's Digest* seems to have minded—if they even knew—that the author of this first piece of puffery, the 1953 article, was a longtime confidant of the American Tobacco Company who had quietly helped that firm navigate the health scares of the 1930s. Clarence W. Lieb, a New York physician, had been a member of a tight industry circle he referred to as "our research council," meeting with Vice President Paul Hahn, Research Director Hiram Hanmer, and others at the company to plan responses to news reports of cyanide, carbon monoxide, lead, arsenic, and acrolein in cigarettes. Lieb had even testified to the "convincing proof" of the merits of "toasting" in a letter to American Tobacco President George Washington Hill, which Hill later used to defend his company against FTC charges of bogus advertising. Lieb had also helped Philip Morris defend its use of diethylene glycol as a "less irritating" additive, and as late as 1953 had written a book identifying "excessive smoking" as two packs or more per day. The flood of new medical evidence soon thereafter made him see the light, however, and by 1957 he had converted to the cause of his former critics, characterizing moderation as futile and smoking as "an enemy of the body . . . an enemy literally unto death." Clarence Lieb is arguably the first great tobacco industry insider, convert, and whistle-blower.[22]

A THERMODYNAMIC IMPOSSIBILITY

"Scientifically, the most effective filter ever developed to free cigarette smoke of impurities"—that's what it said right on every pack of Kents. Lorillard, though, was joined by every other company in making such claims. Some brands even had healthy-sounding names: King Sano cigarettes, for example, were supposed to evoke images of cleanliness, though nicotine deliveries were so low the company eventually went out of business. (Sano's total alkaloids in 1961 were only 0.8 percent, lowest among the top forty U.S. brands.)[23] Cigarette history is littered with brands that failed to keep their alkaloids high enough to ensure "satisfaction," the industry's code word for nicotine. Who today has heard of Cubeb cigarettes, made from the leaves of the Java pepper (in the first half of the twentieth century), or Vanguard cigarettes, made from corn silk and sugar beets (in the 1950s)? Who remembers Bravo cigarettes, advertised in 1966 as "a major breakthrough in safer smoking" with "absolutely no nicotine"? (Made from lettuce, Bravos by 1971 accounted for not even one in a hundred thousand cigarettes smoked in the United States.) Even with big ad budg-ets, low-nicotine brands like Next (Philip Morris, 1989) and Quest (Vector, 2003) have never made much of a commercial dent. People smoke for a reason, and nico-tine-free cigarettes sell about as well as alcohol-free rum or guns that shoot paper bullets.[24]

Of course, the conspiracy not to admit health harms meant it was hard for cig-arette makers to say what exactly these "filters" were supposed to be filtering out. The implication was that dangerous chemicals were being trapped, though specifics were rarely given. The bombast led to suspicion by congressional watchdogs, as in 1957, when the U.S. Congress convened a series of hearings under the leadership of John A. Blatnik, a Democratic congressman from Minnesota, to investigate the industry's "false and misleading advertising." Some of these inflated claims had been punctured by *Reader's Digest,* which had contracted with a chemical testing labo-ratory to find out how much tar and nicotine was actually being removed by these contraptions. Measurements showed that filters were not very effective: filters were doing little to reduce tar and nicotine exposures, especially when cigarettes were smoked down to a very short "butt." Some filtered or king-size versions delivered even more tar and nicotine than regulars—which Clarence Lieb attributed to the use of special high-nicotine Burley. Blatnik's committee heard a broad range of tes-timony (though tobacco executives refused to participate) and concluded that cig-arette manufacturers had "deceived the American public through their advertising of filter tip cigarettes."[25]

Filters did not in fact do what they were widely imagined to be doing, trapping the bad stuff while letting the good pass through. Filtering *per se* was a no-brainer: if all you wanted was to block stuff from entering your lungs, then any complex ob-stacle in the path of the smoke would do. Respirator technology was well developed by the 1950s, and you could even scrub *all* smoke out of inhaled air if you were will-ing to wear a large enough apparatus. You could even just plug up the end of a cig-arette and trap everything; but then you wouldn't really be smoking, just sucking on a dead stick.

The problem was that to actually *smoke* a cigarette, something had to make it past the filter, and it never was entirely clear what that was supposed to be. Purified smoke? Purified of what? What is the "clean" part of smoke? By the 1950s it was starting to become clear that *all* smoke is poisonous; there is no such thing as "clean smoke." Cigarette smoke is just tar and nicotine and gases such as hydrogen cyanide and carbon monoxide; take these out and you don't have much left. And no one seems to have liked the idea of inhaling empty vapors, though a kind of "nicotinized steam" would later be explored in some of the industry's more radical novelties of the 1980s and 1990s (Reynolds's failed Premier and Eclipse cigarettes, for example, discussed in chapter 28).

A closely related difficulty—or really the same rub restated—is that filters have never been very *selective*. Already by the 1930s, in fact, we find this disturbing re-alization at the highest ranks of the cigarette establishment. Hiram Hanmer, Amer-ican Tobacco's powerful research director, wrote to one of his superiors in 1932, pointing out that while a filter could be constructed "which would absorb any de-sired quantity of the constituents of the smoke," this could not be done "without sufficient change in character and flavor as to be readily detected and probably con-demned by the habitual smoker." Hanmer then added an observation that would be key to the filter fraud of all subsequent cigarettes: the drawback of *all* such de-vices, he noted, was that "they cannot be made to absorb selectively or propor-tionally" without the resulting smoking becoming "unbalanced and unsatisfying." Philip Morris in 1958 had a blunter way of putting this: selective filtration of par-ticulates at least was "a thermodynamic impossibility." The difficulty was that car-cinogens were being found in all parts of the smoke; there was no "clean part." Wake-ham made this explicit in 1961, confiding to his superiors that "carcinogens are found in practically every class of compound of smoke."[26]

Scholars outside the industry were never let in on this disturbing little secret—that filters don't really filter—though some of the industry's sharper critics did man-age to come to this same conclusion. In 1939, for example, the great Angel H. Roffo noted that "tar goes wherever the smoke goes" and that it was "very naive" *(una gran simplicidad)* to believe that filtration could destroy the carcinogenic powers of cigarette tar. The AMA's 1953 report on filters came to similar conclusions, noting that when filter tips were replaced by an equivalent length of tobacco no less tar was filtered out. *Advertising Age* in covering this report concluded that "filter tips don't filter much" and that Kent's asbestos filter had actually been "loosened" in the summer and fall of 1952 to allow an easier draw.[27] Which also of course made it easier to inhale the mineral fibers.

The take-home message is that the "filters" attached to the ends of cigarettes re-ally aren't filters in any honest sense of the term. Toxins accumulate in the ends of such devices but are revolatilized as the cigarette continues to be smoked. Which is no different from what happens in "unfiltered" cigarettes. Filtered cigarettes are really no different from ordinary cigarettes with the tobacco more (or less) tightly packed, making it harder or easier to obtain "satisfaction." But it doesn't really mat-ter whether this stuffing is made from ordinary tobacco or some fibrous plastic sub-stitute (as in all present-day cigarettes). Filters prevent a smoker from smoking past a certain point on the rod, but that is hardly "filtration."

"Filters" are gimmicks, pure and simple. Tobacco manufacturers realized this in the 1930s, but the public was never told, apart from those few instances where ex-tra-long cigarettes were advertised as having more "filtering capacity" just by vir-tue of being longer. Axton-Fisher in the mid-1940s, for example, advertised a cig-arette (Fleetwood Imperials) that was supposed to provide "extra filtration" by virtue of yielding smoke "filtered through more tobacco"—provided of course (as the ad cautioned) you didn't smoke farther down on the butt than you would an "old-size cigarette."[28] Similar claims were made for king-size brands such as Pall Mall, which American Tobacco touted as providing extra health protection because they "traveled the smoke further" on the way to your throat ("fine tobacco is its own best filter"). It sounds rather strange today, but king-sizing was actually one of the industry's earliest ways to make a purportedly "safer cigarette"—with no more truth behind this boast than claims for lights, milds, menthols, slims, naturals, or any of the industry's other gimmicks.

CHARCOAL FILTERS

If filters were (and are) a swindle, none of this prevented people—including the general public—from conjuring up creative schemes for new and improved designs. Hope springs eternal, as does hokum. The industry's archives are full of letters from ordinary smokers announcing "breakthroughs" of one sort or another, typically accompanied by an offer to share the invention, usually for a price. The American Tobacco Company received so many mailings of this sort that it opened a file titled "Public Relations, Suggestions, Filter Devices," with entries dating from the early 1930s. People wrote to propose adding iodine or benzedrine to tobacco, or a "carbon monoxide remover," or compounds designed to eliminate the cancer threat or cure some other ailment. Correspondents proposed methods to remove the nicotine or the "bite" of smoke, along with techniques by which cigarettes could be made "self-extinguishing."[29]

Filters were widely regarded as gimmicks within the industry, but the 1950s health scare—and America's love for technical fixes—showed that money could be made from the illusion. And as demand soared and competition increased, innovations in filter designs continued apace, doing pretty much for human health what tail fins did for automotive performance. Cellulose acetate became the industry standard because it was cheap, but countless other materials were explored, along with untold variations on the physical arrangement of the filter's internal chamber. Grooved, crimped, and perforated filters were introduced, including filters boasting single or double barrels of various sorts. Filters sometimes combined paper and cellulose acetate ("dual filtration"), though laminated and honeycombed contrivances were also popular. Lorillard tested an "Aqua filter," and Philip Morris in 1959 tried introducing fungal spores into a filter—by opening and wetting it—hoping that the filaments created thereby might have some salubrious effect. A lot of effort went into crafting names for such devices: in 1964, for example, American Tobacco's advertisers came up with more than twenty different names for the filter that was to accompany its new Durham-L brand (Fortifilter, Twinfilter, Triple Action Filter, etc.).[30] Fancy names helped cover the bluff.

One of the biggest hopes in the 1960s was for filters containing *activated char-*

coal. Charcoal was already known to attract and bind organic molecules of various sorts: carbon atoms are chemically promiscuous, forming bonds with many other kinds of substances. Mineralogists have long torn their hair out over this, since carbon atoms will clamp onto and contaminate a mineral sample being prepared for, say, electron microscopy or X-ray diffraction. Hopes were therefore high that carbon might help sequester some of the nasty stuff from tobacco smoke, and hundreds of different kinds of designs were patented.[31]

The Buckeye Cellulose Corporation in 1963, for example, patented a filter made from "beaten cellulose fibres, a hydrophobic latex, a wet strength resin," and a surfactant containing carbon fibers. Eastman Kodak one year later patented a filter made from crimped cellulose acetate containing "activated carbon bonded with polyvinyl alcohol and methyl cellulose." Other patents specified charcoal blended with thermoplastic polymers, citric acid, or manganese dioxide. A 1952 British patent described a powdered silica gel impregnated with chlorophyll, with activated carbon, pumice, or asbestos listed as possible substitutes for the silica. Other designs incorporated sawdust, methyl acrylate, vinyl acetate, glycol dimethacrylate, and water-insoluble detran.[32] The carbon itself was typically derived from wood of various sorts, but sources ranged from carbonized coconut fibers to charred paper.

Charcoal filters hit the U.S. market in 1958, with Tareyton's "dual action" (charcoal + cellulose) device. Liggett & Myers followed in 1963 with Lark, which did quite well thanks to its hoopla about "low ciliatoxicity."[33] Reynolds hoped for similar success with its charcoal-filtered Tempo one year later, which is also about when Liggett began testing a king-size charcoal filter called Devon. Philip Morris in 1964 introduced its own charcoal filter, the Galaxy, along with a charcoal-filtered cigaretto (smallish cigar) with the ascetic-sounding brand name Puritan ("which need not be inhaled to be enjoyed"). Charcoal filters really only became popular in Japan, however, where by contrast with other parts of the world the distinctive "carbon filter taste" actually came to be liked and, for non-menthol smokers at least, the norm.

EVERYTHING GOOD AND PURE AND NATURAL

Several cigarette companies toyed with the idea of using filters to transport flavorings or even soothing drugs and medications of one sort or another (recall Axton-Fisher's Listerine brand from the 1930s). Filters were built to incorporate flavorants such as coumarin or menthol, or oxidizing agents such as manganese dioxide. And experiments were done to see whether filters could be used to deliver nicotine. A 1969 design led the smoke through a labyrinth with added nicotine, menthol, and sundry other unspecified "medicaments." Nicotine filters—meaning filters designed to *deliver* nicotine—were explored as part of the industry's efforts to develop low-tar smokes that would still have enough of a kick to keep smokers "hooked." Which is why Philip Morris in 1969 patented a filter containing carbon black with adsorbed nicotine: the idea was that tar could be lowered while keeping alkaloid deliveries high—a common hope for the industry (and some public health authorities) in the 1960, 1970s, and 1980s.

Some filters incorporated mechanical devices or novel mineral compositions such as perlite or vermiculite. Still others involved mazelike passageways arranged to force the smoke to follow "a tortuous path." Filters "of the impact type" caused the smoke to accelerate against a surface coated with carbon, and in so-called cross-flow filters smoke was made to pass through layers of a porous material arranged in concentric tubes, with activated carbon sandwiched between each layer.[34] Thousands of patents were awarded for such devices, often drawn to look quite high-tech and intricate, like little satellites or fortifications (see Figure 31).

All of these were essentially gimmicks. A Lorillard brainstorming session from 1976 illustrates this willingness to market illusions:

> How about Old Gold with a new, improved "baking soda" filter? It's crazy, but I thought charcoal filters sounded pretty dirty and unappetizing, when I first heard about them.
>
> We don't know what effect a light sprinkling of baking soda in the filter material would have, but we know what millions of consumers would *think* it might have. Baking soda is associated with everything good and pure and natural—and is even compatible with the idea of oral consumption. After all, it's used for everything from baking biscuits to brushing teeth.[35]

The darker reality was that filtered cigarettes caused illness as easily as non-filtered varieties. In 1962, researchers from the Roswell Park Memorial Institute in Buffalo, New York, published evidence that tar extracts from the smoke of filtered cigarettes caused cancer in laboratory mice.[36] This caused nary a blip on the radar of either health authorities or tobacco researchers, who by that time had realized the nature of "the problem." The biggest consequence, perhaps, was that the scholar responsible for the study, Fred G. Bock, started finding it difficult to get further funding from the industry, given his willingness to admit real hazards.

TOXIN DU JOUR

It would be wrong, though, to imagine that this quest for novel cigarette designs was entirely cynical. The fact is that for more than a decade most tobacco companies kept alive this elusive goal of selective filtration, hoping that if they could not make a cigarette *safe* they could perhaps at least make it somewhat less deadly.[37] A common view was that whatever harm was being done could at least be lessened, by eliminating some specific constituent or careful choice of blends or perhaps by eliminating certain pesticides or fertilizers or finding some new and clever way to manipulate smoke chemistry.

Targets here were numerous, and changed over time. Arsenic, lead, and acrolein were the big fears in the 1930s and 1940s, with benzpyrene coming under suspicion in the 1940s and 1950s. Phenols and nitrogen oxides were hot topics in the early 1960s, which is also about when cigarette designers peaked in their targeting of ciliastats like cyanide and carbon monoxide. Nitrosamines and radioactive isotopes were worries from the 1950s, with episodic cycles of rising and falling interest ever since. Cigarette manufacturers became frustrated with what was sometimes called the "toxin de jour" or "compound of the month"—favorite refrains of Rodgman at Reynolds[38]—but they also felt they had to keep up this half-research, half-charade, hoping against hope for a breakthrough.

And hopes were kept alive by a never-ending stream of mini-breakthroughs that, for a time at least, were touted as solving some piece of this puzzle. Marlboro's cork-tipped selectrate filter, introduced in 1955, was supposed to remove a higher fraction of furfural than of total particulate matter,[39] and similar claims were eventually made for benzpyrene, cyanide, phenols, and formaldehyde. Efforts of this sort intensified in the 1960s, with a rash of new patents. A 1962 patent claimed a method to remove metal carbonyls; a 1963 patent claimed to remove nitrosyls and hydrocarbonyls (via chelating agents). Some of these sound improbable: a 1964 patent, for example, postulated a filter impregnated with "partially dried granules of cheese," preferably Parmesan, Swiss, or Romano. Two years later a patent proposed a filter consisting of active charcoal or clay mixed with oxides of cobalt, copper, zinc, silver, or molybdenum. We don't usually think of the National Cash Register Co. as engaged with cigarettes, but in 1966 that firm proposed a filter using an encapsulating material of gelatin or gum arabic. And charcoal filters kept getting tweaked: the Pittsburgh Activated Carbon Co. in 1966, for example, patented a carbon filter impregnated with monoethanolamine to aid in the removal of carbon dioxide from cigarette smoke. The same firm obtained another patent that year using activated carbon infused with copper sulfate to help reduce acetaldehydes. Other designs incorporated iron or zinc oxide or sepiolite, a clay also used for meerschaum pipes and kitty litter. A German patent of 1971 praised the virtues of granular basalt, boric acid, and sodium metasilicate; and Japan's Tobacco Monopoly Corporation patented a carbon filter coated with polyethylene glycol. Binding agents for such devices included lactose, pectin, polyethylene, polyvinyl acetate, and thermoplastic resins of various sorts. Australia's Wool Research Laboratory explored sheep's wool filters in the 1970s.[40]

All of these had problems. It was sometimes possible to reduce a particular smoke constituent, but this was always accompanied by the elevation of some other. Selective filtration was eventually recognized as a mirage. Industry scientists came to realize it wouldn't work—or at least not without making the smoke unpalatable. And since tobacco itself was recognized as just as good a filter—or rather just as bad—the whole hope for filters as a path to a "safer" cigarette was pretty much in disarray by the end of the 1960s. Epidemiologists a decade later would be showing—through the Framingham study, for example—that smokers of filtered cigarettes were just as likely to suffer from heart disease as smokers of non-filtered cigarettes.[41]

Why, then, were filters so popular? Why did the industry start selling them, and how did they become the sine qua non of smoking?

Filters were put onto the ends of cigarettes for three principal reasons: to lower the cost of manufacturing,[42] to keep tobacco bits from entering the mouths of smokers, and to lure people into thinking that brand Alpha, Beta, or Gamma was somehow safer. These are the real reasons cigarettes have filters—which is also why a number of critics have called for banning them. Filters are major polluters, cluttering beaches, sidewalks, and urinals throughout the world. And since they don't really do what they are supposed to do, why not just ban them? Tom Novotny at San Diego State University has launched such a campaign, stressing that filters are one of the world's single largest sources of trash, measured in terms of number of pieces. Most of the six trillion cigarettes smoked every year have such attachments, and trillions end up on beaches and roadways, clogging sewers and the gullets of beach birds. A million tons of butts are discarded every year. And if tobacco does just as good (or bad) a job at filtering, why not just eliminate them altogether?[43]

FILTERS ARE FRAUDULENT

"Filters" are frauds, a deception built into the fabric of the cigarette. Smokers have been led to believe that bad stuff is being removed, but the fact is that filters really just make it (slightly) harder to smoke—and even that depends on how tightly they are packed. Cigarette manufacturers can allow as much or as little smoke through a "filter" as they like, simply by changing its density. Of course smokers won't buy a cigarette they feel is too difficult to inhale: that's why "easy on the draw" became such a selling point; you didn't want to have to be a vacuum pump to get your nicotine fix. The flipside, though, is that filters were made so loose as to be worthless. Filters that let a lot of smoke pass (meaning all of them) really aren't *filters* in any sense of the term—they're more like smoke speed bumps—and they don't seem to have done anything to reduce health harms.

An alcohol analogy is apt: imagine yourself as a reforming alcoholic, and trying to reduce your intake by running your Jack Daniels through a series of fine-mesh screens before you chug it down. Cigarette filters do about as much—or as little—good.

Or think about drinking through straws of different diameters. Filters are basically like drinking through a somewhat thinner straw: you have to suck a bit harder, but you end up getting the same "satisfaction." Tobacco industry researchers recognized this as early as 1952, when Liggett & Myers's research chief, Frederick R. Darkis, noted the findings of Arthur D. Little, working with the company on filter technology, that "the filters in use at present do not really take anything out of the cigarette." Researchers at Ecusta shortly thereafter concluded that filters just reduced the particle size of smoke while also increasing the volume of vapor-phase poisons.[44] And by offering up an illusion of safety, smokers who might otherwise have quit have been led to keep on smoking.

Filters haven't made smoking any safer, which is why cigarettes still cause about one death per million sticks smoked. One thing that *has* changed since the 1920s, though, is the amount of tobacco in any given cigarette. Cigarettes today contain only about half the tobacco contained in popular brands from the 1920s, which means that on a *per gram* basis cigarettes today are nearly twice as deadly. That is largely because—as we shall see in a moment—cigarettes today are smoked more intensively than cigarettes in the past. Which means that all cigarette makers have really managed to do is to extract more death from every gram of tobacco they put into their products.

20

The Grand Fraud of Ventilation

We must in the near future provide some answers which will give smokers a psychological crutch and a self-rationale to continue smoking.

GEORGE WEISSMAN, DIRECTOR OF MARKETING, TO PHILIP MORRIS CEO JOSEPH CULLMAN III, ON HOW TO RESPOND TO THE SURGEON GENERAL'S REPORT OF 1964

Chief among the things keeping the filter craze going was that it helped sell cigarettes. Many smokers had started worrying about their health, especially after the grim and widely publicized epidemiology and animal experiments of the early 1950s and increasingly after the Surgeon General's report of 1964. The tobacco industry realized that people were willing to switch to filters as seemingly "safer" and did nothing to dissuade them from this myth. Indeed they were its chief architects, championing filters as "cleaner," "more effective," or even "miraculous." The companies were happy to attach such contraptions onto their products, for three principal reasons:

1. Filter materials were *cheaper* than tobacco, which meant that filtered cigarettes could be manufactured at a lower cost than regulars;
2. Filters served sort of like *cigarette holders,* the chief virtue of which was to keep little bits of tobacco from coming off in your mouth; and
3. Filters offered the *illusion of a "safer cigarette,"* helping the companies to move product while also creating the impression they were honestly taking steps to address the health problem.

All this required some fancy dancing, however, since the industry's bluster was that smoking had never been proven to cause *any* kind of harm. Hence this puzzle, at least for the outside world: Why, if there was no genuine evidence of harm, was such a fuss being made about filters? If there was really nothing bad in smoke, then what exactly was being filtered out?

No one ever said directly, though oblique hints were often dropped. Kents were said to remove "harshness and bite," while L&Ms were supposed to filter out "the heavy particles, leaving you a light and mild smoke." Other brands were touted as lowering the tar, nicotine, gas, or "nitrogenous" compounds. The companies rarely went into specifics, preferring instead simply to intimate that filters were the "sensible choice" or "just what the doctor ordered." Brown & Williamson ads featured endorsements by (fictional) astronomers, engineers, scientists, judges, and other idealized eminents, all hawking Viceroy as the "thinking man's filter."

MEDICO-MACHISMO

It is important to appreciate that some within the industry were honest—albeit naive—in hoping that some kind of "magic bullet" might be found to knock out or neutralize the carcinogens in smoke. In the 1950s and 1960s great hopes were held out for this ideal of "selective filtration"—that some Einstein of cigarette design might somehow manage to come up with some new miracle filter, allowing the bad in smoke to be cut out while letting the good pass through. And while nothing heroic was ever found, tiny steps were taken accompanied by the companies' PR trumpets. Lorillard in 1962, for example, claimed that the plasticizers it was adding to filters had enabled it to eliminate many of the *phenols* in cigarette smoke, prompting other manufacturers to start using similar compounds. BAT in 1965 was hard at work on designs incorporating a polyethylene-treated filter "selective for tar relative to nicotine," hoping to keep nicotine levels high while lowering tar.[1]

Great claims were also made for carbon and charcoal granules and other sciency pseudo-breakthroughs. There really was this "quick fix" magic bullet notion, prompted by the examples of penicillin and petrochemical pesticides and the triumphs of military science from the Second World War. Cars and rockets and medical diagnostics were improving, so why not cigarettes? The 1950s were a time of confidence in the power of science to solve human problems, and the examples of jet engines, radar, rocketry, vaccines, antibiotics, and the newly harnessed powers of the atom led to hopes that here, too, technology might come to the rescue. The popular magazine *Science & Mechanics* as late as April 1968 hailed a new tobacco additive, Chemosol, a mix of citric acid and deuterium oxide, as ushering in a new age of "cancer-proof" smoking:

> The violent controversy over smoking and health promises to be ended soon. S&M has learned exclusively of a new chemical compound that takes all the risk out of smoking. It has just been perfected, after two years of concentrated experimentation. In terms of possible health hazards, it provided fool-proof safety for smokers of cigarettes, cigars and pipes. There has been nothing like it before in the history of scientific tobacco research. . . .
>
> By combining Chemosol-mixed tobacco with an activated carbon filter, the ultimate in safe smoking is already within the public's grasp. All that remains is for someone to manufacture and market the product commercially. When this happens, an

estimated 90 million smokers in the United States alone—not to mention those many millions more in other countries around the world—will be able to light up without a loss of flavor. And without fear.[2]

Hopes were also voiced that even if cigarettes might be *causing* cancer, advances in medical science would soon be *curing* it. Not everyone was so naive of course, but we do find this perception that cancer was not such a big deal—or perhaps only an affliction of the constitutionally weak. Hints of this medico-machismo can be found in the popularity of self-experimentation in the labs of the tobacco companies. In June of 1948, for example, the American Tobacco Company had its entire research staff—including Hanmer, Haag, and Larson—breathe vapors containing purified smoke constituents to determine tolerance thresholds. Lucky Strike employees inhaled progressively higher concentrations of acetic acid, nicotine, ammonia, acetaldehyde, and formic acid until a certain "threshold concentration for consistently producing irritation had been determined." The goal was to study the "irritative quality" of such compounds under conditions resembling actual smoking, but some enthusiasts went quite a bit further. Cornelius Rhoads, director of the Sloan-Kettering Institute and a close American Tobacco confidant, volunteered to have his own back painted with tobacco tar (by Wynder) to see whether tumors would develop. (An allergic reaction apparently cut the experiment short.) Such proposals are not common, but they do capture in microcosm the era's oddly macho spirit of self-sacrifice—both for science and for one's corporate sponsor. And some sense of the perceived triviality of cancer, or at least an overconfidence in cures. (Recall John Wayne's braggadocio about how he would "beat the Big C"; he didn't.) Tobacco company employees were often called on to test new cigar or cigarette designs, and in one such series from 1968 several members of American Tobacco's research staff ended up smoking cigars that had been irradiated by a cobalt 60 source to test this as a means of controlling mold without sacrificing taste.[3]

FUMO LOUCO

We saw in the last chapter how hard it was—if not impossible—to design a filter that would cut out, say, benzpyrene or phenols or aldehydes while leaving only "pure, healthy smoke." Cigarette smoke turns out to be so viciously complex that effective filtration is virtually impossible—at least on the scale of a cigarette. Failure was in a sense predetermined, given what it means to actually smoke a cigarette.

Recall again what happens when you light up a Camel or a Marlboro or a Mild Seven. You begin by touching a sulfur match or petroleum flame to the end, while oxygen from the surrounding air is pulled—by suction—through the rod to get the thing burning. Following ignition, the smoker draws further on the cigarette, pulling smoke through the tobacco column and into his or her mouth. Nicotine molecules (about 50 to 150 micrograms per puff) start wafting against nerves at the back of the throat, causing an initial "throat catch" or "throat kick" sensed by the brain within a matter of seconds. Smoke in the mouth is then combined with a larger volume of external air, which is then quickly inhaled into the lungs and transferred by the blood to the brain, creating the nicotine rush that tobacco makers pretty up as "satisfaction." More honest would be "temporary relief from the withdrawal symptoms of nicotine addiction."

Recall also the constitution of the cigarette itself, which is not just chopped leaf with a paper wrap and filter plug. Cured tobacco leaf accounts for only about two-thirds of the mass of a typical cigarette, with the rest being flavorings, moisteners, and the paperlike reconstituted tobacco sheet known as recon or G-7 (up to 30 percent by weight), along with diverse sugars and burn accelerants—plus of course the filter, the paper, and whatever inks may be printed thereupon and glues holding the whole together. Flavorings—including anesthetics like menthol and various pack aromatics—account for a significant fraction of a cigarette's heft: typically about 4 percent.[4] *Burning* turns this all into a complex chemodynamic brew that transmogrifies over time as the hot, newly generated smoke is pulled through the intact portion of the rod. This boils and/or burns the remaining "filler" while also transforming it into thousands of different chemicals, some short lived, some more enduring. Part of this moist, gassy, half-combusted load is then dropped into your mouth—nicotine is a small molecule and migrates easily through thin mucous layers—but most moves on into the catacombs of your lungs, where the tar spray-paints onto the cells lining the interior of that organ. Much of this crud is retained in the lungs, which actually function as tolerably good "filters." Hermann Druckrey in Germany in the 1950s showed that much of the smoke stays in the chest, as indicated by its lowered fluorescence after passage through the lungs.

Filters by some tests lowered inhaled tar and nicotine, but usually only if the "pressure drop" from mouth suction was held constant (a big "if"). Cigarettes could be made to deliver arbitrarily low levels of tar and nicotine simply by tightening the filters—packing them more densely—but the companies quickly found that smokers would not buy cigarettes on which they had to suck too hard to obtain "satisfaction." So the question became, how can machine-measured yields be lowered without making filters so tight that people have to suck like a pump to savor their chosen brand?

One solution was to lower tars as much as possible while maintaining a high nicotine delivery. Lose the cancer, keep the addiction ("satisfaction"). Some early proposals were radical in this regard. In 1958, for example, a Philip Morris scientist wrote to his research director that since "evidence . . . is building up that heavy cigarette smoking contributes to lung cancer" the company should explore an "all synthetic aerosol to replace tobacco smoke." An aerosol of this sort might contain nicotine but "no tobacco tars." Filter designs were also explored that would trap certain particles while permitting "evolution of nicotine off the filter surface back into the mainstream smoke."[5] Many other techniques were used to create low-tar "high-impact" (i.e., high-nicotine) cigarettes—including genetic engineering.

Brown & Williamson in the 1980s, for example, collaborated with a California biotech firm, DNA Plant Technology, to develop a strain of genetically modified tobacco plants containing twice the nicotine of ordinary tobacco. Code named Y-1, these high-nicotine plants were clandestinely grown in Brazil to hide them from the prying eyes of U.S. public health authorities. Local farmers called it *fumo louco*—crazy tobacco—for its large size and high nicotine content. Brown & Williamson would later deny having grown tobacco of this sort, which caused the company all kinds of grief when documents were uncovered showing that by 1990 it had two million pounds of the stuff ready for consumer testing. FDA chief David Kessler and his staff discovered the intrigue in the mid-1990s, prompting federal prosecutors to charge the company's supplier, DNA Plant Technology, with having conspired to smuggle tobacco seeds out of the country. The scandal also helped convince federal authorities that cigarette makers were manipulating the nicotine content of tobacco to keep smokers hooked.[6]

Brown & Williamson's high-nicotine Y-1 scheme has attracted its justifiable share of scorn, but the company was certainly not alone in trying to develop high-nicotine tobaccos. Imperial Tobacco in 1985, for example, had a project to develop "a Canadian High Nicotine Tobacco" to enable "more blending flexibility in developing recipes with low tar-to-nicotine ratios." This was the company's Project T-0576, part of its broader leaf agrology program. RJR-Macdonald (Reynolds's Canadian affiliate) also tried to breed high-nicotine plants, and for similar reasons. The public is often shocked by such revelations, but the fact is that high-nicotine plants were sought as part of this broader effort to lower tar-to-nicotine ratios. The idea was that smokers would not have to smoke so much to obtain a given level of "satisfaction"—meaning less inhaled tar per unit dose of nicotine. Of course there are other ways to think about this: high-nicotine cigarettes might mean the companies could put less tobacco into a cigarette to deliver the same level of "satisfaction," saving on manufacturing costs. Or still less charitably: smokers could still be kept hooked, even if they ended up smoking less. For these and other reasons, elevating nicotine-to-tar ratios became a priority of industry research in the 1970s and 1980s, by which time the companies were clearly thinking of themselves as drug manufacturers, offering nicotine to smokers "in attractive, useful form."[7]

FOUL, ROTTEN RUBBER

A major problem with this high-nicotine, low-tar approach, however, was that people don't seem to like high-nicotine cigarettes. A 1965 study at BAT's Southampton laboratories showed that while it was not hard to elevate the "extractable nicotine" in cigarettes, panelists smoking such cigarettes seemed to hit "a barrier, at about 1 mg 'extractable nicotine', which they were loathe to exceed." Philip Morris's Project Kick failed on precisely these grounds: the goal had been to produce a high-nicotine cigarette for Europe, but panel tests found that the cigarette made smokers "feel ill." Nicotine is a potent drug, and dosages above a certain level—especially when inhaled—are difficult to tolerate. And not very tasty. When smoked alone the alkaloid has "flavor notes" akin to those of burning rubber: "foul, rotten rubber," is how one Reynolds document describes it.[8] That is one reason cigarettes are juiced up with so many different chemical flavorants: you want to cover up this nasty nicotine taste. That is also why it is almost impossible to "overdose" on cigarettes (by smoking them at any rate): you can only smoke so fast, and nicotine inhalation above a certain rate is quite difficult to stomach. The interesting contrast here is with opium or heroin, on which one can easily overdose, especially when injected. If nicotine were injected or ingested rather than inhaled, we would no doubt have many more fatal overdosings. Acute toxicity can and does result when babies swallow a cigarette (it happens more often than you might think),[9] or when tobacco workers handle the leaf improperly ("green tobacco sickness"), or when smoking contests get out of hand (think college parties). But none of these are very common, at least not when compared to more familiar harms from smoking.

A different approach has been to add certain chemicals or physical agents to the paper or the leaf, to help reduce either tar as a whole or specific carcinogens contained therein. Hundreds of different preparations have been tried, from aluminum oxide to various carbon fibers, precious metal catalysts, burn accelerants or retardants—even vitamins, chlorophyll, hemoglobin, and the previously mentioned Chemosol and Parmesan cheese. Chemical accelerants were added to make the cigarette burn faster, which was really just another version of the "less tobacco" cheat. The companies knew that if smokers could get only seven or eight puffs out of a cigarette—rather than the traditional ten or eleven—the robot tar and nicotine numbers would be reduced accordingly.

Eliminating cancer-causing agents from cigarette smoke was intrinsically difficult, however, since smoke is not like polluted water, which can be filtered (or distilled) and come out "clean." The whole point of smoking is *to inhale smoke,* which by its very nature is dirty. Smoke—to repeat—cannot be "purified"; there is no such thing as "clean smoke." Of course it is plausible that certain constituents will be more dangerous than others, and the industry has looked for ways to reduce some of these fouler components—chiefly polycyclics such as benzpyrene; ciliastats such as cyanide or nitric oxide; metals and metalloids such as cadmium, nickel, and arsenic; aldehydes such as formaldehyde; alpha-emitting polonium; or co-carcinogenic phenols or tobacco-specific nitrosamines. Efforts in this direction almost always ran afoul of the fact that blocking one kind of poison meant allowing some other kind to pass. Some of the tar could be blocked, for example, but this would generate more carbon monoxide. Benzpyrene might be eliminated, but this might require addition of questionable nitrates or yield irritants of some other sort—like phenols. Filtration turned out to be a messy many-body problem of near-infinite complexity, quite apart from consumer acceptance. You could always make a cigarette deliver so little "satisfaction" that nobody would want to smoke it: that, again, was the experience with many early filters, which started off too tight and were later loosened to prevent rejection.

That is also why filters were often regarded within the industry as gimmicks and why *perceptions* were so often in the sights of marketeers. In 1962, for example, at a conference at BAT's Southampton laboratories, researchers from the firm's far-flung foreign offices discussed a plan by Sir Charles Ellis to launch a research facility at Harrogate to test the "biological activity" (cancer-causing capacity) of different kinds of smoke. Robert M. Gibb of BAT Canada noted that the industry had been frustrated by having to produce gimmick cigarette designs of one sort or another; the industry needed some means of knowing "not what the facts were but what people thought the facts were" with regard to filters. Explaining "how to sell a gimmick" (i.e., filters), Gibb asserted that in Canada at least "you stated what you thought people wanted to be told, and you made money by doing so."[10]

BAT in this instance was worried mainly about the "threat" posed by Lorillard's announcement of a filter claimed to have successfully reduced phenols in cigarette smoke. Wynder had been making a fuss about phenols since 1960 and had proposed adding catalysts to speed up their destruction (by combustion). Lorillard was the first to respond and by the end of that year was advertising a filter said to be capable of substantially reducing phenols, catching the other manufacturers off guard. The "phenol crisis" was not that smokers were inhaling phenols; that had been known since the nineteenth century, when the stuff was known as "carbolic acid" (physicians had also used it as an antiseptic and an embalming fluid, and Helmut Wakeham at Philip Morris commented on its presence in Lifeboy soap, Scotch whiskey, and hospital disinfectants).[11] The crisis was that a competitor was claiming to have found a way to remove phenol from its cigarettes, violating the "gentlemen's agreement" not to go it alone on tobacco and health. Industry leaders had quietly agreed since the mid-1950s not to make health claims but also to share whatever breakthroughs might come in this realm.[12] The response from the other companies was textbook tobacco misanthropy: not "My God, we're poisoning our customers!" but rather (in effect) "My God, Lorillard is going to capture part of our market!" BAT worried that challenges of this sort would keep popping up, and the organizer of this meeting—Sir Charles Ellis, BAT's chief scientist—asked his colleagues to ponder what other "crises" might be looming on the horizon. (W. W. Reid of Australia's Wills Tobacco Company guessed it might be volatile acids or irritant aldehydes and ketones.) Ellis also speculated that phenols had been highlighted simply because Lorillard had not found a way to remove any of the many other poisons known to be in smoke.[13]

FRAUD ON TOP OF FRAUD

Failing at filtration didn't mean much to the companies, however, since the real goal was *reassurance,* which turned out to be a great success. Half of all cigarettes sold in the United States by 1960 had "filter" tips, a percentage that would continue to climb for decades thereafter, as more and more smokers came to perceive a threat. Competition also increased to deliver ever lower levels of tar and nicotine, as measured on the industry's automatic smoking machines. The Germans had developed such machines in the 1920s, and researchers working for the American Tobacco Company had perfected them in the 1930s. Once every sixty seconds the machines would take a fixed 35-milliliter puff of two seconds' duration, "smoking" the cigarette down to some preordained butt length—originally 30 millimeters and later fixed at 23. Nicotine would then be extracted from the condensed smoke ("tar") and weighed, whence "tar and nicotine numbers."[14]

Some at least within the companies also knew, however, that the tar and nicotine numbers produced by such tests were not reliable indicators of how much smokers would actually inhale. Smokers would smoke a cigarette more or less intensively, delivering higher or lower quantities of tar and nicotine. So long as people failed to recognize this fact and fixated on the (misleading) numbers produced by smoking machines, an opportunity presented itself to game the system, as we find in the brilliant trick of *ventilation.*

To understand ventilation—the punching of tiny holes around the mouthpiece of a cigarette to dilute the smoke stream—we must recognize that there are only so many ways to reduce the tar, nicotine, or gas produced by a cigarette. Nicotine is basically a no-brainer, since the alkaloid is easily removed simply by soaking the tobacco in water or by steam treatments of various sorts. Philip Morris in 1961 had two chief means by which nicotine could be removed: the Rosenthal process, which involved reacting nicotine with "a gaseous compound such as ethyl bromide or chloride," and the company's own "selective extraction method," by which the nicotine in a blend could be reduced to only 10 percent of its original value. Cigarettes were sometimes also redesigned for having *too little* nicotine, typically by altering the blend. In 1978, for example, Philip Morris redesigned its Brunette Extra when an early production run found the nicotine delivery to be "20% too low." Nicotine content is easily altered by choice of leaf blend: a burley blend might contain 5.20 percent nicotine, for example, whereas an oriental blend might have only 0.86 percent (usually measured to within two decimal places). Alkaloid content can also vary according to the conditions under which the plants are grown: hot and dry weather increases the nicotine, for example, whereas heavy fertilizing tends to reduce it. Position on the stalk also matters (the upper leaves are the most potent), as does when the leaf is picked, and so forth.[15]

Cigarette manufacturers have long realized that nicotine-free cigarettes won't sell, however, so rarely has there been much of a push to lower nicotine below what was sometimes called the "weaning" point. (Philip Morris's Next brand is the most important exception: the company developed this 97 percent nicotine-free cigarette in the late 1980s, using supercritical fluid extraction technology, at a cost of around $300 million. The cigarette was a monumental flop.) Tar, however, is a different story. Cigarette makers have never been too happy about the fact that tobacco tars accumulate in smokers' lungs. We're already seen, though, how limited the options were to do anything about this.[16] To reduce *machine-measured* tar you can basically put less tobacco in the rod, or hasten its burn rate, or stuff the cigarette up with a super-tight "filter"—but none of these really work, if by "work" we mean lowering the actual amount of junk delivered into your lungs. Gimmicks of this sort are easily defeated, since smokers can smoke a low-tar cigarette and get a high-tar delivery, simply by pulling harder on the rod or inhaling more deeply or taking larger puffs or smoking farther down on the butt or holding the smoke longer or smoking more cigarettes, and so forth. Tobacco manufacturers certainly *could have* made cigarettes less deadly—by raising smoke pH back above 8, for example, which would have turned cigarettes back into "little cigars"—but why bother when you could make people *think* they were getting a safer cigarette simply by tinkering with the tips?

It may not seem like much, but ventilation is arguably the principal design fraud of modern cigarettes (in contrast to flue-curing, which is the principal design *flaw*). Highly ventilated cigarettes deliver low levels of tar when smoked on a smoking robot, but humans are able to smoke such cigarettes in ways that deliver far more tar and nicotine—by an order of magnitude. Because unlike the machines most human smokers are *addicted* and crave a certain level of nicotine. Humans are also able to defeat the tricks used to ventilate cigarettes—notably by covering the holes punched for this purpose—allowing them to extract higher levels of tar and nicotine than what is advertised on the pack. Ventilation is the chief means by which "light" cigarettes have been made light (ditto for "ultralight"), but smokers are able to extract as much tar and nicotine from ventilated as from regular cigarettes by the compensation mechanisms mentioned above. The first *published* evidence emerged in 1980,[17] but the industry knew about this quite some time earlier while continuing to advertise such products as safer. Which is why ventilation must be regarded as a deceit built knowingly into the cigarette: deceit by design. Ventilated cigarettes—meaning virtually all modern cigarettes—perpetrate a fraud on unsuspecting consumers, who are not likely to know that cigarettes advertised as "low tars" are no less deadly.

Ventilation—also known as "air dilution" or "shunting"—is really nothing new in cigarettes. An early form of the art was popular in vintage cigarette holders, which often came with holes in their sides to "cool" the smoke or let it "breathe." The idea had a medical rationale even in the nineteenth century, since one common theory was that *heat* from the smoke of a pipe might be what was causing all those cancers of the lip and throat. Perforated holders were imagined as helping to cool the smoke, rendering it less harmful. By the end of the nineteenth century patents were being filed for cigarettes with tiny holes punched in the tips, claimed both to improve the quality of the burn and to help prevent disease.[18]

Heat turns out not to be much of a factor in cigarette carcinogenesis, but interest in ventilation continued into the 1930s, principally as a consideration in *how to keep a cigarette lit*. Lorillard researchers in 1933, for example, cautioned that cigarette paper had to be porous to prevent a cigarette from going out between puffs.[19] Keeping a cigarette lit was most often addressed as a matter of smoking convenience, but the methods used—adding oxidizing agents, for example—also made it easier for cigarettes to cause fires. Hundreds of thousands of fire deaths globally are one consequence of this "convenience."

("Spontaneous human combustion" is probably also largely an artifact of the cigarette epidemic: accounts of people burning from no apparent cause multiplied toward the end of the nineteenth century, when cigarettes were becoming fashionable. People were probably falling asleep while smoking, perhaps while overcome with alcohol, and bodily fats could keep the flames alive for long enough to consume large portions of the body.)

Ventilation was sometimes also seen as helping to eliminate certain poisons from cigarette smoke. The American Tobacco Company in the 1930s did a series of experiments to determine how paper porosity influenced tobacco combustion, with the idea being that porous paper might help to eliminate some of the harmful aldehydes known to be in smoke. Hiram Hanmer in 1933 proposed yet another potential use, noting that cigarette paper modified "towards greater porosity" would produce "a dilution of the smoke with air," increasing the mildness of Lucky Strikes. Diluting the smoke in this manner would mean that a single puff would not contain "as great a concentration of the normal components of the smoke." Hanmer wasn't sure whether this would ever prove practical, given that the sensation of smoking might be altered. Similar doubts were raised by Clarence W. Lieb, his Manhattan medical confidant, who believed that paper porosity would adversely affect smoke composition "to a surprising extent."[20]

Porosity by this time (the 1930s) was one of about a dozen physical features of cigarette paper routinely manipulated by cigarette designers—along with thickness, width, weight, whiteness, burn rate, tensile strength, stretch, opacity, texture, spots, pinholes, and a couple of others. Porosity was measured—and adjusted—primarily to ensure a proper rate of burn, so that smokers would have an even and pleasant draw. Reducing tar and nicotine was not yet given much thought, because there wasn't yet much demand for "safer" cigarettes.

Paper porosity comes to be more intensively studied—and manipulated—following the "cancer scare" of the 1950s. Cost was clearly one concern, since porous paper tends to be lighter and therefore cheaper, pound for pound, than heavier varieties. Use of lightweight paper also meant that smokers would burn and inhale less smoke than they would from a heavier paper. Some people at this time still thought that cigarette paper might be causing cancer, and there was this hope that if the quantity of paper smoked could be reduced cigarettes might be made less deadly. The idea also made sense to those who realized that *cigar smokers* don't suffer much from lung cancer. Cigars are not wrapped in paper, though the lesser lung cancer burden as we now know—and must have been known to the industry in the 1950s—stems not so much from how they are wrapped but rather from differences in smoke pH and therefore inhalability. With its high pH (about 8+), cigar smoke is usually too harsh, too alkaline, to inhale.

Reynolds was one of the first companies to boast of using highly porous cigarette paper. An ad campaign from 1959 claimed that Salems had this "revolutionary" new feature, described as "an amazing and exclusive cigarette paper." High-porosity paper was said to allow the smoke to *breathe* and to freshen and "soften every puff." Salem cigarettes were supposed to be "springtime fresh," with the implication that smoke through such a filter could be cleaner even than ordinary air.[21] Other companies were quick to jump on this bandwagon: Lorillard heralded the "Ocean-breeze freshness" yielded by Newport's "super-porous Micropore paper," and Liggett that same year (1960) boosted its Chesterfield Kings as having "air-softened mildness" as a result of "special porous paper," yielding a "cooler, smoother smoke that's mild."

Paper cannot be made arbitrarily porous, however, without compromising its strength. Which is one reason other ways were sought to allow fresh air to "dilute" cigarette smoke—including ventilation by means of tiny slits punched around the filter tip.

PINPRICKS AND LASER SLITS

Slit ventilation starts off innocently enough, as simply one among many cigarette gimmicks. The theory was simple: tiny holes punched in the sides of the cigarette (toward the mouth end) would allow fresh air to mix with the mainstream smoke, lessening its toxic concentrations. Toxic chemicals are still produced, but in theory some fraction of these will not be inhaled—not by the smoker at any rate—but rather released as sidestream smoke. Early versions date from the nineteenth century; I've mentioned cigarette holders, but holes were sometimes also cut into the sides of cigarettes, both to allow an influx of air and to expel or dilute poisons. A patent awarded to a New York inventor by the name of Edward M. Harris in 1890, for example, proposed a cigarette with about a hundred pinprick holes distributed evenly throughout the paper, a design intended to aid in the outflux of "subtle, injurious, and poisonous vapors" from the burning tobacco. These were vapors that, if inhaled persistently, would be "harmful to the throat, sometimes causing cancer" or even heart failure. Harris's "punctured or perforated wrapper" was designed to "deprive cigarettes of their baneful effects and render them innocuous" by allowing fresh air "to commingle with the tobacco-smoke" during its passage through the cigarette while also allowing "egress to any subtle vapors" such as "the oils of creosote" and "the powerful alkaline, nicotine."[22]

In these early years, ventilation wasn't yet so different from paper porosity or even the use of a cigarette holder. American Tobacco's chief chemist in 1927 rejected one such proposal by noting that holes punched in the sides of a cigarette would do little to change smoke deliveries; the effect would be the same as using a perforated cigarette holder and would simply "cause the smoker to draw harder in order to get the amount of smoke he desires." The company also realized that you could achieve the same effect—diluting the smoke—just by putting less tobacco in the rod.[23]

Ventilation was not really taken seriously until the 1950s and 1960s, when tobacco makers revived a specific type of hole punching to reduce apparent tar and nicotine yields—this time knowing full well that the trick did little or nothing to reduce hazards. Philip Morris in 1949, for example, began contracting with outside laboratories to explore "the ventilation principle" as a means to dilute inhaled cigarette smoke. A 1955 report by the same company mentions experiments showing a 46 percent reduction in total smoke solids from three pinholes punched near the mouth end of the cigarette. Smoke could be seen escaping from these (rather large) holes between puffs, so new ways were explored to produce a greater number of smaller holes, using a spark charge delivered by a Tesla coil.[24] Spark puncturing of paper was costly, however, and Philip Morris for a time shifted to the Ecusta Paper Corporation's method of mechanical perforation. Ecusta's machines were able to produce 800 holes per linear cigarette inch, with each hole being the size of a tiny elongated pinprick (.007 × .020 inches). Philip Morris experimented with other designs but quickly realized that cigarettes allowing too much influx of air would frustrate smokers trying to get their nicotine fix. A low "resistance to draw" forced smokers to pull a huge volume of air into their lungs to get a satisfying quantity of smoke, as air whooshed in from all these holes. An added problem was that cigarettes introducing more than about 65 percent "by pass air" were difficult to light—since not enough oxygen was being drawn into the ignition point. Philip Morris explored the pros and cons of different arrangements, deciding that holes placed near the mouth end of the cigarette would produce the most uniform smoke. (Holes punched all along the rod tended to exacerbate the fact that the first puffs on a cigarette are also the weakest.) The technology was also appealing because it reduced machine-mea-sured smoke solids (up to 35 percent) while reducing nicotine by a substantially lower margin (12 percent). A number of different machines were introduced in the 1950s to produce such slits, and by the end of the decade several of the majors were slitting their cigarettes. Spud cigarettes (Philip Morris) in 1958 had air vent per-forations near the filter tip, and Lorillard had its "air-conditioned" Spring brand. By 1960 other ventilated brands in the United States included American Tobacco's Riviera, Brown & Williamson's Life, Philip Morris's Alpine, and Liggett & Myers' Duke.

None of these early ventilated brands made much of a splash. British manufac-turers actually ridiculed the process, commenting (in private correspondence) that similar ideas had been put forward four decades earlier in a children's encyclope-dia (they don't seem to have known about Harris's patent). Lorillard's much-bally-hooed "spark ventilation" they regarded as typical of the Americans' ability "to make the most of very little" and "the height of advertising prowess." Looking today at Lorillard's actual ads leads one to think this a case of British understatement: Lo-rillard had announced its "air conditioned" cigarette in a thousand-word full-page spread in the *New York Times,* effusing over "an amazing electronic process that ventilates Spring through microscopic windows."[25]

More important than Britain's ridicule, however, is the fact that cigarette man-ufacturers already knew that the promise of dramatically lower tar and nicotine yields was not entirely honest, given how smokers would actually smoke such cig-arettes. One prompt for this (private) confession came in 1959, when a physician at London's prestigious University College Medical School, C. N. Smyth, published a letter in the *British Medical Journal* claiming that ventilation holes could make cigarettes less dangerous. The theory was that ventilation would reduce the tem-perature of the burn and redistillation, thereby cooling and reducing the quantity of smoke reaching the smoker.[26] Herbert R. Bentley at Imperial Tobacco summa-rized and commented on Smyth's paper for his superiors, noting that this dilution effect would be achieved only if

> the smoker does not *compensate* for the increased dilution by taking a larger puff than he would with a standard cigarette in order to draw into his mouth the amount of smoke to which he is instinctively accustomed. *In the manufacturers' opinion most smokers would in fact tend to do this.*[27]

Bentley's admission of the reality of compensation ("most smokers would in fact tend to do this") is significant, revealing that prior even to its widespread incorpo-ration into cigarette designs ventilation was regarded as not likely to have any real effect in reducing deliveries. Cigarette manufacturers knew this already in the 1950s—witness Parmele's comment that smokers tend to pull harder on filtered cig-arettes "to compensate for the large proportion of smoke removed"[28]—which is long before most people in the outside world knew that one of the chief means by which cigarette tars would be lowered was dishonest.

The big push for ventilation doesn't come until 1964, however, when the U.S. Surgeon General's report prompted the beginning of the end for ubiquitous smoking. (America's year of per capita "peak cigarettes" was 1963, with consumption topping out at about 4,345 sticks for every man, woman, and child. Total consumption wouldn't peak until 1982, when some 630 billion cigarettes were smoked.) The American Tobacco Company launched its super-low-tar Carlton brand on January 4, 1964; Carltons had been in the works for quite some time, but with the expectation of new health fears from the Surgeon General's report a decision was made to rush the new brand into production. The hope was to exploit "the cancer scare," again turning lemons into lemonade.[29]

Carltons were advertised as using a high-porosity paper, which, when combined with a charcoal filter and "precision air vents," produced a smoke quite low in tar (as measured on an automatic smoking machine—we have to keep this crucial caveat in mind). Carlton was one of the first successful "hi-fi" (high-filtration) brands: a heavy promotion schedule helped of course, but the new brand was also aided by endorsements even by scientists outside the industry, who argued that if you were going to smoke you should at least choose a "low tar" brand. Gio Gori, deputy director of the National Cancer Institute's Division of Cancer Cause and Prevention, claimed as late as 1976—and indeed for some time thereafter—that most people could smoke twenty or more Carlton-type cigarettes per day with virtually no elevated risk from disease.[30] Statements such as this earned him the enmity of consumer advocates but a big reward from the industry: Gori in 1980 left the NCI for an executive position at the Franklin Institute in Chase, Maryland, buoyed by a $400,000 endowment from Brown & Williamson and cozy financial ties to the Tobacco Institute.

The next popular high-filtration brand was True, a cigarette introduced by Lorillard in 1966. True also used ventilation to achieve low apparent deliveries. Ventilated cigarettes by this time were being called "hi-fi" cigarettes—playing off the stereo craze—though there really wasn't much by way of filtration going on. One might as well have said that adding water to fruit juice "filters" it. Ventilation was really just a form of *dilution,* which is desirable only if less of the total product is consumed. And dilution was easily overcome by compensation. Here the analogy with fruit juice breaks down: you might well lower your intake of juice by diluting it, since your stomach gets full. Diluting smoke with ordinary air does not "fill you up," however, because smokers are addicted and cannot satisfy that craving without inhaling a specific dose of nicotine. Cigarette makers knew about compensation, but they also knew that "hi-fi" cigarettes often produced exceptionally high levels of vapor phase chemicals ("gas") such as carbon monoxide.[31] Bottom line: tobacco manufacturers knew that the safety offered by highly ventilated "hi-fis" was an illusion.

Carltons and Trues were made using new techniques for rapid cigarette slitting, techniques quickly picked up and imitated by other companies hoping to capitalize on the low-tar craze. And so by the 1970s most cigarette manufacturers had begun using ventilation to lower (apparent) tar and nicotine deliveries. True was Lorillard's most important low-tar brand, but every company explored and implemented ventilation. Indeed by the early 1980s an estimated 80 percent of American cigarettes were ventilated. Demands of this sort prompted cigarette-machine makers to increase the rate at which they could crank out slit-filter cigarettes. The Hauni company of Hamburg perfected a device using "needle blades," and Molins of London developed a method (in 1973) using lasers. Needle blades were notoriously finicky, however, so Hauni developed its own improved method of punching holes using lasers, which required no physical contact with the cigarette. Electric spark perforation was also improved, and some paper companies specialized in preperforated paper. Speed was key, and some machines used by Philip Morris could perforate cigarette paper at the rate of five thousand linear feet per minute.[32]

There were of course other means to lower tar and nicotine yields. I've mentioned the move to put less tobacco in any given cigarette, mainly by using "puffed" or expanded tobacco or by reducing the diameter of the rod or mixing in nonburnables like glass, ceramics, or inert chalklike materials of one sort or another. Another trick involved increasing the combustion rate of the tobacco by adding chemical accelerants such as sodium or potassium citrate—which would basically burn up the cigarette so fast you'd have less time to inhale its smoke (with increased deaths from fires a pesky side effect). Reconstituted tobacco sheet was also used for this purpose: nicotine was extracted in the course of its manufacture, so low-nicotine sheet could be used to manipulate final yields. All these methods and more were put in place and helped to reduce machine-measured yields. But ventilation was really the only way to push significantly below the 15-milligram tar mark defined by the industry as its arbitrary cutoff for "light" cigarettes. Machine-measured tar deliveries had fallen from about 35 milligrams in the 1950s to about 20 milligrams by the 1960s, but values much lower than this required ventilation.

And so by the 1970s cigarette makers were routinely using filtration, expanded tobacco, blending tricks, burn accelerants, recon, and (especially) ventilation to achieve low tar and nicotine numbers. "Efficiency of filtration" was an expression often used with reference to these lowered deliveries, though this again was misleading, given that ventilation was really just *dilution*—and even then only under the conditions of idealized smoking simulators. Dilution (i.e., ventilation) was commonly measured as the fraction of fresh air compared against the total volume of smoke inhaled through a cigarette: Philip Morris's Project Peter Pan, for example, was an effort from the late 1970s to develop Lark, L&M, and Chesterfield cigarettes for the European market using a filter ventilated to yield 12 percent dilution. Project Gamma was an effort by the same company to produce a Virginia cigarette delivering 4 milligrams of tar at 45 percent dilution. Some cigarettes had dilutions as high as 99 percent—ultra-lows like Philip Morris's Cambridge brand, for example, developed through the company's Trinity Project, which yielded less than .1 milligram of tar on smoking robots.[33] Tar and nicotine levels could in fact be pushed arbitrarily low simply by adding more—or bigger—ventilation slits. Cigarette makers knew that they could increase the "efficiency of filtration" to 50, 80, or even 99 percent just by creating ever draftier cigarettes; they also knew that the process was deeply fraudulent.

HOW WAS VENTILATION FRAUDULENT?

Imagine you are worried about your weight, and someone offers you a "light" or "diet" version of your favorite beer, which turns out to be the same old brew but now accompanied by a special kind of straw through which you are required to drink. This straw has a ring of tiny holes cut around the mouth end, which mixes air in with your beer as you try to suck it up. How would you feel about such a beer being advertised as "light" or "diet"? Imagine further that a testing agency has been established with sophisticated machines designed (by the beer industry) to determine the rate at which one's caloric intake is lowered by such means, so that beers mixed with, say, 50 percent air were classed as "lights," while those with an air-to-beer ratio of, say, three to one were "ultralights." Would that be a legitimate business? (One can of course imagine a straw with so many holes that you don't get anything to drink at all—just air.) And just to complete the analogy: what if the holes on these straws were placed close to the mouth end so people could cover them easily with their fingers or lips, allowing them to imbibe air-free beer, or as much beer as they wanted, with no dilution?

That is very much how ventilated cigarettes work. Most of the "light" and "ultralight" cigarettes sold over the past thirty or forty years have these tiny air intakes, which is the principal means by which cigarettes are made "low tar." You might as well say that whipped cream is "low cal" compared with cream straight from the carton. Which is also why the actual tobacco smoked in today's cigarettes is no safer than anything made a century ago. (On a gram-per-gram basis it is actually deadlier, since the low-alkaline blends introduced with flue-curing allow smokers to inhale. And filters have reduced smoke particle size, producing cancers deeper in the lungs, making them harder to identify and harder to treat.) Cigarette makers learned that by careful placement of these holes they could fool the machines used to measure tar and nicotine deliveries—along with the smokers buying into the whole "low-tar" scam. And the odd fact is that key elements of this deception were revealed to the outside world in the 1980s, when cigarette makers called Brown & Williamson to the carpet for advertising a "99% tar-free" cigarette delivering only a single milligram of tar and only a fifth that mass of nicotine.

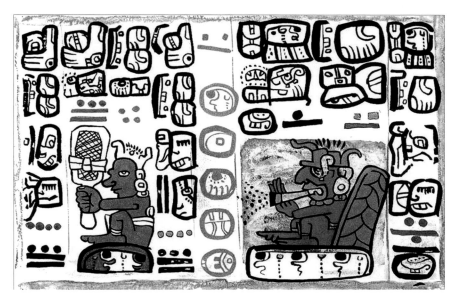

FIGURE 1. Mayan smoking image (and glyphs) from the Madrid Codex, circa 1600. Hundreds of such glyphs are known, with separate symbols for smoking, tobacco leaves, tobacco smoke, and so forth. Exact provenience for this image is unknown, but scholars postulate a seventeenth-century origin in Peten or Tayasal. Enhanced image reproduced by permission from W+D Wissenschaft.

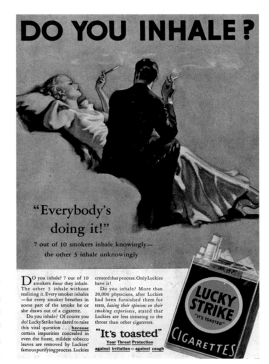

FIGURE 2. "Do You Inhale?" American Tobacco developed this series of ads—drawn by pinup artist John La Gatta—to associate cigarette smoke inhalation with sexual satisfaction.

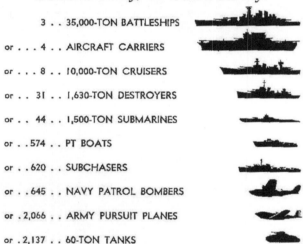

"Sold American"

You're the Man
Behind the Man Behind the Gun!

It takes a lot of money to run a war. And *your* work is paying a goodly part of the bill!

Last year, as a result of *your* production, The American Tobacco Company paid the government more than $310,000,000 in taxes.

With that money, Uncle Sam can buy:

3 . . 35,000-TON BATTLESHIPS		
or . . . 4 . . AIRCRAFT CARRIERS		
or . . . 8 . . 10,000-TON CRUISERS		
or . . 31 . . 1,630-TON DESTROYERS		
or . . 44 . . 1,500-TON SUBMARINES		
or . . 574 . . PT BOATS		
or . . 620 . . SUBCHASERS		
or . . 645 . . NAVY PATROL BOMBERS		
or . 2,066 . . ARMY PURSUIT PLANES		
or . 2,137 . . 60-TON TANKS		

REMEMBER! Every time you help to put together a cigar, a cigarette, or a pack of smoking tobacco—it means money for Uncle Sam, money to build a mighty fighting force to crush the Axis!

FIGURE 3. Tobacco tax patriotism. Tobacco companies in the 1940s bragged about helping to boost the American war effort by generating tax revenues. Much of that braggadocio disappeared in the 1960s, when the industry tried to assume a lower profile. Part of the now-lost rhetorics of gigantism. From *Sold American*, May 15, 1944, Bates 990626163–6450, p. 27.

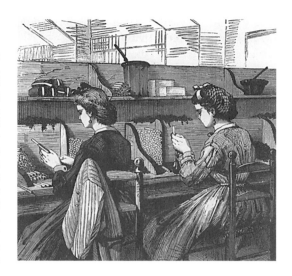

FIGURE 4. Cigarette rollers in nineteenth-century America. Cigarettes were rolled by hand until the invention of automatic rolling machines in the 1880s. The girls and women employed for such purposes would typically roll two hundred to one thousand cigarettes per day, compared with the hundreds of thousands and eventually millions per day cranked out by machines. From Robert K. Heimann, *Tobacco and Americans* (New York: McGraw-Hill, 1960), 211.

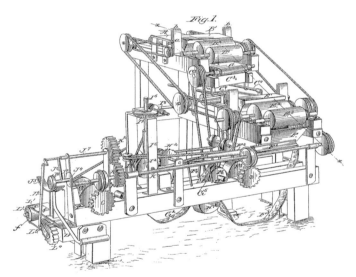

FIGURE 5. Bonsack machine from 1881. James Bonsack's patented cigarette-making machine produced a continuous rod of compressed tobacco, which could then be wrapped with paper and cut to some regularized size. The Bonsack machine revolutionized the manufacture of cigarettes, allowing as many as a hundred thousand cigarettes per day to be extruded. Cigarette making was one of the first examples of "continuous process" manufacturing. From Bonsack's U.S. patent application, granted Mar. 8, 1881 (#238,640).

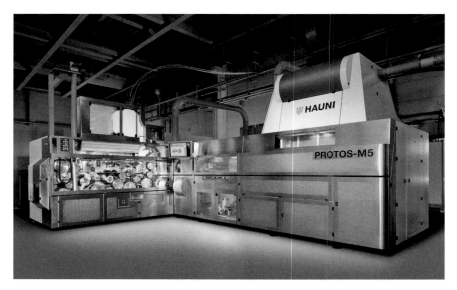

FIGURE 6. Hauni Protos-M5. The Hauni company of Hamburg, Germany, dominates the world trade in cigarette-making machines. Hauni's are the world's fastest cigarette machines, capable of rolling about twenty thousand cigarettes per minute, or 10 million per eight-hour shift. These are some of the deadliest machines ever invented and crucial links in the causal chain joining tobacco leaf and death from smoking cigarettes. From Hauni's website, http.//www.hauni.com.

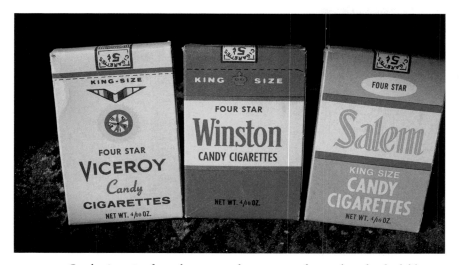

FIGURE 7. Candy cigarettes from the 1940s and 1950s were often packaged to look like the actual smoking article; candy cigarettes from the 1960s and 1970s were more often modeled on real cigarette brands but with names playing off those of actual cigarette brands (Kamel, Winstun, Lucky Stripes, etc.). Cigarette manufacturers encouraged brand infringements of this sort, which trained young children in the gestures of smoking. Private collection.

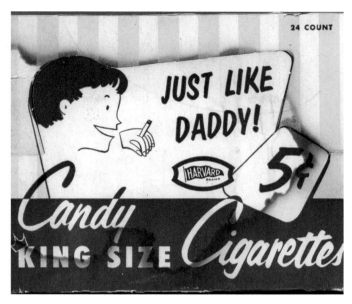

FIGURE 8. "Just Like Daddy!" Harvard brand candy cigarettes from the 1960s. Candy cigarettes were a clever way for cigarette manufacturers to market a kind of tobacco toy to future smokers. Private collection.

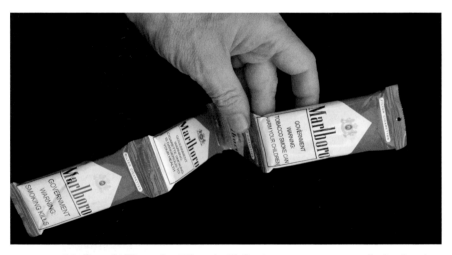

FIGURE 9. Marlboro kiddie packs. When the Philippine government passed a law barring distribution of cigarettes in packs of two, three, or four to restrict youth access, Philip Morris responded by creating dangle packs that could be divided into smaller packs for sale separately. The tobacco industry has been adept at circumventing onerous legislation. In the 1930s, when cigarettes were taxed per stick rather than per pack, the makers of Head Play cigarettes responded by creating packs containing eleven-inch-long cigarettes that could be cut into shorter segments, reducing the tax. Private collection, with thanks to Mary Assunta.

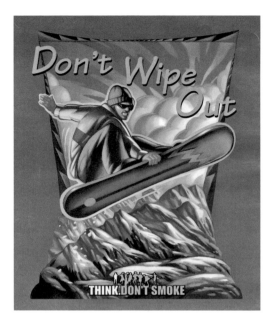

FIGURE 10. "Don't Wipe Out!
Think. Don't smoke." Philip Morris
in the fall of 2000 sent 13 million
of these book covers to American
high schools, with another 13
million planned for distribution
as part of an effort to (appear to)
oppose youth smoking. What do
the billowing clouds remind you
of? How about those leafy brown
mountains or the cool refresh-
ing snow? And what's up with
the snowboard? Notice also the
(non-smoking) teen standing apart
from the crowd—is that what teens
really want? Philip Morris invested
about $100 million in such ads
from 1998 to 2002.

FIGURE 11. "Right Decisions,
Right Now." R. J. Reynolds
launched this campaign in 1991
"to help counter peer pressure an
adolescent may feel to smoke."
Note how the non-smokers
are all younger and playing a
game. The first player cannot
even reach it properly but has
to stand on tiptoe. The boy in
the middle sports a flattop, and
the youngster on the far right is
wearing suspenders. How cool
is that? "Right Decisions" images were sent to 60 percent of
all U.S. junior high and middle
schools, reaching an estimated
three million students.

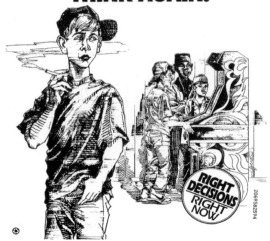

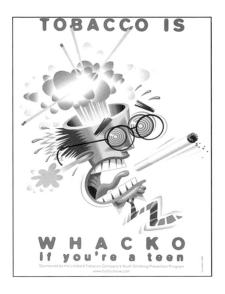
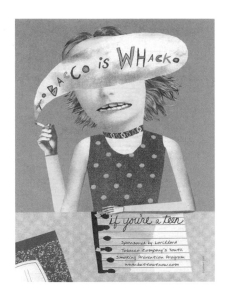
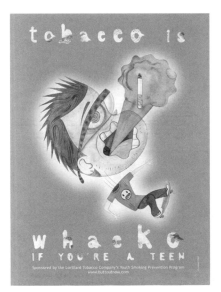
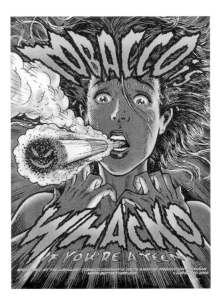

FIGURE 12. "Tobacco Is Whacko If You're a Teen." Lorillard introduced this campaign in 2002 in response to Philip Morris's "Think. Don't Smoke" campaign. Such images do little or nothing to discourage kids from smoking, especially given the insinuation that tobacco is fine for grown-ups. Ads of this sort are of legal value for the industry, which presents them as evidence that they don't want youngsters smoking. Lorillard spent over $13 million on this campaign. Some of these ads appeared in Marvel Comics' "Fantastic Four," 3 (no. 58, Oct. 2002). What are the hidden messages in such ads?

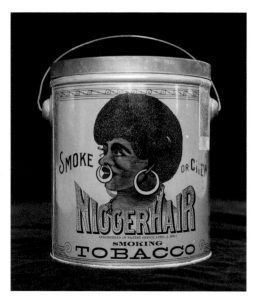

FIGURE 13. Nigger Hair tobacco. Many early tobacco ads were offensive; there was also a Nigger Head tobacco and cigarette packs featuring racist images of Asians and/or Native Americans. Nigger Hair tobacco, made from Kentucky burley leaf "cut in long curly strands," was sold beginning in 1878 by the B. Leidersdorf Co. of Milwaukee, Wisconsin, one of many manufacturers swallowed up by Buck Duke's American Tobacco conglomerate. Ads explained that the brand "got its name from its distinctive crinkly cut." The name was changed to Bigger Hair in the 1940s, but the picture on the pack and tins remained the same. The brand was sold into the mid-1960s, by which time the figure had been labeled a "Fiji Islander."

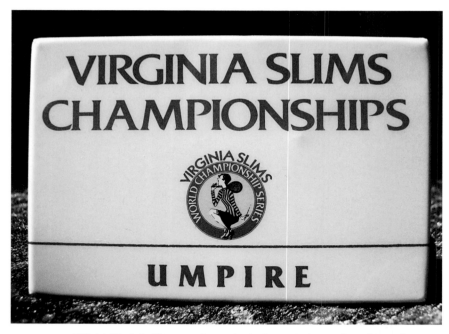

FIGURE 14. Official Virginia Slims tennis umpire badge with the smoking "Ginny." Umpires at Virginia Slims tournaments wore such badges, and brand logos appeared on tickets, napkins, neckpins, notepads, lanyards, press kits, pencils, VIP badges, and banners of various sorts. Philip Morris's Ginny first appears as a silver trophy awarded at the 1973 Boca Raton Virginia Slims tournament, and by 1975 the public was being offered "Ginny Jerseys" through the mail for $6 plus proof of purchase of the cigarette.

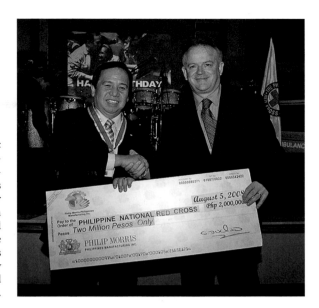

FIGURE 15. Strategic philanthropy. Transnational tobacco companies often support causes such as tree planting or hunger relief to create an appearance of being "good corporate citizens." Here Philip Morris advertises its 2008 donation of money to the Philippine National Red Cross.

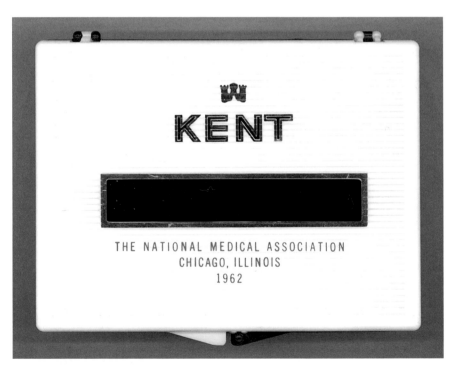

FIGURE 16. Marketing to African Americans. This plastic box of Kent cigarettes was provided as a free sample to African American physicians attending the annual meeting of the National Medical Association in Chicago, August 13–16, 1962. Personal collection.

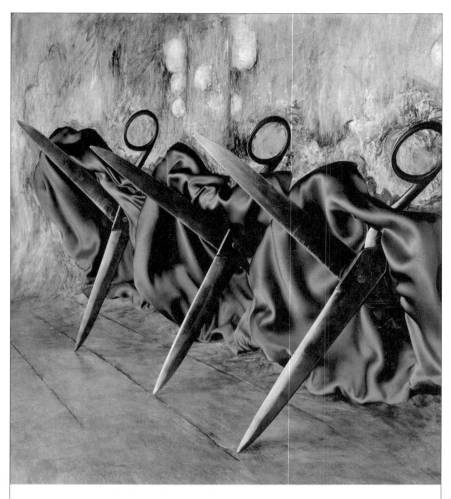

7mg TAR 0·7mg NICOTINE
PROTECT CHILDREN:
DON'T MAKE THEM BREATHE YOUR SMOKE
Health Departments' Chief Medical Officers

FIGURE 17. No words necessary? The semiotics of Silk Cut, a Gallaher brand cigarette widely smoked in Europe. Britain's Gallaher Group began running such ads in 1984, following a British law barring cigarette manufacturers from using words or human images in advertising. Many dozens of such ads were run, which are among the most creative in the history of advertising.

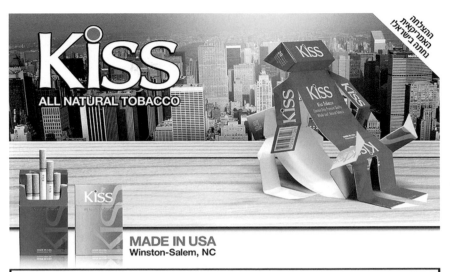

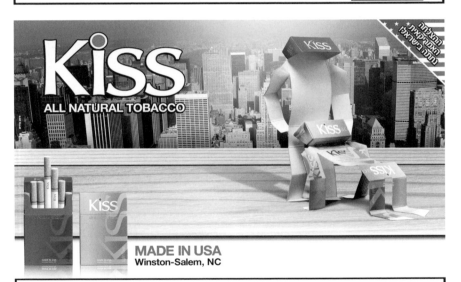

FIGURE 18. Cigarette pack sex. Laws banning the use of human figures in tobacco ads have prompted clever evasions, including this 2007 Israeli ad for Kiss cigarettes showing packs in some rather risqué positions. Russian ads for this same brand in 2011 featured blond teenage girls licking ice cream, with the slogan (in Russian): "If you're not allowed it, but really want it, you can have it."

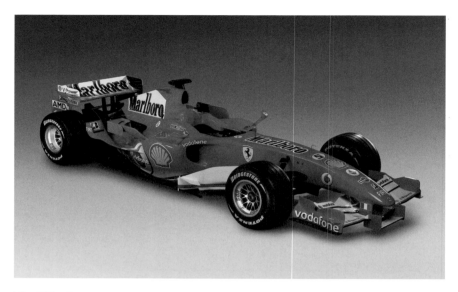

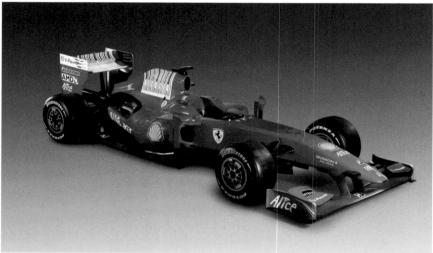

FIGURE 19. Alibi branding. Philip Morris has sponsored Formula One racing for many years, mainly as a way to promote its Marlboro brand. As governments began banning the use of cigarette logos on race cars, the cigarette maker introduced a more abstract "bar code" design similar to the font used in the Marlboro name. The bottom image shows Marlboro livery on the Scuderia Ferrari F1 for 2008; similar designs were included on helmets, uniforms, and so forth. The bar code design was abandoned in July 2010 in response to public outcry about this subliminal advertising. For additional images, see http://www.graphicology.com/blog/2010/4/28/292-the-sneakiest-design-ever.html.

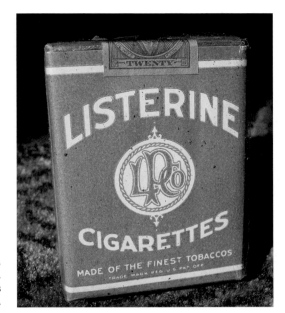

FIGURE 20. Listerine cigarettes.
The Axton-Fisher Tobacco Co.
sold these medicated cigarettes
in the 1930s. Personal collection.

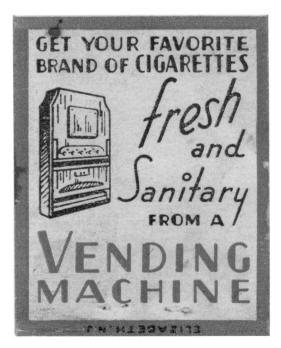

FIGURE 21. Vending machine
ad on a matchbook. Personal
collection.

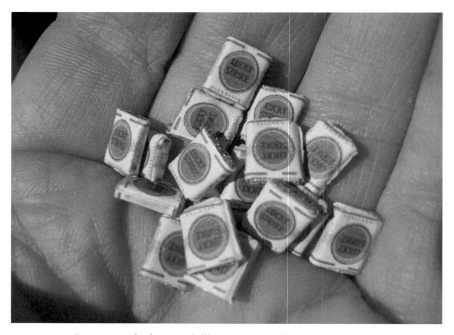

FIGURE 22. Cigarette packs for your dollhouse or toy soldier. Most such toys are miniature versions of genuine brands, prompting us to ask, Who was making these? Does this constitute brand infringement? And if so, why did tobacco manufacturers allow such infringements? Personal collection.

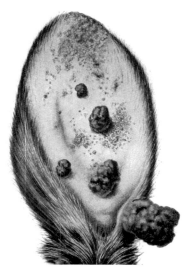

FIGURE 23. Tobacco tar tumors on the ear of a rabbit. Following months of "painting" with cigarette tar, Angel H. Roffo of Argentina was able to produce tumors on the ears of experimental animals. From his *El tabaco como cancerígeno* (Buenos Aires: Imprenta de la Universidad, 1936).

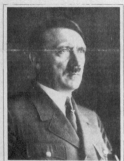

FIGURE 24. "The Führer Has Called Us! And We All Say 'Yes!'" The *Vereinigte Tabak-Zeitungen* was Germany's leading tobacco industry publication in the Nazi era; here in this issue from April 8, 1938, Hitler's annexation of Austria is celebrated.

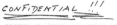

CONFiDENTiAL !!!

RESULTS OF ACCELERATED ANIMAL TESTS

ORIGIN OF CONDENSATE	SEBACEOUS GLANDS			ESTIMATE OF CARCINOGENICITY
	ABSENT	INTACT	VERY FEW LEFT	
Cigarettes rolled in Minn. flax paper	8,8,10	10	12,12	Positive
Cigarettes rolled in Calif. flax paper	10,10,12,12		8,8	Positive
Cigarettes rolled in Rand film	3,8,10		8,10,12,12	Positive
Cigarettes rolled in Burley tobacco leaf	3,8,10,10,12		12	Positive
Cigarette paper alone	10,12	8,8,10	12	Mild
Rand film alone	8,10,10,12		8,12	Positive
Solvent alone		8,8,10,10,12, 12,14,14,16,16		Negative
0.3% Dimethylcholanthrene in the Solvent	8,10,12,12,14, 14,16,16		8,10	Positive

Note: The figures 8,10,12, etc. in each column refer to the number of days of treatment. Thus for instance, in the figures given for condensate from cigarettes rolled in Minn. flax paper, under the "Absent" column the figures 8,8,10 indicate that two of the animals were treated for 8 days and one animal for 10 days.

(June 9, 1953)

FIGURE 25. "Results of Accelerated Animal Tests." The Ecusta Paper Corporation supplied these secret test results to Lorillard on July 1, 1953. Ecusta's secret experiments showed that tars extracted from the smoke of cigarettes caused cancer when painted onto the shaved backs of mice. Data are attached to a letter from Lorillard's J. J. Blanchard, Director of Manufacture, to H. B. Parmele, Director of Research, Lorillard, Inc., July 1, 1953, Bates 00065829 and 00065830.

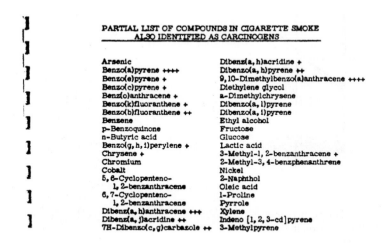

FIGURE 26. Carcinogens in tobacco smoke. Tobacco manufacturers for decades denied that smoking caused cancer, but here a Philip Morris document from 1961, authored by the company's director of research, lists numerous carcinogens known to be in cigarette smoke. The plus signs ("+") indicate potency. From Helmut Wakeham, "Tobacco and Health—R&D Approach," Nov. 15, 1961, Bates 1005069026–9050, p. 9. This is one of millions of documents discovered through litigation in the 1980s and 1990s.

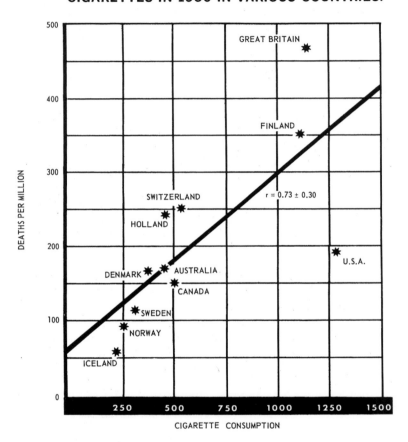

FIGURE 27. Lung cancer mortality as a function of cigarette consumption in eleven nations. Richard Doll in Britain in the 1950s published this chart, showing a consistent relationship between a country's cigarette consumption and its lung cancer mortality twenty years later. Data are for males only. First published in 1955, Doll's chart was reproduced in the 1964 U.S. Surgeon General's report, from which this image is taken (p. 176). From this chart, one can show that one lung cancer death results from every three million cigarettes smoked, with a time lag of twenty years.

A Frank Statement

to Cigarette Smokers

RECENT REPORTS on experiments with mice have given wide publicity to a theory that cigarette smoking is in some way linked with lung cancer in human beings.

Although conducted by doctors of professional standing, these experiments are not regarded as conclusive in the field of cancer research. However, we do not believe that any serious medical research, even though its results are inconclusive should be disregarded or lightly dismissed.

At the same time, we feel it is in the public interest to call attention to the fact that eminent doctors and research scientists have publicly questioned the claimed significance of these experiments.

Distinguished authorities point out:

1. That medical research of recent years indicates many possible causes of lung cancer.

2. That there is no agreement among the authorities regarding what the cause is.

3. That there is no proof that cigarette smoking is one of the causes.

4. That statistics purporting to link cigarette smoking with the disease could apply with equal force to any one of many other aspects of modern life. Indeed the validity of the statistics themselves is questioned by numerous scientists.

We accept an interest in people's health as a basic responsibility, paramount to every other consideration in our business.

We believe the products we make are not injurious to health.

We always have and always will cooperate closely with those whose task it is to safeguard the public health.

For more than 300 years tobacco has given solace, relaxation, and enjoyment to mankind. At one time or another during those years critics have held it responsible for practically every disease of the human body. One by one these charges have been abandoned for lack of evidence.

Regardless of the record of the past, the fact that cigarette smoking today should even be suspected as a cause of a serious disease is a matter of deep concern to us.

Many people have asked us what we are doing to meet the public's concern aroused by the recent reports. Here is the answer:

1. We are pledging aid and assistance to the research effort into all phases of tobacco use and health. This joint financial aid will of course be in addition to what is already being contributed by individual companies.

2. For this purpose we are establishing a joint industry group consisting initially of the undersigned. This group will be known as TOBACCO INDUSTRY RESEARCH COMMITTEE.

3. In charge of the research activities of the Committee will be a scientist of unimpeachable integrity and national repute. In addition there will be an Advisory Board of scientists disinterested in the cigarette industry. A group of distinguished men from medicine, science, and education will be invited to serve on this Board. These scientists will advise the Committee on its research activities.

This statement is being issued because we believe the people are entitled to know where we stand on this matter and what we intend to do about it.

TOBACCO INDUSTRY RESEARCH COMMITTEE

5400 EMPIRE STATE BUILDING, NEW YORK 1, N. Y.

SPONSORS:

THE AMERICAN TOBACCO COMPANY, INC.
Paul M. Hahn, President

BENSON & HEDGES
Joseph F. Cullman, Jr., President

BRIGHT BELT WAREHOUSE ASSOCIATION
F. S. Royster, President

BROWN & WILLIAMSON TOBACCO CORPORATION
Timothy V. Hartnett, President

BURLEY AUCTION WAREHOUSE ASSOCIATION
Albert Clay, President

BURLEY TOBACCO GROWERS COOPERATIVE ASSOCIATION
John W. Jones, President

LARUS & BROTHER COMPANY, INC.
W. T. Reed, Jr., President

P. LORILLARD COMPANY
Herbert A. Kent, Chairman

MARYLAND TOBACCO GROWERS ASSOCIATION
Samuel C. Linton, General Manager

PHILIP MORRIS & CO., LTD., INC.
O. Parker McComas, President

R. J. REYNOLDS TOBACCO COMPANY
E. A. Darr, President

STEPHANO BROTHERS, INC.
C. S. Stephano, D'Sc., Director of Research

TOBACCO ASSOCIATES, INC.
(An organization of flue-cured tobacco growers)
J. B. Hutson, President

UNITED STATES TOBACCO COMPANY
J. W. Peterson, President

FIGURE 28. "A Frank Statement to Cigarette Smokers." This full-page ad appeared on January 4, 1954, in 448 newspapers throughout the United States and may well be the most expensive single-day ad ever run up to that time, costing in excess of $244,000 just for newspaper space. The "Frank Statement" launched the cigarette industry's denialist conspiracy.

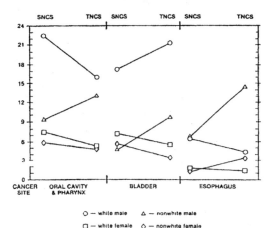

Incidence Rates* per 100,000 Population from
Second National Cancer Survey (SNCS) (1947-49) and
Third National Cancer Survey (TNCS) (1969-71)

○ — white male   △ — nonwhite male

□ — white female   ◇ — nonwhite female

FIGURE 29. Graphic agnotology. Here the Tobacco Institute is suggesting that since cancer trends are chaotic, smoking cannot be to blame. Note that lung cancer is not shown. From the TI's *Smoking and Health, 1964–1979: The Continuing Controversy,* Jan. 10, 1979, Bates 1005057750–7926, p. 104. This document was distributed to the press one day before publication of the 1979 Surgeon General's report, to steal that document's thunder.

Report: G:\Cognos32\Imp4user\User Workspace\K&S Health.imr   Date: 12/9/99
Smoking and Health Issues
Detail Filter: Entry Date Time >= 1999-08-01 and Specific Code = 305

Contact Number	Comments
2494575	Consumer called because his 10 month old daughter ate some filtered tubes. He called Poison Control and they told him not to worry. That they would not hurt her. He wanted to check with us also.
2390277	He smoked for about 50 years and is in good health.
2458976	Consumer is upset with the gov't suing the tobacco companies. He said he thinks the toxic waste is what's causing people to get sick and not the cigts.
2340000	Caller wanted to know if we had data about the long term affects of smoking based on how many cigts. are smoked per day and the risk increase with each cigt. that is added on a per day basis.
2349775	Consumer writes to say we lied to our customers about cigt addiction. He is also angry that "you and the government are hijacking th public...shifting the fines to the user."
2329432	Consumer stated the filter harms people, not the tobacco. She also asked for our website address. Her e-mail address is BLUEKYGRRL@aol.com.
2425928	Consumer heard Rush Limbaugh's talk show. She thinks smoking is not addictive. "Smoking or not smoking is an act of the will."
2430671	Consumer wants a copy of the Tobacco Use/Smoking and Health information on our Web site.
2442578	Caller is upset that people continue to blame every disease on cigarettes.
2408210	The consumer says our PR needs to read these books 'The Nazi War on Cancer', 'Cancer Wars What We Know and Don't Know about Cancer', and 'Racial Hygene' by Dr. Robert N Proctor at Penn State.
2329428	Consumer asked if smoking is addictive.
2400381	(WR) Japan # 9100129 - Consumer claimed cigt had funny odor when smoking and there was a glass fiber-like substance inside of its rod. *RL/NA. (Retrieved the product. He was so anxious and worried about its harmfulness and damage for his health.
2338494	Consumer would like an ingredients list. She heard that filtered cigts. cause cancer and non-filtered cigts. cause emphysema.
2470083	Consumer stated cigt. smoking doesn't cause cancer in everybody. She wants to call the toll free number she heard about to make that comment and to say that she knew Jeffrey Wigand and he was a horrible person.
2440314	He said he has the cure for lung cancer. He said it is caused by a virus. He would like to be paged and leave a toll free number for him to call.
2426078	Caller asked if LUCKY STRIKE was better for you than Marlboro. He hung up when I asked his DOB.
2390305	(SF) Consumer wants coupons. He wanted us to know that he's been smoking for many years and is in good health.

FIGURE 30. Brown & Williamson's telephone log from 1999. The makers of Kool, Viceroy, and Barclay cigarettes kept this record of calls to the company on "Smoking and Health Issues." One cannot read such logs without realizing that many smokers remain ignorant about the health impact of cigarettes. Here the first of eight pages, Bates 06000308–0315.

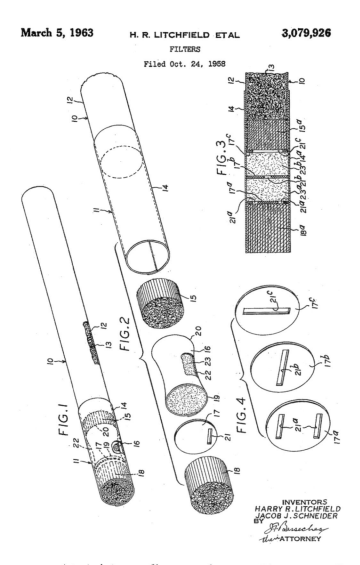

March 5, 1963   H. R. LITCHFIELD ET AL   3,079,926

FILTERS

Filed Oct. 24, 1958

FIG.3

FIG.2

FIG.1

FIG.4

INVENTORS
HARRY R. LITCHFIELD
JACOB J. SCHNEIDER
BY
J. Bassechez
their ATTORNEY

FIGURE 31. A typical cigarette filter patent from 1958. Filters never really worked, if by "worked" we mean made cigarette smoking safer. Thousands of different designs have been contrived, incorporating myriad different additives and physical baffling. This particular device incorporated "fragments of lung tissue of calf, fowl, sheep or hog, preferably in powdered or pulverized form." Countless other designs can be found by searching Google Patents or the industry's internal documents.

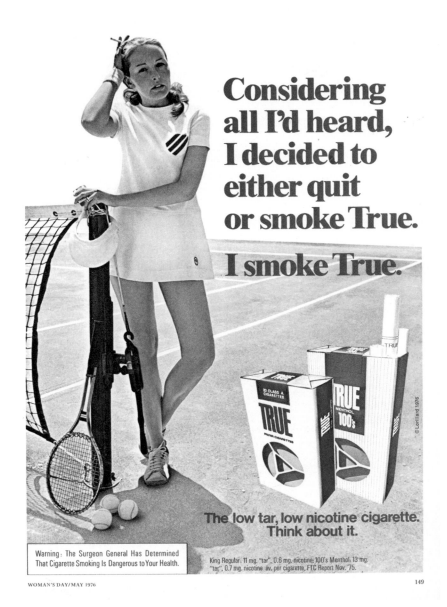

FIGURE 32. "Considering all I'd heard . . . " True cigarettes, made by America's oldest continuously operating tobacco company (Lorillard), were a highly ventilated brand introduced in 1967. The oblique reference here in this ad from 1976 is to diseases caused by smoking, but the companies rarely made such claims explicit.

Founded by Henry E. Sigerist

Gert H. Brieger, Jerome J. Bylebyl   *Editors*

Susan L. Abrams   *Assistant Editor*

Miriam L. Kleiger   *Copy Editor*

Advisory Editorial Board

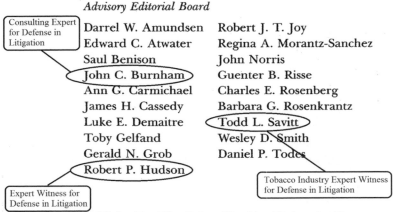

Consulting Expert for Defense in Litigation

Darrel W. Amundsen
Edward C. Atwater
Saul Benison
John C. Burnham
Ann G. Carmichael
James H. Cassedy
Luke E. Demaitre
Toby Gelfand
Gerald N. Grob
Robert P. Hudson

Robert J. T. Joy
Regina A. Morantz-Sanchez
John Norris
Guenter B. Risse
Charles E. Rosenberg
Barbara G. Rosenkrantz
Todd L. Savitt
Wesley D. Smith
Daniel P. Todes

Expert Witness for Defense in Litigation

Tobacco Industry Expert Witness for Defense in Litigation

Published by The Johns Hopkins University Press

Cover: Physic, hand-colored etching by Henry Heath (English, active c. 1824–32). "The cluttered counter in Heath's pharmacy appears in sharp contrast to the many handsome drug jars, show bottles, and rows of attractively labeled drawers. There is also a contrast between the concerned faces of the pharmacist and his client and in the look of extreme boredom shown by the apprentice, contemplating his difficult and lengthy task of manipulating an oversize mortar and pestle. . . ." From *The Picture of Health: Images of Medicine and Pharmacy*, commentary by William H. Helfand (Philadelphia: Philadelphia Museum of Art, 1991), p. 73. Poster reprinted with permission of the Philadelphia Museum of Art: The William H. Helfand Collection.

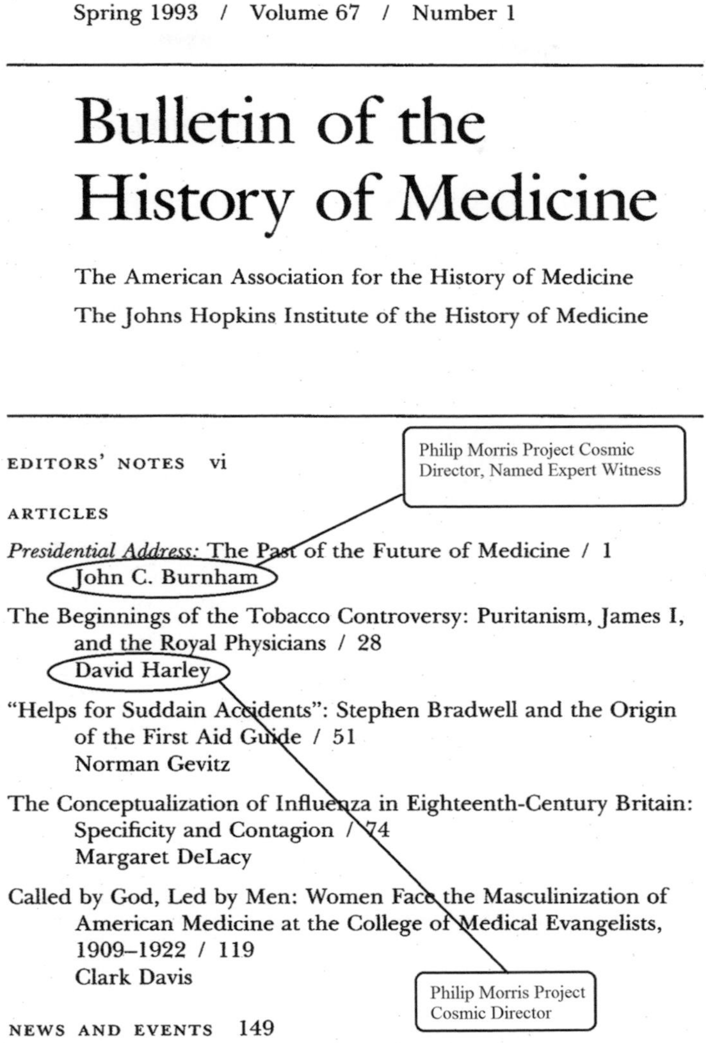

Spring 1993 / Volume 67 / Number 1

Bulletin of the History of Medicine

The American Association for the History of Medicine
The Johns Hopkins Institute of the History of Medicine

EDITORS' NOTES vi

Philip Morris Project Cosmic Director, Named Expert Witness

ARTICLES

Presidential Address: The Past of the Future of Medicine / 1
John C. Burnham

The Beginnings of the Tobacco Controversy: Puritanism, James I, and the Royal Physicians / 28
David Harley

"Helps for Suddain Accidents": Stephen Bradwell and the Origin of the First Aid Guide / 51
Norman Gevitz

The Conceptualization of Influenza in Eighteenth-Century Britain: Specificity and Contagion / 74
Margaret DeLacy

Called by God, Led by Men: Women Face the Masculinization of American Medicine at the College of Medical Evangelists, 1909–1922 / 119
Clark Davis

Philip Morris Project Cosmic Director

NEWS AND EVENTS 149

FIGURE 33. *Bulletin of the History of Medicine,* masthead and table of contents from the Spring 1993 issue, with callouts for scholars working for the tobacco industry. Thousands of scholars have worked for the industry, though such collaborations are often not publicly disclosed. Gerald Grob was offered tobacco money but he refused; they wanted to pay him even while he slept.

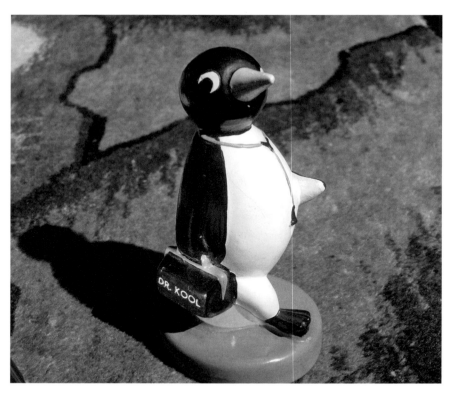

FIGURE 34. Dr. Kool. Paperweights in the form of Brown & Williamson's penguin mascot were sent to physicians throughout the United States as part of an effort to promote this popular menthol brand. Note the doctor's bag and stethoscope. Menthols were introduced in the 1930s in Kool cigarettes but were not very popular until the "cancer scare" of the mid-1950s, when sales of menthol brands skyrocketed. Smokers were given the impression of a cooling sanitary freshness, and regarded menthols as a "healthier smoke." By the 1960s menthols were being heavily marketed to African Americans.

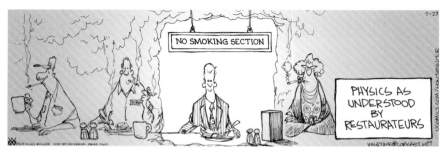

FIGURE 35. Restaurants for many years allowed separate sections for smokers, a practice likened by critics to having "a peeing section in a swimming pool." Municipalities are now banning smoking in conjoined housing and in outdoor spaces where people congregate, since smoke can travel far from its point of origin—in the form of microplumes, for example. Cartoon by David Wiley Miller, 2005. Reprinted with permission.

FRAUD ON TOP OF FRAUD ON TOP OF FRAUD

Brown & Williamson's ultra-low-tar Barclay, launched with great fanfare in 1980, was unusual for several reasons. It was the most expensive launch in cigarette history, with $150 million allocated for advertising and promotion. It was also one of the first cigarettes to make successful use of a toll-free 800 number, which customers could call to redeem coupons for a free carton. And it was the most radically ventilated cigarette, using a design quite different from brands such as True or Carlton. Instead of tiny ventilation slits, the new cigarette had four evenly spaced hollow tubes running lengthwise along the mouthpiece, allowing air to rush in from a ring of holes punched around the filter, like miniature jet intakes. "Channel," "bypass," or "backflow filter" ventilation it was sometimes called.

Other manufacturers were infuriated by Barclay's claim to be delivering only one milligram of tar—which was (rightly) recognized as a deceptive underestimate, a fraud on top of a fraud on top of a fraud we might say. (*Filters* were already fraudulent, *ventilation* added another layer of deception, and Barclay's *bypass filter* was fraudulent even from the point of view of the companies making ventilated cigarettes.) In June of 1981 R. J. Reynolds took the unusual step of appealing to the Federal Trade Commission for a ruling on claims being made for Barclay, explaining how the cigarette had been designed to conceal its actual deliveries. Reynolds attorneys noted that while advertised as yielding only one milligram of tar, the Barclay was really more like a 3- to 7-milligram device, with a comparable exaggeration for its nicotine delivery. The deception was greater even for Kool Ultra 84s: in a series of experiments with its competitor's cigarettes, Reynolds found that this nominally one-milligram cigarette was in fact an 11-milligram device when smoked (on a machine) with all four of its air channels blocked.[34]

Reynolds's complaint was a high-risk proposition, given that virtually *all* low-tar cigarettes by this time were relying on ventilation to achieve their good marks from the FTC's smoking robots—including the "hi-fi" brands marketed by Reynolds itself. Reynolds in the fourth quarter of 1980, for example, had nearly doubled the ventilation of its popular Salem Lights, from 15 to 29 percent (29 percent ventilation means that 29 parts of fresh air are mixed with every 71 parts of smoke). Then again in 1982, the same company increased the ventilation of another of its popular brands from 25 to 41 percent while reducing the weight of the cigarette slightly. A "Strategic Analysis" prepared for the company in 1982 confided that "RJR in the past has tended to lower tar level mainly through air-dilution."[35] Brown & Williamson with Barclay may have waded in too deep, but it's not like the other manufacturers were entirely dry.

The tobacco companies also knew that cigarettes delivered highly variable quantities of smoke, depending on how intensively people smoked them. An unfiltered fifties-style Camel puffed on lightly would deliver far less tar and nicotine than the world's lightest ultralight, smoked to the bitter end in the manner of a seasoned marijuana connoisseur. Some companies even toyed with the idea of making cigarettes with adjustable delivery rates, allowing smokers to choose their own personal level of "satisfaction." Philip Morris and Reynolds in the early 1980s both tried marketing "dial a filter" cigarettes, outfitted with devices that allowed a smoker to close or to open up ventilation channels to adjust their own smoke deliveries—from, say, 3 to 10 milligrams of tar or vice versa.[36] Dial-a-tar gimmicks lasted only a couple of years but weren't really even necessary. They weren't necessary because smokers were already able to extract however much nicotine (and therefore tar) they required simply by adjusting their smoking behavior through the unconscious process known as *compensation.*

COMPENSATION

I've mentioned Lorillard's observation from 1951 that smokers of tightly packed filters tend to pull harder on their cigarettes, to compensate for the reduced smoke flow rate. Also BAT's admission from later in that decade that smokers of ventilated cigarettes would tend to smoke more cigarettes, or to smoke them more intensively, to obtain their accustomed dose of nicotine. German manufacturers had made similar admissions even earlier. In 1940, for example, Peter Schesslitz in Germany's leading tobacco trade newspaper commented on the call for low-nicotine products: "What is the practical consequence of reducing nicotine? If in fact less nicotine is taken in, people will just smoke another cigar or cigarette. For every smoker requires a certain dose of nicotine to be satisfied." Schesslitz's point was that it didn't make sense to reduce the nicotine in cigarettes, since people would just end up smoking more. And so instead he suggested that manufacturers should try to take out whatever in *the tar* might be causing health problems. Nicotine was "the most important constituent" *(wirksamste Prinzip)* of tobacco, which is why nicotine-free tobacco "will never succeed" as a mass consumer good. Nicotine was not the *only* reason people smoke; they also smoke because they like the taste, the smell, and the look. But the comfort, the stimulation they get from smoking—"that comes from nicotine alone."[37]

Some tobacco manufacturers were clearly aware of compensation in the 1940s and 1950s, but the phenomenon is not intensively studied until the 1960s and 1970s, with the push to develop ever lower tar and nicotine yields. Ventilation becomes a crucial element in cigarette design during this period, and cigarette makers start worrying about—and researching—how low nicotine deliveries could be pushed while still keeping smokers hooked. And the companies start trying to better understand the psychology and psychopharmacology of smoking. They also come to appreciate that cigarettes could be designed to be *elastic,* allowing smokers to obtain virtually any level of "satisfaction" simply by smoking their cigarettes more intensively.[38]

Philip Morris had one of the most ambitious efforts of this sort. Helmut Wakeham in the early 1960s had stressed the importance of understanding the psychology of smoking and launched a substantial effort to explore how and why people take up and continue the habit. Smoking behavior was the main focus, but the program encompassed things like why smoking increased one's heart rate, the impact of nicotine on brain waves, and whether smoking helped to reduce stress or aggression—and how best to understand compensation. From the outset the assumption seems to have been that compensation was real: Wakeham by 1969, for example, could report that people who changed to weaker cigarettes "smoked more of each one and/or more cigarets," just as people who changed to stronger cigarettes "smoked less of each one." William Dunn, the company's top psychologist (and Principal Scientist), about this same time commented on evidence accumulated by Philip Morris that since "the smoker adapts his puff, it is reasonable to anticipate that he adapts to maintain a fairly constant daily dosage."[39]

Compensation remained a focus of Philip Morris's Behavioral Research Program into the early 1980s. A crucial precondition for work in this area was the realization—by the 1960s—that most "confirmed" smokers (i.e., most smokers) are *addicted* and smoke to obtain the alkaloid nicotine.[40] Hundreds of testimonials to this effect can be found in the industry's archives. Nicotine was said to be the "primary reason" people smoke, the sine qua non of smoking, and "the substance people desire in their use of tobacco"; nicotine delivery was supposed to be the "dominant specification" of cigarette design, and so forth.[41] Here is some of the (private) language used to define *nicotine* during this period:

"the primary motivation for smoking"	Philip Morris, 1969
"a powerful pharmacological agent"	Philip Morris, 1969
"a potent drug with a variety of physiological effects"	Reynolds, 1972
"a habit-forming alkaloid"	Reynolds, 1972
"the dominant desire"	Reynolds, 1972
"the *sine qua non* of smoking"	Reynolds, 1972
"the goodies"	Philip Morris, 1975
"very basic to the cigarette industry's existence"	Reynolds, 1976
"the psychopharmacologic agent in tobacco"	Reynolds, 1976
"a critical mainstay of tobacco consumption"	Philip Morris, 1977
"the all important pharmacological effect"	Lorillard, 1978
"the most important component of cigarette smoke"	Philip Morris, 1980
"the thing we sell most"	Philip Morris, 1980
"the addicting agent in cigarettes"	Brown & Williamson, 1983
"a product design parameter"	Reynolds, 1990

Corresponding definitions were given for cigarettes, and for smokers. Cigarettes were "the vehicle of smoke" and the act of puffing "an injection of nicotine." Sir Charles Ellis at BAT in 1961 characterized smokers as "nicotine addicts," while others in the industry talked about smokers as "nicotine seekers" who smoked "to maintain a constant level of nicotine in the body." William L. Dunn at Philip Morris asked his colleagues to think of the cigarette pack as "a storage container for a day's supply of nicotine" and the cigarette as "a dispenser for a dose unit of nicotine."[42]

CLAUDE TEAGUE'S CONFESSION— AND THE WHITEWASH OF THE NICOTINE KID

This last-mentioned request, by the head of Philip Morris's Behavioral Research Program, deserves some comment. Dunn—aka "the Nicotine Kid"—was the company's chief psychologist and organizer of a January 1972 conference on the island nation of St. Martin devoted to explaining "why people smoke." Code-named Project Carib, and sometimes referred to as the "Caribbean Caper," the conference brought together twenty-five experts in psychology, sociology, anthropology, and psychopharmacology, many of whom were old industry cronies, to reflect on what Dunn in his opening remarks called "the charm" of tobacco use. The conference itself was not a secret—the proceedings were published[43]—but the published record tells quite a different story from what Dunn et al. were saying about nicotine in private.

In private Dunn talked about cigarette smoke as "a drug" ("It is, of course"), confessing this to his superior, Helmut Wakeham, and adding that this should not go "beyond these walls" given its "dangerous F.D.A. implications." Dunn hoped to be able to predict "whether a trier will become a smoker" and compared smoking to "an injection of nicotine." The difficulty was that a cigarette that does not deliver nicotine "cannot lead to habituation, and would therefore almost certainly fail." Wakeham himself had postulated a two-stage sequence for "Why One Smokes," with novices starting for "psychosocial" reasons whereas "confirmed smokers" continue as "the pharmacological effect takes over to sustain the habit." Wakeham identified "the primary motivation for smoking" as being "to obtain the pharmacological effect of nicotine"; that was indeed his "first premise."[44] Dunn also approved the following description of how hard it was to quit, based on his company's study of the 1969 attempt by the entire town of Greenfield, Iowa, to quit smoking "cold turkey," coincident with the local filming of a movie with that title (starring Dick Van Dyke):

> Even after eight months quitters were apt to report having neurotic symptoms, such as feeling depressed, being restless and tense, being ill-tempered, having a loss of energy, being apt to doze off. . . . This is not the happy picture painted by the Cancer Society's anti-smoking commercial which shows an exuberant couple leaping in the air and kicking their heels with joy because they've kicked the habit. A more appropriate commercial would show a restless, nervous, constipated husband bickering vi-

ciously with his bitchy wife, who is nagging him about his slothful behavior and growing waistline.[45]

Dunn's published conference volume paints quite a different picture. The book
makes only a couple of passing references to nicotine addiction, and gives a white-
washed, cigarette-friendly slant to "why people smoke." Hans Selye from the University of Montreal talked about smoking as a "defensive mechanism" against stress;
smoking was a "diversional activity" that people "naturally turn to" to mitigate the
stimuli of modern life. Hans Eysenck emphasized personality traits: smokers were
"thrill" and "sensation seekers" who smoked more, just as they were "more active
sexually," enjoying sex "in more different positions," with "more prolonged love play."
Norman Heimstra from the University of South Dakota postulated "a beneficial role"
for smoking in the realm of mental health, and Albert Damon from Harvard reported on how Bushmen from the Kalahari Desert saw smoking as increasing "social rapport and kindness toward others." Richard Hickey and Evelyn Harner from
the University of Pennsylvania admitted that smokers smoke to obtain nicotine but
also claimed that the alkaloid worked to alleviate hunger and sharpen mental faculties. Smokers were better drivers and better able to solve mathematical problems.
Hickey and Harner hypothesized that smoking "may be of benefit to some people
in the alleviation of hypoglycemia" and challenged the reigning medical orthodoxy
that smoking could be blamed for women having smaller babies. Much of this is
wrapped in the guise of complex charts and sciencey-sounding language.[46] There
is no mention of the crucial fact of compensation, and no talk of how low-delivery
cigarettes were not likely to be lessening risks. The whitewash is perhaps not surprising, given that the Council for Tobacco Research financed the junket and several contributors were either CTR Special Projects operatives (Hickey, Eysenck, and
Selye, for example) or industry employees (Dunn himself but also A. K. Armitage
from Britain's Tobacco Research Council in Harrogate).

Privately, however, Dunn was admitting that people smoke principally to obtain
nicotine, that most smokers are addicted, and that smokers switching to "light" or
"low-tar" cigarettes will smoke them more intensively to obtain their requisite nicotine fix. In March of 1973 Dunn reported on a Philip Morris study comparing smoking behavior in 1972 to that in 1968, observing that smokers who had shifted to
lower-delivery cigarettes were now smoking "more cigarettes as well as more of the
rod from each cigarette," confirming previous studies suggesting the operation of
a "tar and/or nicotine quota mechanism." Smokers had adjusted their behavior "to
compensate for the decreases in tar and nicotine delivery of their cigarettes."[47] And
smoking was clearly not just a habit. In a 1974 presentation to Philip Morris president Clifford Goldsmith, Dunn commented:

> I'm sure you are aware of our belief people smoke for rewards they get from smoke at
> the pharmacological level. . . . It's simply not an adequate explanation to say that smok-

ing is a habit, or that it is social behavior. . . . If this is true, then we would expect the smoker to seek to take in that amount of smoke that does the job best for him. He is going to regulate his intake to suit his need. . . . We are hypothesizing that the smoker regulates his smoke intake. To suit his dosage needs he'll take in more if the smoke is low in tar, less if the smoke is high in tar. . . . It may be that the Marlboro smoker to-day gets as much from his cigarette as the Philip Morris non-filter smoker got 20 years ago.[48]

The other companies were working along these same lines and coming to similar conclusions. Claude E. Teague in 1972 in an internal Reynolds memo confided:

> In theory, and probably in fact, a given smoker on a given day has a rather fixed per hour and per day requirement for nicotine. Given a cigarette that delivers less nicotine than he desires, the smoker will subconsciously adjust his puff volume and frequency, and smoking frequency, so as to obtain and maintain his per hour and per day requirement for nicotine. . . . Thus, despite the philosophy of our critics, there can be no virtue or logic in reducing per cigarette nicotine level below that desired by the smoker. Additionally, if this be true, and if all leading cigarette brands deliver about the same amount of "tar" per unit of nicotine—that is, all have about the same T/N Ratio—then regardless of which cigarette the smoker choses [sic], in obtaining his daily nicotine requirement he will receive about the same daily amount of "tar." If, as claimed by some anti-tobacco critics, the alleged health hazard of smoking is directly related to the amount of "tar" to which the smoker is exposed per day, and the smoker bases his consumption on nicotine, then a present "low tar, low nicotine" cigarette offers zero advantage [!] to the smoker over a "regular" filter cigarette, but simply costs him more money and exposes him to substantially increased amounts of allegedly harmful gas phase components in obtaining his desired daily amount of nicotine.[49]

In a nutshell: the tar and nicotine values advertised by cigarette manufacturers (from FTC ratings) didn't mean very much. "Low tars" were a fraud, just as "lights" would be in the decades following their introduction in the early 1970s.

THE SPECTER OF WEANING

These were serious matters, especially in the context of falling (machine-measured) tar and nicotine yields. No one really knew how low nicotine could go before smokers would start quitting; compensation obviously had physical limits, but no one knew what these were. That, again, is one reason nicotine pharmacology was given such attention: the fear was that nicotine levels might be pushed below some critical threshold, loosening the grip of addiction. Much of this was discussed in terms of "weaning"—or worse. BAT researchers as early as 1959 worried that lowering the nicotine content of cigarettes past a certain point "might end in destroying the nicotine habit in a large number of consumers and prevent it ever being acquired by new smokers." Claude Teague a decade later talked about the danger of "weaning" as the "long term liquidation of the cigarette industry."[50] This was a worry throughout the 1960s and 1970s—and not just in the English-speaking world.

In 1968, for example, British cigarette manufacturers reported on concerns expressed by the Japanese tobacco monopoly that "if nicotine level goes below 0.7 and tar below 10 mg per cigarette, the consumers would not accept it." This is a crucial aspect of the history of cigarettes, this worry within the industry that if nicotine levels were to fall below some critical threshold people might start to quit. Expressions of concern along these lines can often be found in the industry's archives, along with discussions of how low nicotine levels could go while still keeping smokers hooked. Philip Morris in 1965, for example, in a detailed plan for future cigarette designs, recommended that while *tar* deliveries should be kept below 10 milligrams, *nicotine* deliveries should be kept at 0.7 milligram or above. Teague at Reynolds calculated a "minimum satisfying amount of nicotine" at 1.3 milligrams per cigarette, with a "minimum practical" tar-to-nicotine ratio of about ten.[51] Similar calculations were performed at the other companies. (N.B. These are calculations of nicotine *deliveries,* not nicotine *in the actual rod.* Nicotine in the actual rod was rarely allowed to drop below about 10 milligrams per cigarette, and no cigarette was ever commercially successful with much less than this amount. See the box on page 380.)

Evidence of a deliberate strategy of this sort—keeping nicotine levels above some minimal level while reducing tars—can be found in many industry documents. Philip Rogers and Geoffrey Todd of Britain's Tobacco Research Council visited the United States in 1964, for example, where they learned that Hanmer at American Tobacco had been told that "it was important to keep up the nicotine content of the smoke, while reducing anything that ought to be reduced." Similar views prevailed in England. Brown & Williamson's head of research toured Imperial Tobacco's facilities at Bristol and TRC research labs at Harrogate in 1965, reporting back that "their approach seems to be to find ways of obtaining maximum nicotine for minimum tar." Lots of different methods were being tried for this purpose, including "addition of nicotine containing powders" to tobacco and "nicotine fortification of cigarette paper."[52]

Of course the industry's public posture was rather different. The companies have always insisted that tar and nicotine levels are somehow dictated by the biology of the tobacco plant, when the truth is that these "travel together" only because manufacturers choose this to be the case. Tar-to-nicotine ratios are the result of intentional design and in no sense facts of nature. The common ten-to-one ratio in the machine-measured deliveries of many cigarettes is a result of two rather different decisions: (1) nicotine deliveries are kept as high as they are because to go much below this risks "weaning" smokers from their habit; and (2) tar levels are kept as high as they are because "flavors" are needed to mask the unpleasant taste of nicotine. Deviations from such designs are not difficult to produce, however. Nicotine-free cigarettes were already being manufactured in the nineteenth century, and the

HOW MUCH NICOTINE SHOULD BE ALLOWED IN CIGARETTES?

The new FDA is barred from eliminating nicotine from cigarettes entirely, but nothing prevents it from requiring a drastic reduction in nicotine to sub-addictive, sub-compensable levels. Mandating such reductions will cause people to smoke far fewer cigarettes and will result in dramatically reduced rates of death and disease. How low, though, should nicotine levels be pushed to prevent addiction?

There has never been a commercially successful cigarette with less than about one percent nicotine in the rod. Cigarettes weigh about a gram, so one percent would be about 10 milligrams (mg) in the actual tobacco. Sano cigarettes in 1961 had only about 8 mg, lowest among the top forty brands in the United States, and its failure is sometimes traced to its low nicotine numbers. Drop this to about one milligram in the rod, and we would probably have a cigarette that could not create or sustain addiction. Smoking rates would plummet. One could also, though, build in a larger margin of safety.

Neal Benowitz and Jack Henningfield in a 1994 article in the *New England Journal of Medicine* made a case for allowing no more than 0.4 to 0.5 mg of nicotine per cigarette (in the rod), based on their reckoning that people who smoke only five cigarettes per day are usually not addicted. People who smoke only five cigarettes a day typically have a daily nicotine intake of about 5 mg, which these authors claim would be a threshold below which one could not "readily establish and sustain addiction." Cigarettes today contain an average of about 10 mg of nicotine and deliver about 1 mg to the smoker—meaning a "bioavailability" of around 10 percent. Cigarettes can be smoked more or less intensively, however, and this bioavailability can vary from 3 percent to as high as 40 percent. A (very) light or cautious smoker might draw out only 3 percent of the nicotine in a cigarette, but a (very) determined smoker might extract as much as 40 percent.

Assuming this maximum of 40 percent, how low would the nicotine content of a cigarette have to be to guarantee that a smoker of, say, thirty cigarettes per day would receive no more than 5 mg daily of nicotine? Benowitz and Henningfield point out that if each cigarette contained only 0.4 mg of nicotine, then smokers of thirty cigarettes per day could get only $30 \times 0.4 \times 0.4 = 5$ mg per day. It would therefore be very hard for anyone to become addicted by smoking cigarettes containing only 0.4 mg of nicotine. Cigarettes of this sort could still cause disease, but they would not be cigarettes to which one could become addicted. The tobacco industry has the means to produce such cigarettes: supercritical extraction technologies, for example, allow the removal of up to 97 percent of the nicotine from a tobacco blend.

Food and drug authorities should move quickly to reduce the levels of nicotine allowable in cigarettes. Short of barring cigarettes altogether, it would be hard to name a policy with more dramatic consequences for public health. Millions of lives would be saved, as smokers would be weaned from their addiction. Which is, after all, what most smokers want.

industry has experimented with devices delivering nicotine only, meaning virtually zero tar (recently fashionable "electronic cigarettes" come close to this, though they also typically deliver flavorants and humectants such as propylene or diethylene glycol). The industry landed on the 10:1 tar/nicotine ratio because this was what sold—and was needed to preserve addiction. Nicotine-free cigarettes have never been commercially successful, because they don't create and sustain addiction. And nicotine-only designs tend to be awkward and inconvenient—and usually taste rather foul. And are poor alternatives to quitting.

ENGINEERING ELASTICITY

The principal response to the threat of weaning, however, has been to design cigarettes in such a way that smokers could obtain however much nicotine they wanted, even from cigarettes rated low in tar and nicotine. (Here again the distinction between nicotine *content* and nicotine *delivery* is crucial, since "low delivery" cigarettes usually *contain the same amount of nicotine* as regulars—typically about 10 milligrams in the actual rod—even though they *deliver less* when measured on smoking robots.) Several different methods have been developed to enable this "elasticity," but the most important involve placing ventilation slits close to the mouth where they can easily—and unconsciously—be covered by the smoker's lips or fingers. The phenomenon is known as "occlusion," "hole-blocking," "obturation," or "lip drape" and eventually becomes a key aspect of cigarette design.[53]

When did the industry realize that smokers could use such methods to defeat ventilation? The companies must have known from the beginning that ventilation could be gamed, but the first known studies attempting to quantify this effect date from the mid-1960s. Philip Morris's Project 1600 was an important locus for such inquiries, and the project's 1966 Annual Report makes it clear that smokers of low-delivery cigarettes ("health filter smokers") were adjusting their puff volume—taking larger puffs—to obtain a constant smoke intake. Additional measurements were done the following year, as part of an effort to see whether smokers might be covering up the ventilation holes. William Dunn at Philip Morris supervised a number of such studies, exploring the extent to which "lipping behavior" might be compromising ventilation. Dunn and his colleagues had found that "partial occlusion of air holes" was "likely among many smokers when the holes are placed in an 8 to 10mm band, measuring from the outer end of the tipping." They also commented on how ventilation holes were most commonly being placed at about 8 to 10 millimeters from the mouth end of the cigarette—precisely where smokers could easily cover them up. The take-home message was clear: "We submit these results as further evidence that smokers adjust puff intake in order to maintain constant smoke intake."[54]

Over the next several years Philip Morris produced dozens of internal reports on vent hole "occlusion." William Dunn at Philip Morris was a leader here; in an operation given the code name Project Pandora he and his technical staff designed elaborate setups to photograph smokers as they covered the holes. In one instance the holes were so small that the cameramen had trouble getting clear shots, so they ended up having to mark the holes with ink to see when they were being covered. The researchers didn't want the subjects to know what was being measured, so a "cover story" was invented about the photographers needing something to focus on.[55] Studies of this sort showed that people smoking cigarettes with highly ventilated tips end up unconsciously covering the holes with their lips or fingers, allowing them to extract more nicotine.

The industry regarded this as part of the more general phenomenon of *compensation,* also referred to as "adaptation," "titration behavior," or "self-dosing." And the phenomenon was clearly regarded not as a negative but rather as an aspect of smoking behavior that could be exploited. Cigarettes were in fact *designed* to be "elastic," meaning they could be smoked with different levels of intensity. Elasticity made it possible for smokers to obtain high levels of nicotine even from cigarettes certified as low-yield by FTC standards.[56] So cigarettes designed to yield, say, half a milligram of nicotine when tested on a machine would deliver twice that when smoked by an actual human. BAT made this explicit in a 1977 document discussing "minimum effective nicotine levels": "The minimum effective nicotine level will depend very much on the idiosyncrasies of individual smokers, but we should aim at a cigarette delivering at least 0.5 mg of [machine-measured] nicotine. With appropriate design, including moderately low draw resistance, smokers will be able to obtain up to 1 mg nicotine from such a cigarette."[57] Compensation, in other words, allowed cigarette makers to design cigarettes that would deliver significantly higher yields to people than would be recorded on automatic smoking machines.

That was clearly the virtue of Barclay's radical bypass filter, whose inventor, Robert R. Johnson, actually expressed his pleasure at having found a way to deliver more tar and nicotine than the FTC's machines would record. In a series of memos sent to the company's chief of research and other higher-ups in the company, Johnson waxed enthusiastic about having found "a cigarette that shows low deliveries on machine smoking and much higher deliveries when people smoke it." For Johnson et al. this was clearly not a flaw but a virtue—and an opportunity (hence the patent)—with the key innovation being the "loss of filter ventilation by collapse of tipping into the grooves during hard puffing."[58] The filters were designed to succeed by failing—and by fooling their users.

Cigarette manufacturers collected "delivery data" throughout the 1970s and 1980s, refining their understanding of compensation and how to deal with it. Machines were developed to more accurately simulate human smoking and to compare the smoke inhaled by humans with smoke inhaled by the (less honest) machines used to establish tar and nicotine numbers. In 1975, for example, Barbro Goodman, the scientist in charge of Philip Morris's human smoke simulator program, reported on a study comparing Marlboro Lights and Marlboro regulars: "Marlboro Lights cigarettes were not smoked like regular Marlboros. There were differences in the size and frequency of the puffs, with larger volumes taken on Marlboro Lights by both regular Marlboro smokers and Marlboro Lights smokers." Goodman found that Marlboro Lights "delivered more TPM [total particulate matter] to the smoker" than standardized machines would indicate, suggesting that smokers were taking larger puffs, puffing harder, or performing some other compensatory behavior. Her report concluded that smokers of Marlboro Lights took larger puffs than when smoking Marlboro (regular) 85s: "The larger puffs, in turn, increased the delivery of Marlboro Lights proportionally. In effect, the M 85 smokers in this study did not achieve any reduction in smoke intake by smoking a cigarette (Marlboro Lights) normally considered low in delivery."[59] Goodman's report circulated widely within the company, with copies going not just to her immediate superior, Leo F. Meyer, but also to at least eight others in the company, including Frank E. Resnick, director of the Philip Morris Research Center and later chairman and CEO of Philip Morris USA. This was sophisticated science, using precise measurements, multivariate statistical analysis, and careful controls. The data and graphs alone took up more than ten pages.

Most manufacturers by this time were conducting similar studies. BAT in its Southampton laboratories had a specially designed smoking machine ("puff duplicator") that could be programmed to reproduce the smoking pattern of any given human, complete with variations on puffing size, duration, timing, resistance to draw, and so forth, collecting and measuring the effluent tar, nicotine, and gas.[60] Philip Morris had a sophisticated "Human Smoker Simulator," allowing it to mimic and model any desired human smoking behavior. Imperial Tobacco's machine, interestingly, was known as a "Slave Smoker," a nice complement to their private observation that people who try to quit soon learn they have become "slaves to their cigarettes."[61]

HANGING TOGETHER

Now back to the Barclay squabble. The Federal Trade Commission was convinced by Reynolds's charge of "design defects" in BAT's cigarette and ruled in June 1982 that Barclay's "unique filter design" precluded an accurate measure of tar and nicotine deliveries.[62] The matter didn't rest here, however, as the fraternal infighting was soon dragged overseas. On September 2, 1983, Philip Morris paid for ads to be placed in two leading Dutch newspapers, attacking Barclay's claims (as BAT's awkward translation reveals): "People think that there exists no health danger anymore now, but research in America has proved that smokers, who slightly compress the Barclay filter between their lips, will take in six times as much nicotine and tar as stated on the packing." BAT was infuriated, calling this "the first occasion of which we are aware" in which a competitor had "raised the health issue to gain a competitive advantage." BAT lawyers also accused Philip Morris of breaking the law—by using "comparative" and "misleading" advertising. BAT Chairman Patrick Sheehy wrote to Philip Morris, accusing the Americans of making a "mockery of industry co-operation on smoking and health issues" and inaugurating a "free-for-all" in which the industry as a whole would suffer.[63]

Philip Morris realized it had made a mistake and reassured BAT of its desire for the industry to "hang together," especially when BAT withdrew from INFOTAB, the industry's global information clearinghouse (Philip Morris's local Dutch operations were blamed for the embarrassing ads). BAT for its part knew the situation was "legally and morally dangerous for the industry"; they didn't want to harm IN-FOTAB or the collaborative project more generally, they just wanted to be sure that "all members stick to the rules for the future"—meaning no competition over health claims and no maligning of other companies' products.[64]

Ill will between the companies dragged on for years, however, as BAT kept advertising its Barclay as a one-milligram (tar) cigarette. Following threats of litigation in a number of countries, BAT's American affiliate, Brown & Williamson, finally met with Philip Morris and Imperial Tobacco to try to heal the rift. On January 19–20, 1989, in a hotel room at London's Gatwick airport, Philip Morris expressed itself as still "very unenthusiastic" about the claims being made for Barclay as "99 percent tar free" but also cautioned BAT against publicizing how actual human deliveries could deviate from the numbers indicated on cigarette ads and packs. Philip Morris reminded Brown & Williamson that such comparisons were "*extremely dangerous* for the entire industry," threatening as they did to upset the whole low-tar applecart. BAT finally promised to withdraw its one-milligram claim and Philip Morris withdrew its complaints, to preserve the integrity of the conspiracy not to air any dirty "smoking and health" laundry in public.[65]

The public health community by this time, however, was beginning to recognize the fraudulent nature of low-yield cigarettes. Crucial here was a series of papers from 1980 by Lynn T. Kozlowski, a psychologist at the University of Toronto, who showed that smokers of low-tar cigarettes "sometimes defeat the purpose of the smoke-dilution holes by occluding them with fingers, lips, or tape." Kozlowski and his colleagues examined staining patterns on cigarette butts and found that as many as two-thirds of all low-tar smokers were routinely blocking the slits punched into ventilated filters. Lipstick marks were found covering the holes, and some smokers were observed holding the cigarette with their teeth, allowing their lips to "occlude" the holes. Some even admitted to covering the holes with tape or holding the cigarette with both hands. The team also found signs of hole blocking on spent filters (apart from the lipstick marks): the ends of obstructed filters were typically a homogeneous brown, whereas unblocked filters had a dark spot in the middle surrounded by a less darkened ring (since clean ventilated air rushes in from the edges). Measurements of cigarettes with blocked and unblocked vents showed that smokers could more than double the amount of tar and nicotine they were inhaling—and quadruple their carbon monoxide. Kozlowski et al. followed shortly thereafter with other articles in *Science* and elsewhere, concluding that tar and nicotine deliveries had changed little over time, despite the much-ballyhooed introduction of "light" and "low-tar" cigarettes.[66]

Scientists also started finding that the amount of tar and nicotine actually absorbed by smokers was pretty much the same, regardless of whether one smoked high- or low-tar cigarettes. In 1983 UCSF pharmacologist Neal Benowitz published an article in the *New England Journal of Medicine* on his discovery that smokers were getting just as much nicotine in their bodies, regardless of whether they smoked low- or high-yield cigarettes. Benowitz had been measuring a nicotine metabolite known as *cotinine* in the blood of smokers and noticed that when he tried to correlate cotinine levels with official tar and nicotine values listed for the brands actually smoked there was no distinguishable pattern—meaning no low-tar benefit. Smokers of "high-yield" cigarettes had low levels of cotinine in their blood, and vice versa. This shocking conclusion was announced in the title of his article, as was coming to be the fashion in science: "Smokers of Low-Yield Cigarettes Do Not Consume Less Nicotine." An editorial in the same issue asked, "Are 'low-yield' cigarettes really safer?" The answer was a resounding "No." Scholars henceforth would have to acknowledge what the industry had known for years: people smoking "light" or "low-tar" cigarettes were getting as much tar and nicotine as smokers of regular cigarettes.[67]

This was an astonishing conclusion and spelled the beginning of the end for (public) hopes that low-tar cigarettes would prove less deadly. A generation of public health bureaucrats had credited the industry with making "safer" cigarettes, and some had even worked with the companies to help design such products.[68]

What Kozlowski and Benowitz did not know, though, and could not have known, was that they were basically reinventing wheels fashioned years earlier by the industry. Dunn at Philip Morris, for example, had been exploring compensation since the mid-1960s, in a series of elaborate experiments on smoking behavior conducted as part of the company's Project 1600. By the mid-1960s Dunn and colleagues had found strong evidence that "smokers adjust puff intake in order to maintain constant smoke intake."[69] Compensation was so well known inside the industry that it had many different names: I've mentioned "hole-blocking," "obturation," "lipping behavior," and "self-dosing," but there was also talk of "finger-tip dosage control," "self-medication," "accommodation," "nicotine titration," and a "quota mechanism." The companies also made efforts to quantify the phenomenon and to explore how it might be used to guard against the threat of weaning.

One reason this is significant is that (some) health authorities throughout this time had been advising smokers to switch to cigarettes delivering less tar and nicotine. The 1981 Surgeon General's report advised that people "switch to cigarettes yielding less 'tar' and nicotine," provided they didn't change their smoking behavior in other ways. David M. Burns, a distinguished pulmonologist who had also served as one of the scientific editors of the report, later testified that if those preparing the report had known what the industry knew, they never would have made that recommendation. Jonathan Samet, an epidemiologist (and pulmonologist) who worked on other Surgeon General's reports, put the matter as follows:

> The 1981 Report did not fully take into consideration the phenomenon of compensation, and how smokers smoke to get a certain amount of nicotine, and will even adjust their smoking behavior to get the amount of nicotine they seek or are accustomed to . . . we didn't know in 1981 the extent to which smokers would compensate after switching to a "low tar" and low nicotine yield product.[70]

Samet et al. didn't know, because the industry had never disclosed its extensive work in this area.

MORAL REASONING, TOBACCO-STYLE

Should the industry have publicized what it knew about compensation? Oddly enough, this question was posed as early as 1974 by Philip Morris's principal scientist, Raymond Fagan, who came to a predictable conclusion in a discussion of the company's "moral obligation." The memo is addressed to Helmut Wakeham, Philip Morris's vice president for research, and is one of the few instances in which we find industry scientists engaging in moral reasoning: "Some concern has been expressed concerning the moral obligation of Philip Morris (and perhaps the tobacco industry) to reveal to the FTC the fact that some cigarette smokers may be getting more tar than the FTC rating of that cigarette."[71] Wakeham had mentioned such concerns after a recent speech in New York, and the same question was raised when he spoke again in Richmond. Fagan reassured his boss of the rightness of their silence:

> I believe that there need be no such concern, at least from a position of morality. It is obvious that HEW knows that smokers can vary their intake. . . . The FTC tar and nicotine rating is an indicator of the delivery. The assumption upon which the numbers is based is that the smoker's puffing habits will not change. There is no assumption that the number of cigarettes or that the number of puffs will change. Granting that puffing behavior (puff volume, puff duration, puff interval) remain constant then the cigarette with a lower FTC tar will deliver to the smoker less tar than a cigarette with a higher FTC rating. And that is all the FTC and HEW are trying to do with the publicized numbers.[72]

Actually, that is *not* all the Federal Trade Commission and Department of Health, Education, and Welfare were trying to do with those numbers. The FTC was trying to provide a reasonable measure of how much tar and nicotine smokers could expect to inhale, as part of its statutory duty to prevent "deceptive acts or practices." The numbers were supposed to be relevant to the question of danger. Lower-tar cigarettes were widely thought to be safer cigarettes; the companies had implied as much in advertising, and policy recommendations had been constructed on this basis. Senator Robert Kennedy in 1967 had proposed a federal sales tax pegged to tar levels, and similar bills were proposed in the 1970s by Senators Frank Moss (D-Utah) and Ted Kennedy (D-Mass.). The city of New York in 1971 passed a special tax on high-tar cigarettes, acting on the initiative of Mayor John Lindsay. Governments in other parts of the world were also taking steps to mandate maximum allowable cigarette yields, believing these to be of real health benefit. Britain's High Tar Tax went into effect in 1978, and a personage no less than Sir Richard Doll defended such a tax in 1982. Several Middle Eastern states (Saudi Arabia, Egypt, Iraq, Oman, Bahrain, etc.) passed maximum tar and nicotine standards (typically 15 and 1 milligrams, respectively) in the early 1980s, and the European Union in 1990 enacted similar restrictions, requiring maximum tar yields to drop from 15 milligrams in 1992 to 12 milligrams by 1997.[73] Many people in the public health community had been led to believe that "low tar" meant "safer" and would continue along this false path for years to come.

The tobacco industry likes to confuse this point in court, claiming basically that *everyone knew* that the tar and nicotine figures reported to the FTC were only approximations and could not be used to predict actual smoking behavior. That is not the crucial question, however, nor has it ever been. The question was never whether the harmful effects of smoking depend on how or how much you smoke—that has always been obvious—at least since the recognition of tobacco mortality. If smoking is bad for you, then it is obviously worse to smoke more rather than less. Smoke a cigarette farther down on the butt, or hold the smoke longer in your lungs, or inhale it more deeply, and you will get a bigger dose of poisons. Throw the cigarette down as soon as you light it, and you won't be exposed to much of anything. That much is obvious—a banal truism—and beside the point.

The point is rather that cigarette manufacturers knew from early on that tar and nicotine numbers were *systematically* flawed in the direction of *underestimating* yields, due to compensation. Compensation was not taken into account in the FTC's decision to require publication of tar and nicotine levels; those measurements were mandated to provide an index of what smokers could expect from smoking a particular kind of cigarette. Smokers did not know—nor were they ever told—that these numbers were essentially meaningless.

Fagan, though, reports to his research chief at the world's largest tobacco company that they had no "moral obligation" to inform government regulators that their measurements were flawed. And then goes on to suggest that one way to get smokers to lower their tar intake would be to "teach the smokers to smoke in a manner which gives him less tar." There is no evidence the industry ever took such a step, or even took it seriously. Fagan's memo concludes (bizarrely) by noting that in the history of human health, diseases have more often been conquered by changing the *environment* (he mentions chlorination of water and pasteurization of milk) than by changing *behavior*. The obvious conclusion would be to have cigarette manufacturers stop making cigarettes, but that is not where Fagan takes us. Nor does he ever acknowledge that tobacco was the chief cause of the world's rapidly worsening cancer epidemic and that men like himself were crucial agents in its advance.

AS DANGEROUS AS ANY EVER SMOKED

The cigarettes smoked today are as dangerous as any ever smoked. And as addictive. Total alkaloid levels in virtually all cigarettes remain as high as in the 1950s—kept between one and two percent by weight—since the industry knows this is crucial for maintaining addiction. The billions spent by the industry on research have really just brought us ever more perfect killing kits, dressed in ever more attractive packaging. Smokers who smoke today's filtered, low-tar, or "light" cigarettes are as likely to suffer and die from smoking as earlier generations, a fact at variance with decades of advertised assurances.

That was the shocking conclusion of the National Cancer Institute in its important 2001 publication titled *Risks Associated with Smoking Cigarettes with Low Machine-Measured Yields of Tar and Nicotine*, better known as *Monograph 13*. This carefully researched volume showed that low-yield cigarettes "have not significantly decreased the disease risk" and that, in fact, the shift to such cigarettes "may be partly responsible for the increase in lung cancer for long-term smokers who have switched to the low-tar/low-nicotine brands."[74] Chapters by Kozlowski and Benowitz reviewed the case for compensation and the exploitation of "elasticity"; and a long chapter on epidemiology by David Burns, Jacqueline Major, and Thomas Shanks of UC San Diego, Michael Thun of the American Cancer Society, and Jonathan Samet of Johns Hopkins explained how hopes for a decline in lung cancer from the shift to lower-yield cigarettes had not materialized. The authors cautioned that the reduced particle size of smoke from filtration might even be causing an *increase* in lung cancers in the distant reaches of the lungs, making smoke from low-yield products even more harmful.

NCI publications are not generally given to overstatement, and it is serious business when they charge an industry with deception. The report was immediately endorsed by the American Medical Association, which called for Congress to enact legislation to allow the FDA to regulate tobacco and to protect the lives and health "of all Americans from the specious lies the tobacco industry has spread for decades."[75] *Monograph 13* is significant for what it concludes but also for the kind of sources it used to come to that conclusion. It is the first major U.S. governmental report to use the extensive, formerly secret documents of the tobacco industry to come to an assessment of a health hazard. This is an important breakthrough, this recognition that we can no longer understand disease in the human body without understanding the extent to which some corporate agent, by its decisions or negligence, may have caused that disease. The tobacco industry for decades operated largely in the dark, with unimpeded access to the halls of power and virtual freedom from regulation. That free ride is finally coming to an end, following decades of doubt-mongering and duplicity.

Crack Nicotine

Freebasing to Augment a Cigarette's "Kick"

A cigarette is the perfect type of a perfect pleasure. It is exquisite, and it leaves one unsatisfied. What more can one want?

OSCAR WILDE, *THE PICTURE OF DORIAN GRAY*, 1891

Let us provide the exquisiteness, and hope that they, our consumers, continue to remain unsatisfied. All we would want then is a larger bag to carry the money to the bank.

COLIN C. GREIG, STRUCTURED CREATIVITY GROUP, BRITISH AMERICAN TOBACCO, COMMENTING ON WILDE'S RHAPSODY, 1984

It has always struck me as odd when people are shocked to learn that the tobacco industry has "manipulated" nicotine chemistry. What should we expect? Nicotine manipulation is not even necessarily a bad thing: if you're going to smoke, you'd probably just as soon have your nicotine manipulated as left to chance. Whiskey makers know—and can control—how much alcohol will end up in their product, and drug makers of course calibrate dosages quite precisely. Heroin users die because their doses are unregulated, uncontrolled.

The presumption behind the shock seems to be that tobacco should be as "natural" as possible. And the industry itself has cultivated this image of the cigarette as a folksy, down-home product that is honest, simple, and unadulterated (albeit now "controversial" and "risky"). But tobacco has never been a natural phenomenon, not as used by humans at any rate. Like olives or ayahuasca, tobacco leaves have to be painstakingly cured and processed prior to consumption. For this alone we cannot condemn the cigarette. The real indignity stems from precisely *how* and *why* cigarette makers have manipulated nicotine chemistry—which has been dishonest but also deadly. Cigarettes were designed to *appear* to be safe, when the manufacturers already knew they were not. We've encountered the nested frauds of filtration and ventilation, made possible by a crafty exploitation of compensation. But it's also important to realize that *the chemistry* of tobacco has been manipulated in a deceptive manner, with the goal of keeping smokers hooked. Smokers have been encouraged to switch to brands promising ever lower yields, without being told that the nicotine in those brands has been juiced up chemically to increase its potency. Think of cajoling an alcoholic, "Here, have some vodka, we've taken out some of the alcohol!"—while secretly increasing the potency of those molecules that remain. Nicotine freebasing is comparable, and consequential. This simple chemical trick helped propel Marlboro from obscurity to the world's most popular cigarette—and still today helps keep smokers smoking.

SEX WITHOUT ORGASM

Nicotine, as Claude Teague at Reynolds used to say, is the sine qua non of smoking.[1] People smoke to obtain this simple alkaloid, which stimulates the brain and eventually leaves the hard mark of addiction. Hints of this beguiling twist were recognized prior even to the discovery of the nicotine molecule: Christopher Columbus is said to have observed with regard to his sailors taking up the pipe, "It was not within their power to refrain from indulging in the habit," and King James I in his notorious *Counter-Blaste to Tobacco* worried that "he that taketh tobacco cannot leave it, it doth bewitch." The great French traveler Jean-Baptiste Tavernier wrote from Persia in 1640: "Men and women are so addicted that to take tobacco from them is to take their lives." Mark Twain is famous for his quip that smoking was easy to quit; indeed he had done so many times.

It was not until the twentieth century, however, that the mechanisms by which nicotine railroads the brain came to be deciphered. The British physiologist John Langley was a pioneer in this realm, using nicotine to map the cholinergic peripheral nervous system. In a series of experiments using curare, nicotine, and other psychoactive chemicals, Langley and his collaborators postulated the existence of "receptor" sites in cells that would receive and transmit the chemical instructions involved in all neurotransmission (indeed we still talk today about "nicotinic cholinergic receptors" throughout the body). Lennox M. Johnston of Glasgow, Scotland, in a widely read article in *Lancet* later showed that people injected with nicotine eventually develop a tolerance, and then a dependence, and that people develop cravings when the injections stop. Johnston, much of whose work was "suppressed by smoking medical editors," proposed that tobacco use was "essentially a means of administering nicotine, just as smoking opium is a means of administering morphine."[2]

Cigarette makers would eventually come to realize that *the impact* of nicotine could be manipulated, even while keeping its quantity in any given cigarette fixed. In the 1940s, for example, Lorillard scientists at the company's Middletown, Ohio, branch explored the possibility of adding urea and other alkaline agents to cigarette paper to raise the pH of cigarette smoke. A letter of April 11, 1946, from the company's chief chemist to the head of its Committee on Manufacture noted that a number of different buffers and bases had been added, causing the production of "a volatile base when the cigarette is burned." Sodium bicarbonate, soda ash, caustic soda, and caustic potash all were explored for this purpose, as were compounds such as ammonium phosphate, triethanolamine, and hexamethylene-tetramine. Ammonia was selected as "about the only material that we know of which is easily volatile"; the problem was therefore to find "a compound which contains bound ammonia that will be liberated by heat of combustion."[3]

Here are some of the early glimmers of the "freebasing" revolution that would rock the industry in the 1960s and 1970s, propelling Marlboro to the top of the cigarette charts. There was not yet any point, however—not in the 1940s or 1950s—to boost the potency of nicotine. Tobacco chemists were still looking mainly for ways to make smoke "milder," and acid-base manipulations were done mainly to reduce harshness from corrosive acids or (more often) bases. There was not yet much of a demand for low-nicotine products, and manufacturers felt no urgency to augment nicotine's potency. Tobacco researchers knew that free nicotine could be released by increasing pH, and even knew that free nicotine had a greater physiologic impact.[4] But that was more or less a curiosity, since there was not yet any push to lower yields.

With increasing publicity of the cancer hazard, however, cigarette makers began trying to lower tar and nicotine deliveries and to better understand how nicotine works in the body. Countless schemes were devised to lower nicotine levels—which wasn't terribly hard from a manufacturing point of view. The alkaloid is water-soluble, so a simple soaking will remove most of it from the leaf. (That is one reason hand harvesters sometimes suffer from green tobacco sickness: tobacco leaves wet from the morning dew can transfer nicotine to the skin, causing poisoning or even death for long-term handlers. Contact with sweat on the skin can have a similar effect.) Breeding techniques were also developed to produce low-nicotine plants. Europeans were ahead of the curve in this respect, and by the 1930s Germany's state-financed (pro-)tobacco research laboratory, the Reich Institute for Tobacco Research at Forchheim, had engineered tobacco plants containing very little nicotine: about 0.15 percent as compared with the usual 2 to 3 percent in regular cured leaf. For a one-gram cigarette, this meant 1.5 milligrams of nicotine instead of the usual 20 to 30 milligrams.

Here again—just to remind the reader—we are talking about nicotine *content*, not nicotine *yields* or *deliveries*. The distinction is crucial: content is how much is actually in the cigarette; delivery is how much enters the smoker's body when the cigarette is smoked in some standardized manner, typically on a smoking machine. Deliveries can vary widely, since smokers can smoke a cigarette more or less intensively—which is why regulators when they decide to limit nicotine in cigarettes must focus exclusively on content, not deliveries. Only reducing the actual *content in the rod* below a certain amount will prevent cigarettes from being addictive (see again the box on page 380).

Tobacco manufacturers by the early decades of the twentieth century already knew how to quantify the nicotine in smoke and/or leaf and had developed techniques to raise or lower the concentration to any desired level. Nicotine content of the finished product became part of manufacturing specifications, and was controlled quite precisely. Cigarettes were also starting to become more uniform—from the point of view of physical design—for tax reasons and by virtue of how cigarettes were made and distributed. The widespread use of vending machines required a certain uniformity, for example, as did mechanized production à la Bonsack et al.'s equipment. The standard American "Class A" cigarette by the 1930s was 70 millimeters long and contained just over a gram of tobacco; the nicotine content varied somewhat but was typically kept in the 20- to 30-milligram range. There was no point yet in moving outside this range: higher values would have been too harsh, and significantly lower values would have been considered "low-nicotine" specialty items, or worse.

The American Tobacco Company conducted elaborate tests on nicotine-depleted cigarettes at the end of the 1930s, leading Hiram Hanmer to conclude that "The emasculated cigarette, whether produced by removal of nicotine from tobacco, or the use of nicotine-poor tobacco in blending, gives an insipid smoke which is thin, sharp, and lacking in character." Hans Kuhn of Vienna's tobacco monopoly agreed that a "moderate" level of nicotine was crucial for maintaining a smoker's interest; Kuhn had a piquant way of putting it, comparing cigarettes without nicotine to "a kiss from one's sister." Philip Morris psychologists would later liken nicotine-free tobacco to sex without orgasm.[5]

With the "health scare" of the 1950s, however, many smokers started switching to cigarettes offering lower tar and nicotine. Machine-measured yields began to fall in response, as smokers began to shift to what they imagined to be "safer" cigarettes. Questions started being asked about how low nicotine yields could go before cigarette sales would start to suffer; the fear was that if driven too low, people would simply stop smoking—whence all those worries about "weaning."

This was not a trivial concern. People smoke to satisfy their nicotine cravings, and if they can't satisfy that urge they won't keep on with the habit. Surveys show that most people don't like to smoke and wish they didn't; they smoke only because they feel it is beyond their control to stop. That is why nicotine-free cigarettes have rarely been commercially successful: "confirmed" smokers smoke for the nicotine, and cigarettes without cannot "satisfy." Some people may smoke purely for the ritual or the taste, but that is the exception rather than the rule. Cigarettes without nicotine have never been more than gimmicks and curiosities.

Demand for "low-tar" cigarettes continued to grow throughout the 1950s and 1960s, as increasing numbers of smokers imagined this as a way to reduce their risk of disease. So whereas cigarettes in the early 1950s averaged 35 milligrams of tar (on standardized smoking machines), yields by the 1980s had dropped by about half. Part of the decline was from the introduction of filters, along with new blending tricks and burn accelerants, but most was from putting less tobacco in the rod and from ventilation. For a time at least the hope was basically to keep up the nicotine (addiction) while reducing the tar (cancer); Wynder, Russell, and numerous others had proposed this same solution, that the ideal cigarette would be reasonably high in nicotine but as low as possible in tar.

Nicotine can exist in myriad chemical forms, however, and can be manipulated to deliver a more or less powerful nicotine "kick." There are several different ways to do this, the most notorious of which involves freebasing, the transformation of a molecule from a (bound) salt to a (free) base, typically by adding ammonia or some other alkaline compound. This is one of the most significant developments in the history of modern drug design, and one virtually unknown to the outside world—applied to tobacco at any rate—until the 1990s, when the industry's internal documents first came to light.[6]

From a historical point of view, freebasing essentially reverses the trend toward ever milder, low-pH smoke ushered in with the flue-curing revolution. Flue-curing you will recall involved the lowering of cigarette smoke pH from 8 to about 6, making it less harsh and therefore easier to inhale. Freebasing pushes the pH back up a bit, but the purpose of the manipulation is quite different. Flue-curing makes tobacco smoke *less alkaline* and therefore mild enough to inhale. Freebasing, by contrast, allows the nicotine to *volatilize more effectively,* making more of it more readily available to the body. "Freebasing" is the street word for the trick as popularized in the cocaine trade, but it was actually cigarette makers that invented the process, or at least commercialized it on an industrial scale. Marlboro was its first great beneficiary: indeed much of the success of this global cowboy brand can be traced to this chemical trick.

But to understand how this works, we need to return again to the nature of smoke and how nicotine gets carried into the body.

PARTICLE VERSUS GAS PHASE PARTITIONING— AND FOLK FREEBASING

Tobacco smoke is interestingly complex. It's sort of like a moist gassy dust, or dusty gas, containing thousands of different chemicals in myriad complex and changing physical forms. The first step in simplifying this complexity is to realize that smoke has two physical states or "phases": one composed of *particles* and another composed of *gas*. Tobacco smoke is technically an aerosol in this sense, with most of the soot, tar, and nicotine being in chunky little droplets (12 billion per cigarette by one estimate) suspended in a gas consisting of carbon monoxide and dioxide along with water vapor, nitrous oxides of various sorts, hydrogen cyanide, nicotine in a gaseous state, and other gases not bound to the tiny droplets.[7]

The *particle phase* consists of everything that can be condensed from tobacco smoke when you apply an electric charge to these droplets and pull them down onto an electrostatic filter (also known as a Cambridge filter). This will include all of those tiny charred chunks of matter known as "soot," along with most of the greasy-waxy compounds known as "tar," plus whatever other solids or viscous liquids fall out when smoke is pulled across that electrostatic filter. A 1965 Reynolds document comments on how several different names have been given to this particle phase, including "tars, smoke solids, solids, total solids, particulate matter, total particulate matter, smoke condensate, total smoke condensate and smoke condensables."[8]

The *gas phase*, by contrast, is everything that cannot be filtered out—things like carbon monoxide and cyanide gas. These can be measured by techniques such as gas phase chromatography, developed by tobacco industry chemists in the years after the Second World War. The existence of such chemicals is one key limitation of "filtration" in the cigarette context, and one reason cigarette makers never like to talk about "gas" in cigarette smoke. Tobacco researchers for a time explored gas phase properties of smoke to find out whether they could eliminate some of these nastier constituents; great hopes for such a possibility were expressed in the 1950s, though by the 1960s and 1970s most hopes for "selective filtration" had been abandoned.

Like a number of other compounds in tobacco smoke, nicotine is present in both particle and gas phases. It is a small molecule and can either stand alone as a free base or bind to other compounds in the form of a salt—like nicotine citrate or acetate. In its stand-alone form it tends to move more easily into the gas phase of smoke—because the free base is more volatile.[9] This is crucial for understanding the logic of freebasing, since (1) free (or free-base) nicotine is far more potent than nicotine in the bound or salt form; and (2) how much nicotine ends up in the particle or gas phase has a lot to do with how *acid* or *alkaline* the smoke is. Increase the alkalinity, and you increase the proportion of nicotine in the gas phase. Reduce the alkalinity, and you push the nicotine back into the more inert particle phase. Free nicotine is more easily volatilized and more easily absorbed through bodily tissues. All of which means that by manipulating the pH of tobacco smoke you can influence how potent it will be when you inhale it.

This may come as a surprise to some readers, that smoke can be alkaline or acidic. The crucial take-home fact, though, is that free nicotine packs a more potent punch than bound or salt form nicotine.[10] The physiology is not entirely understood, but free nicotine seems to reach the lungs more efficiently, from where it passes into the blood and then into the brain—whereas nicotine in the particle phase is more easily expelled from the lungs or otherwise slowed in its transit to the brain. The difference may have to do with the fact that free nicotine is more lipophilic—literally, "fat-loving"—allowing it to pass more easily through the fatty membranes surrounding the brain.

The freebasing of nicotine goes back a long time, even prior to the industrial manufacture of cigarettes. A similar chemistry is implicit in what I like to call "folk freebasing," which many traditional cultures use to augment the potency of their preferred alkaloids. No one knows how the practice originated, but rural people in many parts of the world chew tobacco mixed with lime (calcium oxide, not the fruit) to sharpen the punch of the alkaloid.[11] Some cultures even urinate on the tobacco as part of the curing process, with the alkaline urea—an ammonia compound—doing basically the same trick. The freebasing of cocaine hydrochloride into "crack" is based on a similar chemistry: the cocaine alkaloid is far more potent in its free base form than as a salt, so bicarbonate is used to transform cocaine hydrochloride into chemically pure crack cocaine.

How, though, was freebasing discovered by tobacco manufacturers? The basic chemistry behind freebasing was already well known to chemists—including tobacco chemists—by the 1930s and 1940s. I've mentioned Parmele's 1946 discussion of adding ammonia to cigarettes to make the nicotine more volatile, but there are even earlier discussions. American Tobacco Company researchers in 1930 reflected on the fact that "Ammonia has the property of setting nicotine free from its salts. If tobacco contains nicotine in the free state, it will be taken up by the smoke more readily, whereas the salts are not volatile to the same extent and the nicotine will be consumed on burning." German and Russian tobacco experts also knew about the potency of free versus bound nicotine and wrote extensively on this topic.[12]

There was not much practical use for such ideas in the 1930s and 1940s, however. There was not yet any reason to augment nicotine's punch, so the question of free versus bound nicotine was little more than a chemical curiosity. Cigarettes still contained high levels of nicotine—typically 20 to 30 milligrams per stick—and the idea of increasing its impact wouldn't have served any useful purpose. Tobacco manufacturers were far more interested in making cigarettes *milder* and had no reason to give them any extra jolt. Claude Teague in 1954 was typical in still trying to find out how to *reduce* the free nicotine in burley leaf: the harshness (or "strength") of burley was known to come from the "high smoke concentration of free bases," and Teague actually proposed adding organic acids (citric, malic, or succinic, for example) to the tobacco to reduce this alkaline harshness. The proposal was hardly a new one: the Russian tobacco chemist Aleksandr Shmuk had made virtually identical proposals nearly a quarter of a century earlier. For Teague, as for everyone else in the tobacco world up to that point (circa mid-1950s), the quest was for an ever milder smoke, to facilitate inhalation and to comfort anyone worried about "irritation." And to encourage novices.[13]

Chemical priorities changed, however, with the push to develop low-delivery "health reassurance" cigarettes. Cigarette companies in the 1950s and 1960s started wanting to lower tar and nicotine as far as possible without weaning smokers from the habit. So the question became, not just how low can we go, but also how can we squeeze more power out of a given quantity of nicotine? How can we maintain "satisfaction" while lowering (apparent) deliveries? Finding answers to such questions became increasingly urgent, especially after governments started requiring publication of tar and nicotine values (in the late 1960s) from machines in which cigarettes were smoked in some standardized manner. Ventilation was one response; freebasing provided yet another, albeit by accident and through a rather circuitous route, involving ammonia and the processing of tobacco scrap.

CIGARETTE FACTORIES AS PAPERMAKING MILLS

Ammonia has long been used in tobacco manufacturing, long prior even to its recognition as a freebasing agent. The earliest patents go back to the 1880s, when the compound was proposed as a means to eliminate the "bad odor" of fermented leaf. More often, though, ammonia was viewed as an unwanted irritant generated through the curing process. One early rationale (or rationalization) for American Tobacco's much-ballyhooed "toasting" was that heat treating would drive off much of the cured leaf's accumulated ammonia: the goal was to chase a noxious irritant but also to lower the potency of the nicotine delivered to the smoker by keeping more of it in its bound (vs. free volatile) state.[14] Ammonia was occasionally added to tobacco but this had nothing to do with freebasing: I've mentioned deodorizing, but ammonia was sometimes used as a solvent to denicotinize tobacco and for a time even (in the 1950s and 1960s) to neutralize carcinogens such as benzpyrene. But the innovation that led to its use as a freebasing agent came from its role in the manufacture of *reconstituted tobacco*.

Reconstitution is a process whereby parts of the tobacco plant formerly tossed as waste are transformed into a pressed paper sheet, through a technique closely akin to papermaking. "Recon" factories are basically papermaking mills, where huge vats of crushed-fiber tobacco-stem slurry are floated into twelve-foot-wide sheets, which after drying get sprayed with "casings" of various sorts—including nicotine and diverse flavorings and preservatives. One could say that recon is basically to tobacco as plywood is to wood, but the process is really more like papermaking, which is why papermaking unions often represent the workers at such plants (United Paper Workers International, for example).[15]

Ammonia was added to recon beginning sometime in the late 1950s, principally to make fibers from the woody stems and ribs of the tobacco plant more smokable. German tobacco makers had started including these woody stems in cigarettes during the Second World War, as part of an effort to squeeze more smokable substance out of every pound of harvested leaf. This increasing use of stems was actually thought by some (in the 1940s) to be why cigarettes were causing cancer: cigarette makers had traditionally used only the non-woody parts of the leaf, but with efforts to rationalize production a decision was made to use more and more of the tobacco plant—basically everything but the roots and central stalk—to lower costs and speed mechanical processing.

It was not such an easy thing to make these woody parts smokable, however. The stems are very much like wood, which smokes about like, say, cardboard or saw-dust or "brown wrapping paper," as industry chemists used to say. Nicotine can be added, but the resultant smoke is still quite acidic, which is where the ammonia came in. Ammonia was added to neutralize the acid but also to release the pectins in the leaf (and stem), allowing a more effective binding of the fibers required to hold the dried slurry sheet together. Research into this process of *reconstituting* to-bacco (to make recon) intensified in the 1950s, and between 1952 and 1994 at least 231 patents were filed on the process. R. J. Reynolds was a key early player: the com-pany's official historian recalls a 1946 journey by three company managers to the public library in Winston-Salem to research techniques of papermaking,[16] and by the end of the 1950s most of the majors were using at least some recon in their cig-arettes. Some companies had earlier used recon for cigar wrappers, but Reynolds was apparently the first to use it in American cigarettes. The paperlike tobacco sheet is chopped into threads to look much like the chopped leaf itself, and much of what one smokes in a cigarette today is actually recon, which gives the companies a cer-tain flexibility in how to manipulate the final product.

Tobacco manufacturers had hoped that recon would be acceptable to smokers, but no one imagined how seductive it would become. Adding ammoniated tobacco sheet to traditional leaf gave the resulting blend a new and delightful flavor, de-scribed in industry documents as a rich burley or "chocolaty" taste. Even more im-portant, though, were its pharmacologic effects, since ammoniation also gave to-bacco a more powerful nicotine punch, gram for gram. In the health-conscious climate of the 1960s and 1970s, this meant that manufacturers could continue to reduce the (machine-measured) deliveries of cigarettes while still giving them the nicotine kick expected from "full flavor" brands.

CHOCOLATE NOTES

Philip Morris was apparently the first to realize that ammonia could be used to pro-duce this delicious, extra-added kick. The discovery seems to have come about by accident, in the early 1960s, as the company was conducting experiments on the taste and psychopharmacology of ammoniated tobacco sheet. As at Reynolds, am-monia was being added to tobacco sheet to improve its binding properties, giving it the tensile strength needed for processing into cigarette "filler." (A high sheet strength allowed recon to be pulled rapidly through automated machinery for pro-cessing.) Early taste tests were satisfactory, and in 1961 the company set up an experimental pilot plant to manufacture ammoniated tobacco sheet, using the so-called DAP-BL (diammonium phosphate–blended leaf) process.

Philip Morris engineering reports from this period note that the company's new DAP-BL process was economical, eliminating the need for "stem soaking, stem cooking and stem refining," but there were also good signs on the taste front. On November 6, 1962, Philip Morris chemist John D. Hind wrote to the company's manager of development, Robert B. Seligman, commenting on how treatment with DAP had produced a particularly strong "flavor of chocolate," allowing "a much more efficient way of producing the chocolate 'notes' in cigarettes and packages." It took some time to gear up for production, though, and lots of different variations on this DAP-BL process were tried, including the addition of "a methanol-washed lemon albedo" that gave "a favorable flavor variation." Process and equipment testing of pilot runs continued through the spring and summer of 1963, and after ironing out a number of potential kinks a decision was made to start commercial manufacture on October 15, 1963.[17]

Ammoniated tobacco sheet was first incorporated into Marlboros on a large-scale basis in 1964, and it is important to realize how radically this transformed the fate of the cigarette. The factory-scale use of ammoniated tobacco sheet—coincident with the launch of the "Marlboro Country" campaign—worked wonders for Philip Morris and its flagship brand. Marlboro had always been a relatively minor brand and in the 1950s had never garnered even a 5 percent share of the American market. By 1967, however, when Philip Morris secured a patent on its DAP-BL process—making no mention of freebasing, interestingly—Marlboro was well on its way to becoming the world's most popular cigarette. Market share in the United States alone grew from 5 to more than 40 percent from 1965 through 2005, the most spectacular rise of a single brand in cigarette history.[18] Marlboro surpassed Winston as America's most popular cigarette in 1976 and would soon become the world's number one brand. Charts of the brand's market share in the United States show a sharp kink upward in 1964, when the freebased version came on line.

THE SECRET AND SOUL OF MARLBORO

It is impossible to say how much of the success of Marlboro is due to freebasing and how much to the sophisticated marketing of Marlboro Country and the Marlboro Man. Hard-packed and masculine with its bright-red-roof chevron, the brand was perhaps even tough enough to stand up against cancer. (Recall that this manly image was new in 1955, when Marlboro was transformed from a woman's into a man's brand. In its feminine incarnation Marlboros had been "mild as May" with "ivory tips to protect the lips.") Smokers, and especially young smokers, seemed to like the new version's quick jolt, prompting envy and imitation from other manufacturers. Philip Morris would eventually apply its freebasing techniques to several of its other brands—notably its low-tar (and low-nicotine) Merit cigarettes, introduced in 1976 as "a radical breakthrough in cigarette technology." Merit was Philip Morris's hope for a new generation of smokers seeking a "safer" smoke; the new brand advertised a nicotine yield only half of that offered by Marlboro but by virtue of treatment with diammonium phosphate still delivered the same amount of free nicotine to smokers. Brown & Williamson scientists reflected on this in 1980, commenting that "in theory a person smoking these cigarettes [Merit and Marlboro] would not find an appreciable difference in the physiological satisfaction from either based on the amount of free nicotine delivered."[19]

Philip Morris enjoyed a monopoly on ammonia technology for a number of years, but the "secret" and "soul" of Marlboro was eventually found out. (Cigarette makers have a long history of reverse engineering their competitors' brands, to learn what kinds of tricks they might adopt.) Marlboro's success led to intense efforts at imitation, which is how the other companies came to discover the virtues of freebasing. Liggett & Myers in 1971, for example, tried to elevate its smoke pH by adding calcium hydroxide to its blends, with the following rationale: "We are interested in developing a cigarette with increased smoke pH in order to increase the free base as opposed to acid salt form of nicotine in smoke, perhaps giving a more satisfying smoke. If this could be done there could be a reduction in total nicotine in the smoke without a reduction in the physiological satisfaction associated with nicotine."[20] The author of this report knew that the "physiological effect" of nicotine could be increased by altering this ratio of free-base to acid-salt forms; here, too, the goal was to increase the alkaloid's strength while lowering apparent deliveries.[21]

Reynolds was another avid imitator. In 1973 Claude Teague, author of the "Survey of Cancer Research" and now assistant director of research at the company, wrote a long analysis of Marlboro's success, attributing the popularity of this brand, especially among young people, to Philip Morris's use of ammonia technology. Teague explored a number of different reasons for Marlboro's success—along with Brown & Williamson's Kool—with the goal of helping his company close the gap. His conclusion: "the most significant difference between our brands and Philip Morris brands and Kool has been in the area of smoke pH." In this same 1973 report—stamped "Secret"—Teague noted that by comparison with Reynolds's own Winston brand, Marlboro showed "1) higher smoke pH (higher alkalinity), hence increased amounts of "free" nicotine in smoke, and higher immediate nicotine "kick," 2) less mouth irritation, [3] less stemmy taste and less Turkish and flue-cured flavor, and 4) increased burley flavor and character."[22] Seeking to capture this allure, Reynolds began ammoniating its own cigarettes shortly thereafter. In 1974 the company started using ammoniated sheet in the manufacture of its Camel filters, allowing them to deliver 36 micrograms of freebasing ammonia in the mainstream smoke of each cigarette. Reynolds researchers here again reasoned that people were turning to Marlboros because they delivered more free nicotine as a result of ammonia technology.[23]

Brown & Williamson was yet another convert. By 1965 scientists from the company's parent BATCo laboratories in Southampton were well aware that the "strength" or "impact" of a cigarette was related not to total nicotine delivered but rather to the amount of "extractable" or "free nicotine," which varied significantly with smoke pH. Ammonia was an obvious way to manipulate smoke pH, and by 1971 the company had given the code name UKELON to *urea*, an ammonia source recognized as "a way of achieving normal impact from low tar cigarettes." Free nicotine was "more readily absorbed" and therefore more likely to have "a decidedly satisfying effect on the smokers' taste receptors." The company's Project LTS (Low Tar Satisfaction) was designed to exploit this effect, with the goal being to create a cigarette containing "greater levels of 'free' nicotine" in "an enhanced alkaline environment." A 1971 Brown & Williamson document titled "Ukelon Treatment of Tobacco" noted that urea treatment could be "one avenue toward the development of a low-tar, full-impact cigarette."[24]

Brown & Williamson continued research along these lines throughout the 1970s and by 1980 was able to conclude that "we have sufficient expertise available to 'build' a lowered mg tar cigarette which will deliver as much 'free nicotine' as a Marlboro, Winston or Kent without increasing the total nicotine delivery above that of a 'Light' product."[25] UKELON by this time was being used in the company's Kool and Viceroy brands, and we even have some of the recipes detailing how many pounds were sprayed (as "casing") onto the finished blend per hogshead of tobacco. Casing for a ten-thousand-pound batch of the company's experimental MT-768 tobacco in 1989, for example, included the following ingredients:[26]

CELANDO	(= glycerine)	98 pounds
HALWAY	(= honey)	147 pounds
QUASER	(= invert sugar)	319 pounds
GRELANTER	(= propylene glycol)	383 pounds
UKELON	(= urea)	49 pounds
XCF-2273	(= an experimental casing)	7 pounds
HOTANTIS	(= water)	288 pounds

The recipe provides only the code names; I have given here the decoded ingredients in parentheses. We also have the mixing instructions: HOTANTIS (= water) was to be added at 120 degrees Fahrenheit prior to a "drop to solids tank," following which UKELON (urea) would be added and mixed for ten minutes. The special "casing" (flavoring) XCF-2273 was then added along with the glycerine, honey, sugar, and propylene glycol, followed by application to the tobacco at 120 degrees Fahrenheit. This was all part of the company's Project Best, the goal of which was to develop a cigarette to outperform archrival Marlboro. With a key question being: "Is there more NH_3 [ammonia] chemistry in Marlboros"?[27]

This question was of great interest to Brown & Williamson, which is why they hired a corporate intelligence service to investigate how much ammonia Philip Morris was using. In 1985 the Corporate Intelligence Group of a company known as Information Data Search, Inc., reported to Brown & Williamson on the results of a clandestine inquiry into Philip Morris's ammonia usage, pieced together from interviews with chemical suppliers, tobacco growing experts, equipment manufacturers and distributors, fragrance and flavor specialists, chemical engineers, and competing cigarette manufacturers. Brown & Williamson learned by this means that its chief rival was using about 2.5 million pounds of gaseous ammonia per year at its American manufacturing plants.[28]

By this time, however, virtually all the majors had learned how to use ammonia technology—and not just in the United States. In January of 1988 J. S. C. Wong from Research and Development at W. D. & H. O. Wills in Australia reported on his company's efforts to use ammonia to develop a "low alkaloid smoking product without adversely affecting Smoking properties." Wong had reduced the nicotine content in a tobacco blend by water extraction and noted that subsequent exposure to ammonia "restored impact and irritation levels to a similar order of magnitude as those for the unextracted tobacco." Wong also remarked on the "smoother smoke" produced by ammoniation.[29]

New methods to measure nicotine's impact were also developed, including the so-called Woodrose technique, which ranked the subjective impact of a particular cigarette on a scale from 1 (low) to 4 (high). In the early 1970s this was part of an elaborate testing mechanism by which cigarettes would be rated for impact, irritation, and flavor, and on this basis awarded different "amplitudes" or "scores." Impact was basically nicotine "satisfaction," irritation was how much a cigarette bothered your mouth or throat, and flavor was, well, flavor. Each of these was further broken down into subcategories. Irritation could be different in the mouth, nose, or throat, for example; and flavor could be "musty," "earthy," "green/grassy," "dirty," "roasted/toasted," and so forth. Tobacco manufacturers spent a lot of time rating cigarettes in this manner, with test panels assembled to evaluate different blends and additives. Experts were also hired in the area of "sensory science," with the hope of creating some of the same kinds of scales fashionable among wine connoisseurs. Summary instruments of various sorts were developed, including a "Tobacco Aroma Wheel" comparable to what wine critics had in the form of "wine wheels" to evaluate cabernet, pinot, and chardonnay.[30]

Ammonia technology by the 1980s had become routine in cigarette manufacturing. An Ammonia Technology Conference organized by Brown & Williamson at Louisville, Kentucky, on May 18–19, 1989, concluded that ammonia technology was "the key to competing in smoke quality with [Philip Morris] worldwide." Minutes from this meeting reveal that with the exception of Liggett, all U.S. cigarette manufacturers were using some form of ammonia technology by this time. Philip Morris was using DAP recon and urea; Reynolds was using ammonia gas; American and Lorillard were using DAP recon; and Brown & Williamson itself was using DAP recon and urea, code named QUELAR and UKELON, along with half a dozen other tricks under the rubric "Root Technology."[31] Controlled ammonia processing was identified by Brown & Williamson researchers as "the soul of Marlboro":

> Marlboro is a moving target. Its blend alkaloids have markedly increased over the last three years. Humectants levels have increased. We find increasing amounts of two PM additives, urea and propyl paraben, in Marlboro. . . . We stand on our prior conclusion that the soul of Marlboro is controlled ammonia processing of tobacco, with this processing being accomplished during reconstituted tobacco manufacture. PM's band-cast recon most efficiently accomplishes the desired ammonia chemistry, thus it is an essential ingredient in Marlboro.[32]

None of this, of course, was made public, and the companies for many years denied they were manipulating nicotine. Philip Morris was actually brash enough to sue ABC Television—in 1994 for $10 *billion*—for reporting that Marlboro's maker had been "spiking" its cigarettes with nicotine.[33] The irony is that the companies could have made a case that freebasing was simply a way to increase the potency of the nicotine while keeping down the tar; freebasing could have been defended as a means of creating a "safer cigarette." Wynder and others had championed this idea, that nicotine-to-tar ratios should be maximized, keeping the nicotine high and the tar low. The companies never made this argument, because they didn't like to talk about how they were manipulating the chemical properties of smoke. They also didn't want to admit that nicotine was addictive. The companies could have said they were trying to make a low-tar cigarette while keeping "satisfying" levels of nicotine, and some public health authorities might even have hailed this as a noble goal.[34]

Making such an argument, though, would have compromised one of the pillars of the industry's deception, which was that nicotine was simply one of the many "taste" elements in a cigarette and in no way craved by smokers, robbing them of their self-control. The public had been led to believe that nicotine was just one of many natural constituents of tobacco leaf, beyond the control of the manufacturers. Admitting they were juicing up its potency while promising ever lower deliveries would seem to have required admitting addiction, which they were not yet willing to do. Not to their customers at any rate. The official line was always that ammonia was added simply to improve the "taste" of tobacco.

Privately, however, the companies were quite upfront about free nicotine being a more powerful—and dangerous—form of the alkaloid. Free nicotine was always a health and safety concern on the tobacco factory floor, where leaf-processing equipment would routinely gum up from contact with the waxy alkaloid. And to clean such equipment, the companies would often engage in what we might call "de-freebasing," wiping nicotine-clogged machine parts with citric acid to convert the volatile free base into a more harmless (acid) salt. Nicotine in its free base form is extremely toxic, and manufacturers knew that contact with even a few drops could prove fatal—by direct absorption through the skin. Confidential safety protocols for Philip Morris's pilot plant making denicotinized tobacco for the company's Next brand cigarette recognized that "The use of citric acid when decontaminating a piece of equipment serves to convert nicotine free base to the less readily absorbed salt form, at the same time rendering it less volatile." The resulting salt—nicotine citrate—was still quite toxic but now at least had the "advantage" of having "only about one twentieth the rate of skin absorption as free base nicotine."[35]

Another problem with admitting nicotine manipulation stemmed from the fact that cancer is not the only harm from smoking. Smoking also causes heart disease and dozens of other maladies, in which nicotine is not entirely innocent. Nicotine has been implicated in cardiovascular disease—by causing constriction of the arteries—and contributes to death from stroke and possibly even cancer. John Cooke at Stanford has shown that nicotine stimulates blood vessel growth, which means that exposure to nicotine might well promote tumorigenesis, by helping to supply new tumors with oxygen-rich blood. And scholars have shown that nicotine may be involved in blocking some of the enzymatic activities that help to detoxify to-bacco-specific nitrosamines.[36] Pharmaceutical companies even today are hamstrung in their development of new drugs, since nicotine interferes with basic detoxification processes in the body.

The bottom line is that freebasing helped sustain mass addiction. Smokers thought they were buying low-yielding cigarettes, when in truth they were getting just as much nicotine—and in a more powerful form. Freebasing was a response to worries that falling nicotine yields might cause people to quit; the point was to increase the "extractable" nicotine in smoke, delivering a higher nicotine kick per milligram of the alkaloid. The process was deceptive, in that it was introduced into many of the same brands advertised as "light" or "lower yield." So even though tar and nicotine levels measured by automated smoking machines showed steady declines over time, the augmented impact kept customers as addicted as ever. Freebasing facilitated compensation and is best regarded as a form of chemical deception, a subterfuge to keep smokers coming back for more.

POSTSCRIPT

This history—and chemistry—now has regulatory implications, since the newly empowered FDA will probably try to establish some maximum allowable limit to how much nicotine will be allowed in cigarettes, to prevent addiction. The industry will surely resist any such effort, but if some reasonable upper limit is established (see again the box on page 380), the companies may try to game this by reducing the size of cigarettes (to keep a high fraction of nicotine per puff) or raising the pH of the resulting smoke or adding other kinds of chemicals to make sure smokers remain hooked. Regulators will have to guard against industry efforts to increase the potency of nicotine by other means, or even to de-freebase cigar smoke to make it inhalable. The companies may try to exploit nicotine–acetaldehyde synergies, or to add other addictive compounds. Skirmishes of this sort will probably drag on for years, consuming costly financial and intellectual resources, before the courage will finally be found to cut the Gordian knot and ban combustible tobacco products altogether.

22

The "Light Cigarette" Scam

Do you suppose if I continue to smoke Camel Ultra Light Cigarettes and I should develop cancer it will be "Ultra Light Cancer"?

DENNIS J. O'NEIL, WRITING TO R. J. REYNOLDS, 1999

James J. Morgan was one of the most capable marketeers Philip Morris has ever had. After joining the company in 1963, the Princeton graduate (with a B.A. in history) had risen up through the ranks to shepherd, first, the Parliament brand, then Virginia Slims. In 1970, however, he was promoted to market heaven as brand manager for Marlboro, the brand that, as a result of ammoniation and creative cowboy marketing, would soon become the best-selling cigarette in the world. Managing such an important brand was a plum job, and Morgan performed well, judging from his subsequent promotions. By 1994 he was president of the company and its chief executive officer, a position he held until his retirement in 1997—shortly after his shocking claim, under oath, that cigarettes were "much more like caffeine, or in my case, Gummy Bears. I love Gummy Bears and . . . I eat Gummy Bears and I don't like it when I don't eat my Gummy Bears, but I'm certainly not addicted to them."[1]

Morgan's chief innovation was to have introduced the concept of "lights" into tobacco marketing. It is not entirely clear how this idea came to him: when asked about the topic in court he doesn't reveal much. In 1998, in testimony for *Blue Cross and Blue Shield v. Philip Morris et al.*, Morgan listed five great changes in the Marlboro brand: the transformation from a woman's to a man's cigarette in 1955; the introduction of the Marlboro Country campaign in 1962 (complete with music from *The Magnificent Seven*); the end of broadcast advertising in 1971, which led to the company's invention of mega-photolithographic billboards (to advertise the Marlboro Man); and the invention of the "light" branding concept in 1971. This was also about when Philip Morris acquired Miller Beer: the tobacco giant invented "light" beer about the same time it invented "light" cigarettes. I suspect many people will be surprised to learn that the entire concept of light (or lite) as applied to foods,

406

beer, and virtually everything else was a tobacco industry invention, a vehicle to sell cigarettes.

WE DIDN'T SAY "SAFER"

Morgan rejects any suggestion that lights were introduced by the industry to offer smokers some kind of health reassurance. As he describes it, the provocation actually came from New York City Mayor John Lindsay, who had proposed a tax on cigarettes based on their tar and nicotine deliveries. Lights, according to Morgan, were simply a response to this—basically an effort to avoid the tax. Testifying under oath, Morgan claimed that his company had never intended its new branding concept to imply any margin of safety; indeed he says his choice of the word *light* was pretty much arbitrary: "I could have used anything, any word. We didn't say 'was safer.'" Morgan denied that his company was responding to demands from medical authorities or from consumers worried about their health; he also denied that smokers perceived light cigarettes as offering any kind of health benefits.[2]

Internal company documents make it clear, though, that lights were intended to convey an impression of a less hazardous cigarette—and that people perceived them as such. The documents are full of references to "health smokers" and "health filter smokers" preferring light or low-delivery cigarettes. Reynolds in its marketing literature described smokers of "low tar" brands as smoking to "alleviate alleged health concerns," and BAT commented on how smokers "will probably believe that lower deliveries mean less 'risky' products." For Lorillard, low tar numbers were crucial to maintaining "a health cigarette image." Philip Morris's Project Hilton in Germany in 1976 envisioned a cigarette positioned as "very healthy on grounds of its low tar- and nicotine figures"; Project Klaus was yet another effort to target Germany's "health oriented smokers," especially those with the "strongest addiction to smoking." Project Gatwick was a BAT/Imperial effort to develop a "health reassurance" cigarette for Canada using a "visibly different filter" perceived by smokers of Rothmans and Export "as being mild."[3]

Smokers clearly perceived these as "healthier" than ordinary cigarettes. We know this from the many hundreds of references to "health reassurance" in the archives, as well as from internal industry studies dividing cigarette markets into "implicit," "contemporary," and "explicit" "health benefit" segments—according to levels of advertised tar. We also have evidence from the consumer letters, as when a woman from Scranton, Pennsylvania, claimed to have switched to Salem Lights "due to throat and voice problems." Industry marketers appealed to this hope: "With Hilton we offer a truly full flavor cigarette for smokers who would like to smoke healthier but who would never compromise on the taste." George Weissman of Philip Morris had articulated this general strategy shortly after the first Surgeon General's report, emphasizing in a memo to his president and CEO, Joseph F. Cullman III, how important it was for the industry to provide smokers with "a psychological crutch and a self-rationale to continue smoking." Lights were a key part of the effort to fashion such a crutch.[4]

The industry knew it was dangerous from a legal point of view to make such claims explicit, however. Admitting one kind of cigarette was *less* deadly, after all, would implicate others as being *more* deadly and violate the ruse of cigarettes causing no kind of harm whatsoever. Ads therefore, when they implied a health benefit, tended to do so obliquely. One series for Lorillard's True brand announced that everyone "knows the problem" and that Trues were "the solution" (see Figure 32). The problem (cancer? heart disease?) goes unmentioned; the presumption was that people "know." Advertisers reinforced this perception through carefully crafted visual cues. Smokers were portrayed as wearing all white in white rooms, conveying a sense of hospital-like purity and cleanliness. And whereas bright or sunset reds were used for Marlboro regulars, lights were typically cast in soft-toned pastels, with a liberal use of light blues and whites. Ads were sometimes drawn in watercolor, with progressively vanishing images of cowboys and western symbols as you moved from regulars to lights and ultralights. So whereas Marlboro regulars showed large and vivid images of cowboys, lights were usually presented in softer, more distant, scenes in watercolor or gouache. And ultralights might show only a thin line of galloping horses against the distant mountains. Less was supposed to be better—in the ads as in your lungs.

Strategies of this sort are explicit in the industry's internal documents. A 1992 chart of the three principal Marlboro brands, for example, identified Marlboro Reds with "heavy duty" blue-collar macho "real men"; Mediums (Blues) were to evoke the "yuppie"; and Lights were supposed to be "smarter." Advertisers were instructed on how to design ads for these different brands: so Marlboro Reds were to be in sharp focus with close-ups depicting a "single hero" and/or "action shots" with red tints dominant; Mediums would have more shades of blue (and be "product based, not image based"); and Lights were to have a "fuzzier focus" and depict "quieter scenes," incorporating nature and solitude in more "golden earth tones." Lights were also to be "more for women."[5] Color/theme schemes of this sort were carefully scripted, with text, image, tint, and focus all fine-tuned to target specific types of users.

The industry was clearly aware that smokers perceived Light cigarettes as healthier—which of course was the whole point. A 1992 BAT survey found smokers regarding such brands as "the opposite of full flavour. Little taste, low satisfaction, communicating minimal health risks (comparative to full flavour) but less natural and perhaps even synthetic." This same survey—drawing from interviews with smokers in Malaysia, South Africa, and Germany, with input from a BAT French study—found Lights being seen as having "the dimensions of Youth, Modernity striver/achiever," along with this presumption of "minimal health risks." Several other kinds of cigarettes were perceived this way, and not by chance. Menthols had been introduced as a safer (indeed medicinal) smoke in the 1930s, just as king-sizes were in the 1940s, filters in the 1950s, and low tars in the 1960s. Menthols had never been very popular until the so-called health scare of the mid-1950s, however, when market shares began their rapid climb. Focus groups showed that people often switched to menthols when they had a cold or sore throat; studies also showed that even the *names* given to a particular brand were more or less likely to evoke health. In 1964, for example, Lennen & Newell found that the trade name *micronite* was more often regarded as "healthful" than names such as *calgonite, cordite, bakelite,* or *samsonite,* albeit less often than *purite* or *Diet Rite*. Lights were just the latest tactic in this decades-long campaign of reassurance, targeting what the companies called the "concerned," "worrier," or "health" segment.[6]

DIET CIGARETTES?

Light cigarettes were popular from the moment they were introduced. Marlboro Lights hit the market in 1971, but by the end of that decade every major manufacturer in the United States had a "Lights extension." Viceroy Lights appeared in 1972, followed by Winston Lights in 1974, Kent Golden Lights in 1975, and Tareyton Lights in 1976. More than a dozen new Light brands came onto the American market in 1977, making this truly the "year of Lights." New brands that year included Camel Lights, L&M Lights, Old Gold Lights, Kool Super Lights, and half a dozen others in various lengths and styles.[7]

That same year—1977—Philip Morris upped the ante with the world's first "ultra light": an 85-millimeter Parliament. The American Tobacco Co. introduced its own Tareyton Ultra Light in 1979, followed shortly thereafter (in 1980) by R. J. Reynolds's More Ultra Light and Philip Morris's Merit Ultra Light. Viscount by this time in Canada was being sold as a "Super-Mild," a concept introduced in 1978. Lights and ultralights were brand concepts with informally agreed-upon deliveries: "regular" or "full-flavor" cigarettes were supposed to be anything above 15 milligrams FTC tar; "lights" were 7- to 15-milligram tar; and "ultralights" were anything below 7 milligrams. "Lowest tar" and "micro lights" were categories later added for cigarettes in the 1- to 3-milligram tar range. These were never formal rules with any kind of enforcement; nor did they really tell you how much tar and nicotine a smoker would actually inhale, given the phenomenon of compensation and freebasing.

"Slim" and "superslim" cigarettes were supposed to have this same health appeal, attracting health- and fashion-conscious women worried about their weight. Philip Morris launched its Virginia Slims in 1968, trading on the idea that smoking would help keep you from getting fat—which is one reason so many dancers, models, and actors smoked and still smoke. Slims were supposed to be a distinctly female cigarette, with the added implication that slims—and later superslims—were a kind of *diet cigarette*. Ads often dangled this lure by hinting that a "slim" cigarette could keep your figure slim and trim. (Ad for Silva Thins: "I like my figure slim. My men trim. And my cigarette thin.") Slim cigarettes were likened to low-calorie foods: so if you eat slim and smoke slim, you'll keep trim. Small-circumference smokes were referred to as "skinny cigarettes" or even "Reeds" or "Twigs"—brand names considered for a Benson & Hedges cigarette.[8] And ad copy incorporated words like "thin," "trim," and "skinny" to accentuate this purported (and preposterous) low-cal link. Reynolds in one of its ads for its Doral brand featured a young-looking woman explaining how she "lost 650 mg of 'tar' the first week . . . without losing out on taste. . . . I did it on what I call my 'Doral Diet.'" Or as another ad explained: "I'm not too big in the willpower department. But I lost 700 mg of 'tar' the first week on what I call 'The Doral Diet.'"

Logic was not a strong suit in such ads. After all, if smoking really did keep you thin, wouldn't a "light" cigarette have *less* of this effect? Has anyone ever imagined that "full-flavor" cigarettes might make you fat? Oddly enough, that is precisely what many of these ads implied. And the companies often commented on this, when they thought no one would be listening. Documents from Brown & Williamson's secret Project Cirrus describe the "ultra thin" configuration of Barclay Lights as designed to "reinforce low tar attribute."[9] So here was this perfect trifecta: the slim cigarette would keep you thin, thinness would imply low tar or "less" of those bad things in cigarettes, which were sort of like those bad things in food that make you fat. Smokers were supposed to think: slim figure, thin cigarette, low tar, low calorie, "less is more." And forget logic.

Female weight watchers were clearly in their sights in 1987, when Brown & Williamson introduced its Barclay Lights Ultra Thins.[10] The Superslims introduced shortly thereafter were supposed to convey the added impression of being "safer" than other cigarettes by virtue of generating less sidestream smoke. (*Sidestream* smoke comes directly from the lit end of the cigarette into the ambient air, in contrast to *mainstream* smoke, which is inhaled by the smoker.) A market study from 1991 found that while the primary attraction of ultra slims was their "femininity and lightness," smokers also viewed them as "more socially acceptable" and "'healthier' for themselves and those around them."[11]

The sickening reality is that in certain respects cigarettes with low sidestream smoke were actually *more* dangerous—because of how the smoke was reduced. The companies decided that what they really wanted was to reduce the *appearance* of sidestream smoke—meaning its visibility. Industry researchers studied this problem quite intensively in the 1980s—through Projects Lotus, Ambrosia, and Stealth, for example—and found that what mainly determines the visibility of smoke is the size of its constituent particles. Smoke containing large particles is typically more conspicuous, whereas smoke with smaller particles is less so. So to make smoke less visible, cigarette engineers set out to reduce the size of smoke particles—and succeeded to a certain extent.

Success was not achieved without side effects, however, since less visible smoke is no less deadly—and may even be more deadly—for two rather different reasons. For one thing, people may be more willing to expose themselves and others to such smoke, believing it to be less deadly (or not present). More disturbing is the fact that fine particles tend to lodge more easily in the lungs and to penetrate more deeply. The result: doctors are now finding more cancers in the deeper recesses of the lungs, where they are harder to identify and to extract. That is principally from the switch to filter cigarettes, since larger smoke particles are more easily filtered out.[12] But it is also from this effort to make smoke less visible, by reducing smoke particle size. Smokers now tend to get more of these distal tumors—especially adenocarcinomas, which formerly were rare even among smokers. Tumors deeper in the lung also tend to be found at later stages of malignancy, which signals a worse prognosis.

So several different sorts of design modifications have caused cigarettes to actually become more deadly. Counting only those having to do with cancer, this would include (1) flue-curing, which allowed cigarette smoke to be inhaled, generating the world's first epidemic of lung cancers; (2) filters, which reduced smoke particle sizes, allowing tars to penetrate deeper into the lungs; and (3) efforts to make smoke less visible, which further reduced smoke particle size, causing more lung disease and disease of a deadlier kind. This counterintuitive bite-back is common in the world of tobacco, where manufacturers seem to have as their basic operating philosophy: trade in illusions, ignore the health of your customers, and paper over any difficulties with fancy scents and optical tricks. (Chemicals were sometimes put into cigarettes to cover up noxious tobacco odors, part of this effort to make smoking more "socially acceptable.") Greg Connolly of Harvard hit this nail on the head when he compared the industry's odor and visibility manipulations to "adding sugar to rancid meat . . . classic adulteration of a consumer product to conceal the risk."[13]

POPCORN OR PUFFED-WHEAT TOBACCO

We've seen how "low-tar" cigarettes are fraudulent: filters don't really filter, and tricks such as ventilation are easily and unconsciously overcome by the addict. Cigarette makers have used other tricks to lower apparent tar and nicotine yields, including modifications of the blend and burn rate and changes in cigarette dimensions. Smaller cigarettes—simply by virtue of containing less tobacco—will deliver less tar and nicotine when smoked on an automatic smoking machine, because there is less tobacco to burn. One way to achieve this is to reduce the circumference of the rod—and therefore the volume of the tobacco component—but another has been to "lighten" the tobacco by aerating it, puffing it up, making it less dense, so that a cigarette of a given volume will contain less tobacco. The term of art is *expanded tobacco*.

Expanded tobacco (ET) is an important means by which the tobacco companies have tried to make cigarettes appear "safer." Reynolds pioneered this technique in the 1960s: the idea was that by "puffing up" tobacco—typically by exposing it to extreme cold in the form of dry ice, Freon, or liquid propane—you could force air into the leaf and thereby increase its volume, or "filling power." The result was basically a popcorn or puffed-wheat version of traditional leaf which, as with recon, could be used to save on manufacturing costs. Expanded tobacco (also known as G-13 in Reynolds's jargon) is of course less dense, which means that less was needed to fill a cigarette to a given volume. ET saved the companies money, but it also helped to reduce machine-measured tar and nicotine yields, since you were putting less actual tobacco in any given cigarette. So whereas cigarettes from the 1950s typically contained about 1.2 grams of "filler" (tobacco plus flavorings and other additives),[14] cigarettes by the 1970s and 1980s typically contained only two-thirds of a gram, some only half a gram or even less.

The beauty of this system was that it saved the industry money—just like filters. Recall that filters lowered the cost of manufacturing, since cigarettes with plastic tips contain about 20 percent less tobacco. Expanded tobacco had this same cost-cutting virtue—but could also be used to lower tar and nicotine deliveries as measured by the smoking robots mandated by the FTC. Cigarettes containing less tobacco meant less tar and nicotine from any given cigarette—if smoked the same way as a regular (a big "if"). It also meant smoking more *paper* per gram of tobacco. Not that that the latter really mattered much, since much of the modern cigarette (notably the recon) is just chopped and flavored paper onto which nicotine-laden tobacco extracts have been sprayed.

How, though, was expanded tobacco developed?

The idea of pumping air into products to fluff them up goes back to the early years of the twentieth century. Puffed wheat and rice date from prior even to the First World War, though no one seems to have bothered applying such techniques to tobacco until the 1960s. Nineteenth-century governments would surely have regarded it as a form of adulteration—and sleazier even than pumping tobacco full of sugar and the like, since expanding tobacco just adds a bunch of empty air to the cigarette. The process had an obvious economic rationale: ET allowed cigarette makers to fill a cigarette with substantially less tobacco. A new justification emerged in the 1960s, however, since including ET also allowed cigarette makers to lower tar and nicotine deliveries as measured on standardized smoking machines. The first recorded suggestion of this sort is a 1964 "Communication of Invention" by James D. Fredrickson of Reynolds, who proposed reducing the volume of cigarette smoke by "limiting the quantity of tobacco consumed in smoking." The method involved subjecting cured tobacco leaf to a volatile solvent such as hexane, followed by a sudden-shock treatment with steam. Reynolds researchers had found that hexane-extracted stem could be puffed up by this means, allowing a reduction in tar and nicotine numbers when incorporated into a cigarette. Fredrickson in his lab notebook commented that the "economic aspects of the process" would also be attractive, given that "the amount of tobacco in a cigarette would be decreased." Fredrickson later proposed other methods of expanding tobacco—by incorporating an inert gas such as carbon dioxide or Freon into the leaf, which would then be allowed to swell by subjecting it to a partial vacuum.[15]

Philip Morris and Reynolds by the late 1960s were both taking expanded tobacco quite seriously. Indeed it was like a dream come true. Simply by applying certain chemical and physical agents, cigarette makers could take a given mass of tobacco and puff it up to nearly twice its pretreated volume. Cigarette makers could thereby reduce the mass of "filler" in the rod by about half—producing cigarettes containing not even half a gram of tobacco. Here is how Helmut Wakeham described it to his superiors in 1973:

> Tobacco filler expansion is achieved by impregnating the tobacco cells with a volatile expansion agent and then applying quick thermal energy to convert the agent into a gas which blows up or expands the cell. The Reynolds process uses Freon as the agent which works well but has the disadvantage of leaving some foreign Freon residue in the tobacco. The current method used by Philip Morris utilizes the formation of ammonium carbonate in the tobacco cells. On exposure to heat, this compound breaks down to ammonia and carbon dioxide gases which expand the [filler]. There is some excess residual ammonia, but the main disadvantage of this method is that the elevated temperature required to effect the expansion also produces some undesirable changes in tobacco composition.
>
> Consequently, we have been investigating other methods.

The most important of these other methods was the so-called dry ice or DIET (dry ice expanded tobacco) process, which involved freezing and then thawing the leaf or sheet to puff it up. Other methods were tried, including an ammonia–carbon dioxide procedure involving alternating cycles of heat, cold, and exposure to steam, but dry ice comes to be regarded as the cheapest and most effective. Wakeham had a theatrical bent and liked to dramatize the process by handing out a piece of dry ice impregnated tobacco leaf, which when fondled by his audience would warm up and expand before their very eyes.[16]

Like ventilation, expanded tobacco was one of the principal ways by which cigarette makers in the 1970s and 1980s lowered (apparent) tar and nicotine yields. The idea was basically that you would not smoke as much because there would be less tobacco in your cigarette. This was hardly a profound concept, but it did lead to savings for the industry and lower apparent yields. Which is also why it generated such enthusiasm—and kept on generating it for decades. Philip Morris in 1987 increased the capacity of its Munich ET facility from 1,050 to 1,250 kilograms per hour, partly by increasing the temperature of the process. The time required to process a single batch in the company's secret Project Duerer went from nearly four to only two and a half hours. New puffing methods were also developed, including impregnation of the leaf with a volatile organic liquid followed by heating with a hot gas. Stems or leaves were also irradiated with microwaves, causing the tobacco to puff up. Some companies expanded only those varieties of tobacco thought to be more harmful, hoping thereby to lessen the risk of cancer.[17]

Odd as this may seem, then, "light" cigarettes are, among other things, just light-weight cigarettes, cigarettes with less tobacco in them. Most smokers probably have no idea that the actual mass of tobacco in cigarettes has declined substantially over the past eighty or ninety years. In 1922, for example, Class A cigarettes in the United States were required by law—the Tobacco Tax Law—to weigh at least three pounds per thousand cigarettes, meaning an average minimum weight of 1.36 grams per cigarette. Lucky Strike cigarettes in 1921 averaged about 1.27 grams and contained 1.20 grams of tobacco. Cigarettes manufactured since the 1940s, however, have steadily declined in weight. (It is not clear why this 1922 law was not enforced.) The industry used to gauge the weight of cigarettes in terms of how many it took to make four ounces; so for Tareyton Filters in 1956 it took ninety-two to make four ounces, with each whole cigarette weighing 1.23 grams (1.03 for the tobacco and the rest for paper and the filter). Camels were somewhat lighter but still weighed about 1.1 grams and were occasionally measured as heavy as 1.26 grams. Cigarettes have continued to lighten since this time: Tareyton Ultra Low Tar Menthols in 1981 contained only 0.56 grams of tobacco; and Brown & Williamson's super-skinny Capri in 1986 (with a circumference of only 17 mm) contained only 0.40 grams of tobacco. By 1991 an *entire pack* of Virginia Superslims Ultra Low Tar contained only 8 to 9 grams of tobacco—so little that adjustments had to be made in mechanical handling and testing procedures, which had assumed that a pack of cigarettes would weigh at least 10 grams. Even American Lights, a very long cigarette at 120 millimeters, contained only 0.82 grams of filler.[18]

THE VANISHING CIGARETTE? TOBACCO IN SELECTED U.S. BRANDS

Year	Cigarette	Tobacco Content
1921	Lucky Strike	1.27 grams
1922	"Class A" Cigs (Tobacco Tax Law)	1.36 grams
1932	Lucky Strike	1.05 grams
1956	Pall Mall	1.20 grams
1956	Tareyton Filter	1.03 grams
1972	Benson & Hedges	0.91 grams
1974	Chesterfield 101 filter	0.85 grams
1974	Old Gold	0.74 grams
1981	Tareyton Ultra Low Tar Menthol	0.56 grams

1980	Carlton 83's (box)	0.50 grams
1987	Capri 100 Ultra Slim	0.40 grams
1993	Marlboro Lights	0.67 grams
1993	Virginia Slims Superslims (box)	0.42 grams
2010	Marlboro Lights	0.65 grams
2010	Marlboro 72s	0.52 grams

The point is that cigarettes today contain significantly less tobacco than cigarettes from the pre-1950s era. Light cigarettes are light because the manufacturers have punched little holes in the sides, allowing fresh air to dilute the smoke, but also because they use this new kind of tobacco, or rather the same old kind subjected to "puffing" or "expansion" (or "swelling"). Expanding tobacco gives it greater filling power, but the end product is no different. Light cigarettes are "light," if you believe that cream by virtue of being whipped has fewer calories or that cotton candy is less likely to rot your teeth than ordinary sugar.

There is one further point that should be made in this context. Epidemiologic studies show that people are still dying as often from smoking on a per cigarette basis, which means that cigarettes today—since they contain only about half the tobacco they once did—are about twice as deadly on a per-gram basis as cigarettes in the past. Despite all the trumpets and drums and hand-waving from the industry's admen and lawyers in court and despite reassurances in the guise of filters, "low tars," and "lights," modern cigarettes are no less deadly than those of a bygone era. Indeed on a per-gram basis they may well be deadlier than at any previous time in history. All the industry has really managed is to extract more death and suffering from any given mass of tobacco, and to wrap the whole mess up in shiny packs full of lies.

COLOR-CODING SCHEMES

In court, when charged with having conspired to defraud consumers by means of this "Light" label, the industry typically blames the public health community for insisting that low-tar cigarettes would be safer. And it is true that for several decades a number of health authorities did recommend that smokers switch to low-delivery brands. The peak of this insistence came in the 1970s, when the tobacco industry and the U.S. Public Health Service collaborated in an effort to explore how "less harmful" cigarettes might be designed, through a body known as the Tobacco Working Group, set up in 1968.[19] The retreat from advocating "reduced harm" cigarettes did not really come until the 1990s, when health authorities realized (mainly from the release of internal industry documents) that the industry had no reason to believe lights were any safer—because of compensation. I've mentioned the pioneering work of Kozlowski and Benowitz, but we cannot really talk about a consensus until 2001, when the National Cancer Institute published its *Monograph 13*, combining evidence from epidemiology, biomarker studies, marketing research, and the industry's own archives to show that lights were no safer.

More recently, the different companies have begun to diverge over what to admit. Philip Morris now admits that lights or low tars were never any safer but refuses to admit it had ever implied such a thing. Contrary to mountains of evidence from the archives,[20] the company also denies that smokers ever *imagined* them to be safer. Reynolds admits that lights may not have been safer, but they also like to stress that many people *outside* the industry also used to think this—including people from the public health community. The industry here as always tries to diminish its own responsibility (and culpability) by casting itself as a kind of neutral innocent, buffeted by the forces of consumer demand and public health admonishments. The industry was not a leader but a follower; their hands were tied. Such is the claim at any rate.

Fortunately, however, the courts have begun to see through this ruse. In the summer of 2006 federal court Judge Gladys Kessler ruled in *United States v. Philip Morris* that the industry had deliberately tried to deceive consumers with its "lights" campaign. Justice Department lawyers had accused the industry of violating the Racketeer Influenced and Corrupt Organizations (RICO) Act—the statute created to punish organized crime—and the court was harsh in its condemnation. In one of the most detailed legal judgments in history—the "Final Amended Opinion" runs to 1,600 pages—the court ruled that the companies had committed fraud and racketeering on a scale of massive proportions. The conspiracy ("enterprise") had lasted over half a century and was ongoing. The companies were found to have

"Falsely Denied that They Market to Youth,"

"Falsely Denied that They Manipulated Cigarette Design,"

"Falsely Represented that Light and Low Tar Cigarettes Deliver Less Nicotine and Tar,"

"Falsely Denied that ETS [Secondhand Smoke] Causes Disease," and

"Suppressed Documents, Information, and Research"

The court also commented on the conspiracy to represent light and low-tar cigarettes as safer, when the reality known to the companies was that these offered no clear health benefit over regulars. The industry falsely marketed lights as less harmful "in order to keep people smoking and sustain corporate revenues." Hundreds of pages are devoted to proving such charges. The marketing of lights was a calculated deception, a ruse to keep profits high even if it costs smokers' lives.

Lights branding of cigarettes in the United States is scheduled to become a thing of the past. Judge Kessler in *United States v. Philip Morris* ordered the companies to stop using descriptors such as "light," "mild," or any other terms to convey health claims,[21] a ruling upheld in July 2010, when the U.S. Supreme Court refused to hear the industry's request for an appeal. The tobacco industry is now officially a racketeer; that is the law of the land. The FDA has also ruled that explicit "light" labels must disappear, effective June 2010. The Framework Convention on Tobacco Control (not yet ratified by the United States) asks all its member nations to avoid using labels such as "Light" or "Mild" in advertising (or on packs), and Brazil, Canada, and most countries in the European Union have already banned such terms. Brazil in 2001 banned *all* tobacco advertising using health-related terminology— including "light" and "mild"—though cigarette makers have also had plenty of time to develop alternate ways to convey this same message of reassurance.

Indeed the industry has long known that *color codes* can be used to differentiate brands and to insinuate this same sense of safety. So instead of Marlboro regulars, lights, and ultralights we will have Marlboro reds, golds, and silvers; or something along these lines. Menthols will no doubt be greens or blues. Brazilian cigarette makers have already introduced such codings, and other countries surely will follow. Tobacco marketers have been building up the public's appreciation for "color perception" since at least the 1970s; a 1978 Brown & Williamson marketing report put it at follows: "Light colors connect with light tasting. Combinations of yellow, orange and red now equate to smoking enjoyment. Merit's brown projects a slightly stronger taste. Certain blues are contradictory to smoking enjoyment and can denote strength and coldness. Other blues are prestigious though in a passive sense."[22] The industry has been working for quite some time along these lines, which means that when "light" labels are finally lost, the companies will already have moved on to color-coded surrogates. We've already seen how manufacturers barred from using text or human images were able to turn to subtler visual cues: a sliver of cut purple silk, a Camel waiting for a bus (see again Figure 17). BAT as recently as 2008 was giving stores in Mauritius a new coat of paint—in favored cigarette brand colors.[23] We can expect tobacco manufacturers to try to carry on the lights fraud via color codings, which is why critics call for plain packaging with nothing but a plain-font brand name on the pack—and graphic warnings. A heated battle is now being waged in Australia over precisely this question of whether the government has the right to mandate plain packaging.

The industry of course is nimble, and has a long history of anticipating (and thwarting) its critics. Which is why we can still count the number of cigarettes smoked per annum in the trillions. The light cigarette scam and its survival through color coding was not the industry's first duplicitous triumph, nor will it be its last.

23

Penetrating the Universities

Only a knave or a fool can support [the] tobacco industry. It is dastardly. This is the Age of the Hollow Man. Let it not be known as the age when our finest thinkers sell out.

CHARLES B. HUGGINS (NOBEL LAUREATE) TO CLARENCE COOK LITTLE (CTR SAB CHAIR), JANUARY 17, 1968

Those who can make you believe absurdities, can make you commit atrocities.
VOLTAIRE

In 1963 Senator Maurine B. Neuberger of Oregon wondered whom future historians might indict for "our failure to find even a partial solution to the problem of smoking during the first 10 years after its dangers were revealed." There was plenty of blame to go around, and the distinguished senator pondered the options:

> The tobacco industry, for its callous and myopic pursuit of its own self-interest? The government, for its timidity and inertia in failing to formulate a positive program of prevention? The medical profession, for abdicating its role of leader in this crucial area of public health? Or is the individual—smoker and non-smoker alike—incriminated by his failure to accept responsibility for his own and his society's well-being?[1]

Nearly fifty years have passed since Neuberger's queries, and our answer must be "all of the above"—and more. The senator makes no mention of those many journalists, advertisers, and PR agents who so faithfully served the industry, nor of the farmers and trade unionists who went along with the doubt campaign. She doesn't mention the myriad providers of paper, filters, and flavorants to the industry, who must have known their ultimate fate. And there is no mention of those legions of lawyers who, like those at Shook, Hardy and Bacon or Covington & Burling, provided intimate counsel to the industry, directing research, cultivating experts, shredding or sequestering documents, and aiding and abetting in other ways the denialist conspiracy.[2]

Also absent from Neuberger's list, however, is *academia,* which is striking given how thoroughly our colleges have been captured. Thousands of scholars have worked as consultants for Big Tobacco, and many hundreds have worked as witnesses in

litigation. And not just in the United States, but all over the world. This massive—
and deadly—collaboration is little known, a virtually undiagnosed black mark on
modern scholarship.

OFF-TOPIC DATA CHAFF AND QUID PRO QUO

We've already seen how the Medical College of Virginia by the 1940s was "sold
American": especially through its Department of Pharmacology, the college supplied the industry with talent for more than seven decades, as it still does today. But
the MCV was not alone in providing help. Dozens of world-class universities have
serviced the industry, defending cigarette makers in court or in hearings, spewing
off-topic data chaff to distract from looming harms, lending the imprimatur of in-
tellect to the world's deadliest business enterprise. Professors from places like Harvard, Yale, Johns Hopkins, Stanford, UCLA, and other beacons of learning have been
happy to serve, and in a variety of capacities. Taking money from the industry's distraction organs (CTR, CIAR, etc.) has been the most common, but scholars have
also appeared for the industry in films or on television, along with evaluating grants,
organizing symposia, publishing books and articles, and countless special arrangements. Scholars serve as expert witnesses for the industry in court or before Congress and write briefs for lawyers, advising them on everything from soft spots in
statistical reasoning to tricky ways to challenge a cancer diagnosis.

Prior to the 1990s, in fact, there seems to have been little reluctance to take such
funds. Harvard administrators in 1964 actually solicited money from Reynolds, offering that such donations (for medical research) would be of "incalculable value"
in demonstrating the "interdependence of good health and industrial achievement."
Here is how Harvard approached the Camel coterie:

> By making a major unrestricted grant for teaching and research in the medical sci-
> ences at Harvard, the R. J. Reynolds Tobacco Company would enjoy enormous pub-
> lic relations benefits, starting with the initial announcement of the gift and continu-
> ing, for generations to come, with the association of the R. J. Reynolds name with a
> steady stream of advances in medical knowledge. The Company would set an exam-
> ple of incalculable value in demonstrating the interdependence of good health and
> industrial achievement.[3]

Reynolds for its part agreed that academic investments would be wise "in the matter of the Company's 'public image'"—and so on October 8, 1964, gave $50,000 to
the illustrious East Coast university. Harvard Medicine Program Officer Lawrence
O. Pratt was gratified, assuring the company of the university's intent "to create with
your initial gift the R. J. Reynolds Teaching and Research Fund" for Harvard:

> The creation of such a fund will have a number of advantages. We will be able to uti-
> lize income from the Fund to support basic research in fields that hold special inter-

est to your company. Because the gift is unrestricted, the Dean of the Harvard Medical School will be able to utilize these new resources, like a good quarterback, in ways which promise maximum yardage in advancing knowledge.[4]

Reynolds later worked with other Harvard deans, including Robert H. Ebert, who succeeded George P. Berry as dean of the medical school in 1965. Dean Ebert was equally appreciative, praising the makers of Camel cigarettes (in 1970) for providing "a significant part of the unrestricted capital available to the Medical School for teaching and research purposes." Ebert invited the cigarette maker to visit the Harvard campus: "We would welcome the opportunity to demonstrate how the Reynolds Fund is contributing to progress of medical science and education." Reynolds was agreeable, noting that Dean Ebert had long had an interest in lung infections—and smoked a pipe.[5]

Gifts of this sort were often "unrestricted," but donors clearly expected some kind of payback. Within a matter of weeks after announcing its first big grant to Harvard, for example, Reynolds had one of its attorneys ask Professor A. Clifford Barger from the medical school to testify on its behalf before a congressional committee investigating smoking. Barger soon thereafter began reviewing grant applications for the CTR and started dipping himself into this pot, receiving Special Project funds after gaining the approval of "all six General Counsel" of the industry. Barger was attractive to the companies because, as lawyers working with Shook, Hardy and Bacon explained, when it came to heart disease Barger "believes that his experimental work shows that stress and not smoking is involved." This was music to the industry's ears, which is why David Hardy in 1969 recommended increasing Special Project money for Harvard in the hope again that "Dr. Barger might consider giving us a statement for hearings." The rationale was familiar: "Dr. Barger is, we believe, sympathetic to our cause insofar as heart disease is concerned, and he feels that stress and other factors are of much greater importance than the unproved case against smoking." Barger received $30,000 that year in Special Projects money, plus another $150,000 in 1972 in regular CTR funds to determine, among other things, "whether nicotine enhances performance of the squirrel monkey." The professor by this time had a big team of Harvard scholars working on the industry's dime—the psychiatrist Peter B. Dews, for example, but also J. Alan Herd from physiology, Roger T. Kelleher and William H. Morse from psychobiology, and several research and technical assistants as well. Barger also had a cozy relationship with the CTR, reviewing and approving grant applications by colleagues who were also reviewing and approving his own applications. As late as 1984 Barger was still presenting lectures to RJR's Board of Directors, reassuring them that heart disease had "unknown" causes despite "many suspects." His colleague Peter Dews as recently as 1994 was advising Philip Morris on "scientific points regarding nicotine addiction" to address claims raised in litigation, while serving also as a member of Reynolds's Scientific Advisory Board. Dews in at least one instance traveled to Philip Morris headquarters in New York to deliver a lecture (to the Board of Directors) on legal matters so sensitive that even today the speech remains "privileged content" and barred from public inspection.[6]

It would take many thousands of pages to chronicle the full extent of Big Tobacco's penetration of academia; the scale of such collaborations is simply too vast. From 1995 to 2007 alone, University of California researchers received at least 108 awards totaling $37 million from tobacco manufacturers for training, service, and research. From a global point of view most such collaborations have been in the realm of agriculture: tobacco companies rely on experts to improve tobacco yields, and thousands if not tens of thousands of scholars have been harnessed for this purpose. Here I shall restrict my focus to health-related collaborations, which present us with the most disturbing breach of academic integrity. Given limitations of space I shall highlight only a few examples from some of our more prestigious universities, organized more or less chronologically.

A FEELING OF GOODWILL

The 1930s was a turning point in tobacco–academic collaborations. Outside expertise was needed to solve certain technical problems, but the companies were also beginning to realize that university ties could burnish the industry's prestige and credibility, both of which had suffered from the first great wave of "health scares" centering around publicity of poisons in tobacco—notably lead, arsenic, and carbon monoxide but also poisons produced by the use of humectants (including acrolein) and nascent cancer grumblings. A. L. Chesley, American Tobacco's top scientist in the pre-Hanmer era, as early as 1931 had pushed the company to use its talents to help "withstand the assault" of competitors and anti-tobacco propagandists; the goal was to make the company's research department "the leader in this field" so that anyone wanting to know about tobacco "will think first of asking us for such information." AT&T's Bell Laboratories was to be a model, but external research contacts were also to be cultivated. Chesley's recommendation: "We should establish a feeling of good will, probably by research work, with several of the leading colleges, such as Columbia, Johns Hopkins, the University of Iowa, and some University on the Coast. . . . "[7]

American led with its MCV collaboration, but by the 1940s most of the companies had joined in the action. Lorillard funded a graduate fellowship (in tobacco chemistry) at Ohio State in 1946, by which time the company was also paying *JAMA* editor Morris Fishbein large sums to promote its cigarettes. C. L. Albright from the physics department of the University of Richmond studied the extent to which Pall

Mall stained the fingers (in 1940), while Philip Morris funded the Mellon Institute of Industrial Research to improve methods for measuring acrolein in cigarette smoke. Brown & Williamson in 1947 established a fellowship at the University of Louisville to research the chemical constituents of tobacco leaf, and Lorillard in 1946 funded yet another postdoctoral fellowship, this time in physiology, "to study cigarette smoke from the standpoint of throat irritation." This last-named initiative was made urgent by the publicity given to Angel H. Roffo's demonstration of a cigarette–cancer link in the 1946 issue of *Reader's Scope*.[8]

Universities were not always proud of such arrangements. Ohio State's contract with Lorillard barred the tobacco giant from using its name in advertising, for example, and Yale was not entirely pleased with its appearance in a series of Reynolds ads extolling nicotine's wondrous power to raise one's blood sugar. Professor Howard W. Haggard's work had been cited in a series of ads that ran in 1,100 newspapers in the spring of 1934; neither Haggard nor Yale had approved the use of their names, however, and there was the added complication that the professor was already under contract with several other tobacco firms, endorsing other tobacco products. Haggard and his colleague Yandell Henderson, from Yale's Applied Physiology Laboratory, were on the payroll of at least three different cigarette companies by this time. For Brown & Williamson, for example, they had been investigating the toxicity of the menthol added to Kool cigarettes, concluding in a letter to the company's law department that the compound was "entirely without any harmful effect whatever, either general or local, upon those who consume these cigarettes." Haggard and Henderson also suggested mentholating *the paper* in the packaging just prior to transport (to avoid evaporation), an idea later taken up by a number of cigarette makers. Haggard had also helped certify the cleanliness of American Tobacco's facilities, but it was not always easy to entice such collaborations. William Esty, head of Reynolds's chief advertising agency, in 1934 reflected candidly on tobacco's difficult relations with academia:

> Nearly all scientists and college professors have an instinctive distrust of business men, especially advertising men. There is some justification for their feelings, since in the past their confidence has been so often betrayed by commercial interests. Professor Haggard especially has reason to distrust tobacco companies and advertising men. He was one of the party which was taken on a special train for a junket to the Lucky Strike factory. Like the others in the large party, he was promised a $1,000 fee simply to inspect the factory and report on its sanitary conditions. The party of visiting scientists was whisked through the factory in a perfunctory way, then entertained at a barbecue and mint julep spree and poured back on the special train. Professor Haggard wrote a letter to the American Tobacco Company stating that he found sanitary conditions to be very good in the factory, then the Ethiopian in the wood pile emerged. American Tobacco Company sent him a long statement to sign, in which he commended their toasting process and other features, obviously to be used in Lucky Strike

advertising. Properly resentful, Professor Haggard returned the statement unsigned and said he would return their check if his first statement was not satisfactory.[9]

Esty realized that such men had to be approached carefully, and subsequently looked for scholars more favorably disposed to business enterprise.

The industry vastly increased funding for scholars in the 1950s and 1960s, following proof and certification of the lung cancer hazard. In 1955 alone the TIRC offered fellowships to seventy-nine medical schools, with only two refusing the money. Trolling wherever they could for support, the companies offered lucrative stipends and retainers to keep scholars in their pockets. Herbert Arkin, for example, was a City College of New York statistician hired by Philip Morris in 1950 to analyze the extent to which different brands of cigarettes irritated the throat. Philip Morris scientists had gathered the data, using "a colorimeter and photo electric cell" to gauge the reddening of tissues at the back of the throat. Crunching company-supplied numbers, Arkin found that whereas Lucky Strikes caused significant irritation, Philip Morris cigarettes produced none (big surprise). Arkin was later hired to dispute Hammond and Horn's studies financed by the American Cancer Society and published an article in *Current Medical Digest* warning that the methods being used to link smoking and cancer were "fraught with dangers of misinterpretation." Newspapers publicized his skepticism, with headlines announcing, "Prof. Questions Cigaret–Cancer Link" and "Smoking, Lung Cancer Link Questioned." Quotes from Arkin and other industry-financed skeptics were later used by Lorillard at FTC hearings to defend its Old Gold advertising.[10] Dozens of other scholars were paid for similar services, and by the end of the 1950s it was hard to find a serious scientific doubter who had not taken money from the companies.

What we really see from this point on is the emergence of two scientific communities, one independent of the industry recognizing the reality of tobacco harms and one dependent on the industry servicing its various technical, legal, and political/PR needs. The distinction is not really captured by "leaders" versus "laggards," since many of those co-opted were bright lights in their own fields. Which is also why it's not really right to talk about science versus pseudoscience. The science supported by the industry was typically not of a particularly low quality but rather simply irrelevant to the question of whether tobacco caused harms. The genius of the industry was to create a new kind of science in its macro-sociologic aspect, which I like to call *distraction science* or *red herring research*. Science of this sort could be advertised as "related" somehow to smoking and health while never running the danger of implicating smoking in any kind of harm. Decoy research could be used to distract attention from the "main issue"—the deadly harms of smoking. Much of this was basic research in molecular or cell biology and the like, one purpose of which was to allow the industry to say, "Look how much research we are funding!"

"Alternative causation" was a focus of much of this research, and scholars were employed both to conduct such research and to summarize its value for litigation. Richard E. Shope, a distinguished virologist at the Rockefeller Institute for Medical Research, worked for Philip Morris attorneys in the late 1950s, for example, preparing an analysis of "The Possible Role of Viruses in Cancer" for use in litigation.[11] Work of this sort was needed to buttress the claim that tobacco was only one of many possible causes of cancer and that we might as well blame a virus of some sort, or stress on the job or air pollution, or even baldness or bird mites (birds fluff their feathers, releasing lung-infesting mites). The utility of such arguments was typically higher if the industry's hand in generating them could remain hidden, which may be why Shope failed to disclose his industry connection when he wrote a guest editorial titled "Koch's Postulates and a Viral Cause of Human Cancer" for *Cancer Research*. Robert Koch had developed criteria for disease causation in Germany in the 1880s, as part of an effort to formalize how to identify infectious disease agents. The idea was that if a germ of a particular sort really does cause a particular disease, then one should be able to find that microbe in the body of the afflicted patient. For complex diseases such as cancer, however, Koch's postulates were not terribly useful. Cancers are most often not caused by germs, and the same effect might have many different causes. As summarized by Shope, however, the first of Koch's postulates required that "the investigator should find the agent in every case of the disease."[12] The Rockefeller virologist seems not to have realized that cancer was different: tobacco could be causing a disease even if it could also arise by other means. Lung cancer could derive from exposure to radioactivity or coal tar or metals or a number of other bodily insults, including smoking. The disease is basically a train wreck in the DNA of your lungs, without one single type of exposure being the cause-all in every instance. Shope was myopic on this point, and seems not to have realized that causal models developed for microbial disease were inadequate for understanding chronic, slow-acting, DNA-scrambling diseases caused by toxic pollutants.

Shope was a relatively benign collaborator, but Harry S. N. Greene, chairman of Yale University's Department of Pathology, was closer to what we could call a tobacco hack—a hired gun paid to appear as a witness in regulatory hearings. In 1965 testimony before the U.S. Congress Greene dismissed Wynder et al.'s celebrated mouse-painting studies, claiming that cancer had also been produced in mice "by a variety of common innocuous substances such as salt, sugar, egg white, and cellophane." Epidemiology was also not to be trusted—because it was based on "statistical judgment." Greene had earlier reassured lawmakers at the Blatnik hearings, "If I have a bad cold coming on I smoke a lot of cigarettes and usually wake up in the morning without a cold." The man may have felt a certain bitterness from having failed to produce tumors by means of tobacco extracts placed under the armpits of mice, and we should probably not overlook the fact that by the time he was testifying for Blatnik he had already been smoking for some forty-odd years. British tobacco manufacturers in 1958 recognized Greene as quite out of step in refusing to admit health harms, listing him as one of only a handful of serious scholars still willing to deny any causal link.[13] Industry headhunters scoffed when his name was put forward as a candidate for the job of scientific director at the CTR—the job C. C. Little eventually took—calling him "crazy."

MORE ON HARVARD'S ENGAGEMENTS

Whereas some kinds of co-opting were planned to be invisible, others were supposed to be quite up front, allowing the industry to *brag* about the collaboration. Sponsored research channeled through the TIRC/CTR was displayed in artfully prepared "annual reports," for example, and the industry's many other high-price gifts and grants were always widely publicized. But some collaborations were supposed to be more circumspect.

The University of Kentucky in the 1960s, for example, established a Tobacco and Health Research Program in Lexington headed by Gus W. Stokes, associate dean of the school's College of Agriculture. The program was supposed to assess "the nature and magnitude of the relation of smoking to health," but even Philip Morris recognized this as a stretch, given the absence of any kind of "epidemiological unit which might approach the statistics." Stokes directed the program into the 1970s, when it was renamed the Tobacco and Health Research Institute with new financing from a half-cent per-pack tax on all cigarettes sold in the state. Industry-friendly research was organized with support from Brown & Williamson, which both bankrolled the institute and helped vet grant applications. In this instance, however, the tobacco maker asked *not* to be identified as a sponsor; the university was also not to identify "any information supplied by Brown & Williamson" as coming from the company.[14] Publicity of industry-sponsored research has always been carefully stage-managed, given the dangers of exposing inconvenient truths.

Lawyerly influence was also felt at Harvard's Tobacco and Health Research Program, established via hefty grants from the companies in 1972. The program was actually the brainchild of the Tobacco Institute, which approached Gary L. Huber, chief of respiratory diseases at Boston City Hospital's Harvard Medical Unit. Huber had always been willing to play ball with the companies, pleasing them with his willingness to defend the "constitutional hypothesis" and the possibility of a "safe" cigarette. Huber thought it significant that some people must be more vulnerable to harms than others and at one point confessed to his Reynolds handlers, "As a chest physician, I would like to know which of my patients I should ask to stop smoking." The Harvard project made the industry look good and so was handsomely endowed, absorbing $7 million over an eight-year period. Research topics ranged from animal models for emphysema to smoke chemistry, experimental filters, and human smoking behavior, but the industry seems to have been caught off guard in 1978 when Huber announced, on the basis of human experiments, that low-tar cigarettes probably were no safer and might even be *extra* dangerous insofar as smokers "consistently held the smoke from the low tar cigarettes in their lungs a longer time in an apparent effort to extract more satisfaction from them." This was clear evidence that "low tar" didn't necessarily mean "safer"—and a deep challenge to the industry's principal business strategy of health reassurance. Charles Waite, medical director at the Tobacco Institute, when confronted with these findings conceded that people smoke "for nicotine" and "self-regulate their own dose levels" but derided Huber's experiment as "artificial" and flawed by virtue of using too small a sample size. Waite also claimed that the companies had never implied that low tars were any safer—which was also not entirely accurate.[15]

Huber's Harvard program fell on hard times after this point. Tobacco industry lawyers had always supervised his work, but attorneys from Lorillard, Shook, Hardy, and Brown & Williamson now started cautioning that he was "getting too close to some things." As Huber's relationship with the industry soured, his money faucet was turned off. By 1980 the industry had decided his work was not worth the embarrassment; his Harvard grant was axed, the program closed. Huber many years later learned (or so he claimed) that he had been used as a pawn in the industry's doubt-mongering campaign, wasting fifteen years of his career to discover what the companies already knew from work in their own laboratories. Attorneys suing the industry showed him documents demonstrating his role in this scheme, and he agreed to testify against his former benefactors in court, exposing their duplicitous manipulation of science.[16]

Harvard has had many other engagements with the industry. The physical anthropologist Carl Seltzer in the 1950s tried to correlate propensity to smoke with body type, and the 1964 Surgeon General's report has an entire chapter on "The Morphological Constitution of Smokers" featuring Seltzer as an authority. (Nonsmoking Harvard sophomores supposedly had anatomic traits tending toward "the extreme masculine form.") Seltzer liked to play up his Harvard connection even though he never held a permanent position, living mainly off tobacco industry contracts run through either the Peabody Museum or the School of Public Health. Seltzer testified for cigarette makers in numerous public hearings and in 1972 appeared as a nerdy white-coat in the Tobacco Institute's denialist film, *Smoking and Health: The Need to Know.* Seltzer here characterized smokers as "more aggressive, outgoing, extroverted people—hard driving, full of tension," implying that personality traits such as these might well be causing them both to smoke and to succumb to heart disease. His bottom line: "We do not know whether or not there is a causal relationship between smoking and heart disease."

Harvard atoned for some of this in 2002, when its School of Public Health decided henceforth to refuse all sponsored research from the industry. Right-minded universities were starting to wake up to the dangers of such collaborations: more than a dozen banned tobacco-industry sponsorship in the 1990s, and in the new millennium these were joined by the Karolinska Institute (which hands out the Nobel Prize in medicine), Johns Hopkins, Emory, the University of Berlin, and several dozen others—many of which are in Australia, which has one of the world's strongest tobacco prevention movements. Several of these schools had suffered public relations embarrassments when concerned journalists exposed their faculty as having aided and abetted the world's largest industrial killer.[17]

SPONGING UP FOR BIG TOBACCO:
SAFE TOPICS AT WASHINGTON UNIVERSITY

Academic collaboration takes many different forms,[18] and in some instances the school owes its very existence to cigarette philanthropy. Duke University in Durham, North Carolina, fits this bill, but so does the Bowman Gray School of Medicine in Winston-Salem. Bowman Gray Sr. was R. J. Reynolds's powerful president (from 1924 to 1931) and later chairman of the board (1931–35), steering the company through its turbulent post–trust bust years. When Gray died in 1935, a bequest of $750,000 from his estate was granted to Wake Forest School of Medicine on the condition that it relocate to Winston-Salem, a hundred miles to the west, where it joined with the local Baptist Hospital to become a four-year medical college. Bowman Gray for more than half a century was one of only two American medical schools named for a tobacco magnate (Duke was and remains the other). Bowman Gray changed its name to Wake Forest University School of Medicine in 1997, feeling perhaps that a medical school honoring a tobacco baron might not be in the best interest of public relations. No such taint seems to have attached to the Weissman School of Arts and Sciences at Baruch College, named for Philip Morris President and CEO George Weissman (and his wife), or to Wills Hall at the University of Bristol, honoring W. D. & H. O. Wills, the British tobacco magnates. One wonders whether students or even faculty know what line of work their benefactors were in.[19]

Bowman Gray's scientific collaboration began in 1944, when a Tobacco Research Laboratory was established at the school with financial support from R. J. Reynolds. Nicotine metabolism was one early object of study, with the quest being to show that "even in heavy smokers" there was "no significant accumulation of nicotine in the blood." Bowman Gray scholars later did radioisotope tracer work for cigarette manufacturers. The industry's funding of such research was often not disclosed in publications: in 1948, when scholars from the school's Tobacco Research Laboratory published on nicotine metabolism, the authors credited only the "Medical Relations Division of William Esty and Company, Inc.," failing to reveal that the laboratory itself was a Reynolds creation. So, too, though, was the Medical Relations Division of Esty, Reynolds's principal advertising agency, which had coughed up such wonders as the "More Doctors Smoke Camels" campaign.[20]

Washington University in St. Louis has been another big sponge for tobacco money. Chancellor Thomas H. Eliot announced an initial $2 million grant in the spring of 1971, noting that this was the largest tobacco industry grant ever awarded to a single institution. Millions more were eventually funneled into the School of Medicine, turning it into a hotbed of cigarette-friendly activism. The nominal purpose was to support basic research in tumor immunology, but the underlying goal was to generate good PR and political allies. President Nixon had declared war on cancer that year, and the Tobacco Institute wanted to be able to claim it was doing its part to help promote "early detection, treatment and possible prevention of cancer in man." Newspapers reported glowingly on the collaboration, and Chancellor Eliot and TI President Horace Kornegay joined in praising the alliance as helping to "broaden man's basic understanding of cancer." The expressed goal was to better grasp the biochemistry of tumors, with the hope that cancer-specific antigens of the lung might be identified that could be used to help develop "blood tests to detect early lung cancer."[21]

The irony of Big Tobacco spending millions to explore lung cancer treatment and prevention seems to have been missed by Washington University's faculty taking the cash. The goal was clearly more than cancer cures; the industry also hoped to generate good PR and academic allies. Project director Paul E. Lacy, a distinguished pathologist and "father of islet cell transplants," in 1978 agreed to write to Congressman John E. Moss, commending his cigarette benefactors for their "remarkable foresight and generosity" in supporting research. Lacy was equally effusive in correspondence with the Tobacco Institute, praising the "wisdom and vision of the Tobacco Companies and Tobacco Associates," sentiments also echoed by the university's new chancellor, William H. Danforth. Lacy outlined the kinds of questions made researchable by the industry's "vision":

> The understanding of the basic cause of cancer in Man will be accomplished by determining the biochemical changes induced in cells by a viral agent or a chemical agent. Do the viral and chemical agents produce the same biochemical changes leading to cancer? Does a chemical agent pave the way for the action of a viral agent? Do both of these agents affect the repair mechanism for DNA in the cell?[22]

These were all of course "safe" topics, with tobacco conveniently overlooked in all this talk of viral and biochemical causation. Lacy's codirector, a pathologist by the name of Lauren V. Ackerman, offered an equally friendly vision of cancer research, stressing the dangers (!) of treating man "as an experimental animal":

> The ultimate purpose of cancer research is to develop a means of eradicating cancer in Man. If cancer is to be eliminated by removal from the environment—this ever growing list of potential carcinogens—then the only practical resolution of the problem would be to treat mankind as an experimental animal, house them in a sterile environment, destroy the basis of their society and deprive them of their present human

rights. Fortunately a new era is evolving in cancer research which provides some rays of hope towards achieving the ultimate objective of cancer research—the era of immunology of cancer.[23]

This was an oddly common worry, that nailing down cancer hazards would require the forcible isolation of smokers from non-smokers to see which developed cancer. The industry's approach was presented as more sober, more "cautious," more cellular.

Newspapers like the *St. Louis Globe-Democrat* swallowed this line, that tobacco firms were "Helping in [the] Fight against Cancer":

> For nine years, a prestigious group of researchers at Washington University has been quietly working with millions of dollars from the nation's leading cigarette manufacturers in an effort to untangle the cellular snarl of cancer.
>
> Through a better understanding of how cancer develops, they say, scientists may eventually be able to develop "gene therapies" through which the devastating disease could be prevented—or its victims cured.
>
> At a time when many are groping for quick answers and magical cures, the Washington University team, led by the highly-esteemed Dr. Paul E. Lacy, is slowly and meticulously studying the behavior of genetic material and the intricacies of intracellular interactions.[24]

Washington University by this time was returning the favors. Professor Theodor D. Sterling from computer science was twisting biostatistics to exonerate tobacco, and Professor Joseph H. Ogura from otolaryngology was receiving $24,000 to carry out CTR Special Project 77, authorized to demonstrate "the significance of air pollution and nasal obstruction as influences on the development of lower airway disease."[25] (Not tobacco, in other words.) The historian of medicine Kenneth Ludmerer from the School of Medicine would later become one of the industry's principal defenders in court (see chapter 24).

WYNDER'S TAINT

There is a certain irony in Washington University's collaboration, given that this is where Wynder and Graham had conducted their pioneering lung cancer epidemiology, published in 1950. The irony loses part of its punch, however, once we realize how closely Wynder himself ended up working with Big Tobacco. We saw in chapter 13 how much of Sloan-Kettering's research in the early 1950s—including some of Wynder's work—was industry sponsored, through monies clandestinely channeled from the American Tobacco Company via the Damon Runyon Memorial Fund. Sloan-Kettering continued to take funds from the industry in the 1960s and 1970s thanks to its tobacco-friendly director, Frank L. Horsfall, who thought cigarettes were getting "undue blame" for cancer (and liked the man-sized taste of

Marlboros). Wynder in the mid-1970s expanded the research facility he had founded—the American Health Foundation—with financial aid from Philip Morris and even allowed the tobacco-allied firm of Ruder & Finn to handle public relations. Ruder & Finn sanitized press releases issued by the foundation, allowing the firm to boast to Philip Morris, "we have handled it so there is not one single mention of the problem of smoking and health." Wynder ended up taking around $6 million from the industry over a period of several decades, during which time he supported efforts to make a "safer" cigarette and other smoke-friendly causes, denying even the secondhand smoke–cancer link. Wynder had made it clear—from the mid-1950s—that he wanted not to eliminate but rather only to "improve" cigarettes: as Philip Morris gleefully summarized it, he was not really "anti-tobacco" but rather "pro-improved tobacco."[26]

Wynder never publicly acknowledged taking money from the industry, even though in at least one instance he seems to have allowed Philip Morris to ghostwrite a paper later revised for publication under his name. (Linking dietary fat and lung cancer, the paper fit nicely with the industry's "alternate causation" obfuscation.) The industry also recognized Wynder as an ally in the secondhand smoke arena, characterizing him as a scholar who, despite being "against us on the primary issue" (i.e., death from mainstream smoke), might nonetheless be willing to "speak up in our favor on the ETS issue," helping thereby to marginalize "the more rabid or silly antis." Philip Morris's funding for Wynder started drying up in the mid-1990s, when colleagues at his facility showed that exposure to sidestream smoke resulted in measurable levels of carcinogens in the bodies of non-smokers. Nicole Fields and Simon Chapman in an important review of this history have concluded that Wynder's collaboration threw the companies "a decades long public relations lifeline." And that even in retrospect, toward the end of his life, Wynder "realised the insidious effect of tobacco industry research support but failed to acknowledge this may have applied to his own association with the industry."[27]

TOBACCO LARGESSE AT UCLA

UCLA has been another significant recipient of tobacco largesse. The university had taken tobacco money before, but a new level of involvement began in 1974, when the School of Medicine was awarded a multimillion-dollar grant to establish a "Program on Tobacco and Health." As with all such projects, industry lawyers (notably Shook, Hardy and Bacon) played a key role in the decision to fund—with the companies also conceding that the decision "should be based more on public relations than on purely scientific grounds." The project involved a number of distinguished faculty in the medical school, with topics including immunotherapy, early detection, the impact of silica dust and other environmental pollutants on bronchial ciliary function, and "a possible relationship between tobacco and disease, particularly lung cancer." The goal was to advance our understanding of "complex inter-locking systems which defend our airways against foreign invaders," but one sen-tence in the proposal must have caught the tobacco man's eye: Martin J. Cline, UCLA's Bowyer Professor of Medical Oncology and chief of hematology-oncology, in a letter outlining his planned course of study reassured the makers of Kool, Viceroy, Raleigh, and Barclay cigarettes that "we have no strong scientific evidence that tobacco is causally related to cancer."[28]

Flush with tobacco money, Martin Cline et al. studied how the lung defends it-self, giving little attention to the primary agent known to be attacking it. Over $2 million had been shoveled to UCLA by 1979, with another million approved for an extension beginning that year. And Cline repaid the favor by helping the industry with its legal defense. Shook, Hardy and Bacon flew him to Kansas City to lecture its lawyers on cancer causation, and in 1997 he appeared as an expert witness for the defense in *Broin v. Philip Morris,* a class action suit brought by flight attendants suffering from maladies caused by exposure to secondhand smoke. Cline here testified that while smoking might well be a "risk factor" for certain diseases, it could never be conclusively determined to be causal in any given individual—even those who smoked three packs a day for twenty years. Cline also denied having any knowl-edge of smoking being addictive.[29]

Tobacco collaborators at UCLA have attracted their fair share of criticism from public health advocates, and for understandable reasons. An epidemiologist by the name of James Enstrom has taken much of this heat, by virtue of having been so willing to carry water for the industry. Enstrom, with a Ph.D. in physics from Stan-ford, first came to the industry's attention in 1974, following widespread media hoopla surrounding his work casting doubts on whether tobacco abstinence alone could account for the low cancer rates of Mormons. The Tobacco Institute in its *Newsletter* commented favorably on his work, especially his view that there must be "some other factor beyond not smoking or drinking" behind Mormon longevity. Anne Duffin, a senior executive (and Special Projects director) at the Tobacco In-stitute, sought him out and in the spring of 1975 invited him to apply for a CTR grant, which he did with Lester Breslow as principal investigator (Enstrom was never a tenured member of the faculty). Enstrom asked Duffin to put in a good word for him at the CTR, adding that he was "distressed" about the one-sided nature of the evidence being presented on tobacco and cancer:

> It is hard for me to understand how the rising cigarette consumption during this cen-tury could, by itself, be having a serious adverse [effect] on the health of Americans, when the age-adjusted death rate from all causes has steadily declined by about 1% a year for at least the last 40 years, including declines in every age group.[30]

Duffin politely declined to intervene on Enstrom's behalf, explaining that a letter from her would be inappropriate since "the Council and the Institute have always operated autonomously, each assiduously avoiding the other's areas of responsibility within the tobacco industry." She did express her hope he would publish his "doubts in the cigarette hypothesis." She also blind copied her encouraging words to Robert C. Hockett, research director of the CTR, with an attached comment: "Bob—Enstrom and I have exchanged info sporadically since we met at an epidemiologic meeting last yr. Soft soap here, I'm afraid!" So much for "assiduously avoiding each other's areas of responsibility"![31]

Enstrom was attractive to the industry as a classic "we need more research" skeptic. From the 1970s into the 2000s he published a steady stream of articles challenging the significance of tobacco to health. The documents reveal a certain combative streak and sense of an uphill fight, as in 1997, when Enstrom requested $150,000 from Philip Morris's director of scientific affairs to explore the health effects of environmental tobacco smoke (ETS), insisting that a "substantial research commitment" was required "to effectively compete against the large mountain of epidemiologic data and opinions that already exist regarding the health effects of ETS and active smoking."[32]

Contrarian epidemiology of this sort has infuriated mainstream epidemiologists, but it has also raised the ire of a larger body of scholars who worry that Big Tobacco's funding has so fundamentally compromised the scholarly enterprise that the only solution is to refuse all tobacco corporate sponsorship. Federal Judge Kessler in her 2006 ruling in *USA v. Philip Morris* commented on the flawed nature of Enstrom's work, much of which was "litigation oriented"; the court also noted that the cigarette makers had gone so far as to organize a scientific collaborator for the man— Geoffrey C. Kabat, a long-standing Wynder sidekick—who went on to coauthor further denialist papers with Enstrom, including a much-criticized 2003 article in the *British Medical Journal* that found it "premature to conclude that environmental tobacco smoke causes deaths from coronary heart disease and lung cancer." It may seem strange to hear a federal court weighing in on an epidemiologic dispute, but such has been the power of the industry to corrupt science that even distinguished peer-reviewed journals have not escaped the taint. Enstrom continues even today to defend his work against the medical mainstream, aided by a total of at least $1.4 million in research support from the tobacco racketeers along with an undisclosed sum from years of private consulting for their co-conspiring legal arms.[33]

UCLA's dance with the devil got more press in 2007, when the university was found to have accepted a $6 million grant from Philip Morris to compare how children's brains and monkey brains react to nicotine. Researchers defended the project as potentially of use for improving cessation methods, but the question then of course was, why would Philip Morris want to help people quit? And how could we ever be sure that research along these lines would not be used by the industry to design more addictive cigarettes? Skepticism was also directed at the fact that vervet monkeys were being used in these experiments: the monkeys were being fed liquid nicotine and later killed and dissected to understand how nicotine was affecting the primate brain. Teenage smokers were also enrolled in the study, with children as young as fourteen having their brains scanned to look for CNS effects.[34] And parents were not told this was research sponsored by the cigarette industry. (The secrecy surrounding the project was such that UCLA refused even to provide a full copy of the grant to the chairman of the UC Board of Regents.) Much of the public's attention was diverted when animal rights activists damaged the home of one of the investigators, but the more fundamental ethical issue remains: Should Big Tobacco be funding research into children's brains? And should primates be sacrificed for this purpose?

We don't yet have a good history of animal abuse in the cigarette industry. The topic deserves further study, as does the larger question of whether universities should be taking such money in the first place. Dozens of universities now have policies refusing tobacco industry–sponsored research, and several granting agencies now require such a policy as a condition for scholars or even institutions to apply for grants. Judge Kessler's 2006 finding (upheld on appeal) that the industry has violated federal RICO racketeering laws may embolden such refusals: universities are not obligated to take money from everyone who offers it, and many of our finest have recognized this danger to scholarly integrity. Academic freedom is often invoked by those wanting to continue such relationships, but this is a hollow defense given the corruption involved in taking money from Big Tobacco. Universities do not have to take money from racketeers. Judge Kessler identified the industry's sponsorship of research as central to the industry's ongoing conspiracy to defraud the American public, and it is not such a big step from this to realize that scholars should not be in bed with such knaves.

DIE LUFT DES TABAKS WEHT

Harvard, Washington University, and UCLA have come into focus, but singling out these institutions may be a bit unfair, given that scholars throughout the world have gorged themselves on tobacco money. Indeed it may well be the rare institution that has *not* at one time or another dipped into this pot.

At Stanford University where I now teach, for example, at least eighteen faculty members have received monies (in the form of sponsored research) from the Council for Tobacco Research, with at least two of these—Judith Swain and Hugh McDevitt from the medical school—serving on its Scientific Advisory Board. Stanford pharmacologists were assisting the industry with its diethylene glycol studies as early as the 1930s, and by 1954 Bay Area newspapers were reassuring readers that "Stanford Tests Hint Cigaret Smoke May Prevent Some Cancer in Mice"—referring to the work of A. Clark Griffin, a Stanford biochemist who was also part of the American Tobacco–Runyon Fund–Sloan-Kettering circle.[35] Stanford scholars received

support from the TIRC/CTR throughout its forty-odd years of scientific misdirec-
tion, in addition to grants from the Center for Indoor Air Research and grants provided directly from the companies. The CTR and CIAR were dismantled under the
terms of the 1998 Master Settlement Agreement, but Stanford professors continued to get money from Philip Morris's External Research Program (PMERP)—
which was really just the CIAR revived. And it was not until 2007 that the university's last recipient of tobacco money, John P. Cooke, a professor of cardiovascular
medicine, agreed to give up his Philip Morris grant in response to concerns that I
and other professors—notably Hank Greely, Bernd Girod, and Robert Jackler—
had raised about the ethics of such collaborations. Stanford's Faculty Senate was
split over whether to expressly *bar* its scholars from accepting such funds, but the
issue was rendered moot shortly thereafter, in the fall of 2007, when Philip Morris
terminated its External Research Program, realizing that the negative publicity
outweighed any public relations value. (Funding in some instances was simply
continued by the Philip Morris company without any links to the now-defunct
PMERP.)[36]

Stanford researchers have also done contract work for the companies and served
as expert witnesses on their behalf.[37] A remarkable example of the former is a 1996–
97 grant from R. J. Reynolds to the university's Aviation Safety Laboratory, designed
to test the hypothesis that "nicotine enhances performance in non-smoking pilots."
In an experiment designed by Martin S. Mumenthaler and Jerome A. Yesavage from
Stanford's School of Medicine (Department of Psychiatry), sixteen licensed aircraft
pilots were given nicotine polacrilex gum or a placebo and tested for performance
on a Frasca 141 flight simulator. These nicotinized pilots were measured twelve times
per second for physiological variables and scored on twenty-three flight performance criteria, then compared against an unexposed group of controls. Mumenthaler's study was part of a larger Reynolds ploy to foster research into what they
called the "positive aspects" area, meaning science that would spotlight the sunny
side of smoking. And Reynolds must have liked the study's conclusion that nicotine "may improve overall flight performance in non-smoking aviators." Reynolds
sponsored research for PR or commercial purposes; the whole point was to find
"positive aspects" of smoking that could be disseminated "to both scientific and lay
audiences." And the company was delighted to be able to report its Stanford collaborators as having shown that "nicotine enhances performance of airplane pilots."
These words appear on Reynolds stationery with a reminder on the bottom of every
page: "We work for smokers."[38]

Another Stanford project involved Paul Switzer, a professor in the Department
of Statistics hired to undermine the U.S. Environmental Protection Agency's classification of secondhand smoke as a "Group A carcinogen." The EPA had come to
this conclusion in the fall of 1990, following which it circulated a draft report to obtain comments from interested parties. Switzer was hired along with a string of other

scholars to evaluate the report, and the industry got what it paid for. Switzer denounced the EPA's report as highly flawed and "problematic," peppering his critique with pejoratives like "astonishing," "equivocal," "deceptive and pointless," and "serious difficulties." The Stanford statistician accused the EPA of imprecision, inconsistency, faulty interpretations, improper extrapolations, use of "crude and disputable" estimates of exposure, bias from confounding and misclassification, improper treatment of publication bias, reliance on inconsistent or improperly recorded data, and several other flaws.[39]

Switzer was well paid for his services, receiving a total of $647,046 from CIAR and other grants in one two-year period. He was also paid handsomely for private consultations with cartel law firms. In one three-month period in the fall of 1991 he received $26,900 from Covington & Burling for consulting on "health effects of exposure to ETS in the workplace" and an analysis of "epidemiology of spousal smoke exposure and lung cancer." An invoice for the second half of 1995 records his earning $39,280 for further "professional and consulting services" with the same firm, including at least one trip to Paris (Switzer was then billing $265 an hour for work in his office and $395 an hour for travel). Richard Carchman, director of scientific affairs for Philip Morris USA, was his principal contact, though Covington & Burling was usually cutting the checks. And the industry made good use of his work, principally to thwart the enactment of smoke-free indoor air laws. Switzer's belittlement of the EPA was prominently featured in industry propaganda, including a 1991 Philip Morris brochure titled "Environmental Tobacco Smoke: Rush to Judgment," in which the Stanford statistician was the first of several authorities cited:

"I looked at [the draft report] . . . and thought to myself, How would I have graded it? . . . With all due respect to all the work put in, I would not be able to give it a passing grade."

> Dr. Paul Switzer
> PROFESSOR
> DEPARTMENT OF STATISTICS
> STANFORD UNIVERSITY[40]

Also crucial to this story is the fact that academic collaborations of this sort, even when theoretically public, are commonly unnoticed by colleagues. Trevor Hastie, chair of Stanford's Department of Statistics, had no idea his colleagues had been working for the tobacco industry, earning many hundreds of thousands of dollars, until I brought this to his attention in 2007. He was understandably shocked.

I myself, though, was shocked to learn that several of my closest colleagues had been ensnared. I moved to Stanford in the summer of 2004, and it was several years before I learned that Timothy Lenoir, chair of Stanford's Program in History and Philosophy of Science, had helped Philip Morris prepare its defense for a laryngeal cancer case and that Robert McGinn, director of Stanford's Science, Technology, and Society Program, had provided an expert report to help Brown & Williamson keep its internal documents from becoming public. Imagine the gravity of this situation: Lenoir's testimony helped perpetuate the myth that scientists were slow to recognize tobacco's role in causing cancer; and if McGinn had prevailed—or rather the firm that hired him—many of the archives on which this book is based would never have seen the light of day. What price to trumpet darkness?[41]

ENRICHING STATISTICS

Many people I suspect will be surprised to learn how close such collaborations have been—and how far reaching. Consider again the case of statistics. I've highlighted Paul Switzer, but the fact is that *hundreds* of statisticians have worked for the industry, either as experts on staff for a brand name manufacturer or as consultants to the companies or their law firms or as witnesses at hearings or in court. This includes some rather distinguished scholars. Joseph Berkson at the Mayo Clinic in Minnesota, for example, was paid handsomely for his services (in the 1950s), as was Ronald A. Fisher, the eminent biostatistician and eugenicist. Prior to the 1960s, in fact, Berkson and Fisher were two of the most ardent critics of the "cigarette hypothesis": Sir Ronald because he was a "blame-it-all-on-the-genes" hereditarian, and Berkson because he couldn't imagine a single factor (like tobacco) causing so many different kinds of disease. Rumors swirled after Fisher's death in 1962 that he had either reversed himself on his deathbed or explained away his truculence as opportunism. David Daube, the Oxford biblical scholar, recalls Fisher telling him shortly before his death that his defense of tobacco was simply "for the money."[42]

Statisticians have often testified for the industry at hearings. K. Alexander Brownlee, a Fellow of the Royal Statistical Society and author of two textbooks on statistics, in 1969 testified at congressional hearings that even if all smokers were to stop smoking tomorrow, "it really would not make any difference. They would still have the same death rate from lung cancer." Leo Katz, a Michigan State statistician, at these same hearings testified there was not yet sufficient evidence to demonstrate "that smoking causes any disease"; Katz blasted the "contrived semantics" of the Surgeon General's report and claimed to have detected an "almost unanimous criticism" by statisticians of its "extralogical argumentation." Theodor D. Sterling, the Special Projects operative from Washington University, at this same venue characterized efforts to quantify harms caused by smoking as "meaningless" and "beset by errors"; multivariate data in his view could be "made to show almost anything" and had certainly not demonstrated any health harms from smoking. With garbage of this sort clogging public hearings, is it surprising that cigarette makers have been treated with kid gloves by lawmakers?[43]

Far more common, though, has been the provision of private technical expertise, kept quiet. A quick search of the archives reveals numerous academic statisticians serving as consultants to the industry: Alan S. Donnahoe from the University of Richmond, Joseph Fleiss from Columbia, Jean D. Gibbons from the University of Alabama, Richard Hickey from the Wharton School, John and Elisa Kapenga from Western Michigan State, Kenneth Mullen from the University of Guelph, J. E. R. Frijters from Wageningen University in the Netherlands, Daniel Barry from University College in Cork, Carl A. Silver from Drexel, J. B. Spalding from the University of North Texas, Edwin Wilson from Harvard, Arnold Zellner from the University of Chicago, Nathan Mantel from George Washington University, just to name a few.

Most work of this sort is technical and kept far from the prying eyes of the press, but some has been deployed to sensational effect. Darrell Huff, author of the wildly popular (and aptly named) *How to Lie with Statistics,* was paid to testify before Congress in the 1950s and then again in the 1960s, with the assigned task of ridiculing any notion of a cigarette–disease link. On March 22, 1965, Huff testified at hearings on cigarette labeling and advertising, accusing the recent Surgeon General's report of myriad failures and "fallacies." Huff peppered his attack with amusing asides and anecdotes, lampooning spurious correlations like that between the size of Dutch families and the number of storks nesting on the rooftops—which proves not that storks bring babies but rather that people with large families tend to have large houses (which therefore attract more storks). Huff also pointed to the selection bias in the high rate of breast cancer among Chinese men compared to Chinese women—explainable by the reluctance of females to report their maladies. Senator Neuberger moderated the hearings and was flabbergasted by Huff's remarks: "Do you honestly think there is as casual a relationship between statistics linking smoking with disease as there is about storks and Chinese and so on?"[44] Neuberger probably had no idea how carefully lawyered Huff's words were, or how much he was being paid for his debunkery. That same year Huff was also paid to produce an industry-friendly bulletin outlining his views on tobacco and health, with the industry's powerful Ad Hoc Committee reserving rights to allow or disallow publication.[45] And he was later paid to expand his views into a book-length treatment of the topic. Huff in 1968 was paid $10,000 plus expenses to work on his manuscript, and a contract was secured with Macmillan, though the book seems never to have appeared. Huff was a very good catch for the industry, given that his *How to Lie . . .* was—and remains—the most popular book on statistics ever written.[46]

Law firms representing the industry have also had professional statisticians on staff—as have the Tobacco Institute and the various manufacturers. Geoffrey Todd for many years was Imperial Tobacco's top statistician, and in 1968 the firm had "six graduate statisticians" working on mouse experiments and agricultural projects at the company's Bristol laboratories. Philip Morris has had numerous statisticians on staff: John E. Tindall rose to the rank of senior scientist, for example, by helping the company crunch numbers on smokers' perceptions of nicotine deliveries, advertising's impact on sales, "mucociliary studies on cats," and "chronic smoking in cynamolgus monkeys." Academic statisticians are sometimes invited to the companies as visitors: Philip Morris in 1988 paid John and Elisa Kapenga to come to Richmond as "visiting scientists"; and Reynolds had earlier hired H. Alan Lasater from the University of Tennessee, Knoxville, to help with its secret Project Cal (the low-smoke Premier cigarette). Statisticians provide training for tobacco staff: in 1995, for example, Philip Morris hired Daniel Ennis of Richmond's Institute for Perception to present a series of "Statistics Courses" (co-taught with Kenneth Mullen); . Abbott Associates has also been used for this purpose. Tobacco law firms have sometimes even supported graduate students. In 1979, for example, Bernard G. Greenberg of the University of North Carolina (UNC) contacted Marvin Kastenbaum to see if the Tobacco Institute would be willing to support Joseph M. Janis, a student working on a project stemming from Greenberg's litigation work for the industry. The project was handed over for approval to the CTR's lawyers—which is how Janis's Ph.D. dissertation (questioning the lung cancer–tobacco link) became a CTR Special Project. Janis by 1981 had received more than $25,000 from the industry for his dissertation, which was used in legal strategizing by the industry to combat "the primary issue" (cancer causation). As dean of UNC's School of Public Health, Greenberg also helped secure a job for his tobacco-friendly protégé at that university.[47]

Organizational charts in the archives show that Reynolds in the 1980s had at least seven statisticians working in its brands R&D department, with at least five additional statisticians in its technical services department and another six or seven in marketing and marketing research. Brown & Williamson had a comparable crew, as did most European manufacturers. Reemtsma had a team of statisticians under Rolf Kröger, and Germany's powerful Verband der Cigarettenindustrie worked with a number of statisticians, including Wolf-Dieter Heller of Karlsruhe University, who in 1984 let BAT consultants ghostwrite a paper for him attacking Trichopoulos's work on secondhand smoke. Britain's Tobacco Research Council had a statistical subcommittee handling such matters for British tobacco makers; and Peter N. Lee from Britain's Tobacco Advisory Council headed a similar body: the Tobacco Statisticians' Working Group, set up in 1982. No major tobacco manufacturer can operate without statisticians.[48]

Statisticians have serviced the industry in other ways. In 1981, for example, a team of statisticians led by Nathan Mantel of George Washington University was hired to criticize Takeshi Hirayama's paper showing a lung cancer risk in Japanese women exposed to secondhand smoke. The team—which included Alvan R. Feinstein of Yale and Chris P. Tsokos from the University of South Florida—found a "mathematical error" in Hirayama's work, which the Tobacco Institute publicized with an extraordinary media blitz. Hundreds of newspapers throughout the country carried the story, with very few recognizing that cigarette makers had paid for the poke. (The tobacco press described Mantel et al. as "three independent

statisticians," when the reality was that all three had taken money from the tobacco industry—and Feinstein was a Special Projects operative.) The Tobacco Institute managed to dominate media coverage of this story: in a six-week period
in the summer of 1981 Mantel's "error" report was covered in 469 U.S. newspapers with nearly 57 million "potential impressions."[49] During which time the industry's own scholars—notably Fritz Adlkofer from the German Verband der
Cigarettenindustrie—were admitting, albeit quietly, that Hirayama was "correct"
and Mantel et al. "wrong."[50]

Several other statisticians received CTR Special Projects monies; those we know
about include Ingram Olkin at Stanford, Theodor Sterling from Washington University, George Saiger at Columbia, Jacob Yerushalmy from UC Berkeley, and
Roberto Bacchi from Hebrew University in Jerusalem. Edwin Wilson, a Harvard
statistician, was an early member of the Scientific Advisory Board of the TIRC, and
many statisticians received TIRC/CTR or CIAR grants.

The Tobacco Institute itself for many years had a "Department of Statistics," a
position one might compare to the Department of Geology at the Institute for Creation Research. Professional statisticians seem not to have regarded department
head Marvin A. Kastenbaum as tainted or beyond the pale; indeed in 1975 the Stan-
ford-trained statistician was invited to deliver an after-dinner speech at the annual
meeting of the American Statistical Association, the nation's premier professional
body, which Kastenbaum entertained with lawyered stories about how foolish it was
to blame cigarettes for any kind of disease. He also mocked the "priesthood" of public health scientists trying to grapple with an "alleged" increase in lung cancer rates.
Kastenbaum compared worrying about lung cancer to worrying about toxoplas-
mosis from exposure to cats and pulmonary fibrosis from exposure to parakeets.
His speech is a swamp of technical trickery and nitpickery—but it was also clearly
a coup for the Tobacco Institute, securing as it did the embrace of the country's most
distinguished assembly of professional statisticians.[51] It is disturbing enough to have
statisticians shilling for the industry but perhaps just as disturbing that he was invited to deliver such a speech in the first place. In 1955 perhaps, but in 1975?

Statisticians have also assisted the companies with their legal defense in court.
Here are some of those who have taken this bait, along with some of the cases for
which they have testified:

Edwin Luther Bradley Jr., University of Alabama: *Broin v. Philip Morris*
(1997); *Acton v. Reynolds* (1999); *Butler v. Philip Morris* (1999); *Seaborn v.
Reynolds* (2000); *Anderson & Anderson v. Lorillard and Philip Morris*
(2000); *Tompkin v. American* (2001); *USA v. Philip Morris* (2005)

Richard C. Clelland, University of Pennsylvania: *Cipollone v. Liggett* (1987)

Eugene P. Ericksen, Temple University: *Reed v. Philip Morris* (1997); *Richardson v. Philip Morris* (1997); *Brown v. American* (2000)

Jairus D. Flora, Midwest Research Institute: *Sulcer v. Reynolds* (2009); *Walden v. Reynolds* (2009)

Bernard G. Greenberg, University of North Carolina: *Green v. American* (1964)

R. Garrison Harvey, Wecker Associates: *West Virginia Laborers v. Philip Morris* (1999); multiple Engle progeny cases

Maxwell W. Layard, University of California: *AFCO v. TIA* (1990)

Leo Katz, Michigan State University: *Thayer v. Liggett* (1969)

Lynn R. LaMotte, Louisiana State University: *Texas v. American* (1997); *Oklahoma v. Reynolds* (1998)

Paul Levy, University of Illinois at Chicago: *Dunn and Wiley v. RJR Nabisco* (1998)

Brian P. McCall, University of Minnesota: *Minnesota v. Philip Morris* (1998)

James T. McClave, Infotech: *Florida v. American* (1997); *Washington v. American* (1998); *Boeken v. Philip Morris* (2001); *St. Louis v. American* (2009); *Soffer v. Reynolds* (1998)

Daniel L. McGee, Florida State University: *Piendle v. Reynolds* (2010)

Kenneth Duncan MacRae, University of Surrey: *Marsee v. U.S. Tobacco* (1986); *U.S. Tobacco v. Ireland* (1990); *Aho v. Suomen Tupakka Oy* (1991, 1999)

M. Laurentius Marais, Wecker Associates: *Henley v. Philip Morris* (1998); *Bullock v. Philip Morris* (2002)

Ronald G. Marks, University of Florida: *Broin v. Philip Morris* (1997); *Mehlman v. Philip Morris* (2001)

Nancy Mathiowetz, University of Maryland: *Oklahoma v. Reynolds* (1998); *Blue Cross of New Jersey* (2001); *Bullock v. Philip Morris* (2002)

Irwin Miller, Wesleyan University: *Thayer v. Liggett* (1969); *Cipollone v. Liggett* (1987)

Jacqueline Oler, Drexel University: *Burton v. Reynolds* (1996)

Donald B. Rubin, Harvard University: *Texas v. American* (1997); *Florida v. American* (1997); *Mississippi Tobacco Litigation* (1997); *Ironworkers v. Philip Morris* (1998); *Minnesota v. Philip Morris* (1998); *Washington v. American* (1998); *Northwest Laborers v. Philip Morris* (1998, 1999); *USA v. Philip Morris* (2003, 2005)

Herbert Solomon, Stanford University: designated in *Haines v. Liggett* (1992); consulting for *Cipollone* (1987)

Brice M. Stone, Metrica: *Mississippi Tobacco Litigation* (1997); *Florida v. American* (1997)

Larry Tonn, Tonn & Associates: *Texas v. American* (1997); *Oklahoma v. Reynolds* (1998)

Richard Tweedie, Bond University: *AFCO v. TIA* (1990)

William E. Wecker, Wecker Associates: *Broin v. Philip Morris* (1997); *Florida v. American* (1997); *Mississippi Tobacco Litigation* (1997); *Texas v. American* (1997); *Washington v. American* (1998); *Engle v. Reynolds* (1998); *Blankenship v. Philip Morris* (2000); *Whiteley v. Raybestos-Manhattan* (1999, 2000); *Blue Cross* (2000); *Scott v. American* (2000); *Minnesota v. Philip Morris* (1998); *Lucier v. Philip Morris* (2003); *Falise v. American;* and *USA v. Philip Morris* (2005)

Finis R. Welch, Texas A&M: *Texas v. American* (1997)

Janet T. Wittes, Statistics Collaborative, Inc.: *USA v. Philip Morris* (2005)

George H. Worm, Clemson University: *Texas v. American* (1997)

Arnold Zellner, University of Chicago: *Mississippi Tobacco Litigation* (1997)

Statisticians serving in this capacity have typically been asked to challenge the methods used to estimate health harms, medical costs, or some other pillar in the injured party's argument. William E. Wecker, for example, who runs a consulting firm in Novato, California, has testified in more than a dozen such trials, arguing in each case that something other than tobacco might be to blame for a person's death or malady. Wecker has made a career of exculpatory testimony even outside the tobacco realm, arguing that metallic lead is less stupefying than people think and that manufacturing defects are unfairly blamed for auto accidents. Wecker has taken money from both Big Lead and Detroit (GM) via the law firm Kirkland and Ellis, which represents both industries. Plaintiffs' attorneys in tobacco litigation have drawn attention to these parallels, with the common thread being this shifting of blame onto "other factors"—or something about the victim's constitution or behavior.[52] Wecker has been joined in this effort by at least two other statisticians from his firm: Laurentius Marais and R. Garrison Harvey have testified in more than a dozen trials for Big Tobacco. Harvey in the first decade of the new millennium pulled in more than $2,750,000 for his tobacco work, constituting about 22 percent of the Wecker firm's entire business.[53]

Donald B. Rubin, the John L. Loeb Professor of Statistics at Harvard, has been one of the most successful witnesses for the cartel—and one of the most highly paid. In 1997 he was charging $1,000 per hour for consulting and $1,250 for testimony, which he later raised to $1,250 for consulting and $1,600 for testimony. Between 1997 and 2002 Rubin claims to have earned $1.5 million to $2 million working for the industry, and in *USA v. Philip Morris* alone he billed another "several hundred" hours. Rubin typically testifies that the models used by plaintiffs to calculate the health costs of smoking or industry misconduct are inappropriate or contain "fatal mistakes" that, once exposed, give defense attorneys some grounds for tossing the baby out with the bathwater. He has also testified that the industry's long history of lying makes no difference in how many cigarettes are consumed. Rubin, interestingly, is one of only a handful of scholars working for the defense to have publicly defended such work, which he says is simply "defending the importance of honest and competent statistics, that is all."[54] Rubin has also testified, though, that he has only a "layman's" understanding of causality when it comes to smoking. That is typical, this expression of expert ignorance, in effect: "I only know what I was asked to know, nothing more."

What is remarkable about such testimony is how closely it follows the industry's legal line. Indeed nothing makes a tobacco industry witness more uncomfortable than being asked whether smoking causes disease. There are many examples, but consider this testimony of Lynn R. LaMotte, professor of statistics at Louisiana State University, testifying under oath in 1997 for the defense in *Texas v. American Tobacco*:

> Q: Do you have—well, first of all, do you have an opinion as to whether or not cigarettes cause disease?
>
> A: I—I have an impression. I don't—I wouldn't want to call it an opinion, but I have, you know, a general uninformed impression. If I want to call it all opinion, I need some—I need some basis in fact for it, but I have a general impression that—what was the first question?
>
> Q: Let me rephrase it. Dr. LaMotte—
>
> A: Yes.
>
> Q: —do cigarettes cause disease?
>
> A: Okay. So the question is, do I have an opinion as to the truth of that statement; is that correct?
>
> Q: However you want to answer it.
>
> A: I have a general, casual, uninformed lay impression that I think is probably a fairly general impression, that smoking cigarettes may lead to some sort of health deficit.
>
> Q: Well, let me ask you the question in a simple question. And you can say yes, no, or, I really don't know. Do cigarettes cause disease?
>
> A: I'm trying to answer that. I have the—I have an uninformed impression, not anything that I have looked into actively, that—that smoking cigarettes may lead to some kinds of diseases.
>
> Q: Do you have any evidence to the contrary? You seem—the reason I'm asking you is you seem to be waffling—and I don't mean to be critical, but you seem to be trying to dance around the issue of whether cigarettes cause disease. And I'm just trying to find out if that's true or false, in your mind. That's all I'm asking about is [what's] in your mind.
>
> A: Let me explain the source of my discomfort. I'm here as an expert on statistics

and it appears that you're asking my personal opinion, which I'll be glad to give you, but—

Q: Okay. Please.

A: I want to be sure that it's recognized that that's not even an opinion. It's simply a general impression, totally uninformed, without any sort of active effort by me to verify whether there's any truth to it or not. I have a general impression that smoking in some degree is associated with certain diseases. That's—you know, I have that general impression. It's not informed, not expert. I haven't actively tried to solve—to verify whether it's true.

Q: Third time I'm going to ask you the same again. Do cigarettes cause disease?

A: It is my general uninformed impression, without any sort of active effort to determine any scientific way—I don't have any knowledge as to any specific knowledge of what I regard as hard evidence either way, but it's my general impression that smoking cigarettes, stated fairly loosely, may lead to some diseases.

. . . . .

Q: So if I gave you a true or false test—you're a professor. You've taken lots of tests and given lots of tests, right? So if I gave you a true or false test and asked you to answer it true or false or I don't know—I'll give you three answers. And the question is, in your view, Dr. LaMotte, do cigarettes cause disease which results in increased health care costs to treat those diseases?

A: I would have to answer I don't know.[55]

Plaintiffs' lawyers confronted by the industry's "common knowledge" defense should take notice of such opinions and have them read before any jury trying to figure out whether we can expect young smokers to have understood what was in store for them, forty or fifty years down the road, if they continued smoking. If the industry's own experts don't even know that cigarettes cause disease in 1997, why would we imagine ordinary teenagers just starting to smoke to be so much better informed? Why should we expect them to know so much more than a professor, offered by the manufacturer decades later to testify as an expert witness? Of course knowledge may not be the real issue here: Gabriel DiMarco, vice president for research at R. J. Reynolds, once grumbled to senior lawyers at his company that "our medical/scientific witnesses will say whatever we want them to say."[56]

SHOWERED WITH HONORS

I don't know which is more disturbing: the harnessing of statisticians by the industry or the willingness of so many scholars to service the industry in this manner. Are statements such as those quoted above consistent with professional ethics? Are statisticians as a group proud of such collaborations? And if not, why have we seen so few scholarly critiques or exposés of such services? Do they even know it is going on? Where is the collective conscience of the profession? Or should we rather regard such activities as private matters, nobody's business, properly governed only by personal conscience? The American Statistical Association's website does list "Ethical Guidelines" adopted in 1999, one article of which asks statisticians to "provide only such expert testimony as you would be willing to have peer reviewed." But what is the force of such an admonition? Has there ever been any attempt to sanction a colleague for violating such a provision, or to subject such testimony to peer review? And what if a discipline is so thoroughly suffused with tobacco money that one cannot be sure one's peers are not on the take? Could this mean that "peer review" becomes compromised? Something close to this, as we shall see, is the present plight of professional historians, the most benighted of all disciplines in this respect.

Of course we can and should raise such questions for *every* academic discipline—and not just for tobacco work. The tobacco case is particularly egregious, however, given how many different disciplines have been ensnared. A 1999 list of Philip Morris witnesses for the industry includes experts on addiction (e.g., George Seiden), advertising (Timothy P. Meyer), biomedical ethics (Kevin Wildes), cardiology (Malcolm P. Taylor), communications and polling (Dexter Neadle), computer science (Stephen Murrell), diagnostic radiology (David Rosenbach), epidemiology (Robert Verhalen), fire causation (Donald F. Pisculli), hypertension (Suzanne Oparil), insurance underwriting (Jay C. Ripps), law and legal ethics (Martin H. Redish), lobbying (Karl Rove), marketing (Richard J. Semenik), maternal smoking (Jack McCubbin), oncology (Joseph F. Laucius), otolaryngology (John S. Knight), pathology (Emanuel Rubin), pediatrics (Percy Luecke), product integrity (Richard P. Solana), pharmacology (Peter Putnam Rowell), propaganda and persuasion (Thomas M. Steinfatt), psychology (Cecil R. Reynolds), pulmonology (Stephen E. Jacobs), sociology (Rachel Volberg), and toxicology and risk analysis (Andrew Sivak). The individuals named here are sampled from one single document, but some fields have had *dozens* of servicing experts.[57]

One thing that has made such collaboration possible—and easy to conceal—is that when scholars work for the industry, either as consultants or as witnesses, this is rarely divulged to their colleagues. Services of this sort may be nominally public—recorded on some transcript stored in a courthouse—but little publicized. "Public in a copy of one" is how one might think about it. So a cardiologist may be working for the industry while colleagues know nothing about this. A historian may be president of a professional association, with few of its members aware of his or her legal work. This makes it possible for scholars to collaborate with the industry with little or no consequences for their reputations—because colleagues will rarely even be aware that activities of this sort are going on. Which is why we need to shine light on this process: scholars should be held accountable for their public and political engagements, and I would endorse a policy requiring all scholars to disclose all consulting arrangements on university-sponsored websites. And if scholars are not proud of what they are doing or worry about being "outed," then perhaps they should not be doing it in the first place.

The reality has been that, far from being censured or shamed, scholars working for the tobacco juggernaut are very often showered with honors and awards. In an earlier chapter I reviewed the honors won by the cardiologist Suzanne Oparil, but collaborators in many other fields have been similarly fêted. Bernard G. Greenberg, the Special Projects operative and first statistician ever to testify for the industry in court,[58] in 1981 won the O. Max Gardner Award, given annually by the Board of Governors of the University of North Carolina to a faculty member who has made "the greatest contribution to the welfare of the human race." Kenneth Ludmerer was named a Master of the American College of Physicians in 2005, after testifying in more than a dozen trials for the industry. Ludmerer also won the Nicholas E. Davies Memorial Scholar Award for "outstanding contributions to humanism in medicine" and in 2001 won the first Dean Tosteson award, with the Harvard pulmonologist Stephen Weinberger as head of the prize committee. Should lung doctors be giving prizes to scholars who earn hundreds of thousands of dollars defending Big Tobacco?

Other collaborators have had prizes, professorships, or even buildings named for them. The Morris Fishbein Professorship at the University of Chicago honors a long-standing friend of tobacco, as does the Clarence Cook Little Hall at the University of Maine. The John C. Burnham Early Career Award given out by the *Journal of the History of the Behavioral Sciences* honors a former Philip Morris Project Cosmic director (see chapter 24), and Burnham himself in 2009 won the Lifetime Achievement Award from the Society for the History of Psychology—part of the American Psychological Association. The Arnold Zellner Doctoral Prize, awarded to students at the University of Chicago's Booth School of Business, honors a man who testified for the industry in court as an expert witness. Many other prizes have been awarded in the name of scholars who have worked for Big Tobacco—or sometimes even influential tobacco lawyers. The H. Thomas Austern Memorial Writing Competitions—open to students of law throughout the United States—honor a man who became wealthy helping Big Tobacco defend its legal interests. The prize committee's website (organized by the Food and Drug Law Institute) describes Austern as having practiced "food and drug law for over fifty years at the firm of Covington and Burling" but leaves off any mention of the fact that Austern was also a major architect of tobacco's legal strategy. Winners of such handsomely endowed prizes might be surprised to learn where the money came from.

ROCKEFELLER'S SEITZ AND LEDERBERG

When it comes to sponsored research, part of the problem has been that university administrators often don't seem to know much about how the industry operates and what it means to collaborate with such entities. I've mentioned the growing number of institutions refusing such ties, but the more common pattern has been to welcome tobacco's easy money. The archives are full of letters from administrators bowing down before these mighty dispensers of cigarette largesse. In March of 1980, for example, Rockefeller University's executive vice president wrote to Ernest Pebbles, chief counsel of Brown & Williamson, expressing his gratitude for the company's recent gift:

> Dear Ernie:
> Please forgive my delay in writing formally to thank you again for arranging with Mr. Shinn [from Shook, Hardy and Bacon] to visit the campus with Jack Roemer [Reynolds's general counsel] on January 3, joining us for lunch and visits both to our Hospital and to Dr. [Norton D.] Zinder's laboratory. Dr. [Joshua] Lederberg sincerely regretted that he was not able to return from the West Coast prior to your visit then, and so he was delighted that he could meet you on February 6.
> I hope that during these recent meetings we have conveyed an overall perspective on the missions that the University—earlier the Rockefeller Institute—continues to fulfill in the development of biomedical research in the U.S. . . . In any case, now that B&W is a major partner in our work—and many thanks again for so quickly arranging the generous grant of $90,000—we look forward to frequent exchanges on many subjects of mutual interest. . . . We look forward to welcoming you back to the campus often.[59]

Rockefeller President (and Nobel laureate) Joshua Lederberg was equally thrilled to have Big Tobacco on campus, writing to Reynolds's CEO ("Dear Paul") to express how "tremendously grateful" he was for the company's "extraordinary generosity." Six years later Lederberg wrote to the top lawyer for Brown & Williamson, maker of Viceroy and Kool cigarettes: "I know you will share our pride in the caliber of scientific endeavor made possible by your partnership with us in the expansion of knowledge for human benefit. . . . Your company's support has been a source of much encouragement to us all." Lederberg listed some of the uses to which this money was being put, including the study of illness from parasitic infection (in global terms "the leading health problem"); purchase of a nuclear magnetic resonance spectrometer; and expansion of a dermatology center exploring "carcinogenic damage that may result from the toxic effects of atmospheric oxygen and from exposure to chemicals, drugs, and ultraviolet irradiation." Cigarettes of course go unmentioned, and the tobacco men must have been pleased to see this friendly neglect.[60]

Of course one could argue that Rockefeller was just taking the industry's money in order to advance the cause of basic science. And what harm could there be in that? (A senior Stanford medical colleague of mine likes to say that the only problem with "tainted" money is that there "'taint enough of it.") Collaborations of this sort, though, allow tobacco manufacturers to advertise themselves as responsible corporate citizens, promoters of science and the noble goals of medical research. Such was the case in 1975, when the makers of Camel cigarettes established the R. J. Reynolds Industries Postdoctoral Fellowship at Rockefeller, endowed with a gift to the university of $300,000. That same year an additional $2.5 million was promised to establish a five-year R. J. Reynolds Fund for the Biomedical Sciences and Clinical Research on campus, characterized by the company as "an effort to achieve progress in understanding the basic causes of the principal diseases afflicting mankind." As explained in company documents, however, the goal was also "to furnish tangible evidence of the Company's commitment to good citizenship on a major national scale in a field of great potential benefit to mankind."[61]

Rockefeller's enthusiasm for such arrangements becomes clearer, once we understand the personal devotion of Lederberg's predecessor to the tobacco cause. Frederick Seitz, president of Rockefeller from 1968 to 1978, was a powerful figure in American science, serving as both president of the National Academy of Sciences (1962–69) and a member of President Richard Nixon's Science Advisory Board (which must have helped him win the National Medal of Science—for his work in solid-state physics). Seitz was also, though, an enthusiastic advocate for R. J. Reynolds and its denialist cause—and later a vociferous denier of global warming.[62] The man had zero medical credentials, but that didn't prevent him from being hired (in 1979) to head Reynolds's new Medical Research Committee (MRC), the chief conduit through which the Camel makers dispensed funds for external medical research. Seitz was joined on this committee by Alvan Feinstein, the well-heeled CTR Special Projects operative at Yale, and Leon Golberg, a corporate confederate from the Chemical Industry Institute of Toxicology in North Carolina.

Seitz's job as head of the MRC was basically to help decide how to turn a sliver of Reynolds's profits into "basic research in the field of degenerative diseases." None of this work implicated tobacco in any kind of illness.[63] Kenneth Moser at San Diego was exploring a causal role for fungi in lung disease; Joseph Post at NYU was studying hormone therapies for breast cancer; and Hidesaburo Hanafusa at Rockefeller was probing "certain virus-induced cancers in fowl." Seitz knew that "only a few human cancers seem to be linked to virus infections," but he also informed his paymaster that research along these lines had produced a "detailed working model of a cancer-causing system at the molecular level." Seitz reviewed other work funded by Reynolds: on cellular membranes and stem cells at Colorado's School of Medicine, on chromosomal markers for genetic diseases at Rockefeller, on viral diseases at the Wistar Institute, and similar work at Duke, the University of Utah, the Eleanor Roosevelt Institute for Cancer Research in Denver, and so forth. All perfectly respectable science, and perfectly irrelevant (or worse) to the problem of tobacco and disease. Seitz characterized Reynolds-funded work at the Southwest Research Institute (San Antonio) on pedigreed baboons as showing "high promise of adding to our store of information regarding the relative influence of diet and genetics on the development of arteriosclerosis," deflecting attention from tobacco. Seitz sometimes recommended support for projects already funded by federal agencies: a Columbia University effort to establish blood biomarkers "to single out individuals who are at special risk for contracting emphysema," for example, Seitz urged as exceptionally fund-worthy. Seitz himself profited handsomely in this capacity: *Vanity Fair* in 2006 reported his having earned about $585,000 from Reynolds for his work as a company adviser.[64]

Joshua Lederberg continued this friendly relationship with Tobacco in 1978, when Seitz retired as Rockefeller's president. The archives preserve a record of President Lederberg telling Brown & Williamson about his desire to see research into "the effect of depriving people of cigarette privileges when they are under stress." Brown & Williamson by this time was providing hundreds of thousands of dollars to Rockefeller, and Lederberg himself was quietly servicing the company as a paid consultant—while serving as Rockefeller's president. We don't know much about what he was doing; it apparently had something to do with the FTC's ongoing investigation of the Barclay filter. We do know that the very existence of this consulting arrangement was to be held in "absolute confidentiality." Rockefeller academics would continue chumming around with tobacco executives for quite some time: on April 1, 1988, for example, Reynolds flew half a dozen of its corporate higher-ups (by private jet) to Manhattan to explain to Lederberg, Seitz, and others at the university the virtues of the company's new "smokeless" Premier cigarette.[65]

NAÏVETÉ AND GREED

I've cited ingratiating letters from Lederberg and Seitz to cigarette makers, but *hundreds* of such letters from university administrators are preserved in the tobacco archives. Collaborations of this sort were made possible by a confluence of political naïveté and greed. These were surely not ignorant men, but perhaps we should not overestimate their understanding of the sociology of knowledge and the potential for bias. An overly narrow conception of the nature of science could well have led some of these scholars to fail to see their role as pawns in larger schemes of knowledge management. Or maybe it's better just to talk about naïveté and greed. University administrators may well have failed to see any harm in taking such money, imagining perhaps that in moving from cigarette profits to research funds, the lucre of the Camel men was cleansed of its questionable origins. No one was ever forced to take such money, after all, and recipients were nominally free to do with it as they wished. This is a very narrow view of how science works, however. Research relationships build up, there are incentives to please, PR comes into play, and there is a *subject matter skew* to what gets funded, altering the balance of research priorities on campus. Scholars taking such funds may be free to research whatever they want, but the companies make sure that money only goes to topics (and scholars) judged harmless or even helpful to the cigarette cause. And hand-shakes of course make good photo ops, and the industry garners laurels.

The industry sponsors academic research because it polishes its reputation, pro-viding it with a semblance of authority and legitimacy. In a nutshell: How can we be so bad if Stanford and Harvard and UCLA are helping us? The names of such insti-tutions are used for public relations purposes. In 1988, for example, the Tobacco In-stitute published a brochure titled *In the Public Interest: Three Decades of Initiatives by a Responsible Cigarette Industry,* citing sponsorship of University of California scholars as evidence of its corporate responsibility. In a section titled "Scientific Re-search" we learn that UCLA's School of Medicine had been given a $2.75 million grant to investigate "lung defense mechanisms including early detection and treatment of cancer." The Council for Tobacco Research issued a press release celebrating this same grant, citing it as evidence of the industry's honest and sincere "efforts over the past two decades to resolve questions about smoking and health." E. A. Horrigan, RJR's chairman of the board, had made similar arguments in a 1984 publication titled *An Open Debate.* In a section of this glossy brochure labeled "No Scientific Proof," Hor-rigan claimed that evidence of a smoking–disease link had been based only "on sta-tistical studies, not on scientifically established proof of cause." The brochure also claimed that the industry was trying to find answers by financing "independent re-search at such institutions as Harvard University, the University of California at Los Angeles, Washington University and other top centers of scientific research."[66]

Of course it is not just the *name* of the university that is coveted; there is also the desire to win friends and stockpile useful facts and solve certain legal or PR prob-lems or otherwise strengthen the ability to sell cigarettes. Why did Reynolds in the mid-1970s give the University of Washington in Seattle $2.8 million for a five-year project on cardiovascular disease? The industry's archives reveal a desire to exer-cise "influence on the scientists and doctors there," and specifically to use such con-tacts to spread the word that "tobacco people are not ogres." Why did Philip Mor-ris give the psychiatrist Redford Williams at Duke $4.75 million? They liked his idea of heart attacks being more common among "angry" people—because "hostiles" secrete more of certain hormones that can also cause heart attacks.[67] The industry has long had this goal of funding not just skeptics or sycophants, or persons skilled in scientific sleight of hand, but also scholars who have some way of making nico-tine look good.

Similar goals were in play when Philip Morris sponsored John P. Cooke's work at Stanford. Cooke, a distinguished cardiologist, was an early recipient of money from the company's External Research Program, an organization set up in 2000 to continue the work of the Council for Tobacco Research and Center for Indoor Air Research (in violation of the 1998 Master Settlement Agreement—so ruled the court in *USA v. Philip Morris*). Cooke had been doing experimental work showing that nicotine promoted angiogenesis—growth of new blood vessels—which for a time looked like it might have commercial prospects in the form of nicotine-coated stents. The theory was that nicotine would help promote the growth of new blood vessels, speeding the recovery of people who had undergone heart surgery. Philip Morris liked this idea of a therapeutic use for nicotine and authorized a multimillion-dollar grant to support Cooke's research. The work was clearly of public relations value, which is why the *Tobacco Reporter* published an article extolling the Stanford professor's work on what it called the "Healing Weed":

> The news has been conveniently ignored by tobacco's adversaries, but recent studies indicate that, aside from its well-known risks, the golden leaf may have some health *benefits*. More and more research is showing that certain tobacco compounds offer protection against medical disorders, such as brain diseases like Parkinson's disease and Tourette's syndrome.
>
> Much like the rainforests have been a plentiful source of compounds for developing new pharmaceuticals, tobacco fields could be the next gold mine for the pharmaceutical industry.

The article goes on to describe how Cooke et al.'s research proves that "certain tobacco compounds have therapeutic qualities," allowing us to conclude that *Nicotiana* is "not merely the 'evil weed' that some public health activists make it out to be."[68] Cooke would later defend the right of faculty to collaborate with the industry as a basic academic freedom but only after he himself decided to turn down future funding from the tobacco maker, to avoid all appearances of impropriety.

BERGER'S ENTANGLEMENT

The TI, CTR, CIAR, and PMERP were well-oiled vehicles for the industry's doubt-mongering in the United States, but other kinds of academic front groups have been established in other parts of the world. In 1988, for example, when nicotine addiction was coming under attack as comparable to heroin and cocaine addiction, Philip Morris responded by setting up an organization called ARISE—for Associates for Research into the Science of Enjoyment—composed principally of European scholars dedicated to defending smoking. Self-advertised as "apolitical," the true purpose of the group was to challenge efforts to regulate tobacco use, and to do so using "third parties" to hide the industry's involvement. ARISE began by hosting a series widely advertised workshops: on "Addiction Controversies" in Florence in 1988, on "Pleasure: The Politics and the Reality" in Venice in 1991, on "Pleasure and Quality of Life" in Brussels in 1993, and on "Living Is More than Surviving" in Amsterdam in 1995. Conferees' papers and opinions were splashed about the press and published to further spread the message, albeit with no acknowledgment of the role played by the tobacco industry as the primary instigator and sponsor.[69]

The whole point of ARISE was to reclaim smoking as a vital and even healthful part of human life. David M. Warburton, a psychopharmacologist at the University of Reading and "worldwide co-ordinator" of the group, warned about health educators becoming "the new high priests of pleasure control with epidemiologists as their oracles." Warburton insisted that "moderate" consumption of coffee, alcohol, and cigarettes could actually lengthen life: "There is clear scientific evidence that a cup of coffee, a glass of wine, a cigarette and a few pieces of chocolate make people calmer, more relaxed and generally happier. Medical evidence shows that happier people live longer, so moderate indulgence can only be beneficial."[70] Other ARISE associates made similar claims. Petra Netter, a psychologist from the University of Giessen, claimed that "Pleasurable experiences resulting from the use of food, wine, coffee, smoking, tea, cola drinks and chocolate are beneficial when used in moderation."[71]

The more common ARISE bluff, though—and this is a frequent industry refrain in the 1980s and 1990s—was that the steps being taken to protect against exposure to secondhand smoke constitute an intolerable infringement of basic human liberties. Timothy Evans, a political sociologist from London's Adam Smith Institute, railed against "the proliferation of campaigns designed to restrict personal freedom and individual choice," especially those targeting the "alleged dangers associated with alcohol, tobacco, caffeine and an increasing range of foods." Frank van Dun, a legal philosopher at Maastricht University, held that the use of "political means for the prevention of disease requires totalitarian control over the lives of people." John Luik of the Niagara Institute in Canada took a similar stance, denouncing "neo-puritans and the health paternalists" for meddling in our lives; he also denied the reality of *addiction,* characterizing it as "an ideology." (Luik later went to work for Forces International, a smokers' rights citadel whose website still lists him as a "researcher.") Luik still today says it is wrong to think of tobacco use as causing people to have "no control"; people can and do quit, which he takes as proof that smoking cannot be addictive. Luik is a skilled conjurer, but he also attacks a straw man. No one says an addiction is *impossible* to overcome: people can have a disease, after all, and still be cured—which doesn't mean they were never sick. Even the most highly addicted smoker can quit if sufficiently draconian measures are imposed—but that doesn't mean that addiction is just "an ideology." Luik insists that defending smokers' rights doesn't necessarily make one a tool of Big Tobacco, but the example he himself sets is hardly convincing, given his long and cozy history with the industry.[72]

Project ARISE included twenty scholarly "Associates" from university faculties all over northern Europe and America. The point was to amplify the voices of academics willing to celebrate the joys and benefits of smoking, spreading the good news that smoking was really not so different from enjoying an occasional cup of coffee or piece of chocolate. And Associates were well paid for their services. Philip

Morris from 1991 to 1993 paid David Warburton $250,000 for his work on "smoking psychology," part of the company's larger Project Cosmic (see below.)[73]

These were not uninfluential figures. Indeed, the industry has often been able to capture trend-setting savants to get across its message. One remarkable case is the employment of Peter L. Berger, a Rutgers University sociologist, to fight for the tobacco cause. Berger had become something of a trendy maverick in 1966, when he and Thomas Luckmann published *The Social Construction of Reality,* arguing that facts are very much social constructs and that how we see the world depends on the groups to which we belong and how we are socialized. Berger seems to have come to the attention of tobacco manufacturers in 1977, when he published an article lamenting the success of "antismoking forces" in pushing through laws restricting smoking in public places. Philip Morris et al. liked his denigration of the clean-air movement as "potentially totalitarian," especially his characterization of smoke-free legislation as "another step in a long-term campaign of stigmatizing and even criminalizing smoking." He admitted to having "no competence with regard to the medical questions at issue," but he did claim to know something about the broader social and cultural context, including the "aggressiveness" of anti-tobacco campaigns. Berger was clearly personally annoyed (as an avid cigar and pipe smoker), but he also lamented the "demeaning" segregation of smokers. In 1982 he testified before a U.S. Senate committee investigating whether to strengthen warnings on cigarettes and attacked such proposals as dangerously paternalistic, carrying "the disturbing implication that the American public actually consists of child-like individuals." Five years later he participated in an industry-financed conference organized to undermine the science demonstrating a cancer hazard from secondhand smoke. Berger here complained that faith in the Surgeon General had led people to swallow a load of anti-tobacco claptrap; he also cautioned that anti-smokers had come to have vested interests: they were no longer "a little band of lonely zealots" but rather part of a well-organized "international antismoking conglomerate." The anti-smoking movement was also "elitist," pursuing a "quasi-religious quest for immortality . . . for the fountain of youth." Smoking restrictions he compared to the "prohibition of certain types of cuisine (say, Italian restaurants)" and other "totalitarian encroachments." Berger even played the Nazi card, declaring "Anti-smoking" to be "the new anti-Semitism."[74]

The industry of course loved his conception of ideologies being on both sides of a purported smoking "debate," parsed as freedom versus tyranny. Berger was also useful in that his industry-friendly articles—his quasi-autobiographical "Furtive Smokers" published as the cover story in *Commentary* in June of 1994, for example—didn't reveal his having taken tobacco money.[75] The industry has always liked to exercise its influence through carefully cloaked "third parties," and Berger was apparently willing to play and profit from this game. His trendy constructivism also fit nicely with the industry's denialist agenda: if all facts are constructs and truth is really just a contest of authorities, why should we believe the Surgeon General over the Tobacco Institute?

Berger remains one of the world's most-cited sociologists; his *Social Construction of Reality* alone has more than twenty thousand citations in Google Scholar, though I doubt very much that those who so honor him know about his entanglement with Big Tobacco.

INTIMATE RELATIONS

U.S. tobacco manufacturers from 1954 through 1998 funneled much of their sponsored research through the Council for Tobacco Research, and from 1988 to 1998 through the Center for Indoor Air Research, the comparable body designed to distract from secondhand smoke hazards. Both were ordered disbanded by the Master Settlement Agreement, but Philip Morris resurrected the CIAR in 2000 as the Philip Morris External Research Program, which operated into 2008. The companies still fund academic research, though it is important to realize how different this is from the work of legitimate research foundations. A grant from Reynolds or Philip Morris is not like a grant from, say, the Ford Foundation. An application submitted to the Ford Foundation is not run by the legal department of the Ford Motor Company—which is more like what happens in the tobacco context. Tobacco grants are approved by damage-control experts at the companies, which means that tobacco money is more like development research—or a kind of advertising. So when Stanford takes money from Philip Morris, this is really not so different from putting up a giant Marlboro billboard on campus. The industry supports research to help it sell more cigarettes, or to boost itself in the eyes of cultural and political elites. And scholars who take this money are facilitating these efforts.[76]

Of course there are other ways the companies exercise influence in academe. Professorships have been established: Northern Illinois University in DeKalb has a Philip Morris Professor of Sales, and the University of Kentucky has a Philip Morris Professor of Plant and Soil Sciences and a Philip Morris Professor of Management Information Systems. VCU has a Philip Morris Endowed Chair in International Business, and Yale has a Philip Morris Chair in Marketing. The University of Kentucky hosts the Philip Morris Agricultural Leadership Development Program (to develop "leadership skills of young, active, burley tobacco farmers") and administers the company's Outstanding Young Farmer Awards.

North Carolina State in Raleigh has long had intimate tobacco relations—which is hardly surprising given the crop's importance to the state. The university has always helped farmers with planting problems and by the 1950s was serving tobacco scientists through its Tobacco Literature Service run out of the D. H. Hill Library. Since 1978 the university has had at least fourteen Philip Morris Professors. A quick check of the university's website reveals a Philip Morris Professor of Agricultural and Resource Economics, an R. J. Reynolds Professor of Mechanical Engineering, a Philip Morris Professor of Plant Pathology, a Philip Morris Professor of Crop Science, a Philip Morris Professor of Economics, and a Philip Morris Endowment for Extension. The Philip Morris Endowment stipulates that the tobacco giant "recognizes the important role of North Carolina in the production of an adequate supply of high quality flue-cured tobacco"; Marlboro munificence also "assists the University to retain highly trained and competent tobacco specialists in key roles to work with county extension staffs to assure continued successful tobacco production in the state."[77] North Carolina State also has a number of professorships funded through a gift of ten thousand shares of R. J. Reynolds stock in 1950. The William Neal Reynolds Professorship, named for the brother of the original RJR, remains the highest honor bestowed by the university. Brown & Williamson has also supported the university's pesticide laboratory.

Prizes and fellowships are another avenue of influence. Florida, Georgia, and North and South Carolina in the 1980s were targeted by Philip Morris with its Young Farmer Awards, leadership seminars, and extension specialist trips, with a monetary value exceeding $400,000. Philip Morris–funded activities included "three endowed extension professorships at NCSU, undergraduate scholarships, graduate fellowships, a young farmer short course, and support for the Multiple Cropping/Irrigation Park" in Georgia. Apart from research, Philip Morris also supports reunion seminars, trips to tobacco-growing regions in Brazil, Philip Morris fellowships, and a Philip Morris prize.[78] The University of Georgia has received similar funding, and Clemson in South Carolina has received money from Philip Morris to support seminars on agricultural technology, training in computer technology, and tuition and graduate fellowships for tobacco country extension agents.

Not all such benevolence goes to the tobacco-growing South. Philip Morris in the 1970s offered fellowships at places like Columbia University, where Stanley Schachter used the industry's money to support graduate students working on smoking psychology.[79] And in 1985 Philip Morris approved payment of $275,000 to the City University of New York's Baruch College to sponsor "the Philip Morris Incorporated Distinguished Visiting Professor in Business and Society" and "the Philip Morris Incorporated Lectures on Business and Society" in honor of George Weissman, the company's former president.[80] Similar support has been extended to universities abroad. More than a hundred researchers in Austria, Germany, and Switzerland have received the Philip Morris Prize since it was established in 1983— basically the Nobel Prize of the tobacco world—with winners taking home about $100,000. (The prize is awarded in all fields of science except for medicine, interestingly.) Nyenrode University in the Netherlands has had a Philip Morris Professor of Strategic Entrepreneurship, and there are now several Philip Morris Professorships at the Czech Republic's famous Charles University in Prague.

Philip Morris has often given code names to European collaborations. Project

Claude Bernard was the name given to the industry's support of Jean Pol Tassin's neuropharmacology at the College de France; Project Galileo supported John Gorrod's work on nicotine metabolism at King's College in London; and Project Paracelsus supported Berthold Schneider's biometrics at the University of Hanover. Projects Broca and Descartes supported Robert Molimard's Laboratory of Experimental Medicine at the University of Paris. There are dozens of projects of this sort, with code names including Bacon, Concarneau, Fermi, Franklin, Gauss, Harvey, Kepler, Leibniz, Lavoisier, Newton, Pascal, Rous, and Versin. All were part of Philip Morris's plan to identify and support "potential witnesses or scientists able to help in finding witnesses." Scholars were also chosen for their ability to help present smoking or nicotine in a favorable light, as when Jean-Marie Warter, Gabriel Micheletti, and Béatrice Lannes at the University of Strasbourg were funded to document the beneficial effects of smoking for people suffering from Alzheimer's (Project Cajal).

(Alzheimer's has been one of the few diseases shown—in rats—to respond positively to nicotine—Parkinson's is another—and both of these get mentioned by tobacco lawyers in litigation, to make it sound as if smoking has benefits as well as risks. Neglected is the fact that even the industry's own archives describe such studies as "small," "poor," and lacking in proper controls; ignored also is the fact that many Alzheimer's patients end up quitting when their matches are taken away—to prevent them from accidentally starting a fire.[81] Janine Cataldo at UCSF recently surveyed forty-three published articles on the smoking–Alzheimer's link and after controlling for tobacco industry affiliation found that smoking actually *increases* one's risk of contracting the disease. Cataldo's study is significant from a methodological point of view, in that an effort is made to distinguish tobacco-tainted from tobacco-free research.[82] This is a growing trend in tobacco-free scholarship, recognition that publications on tobacco health hazards cannot be relied on without controlling for the possibility of an industry-friendly skew.)

Academic collaborations have been established in other parts of the world. In Australia grants have been made available through the Smoking & Health Research Foundation, formerly known as the Australian Tobacco Research Foundation, an industry group. Fellowships have also been offered through the Rothmans Foundation, set up by the makers of Winfield cigarettes. Many Canadian universities accept research grants and donations from the industry, but tobacco industry officials sometimes even hold senior academic appointments, ranging from governor, president, and chancellor to positions in teaching hospitals and in university development. A 2002 study of this phenomenon found twenty-six instances of tobacco industry officers and directors holding university appointments in Canada between 1996 and 2001. Academic funding has also been pervasive in Britain—and scandalous—where scholars have actually been paid by the industry to research "corporate responsibility."[83] Scholars have been organized to dispute the hazards of secondhand smoke, through an elaborate network of "ETS Consultants" established by Philip Morris in 1987. Dozens of scholars from Europe and Asia were harnessed for this purpose, with the goal of going "beyond the establishment of a controversy concerning an alleged ETS health risk" and actually working (as one Philip Morris executive put it) "to disperse the suspicion of risk."[84]

In Germany, relations between the tobacco industry and academia have been so close that it is hardly even fair to talk about "penetration" or "conflict of interest." The Verband der Cigarettenindustrie for many years was the principal industry–academy go-between, attracting hundreds of academics to shill for the industry. In 2008, however, the head of Germany's prestigious Institute for Heart Research in Berlin came under fire for accepting a large grant from the Philip Morris Foundation. The recipient claimed that the money was in no way influencing his research, overlooking the multipurpose nature of such grants. The point is only partly to secure industry-friendly results; it is also to gain prestige, establish allies, and create a stable of thankful experts willing to help in some time of need. The companies fund such research to help them survive in the political arena. Recognizing this broader purpose, Dean Martin Paul of Berlin's famous Charité, the largest medical school in Europe, barred all academic contacts with the industry in the early years of the new millennium. Collaborations continue at many other European institutions, however, perpetuating the banality of smoking.[85]

The penetration is even deeper in Asia, where there is not a great deal of independent tobacco scholarship. Transnationals such as Philip Morris have provided scholarships to students in Singapore and in other Asian nations, and we can expect such ties to grow with globalization. In China, tobacco research is almost entirely in the hands of a governmental elite trying to get more people to smoke. The Zhengzhou Tobacco Research Institute in Henan is the largest such institute in the world, with a staff of 281, including seventeen professors. Scholars throughout the country aid and assist the monopoly with technical expertise, while farmers labor to produce the millions of tons of leaf and flavorings needed to supply a third of the world's smokers. As of 2010 there are perhaps fifteen people making their living in China trying to curb tobacco use, while 15 *million* make a living doing everything they can to keep people smoking. Tobacco prevention is not yet taken seriously, though that could change very fast once China's leaders realize how much damage is being done to national prosperity. Smoking may continue for another few decades in China, but it won't be around forever.

ABUSE WITH A VELVET GLOVE

Scholars who worry about academic integrity often focus on theft of intellectual property or falsification of data or improper disclosure and the like. In the case of tobacco industry sponsorship, however, the bias is typically more complex and indirect. The industry does not ask researchers to falsify data or to come up with some preordained conclusion, and they don't usually interfere with a scholar's freedom to publish—indeed they *want* to see industry-friendly research in print. There are of course such abuses, but that is not how the industry ordinarily exercises its influence. The pattern has been to finance large numbers of scholars, with additional awards then going to those who come up with results the industry can live with. As if you were to sow a field with seeds and then to select and nurture only those flowers that grow in the colors you find pleasing. Scholars who pass such tests are then further cultivated and if all goes well will be invited to testify at hearings or in court as expert witnesses.

We saw in an earlier chapter how the industry supports academic research to create what they've called a "stable of experts" for use in litigation or some other public or PR capacity.[86] Not everyone who works for the industry ends up defending it, but even a 5 or 10 percent harvest can still suffice. The tobacco archives contain *hundreds of thousands of pages* of transcripts of trial testimony and depositions of scholars working for the industry, and from all branches of academia. Many of these scholars are from leading research universities; almost all have either a medical degree or a nonmedical doctorate. Many were originally grantees of the CTR or the CIAR, which operated as hothouses for cigarette-friendly expertise. The archives contain long lists of potential experts, along with people whom the companies believe can direct them to others willing to serve.[87] The industry trots out such experts in litigation or regulatory hearings, using them to produce a string of denials, qualifications, rationales, diversions, or whatever else might be needed to exculpate the industry's conduct, past or present.

The bias created by tobacco-sponsored research is therefore different from what is commonly imagined. The industry creates bias in the *aggregate* pattern of research rather than (only) in any one scholar's work. This is notorious in the case of secondhand smoke science, where the industry for many years was able to fund the work of skeptics, producing what amounts to "noise" in the smoke–disease signal. Deborah Barnes and Lisa Bero from the University of California studied this impact of sponsorship on hazard assessments for secondhand smoke and found that scholars taking the industry's money were far more likely to find *no evidence* of a health threat.[88] Brown & Williamson's Director of Scientific Issues later twisted this same disproportion to dispute the reality of risk: "I do not believe that the evidence on secondhand smoke is very convincing. If you look, for example, at the studies on lung cancer, you find that the vast majority of those studies—around 80 percent or so—do not report a significant increase in risk, so from my perspective, I think we have to seriously question a lot of the claims that have been made on environmental tobacco smoke."[89] The industry's modus operandi by this time was familiar: you basically fund lots of research to dispute a hazard, then cite this same research to say that lots of scholars dispute it.

Of course there are always dissenters and laggards in any scientific community, and not just quacks and charlatans but also respectable scholars who, for one reason or another, are not up to date on the relevant research. The industry gives trumpets, drums, and dollars to these laggards, to make it all seem like honest controversy. This is abuse with a velvet glove: as if the Catholic Church had not thrown Galileo in prison but rather had simply hired, fêted, and funded all manner of diehards and skeptics to march in step with those who held the earth to be the center of the universe.

Tobacco industry sponsorship has been corrosive of honest intellectual inquiry on a scale that is difficult to comprehend. Tobacco expertise for many years was dominated by the industry, as it still is in many parts of the world. Entire scientific societies have been formed to sabotage the science showing harms of one kind or another, and several scientific journals owe their existence to the industry's need for "friendly research" (*Tobacco Science* but also more scholarly organs like *Indoor Air*). The industry is not just *corrupting* academia; they are also *creating* it. All businesses want to succeed, of course, and in this respect tobacco is no different. What is different is the extent to which Tobacco has been willing and able to obstruct popular and scientific knowledge, jamming the scientific airwaves with noise. We are talking about racketeers with academics as accomplices—and a breach of academic integrity more serious—and deadly—than anything since the horrors of the Nazi era. Cigarettes should be banned, if for no other reason than to end the corruption of science caused by the industry's drive to continue its deadly trade.

To repeat: collaboration with the tobacco industry is one of the most deadly abuses of scholarly integrity in modern history. Abuses of the Nazis and Soviets are better known and more immediately murderous, but the mortal force of cigarettes is so vast, and so easily avoidable, that the comparison is not inappropriate. A hundred million people died from smoking in the twentieth century, and we are now on a pace to have many times that in the present century. Academics would have blood on their hands but for the fact that most tobacco deaths are bloodless and distant from the acts that first set mortality into motion. Comparisons could be made to prostitution, but that would insult a trade that does not kill half its clients. It also usually takes decades for smoking to kill, rendering the deaths seemingly faint and uncertain on the horizon. But the mortality is no less real and no less nefarious.

24

Historians Join the Conspiracy

The abuse of history is infinite in its variety.
ANTOON DE BAETS, *RESPONSIBLE HISTORY*, 2008

The tobacco industry cannot do what it does without help. Grave misdeeds require accomplices, and in the cigarette world a continual rewriting of the past is key to the industry's survival. Time and again the companies have been forced into court and come out smelling like a rose. They cannot do this alone, however; they need experts willing to help.

Scholars can be a remarkably compliant lot, and my own field of history is no exception. Indeed they have much to atone for. Since the early 1990s more than fifty professional historians have testified for the industry in court (see the box on page 460), earning millions of dollars for presenting lopsided, biased, and historically impoverished accounts of cigarette history. A more shadowy band of historians has worked alongside these experts as consultants, preparing reports and doing archival work, sometimes while being groomed for promotion to the rank of expert witness (see the box on page 464). Some of these historians sign confidentiality agreements, including agreements not to publish on the topic under investigation (James H. Jones, author of the classic history of the Tuskegee syphilis experiment, signed such an agreement when he worked for the industry.) The industry wants to control this work and generally doesn't want its "experts" to expose their labors to peer review.

Of course the industry has long relied on scholars to polish its image. Clarence Cook Little was chosen to head the Tobacco Industry Research Committee in 1954 not just because he could organize a face-saving research enterprise but also because he presented a friendly face to the public, including regulators, juries, and judges. And we've already seen how scholars from virtually all walks of academic life have served this purpose—including hundreds of physicians. Their job has been

HISTORIANS WHO HAVE TESTIFIED AS EXPERT WITNESSES FOR THE DEFENSE IN AMERICAN TOBACCO LITIGATION, 1986–2010

Compiled with Louis M. Kyriakoudes

Ambrose, Stephen E. (deceased). Testified in *Covert v. Liggett Group* (1994); deposed in *Florida v. American Tobacco* (1997), designated in *Haines v. Liggett* (1997).

Bean, Jonathan J., Southern Illinois University. Designated in *St. Louis v. American Tobacco* (2004), named as an expert in *Schwab v. Philip Morris*.

Berman, Hyman, University of Minnesota. Deposed for and testified in *Minnesota v. Philip Morris* (1997 and 1998).

Breeden James O., Southern Methodist University. Expert report submitted in *Allgood v. Reynolds* (1994).

Burnham, John C., Ohio State University. Designated for *Dewey v. Reynolds* (1986); expert disclosure for *Cipollone* (1986).

Burns III, Augustus M., University of Florida (deceased). Deposed for *Florida v. American Tobacco* (1997) and *Engle v. Reynolds* (1998).

Carstensen, Fred V., University of Connecticut. Deposed for and testified in *Cipollone v. Liggett* (1987 and 1988) and deposed for *Izzarelli* (?) and for *Bifolck v. Philip Morris*.

Chesson, Michael B., University of Massachusetts, Boston. Provided affidavit in *Longden v. Philip Morris* (2003).

Cobbs-Hoffman, Elizabeth, San Diego State University. Deposed for and testified in *Boeken v. Philip Morris* (2001); deposed for *Patterson, Evers,* and *Martin* (2009, *Engle Progeny* cases).

Dibacco, Thomas V., American University. Listed for *Richardson v. Philip Morris* (1997); deposed in and testified for *Eastman v. Brown & Williamson* (2003); deposed in *Blue Cross v. Philip Morris* (2000), *Engle v. Reynolds* (1999), and *Katz v. Reynolds* (2010).

Drobny, John, president, IHG, Inc. Disclosed as "Expert Historian" for *Texas v. American Tobacco* (1997).

English, Peter Calvin, Duke University. Testified in *Blue Cross v. Philip Morris* (2001); expert report and deposition for *USDOJ v. Philip Morris* (2001); deposed for *Bullock v. Philip Morris* (2002); designated in *Haines v. Liggett* (1992), etc.

Ford, Lacy K., Jr., University of South Carolina, Columbia. Testified in *Raulerson v. Reynolds* (1997), *Jones v. Reynolds* (2000), *Kenyon v. Reynolds* (2001), and *Allen v. Reynolds* (2003); deposed for *Blankenship v. Philip Morris* (2000), *Engle v. Reynolds* (1997, 1999), and *Medical Monitoring* (2000); deposed for and testified in *Karbiwnyk v. Reynolds* (1997), *Engle v. Reynolds* (1997, 1999), *Little v. Brown & Williamson* (2000), and multiple *Engle Progeny* cases (2008–11); designated in *St. Louis v. American Tobacco* (2004); cross-noticed for *Keegan v. Reynolds*.

Graham, Otis, University of North Carolina, Wilmington. Testified in *Kotler v. American Tobacco* (1990); deposed for *Texas v. American Tobacco* (1997), designated in *Haines v. Liggett* (1992).

Green, George D., University of Minnesota. Retained as expert witness in *Minnesota v. Philip Morris* (1997); deposed on August 26–27, 1997, and expert report submitted on December 8, 1997.

Greenwood, Janette T., Clark University. Expert report for *Donovan v. Philip Morris;* disclosed as an expert witness for multiple *Engle Progeny* cases.

Harkness, Jon M., University of Minnesota. Testified in *Boerner v. Brown & Williamson* (2003).

Harvey, Paul, University of Colorado, Colorado Springs. Deposed for *Coolidge v. Philip Morris* (2004); named an expert in *Alan Nichols v. Asbestos Corporation Ltd.* (2008) and *Koballa v. Reynolds* (2010).

Hilty, James, Temple University. Testified in *Carter v. Philip Morris* (2003).

Hoff, Joan, Ohio University, Athens; Montana State University, Bozeman. Testified in *Rogers v. Reynolds* (1996), *Dunn v. Reynolds* (1998), and *Tompkin v. American Brands* (2001); deposed for *Dunn v. Reynolds* (1997 and 1998), *Tompkin v. American Tobacco* (2001), and *Engle Progeny* cases (2009 and 2010); deposed for and testified in *Whiteley v. Raybestos-Manhattan* (1999 and 2000) and in *Barbanell* (2009, *Engle Progeny* case).

Hudson, Robert P., University of Kansas (deceased). Deposed in *Allgood v. Reynolds* (1994).

Judd, Jacob, Lehman College. Expert report filed in *Standish v. American Tobacco* (2003); testified in *Rose v. American Tobacco* (2003).

Lenoir, Timothy, Duke University (formerly Stanford). Expert report and deposed for *Tune v. Philip Morris* (1998, 2001).

Lipartito, Kenneth James, Florida International University. Named an expert witness in *Engle Progeny* litigation.

Lowery, Charles D., Mississippi State University. Deposed for *Mississippi AG* (1997).

Ludmerer, Kenneth M., Washington University. Trial testimony in *Kotler v. American Tobacco* (1990); deposed for *Cipollone v. Liggett* (1991); expert report for *Unkel v. Liggett* (1994); deposed for *State of Mississippi Tobacco Litigation* (1997), Florida State Attorney General's case (1997), *Engle v. Reynolds* (1998), *State of Washington v. American Tobacco* (1998), *Blankenship v. Philip Morris* (2000), and *Scott v. American Tobacco* (2000); trial testimony in *Williams v. Philip Morris* (1999), *Apostolou v. American Tobacco* (2000), *Anderson v. American Tobacco* (2000), and *Boeken v. Philip Morris* (2001); deposed for *Tompkin v. American Tobacco* (2001) and *Harvey v. ABB Lummus Global* (2002); deposition and expert report for *USA v. Philip Morris* (2002); listed for *Engle v. Reynolds* (1997) and for *Crayton v. Safeway* (2000).

Martin, James Kirby, University of Houston. Deposed in and expert report for *Burton v. Reynolds* (1996); deposed and testified in *Ironworkers v. Philip Morris* (1999) and in *Falise v. American Tobacco* (2000 and 2001).

Martinez-Fernandez, Luis, University of Central Florida. Testified in *Eli Rogelio Figueroa Cruz v. Reynolds* in Puerto Rico (2002); deposed for and testified in multiple *Engle Progeny* cases.

May, Glenn A., University of Oregon. Testified in *Williams v. Philip Morris* (1999).

Michel, Gregg L., University of Texas at San Antonio. Deposed for and testified in *Campbell v. Reynolds* (2009); deposed for *Walden* (2010) and *Webb v. Reynolds* (2010); work for Jones Day since 2003.

Miller, Donald L., Lafayette College. Expert report submitted for *Gerrity v. Lorillard* (2005).

Morgan, H. Wayne, University of Oklahoma. Testified in *Oklahoma-AG* (1998).

Norrell, Robert Jefferson, III, University of Tennessee. Testified in *Newcomb v. Reynolds* (1999, 2003); deposed for and testified in *Karney v. Brown & Williamson* (1998, 1999) and *Scott v. American Tobacco* (2000, 2003); earlier work for litigation in Alabama, Florida, and Louisiana; deposed for and testified in multiple *Engle Progeny* cases (*Martin v. Philip Morris*, 2009)— twelve depositions altogether by 2009.

O'Donnell, Edward T., Hunter College, CUNY, and now Holy Cross College. Expert witness report prepared for *Small and Fubini v. Lorillard* (1997); scheduled for deposition in *Zito v. American Tobacco* (1997).

Parrish, Michael E., University of California, San Diego. Testified in *Miele v. American Tobacco* (2003); deposed for *Barnes (Arch) v. American Tobacco* (1997), *Frosina v. Philip Morris* (1997), *Washington v. American Tobacco* (1997), and *Boerner v. Brown & Williamson* (2003); deposed and testified for *Henley v. Philip Morris* (1998, 1999); affidavits for *Stewart-Lomantz v. Brown & Williamson* (1996), *Frosina v. Philip Morris* (1997), *Small and Fubini v. Lorillard* (1997), and *Tabb v. Philip Morris et al.* (1998). Listed for *Engle v. Reynolds* (1997).

Parssinen, Terry M., University of Tampa. Testified in *Arnitz v. Philip Morris* (2004) and in *Engle Progeny* cases.

Roberts, Randy W., Purdue University. Disclosed as an expert in *Walden v. Reynolds* (*Engle Progeny* case); deposed for *Budnick, Allen, Hetzner, Haldeman,* and other *Engle Progeny* cases (2010).

Rose, Mark H., Florida Atlantic University. Disclosed in *Brown v. Liggett* (2003).

Rosenberg, Nathan, Stanford University. Testified for the industry in 1988 hearings as a "technology policy witness," part of an effort to "ensure smooth introduction of alpha free from federal government interference or regulation."

Sansing, David G., University of Mississippi, Oxford. Testified in *Boerner v. Brown & Williamson* (2003); deposed in *Mississippi Tobacco Litigation* (1997); deposed for and testified in *Horton v. American Tobacco* (1990) and *Wilks v. American Tobacco* (1993); testimony and/or deposition in *Carter v. Philip Morris, Grinnell v. American Tobacco,* and *Schuts and Walton,* inter alia.

Savitt, Todd, East Carolina University (Medical Humanities). Expert report for *Ierardi v. Lorillard* (1991).

Schaller, Michael, University of Arizona. Disclosed for *Arizona v. American* (1998), *Sweeny v. Philip Morris* (1999), and *Simon v. Philip Morris* (2000); testified in *Apostolou v. Philip Morris* (2000), *Reller v. Philip Morris* (2003), *Lucier v. Philip Morris* (2003), and *Frankson v. Brown & Williamson* (2003); deposed for *Selcer v. Reynolds* (1998), *Grill v. Philip Morris* (2010), and *Engle Progeny* cases (2008); trial testimony for multiple *Engle Progeny* cases (2009–11).

Sharp, James Roger, Syracuse University. Expert report for, deposed for, and testified in *Mehlman v. Philip Morris* (2000 and 2001); testified in *Anderson v. American Tobacco* (2000) and in *Engle Progeny* cases.

Skates, John Ray, Jr., University of Southern Mississippi. Deposed in *Mississippi Tobacco Litigation* (1997).

Snetsinger, John G., California Polytechnic State University, San Luis Obispo. Deposition in *Bullock v. Philip Morris* (2002).

Stueck, William, University of Georgia. Expert disclosure and affidavit submitted in *Eiser v. Brown & Williamson* (2002); affidavits in *Mash v. Brown & Williamson* (2004); deposed for *Alexander v. Philip Morris* (2010).

Tulchin, Joseph S., Woodrow Wilson Center, Washington, DC. Testified in *Widdick v. Brown & Williamson* (1998).

Wilson, Theodore A., University of Kansas. Deposed for *Barnes [Arch] v. American Tobacco* (1997), *Chamberlain* (1999), *Clay v. Philip Morris* (1999), *Smith* (1998), *Thompson v. American Tobacco* (1999), *Blankenship v. Philip Morris* (2000), and West Virginia's *Medical Monitoring* cases (2000); expert report (2001) and deposition (2002) for *USDOJ v. Philip Morris*; affidavit for *State of Florida* litigation, etc.

to display their expertise in ways that will exculpate the industry, to make black appear white and vice versa. Whatever is needed.

Historians, though, have come to play a special—and especially disturbing—role in this context. The tobacco industry has been funding historical work for decades, long prior to the "second wave" of litigation in the 1980s[1] and prior even to the Second World War. Much of what we think we know about tobacco's history is an artifact of such investments: tobacco manufacturers like us to think of theirs as an ancient and honorable art; tobacco is the East for the West and the West for the East—whence all those images of camels and liberty. Tobacco is patriotic: America's founding fathers grew the precious leaf, after all, and tobacco leaves are carved atop Latrobe's columns for the Capitol building. And what could be more American than the Marlboro Man on the open range? Historians are used to help craft and maintain this image of a world we cannot do without—which is one reason

HISTORIANS WHO HAVE SERVED AS EXPERT CONSULTANTS FOR THE TOBACCO INDUSTRY WITHOUT TESTIFYING (PARTIAL LISTING)

Abrams, Richard M.	University of California, Berkeley
Black, Gregory D.	University of Missouri, Kansas City
Clune, John J., Jr.	University of West Florida
Engelmann, Larry	San Jose State University
Ettling, John	University of Houston; SUNY Plattsburgh (president)
Grill, Johnpeter H.	Mississippi State University
Harp, Richard	University of Kansas (Engl. dept.) ·
Harley, David	formerly of Oxford University
Herken, Gregg	University of California, Merced
Hook, Ernest B.	University of California, Berkeley
Jenkins, Robert L.	Mississippi State University
Jones, James H.	San Francisco, formerly University of Houston
Kargon, Robert H.	Johns Hopkins University
Klein, Herbert	Stanford University
Kline, Benjamin	San Jose State University
Kushner, Howard I.	Emory University
Lankevich, George J.	Bronx Community College, Manhasset
Means, Richard K.	University of Alabama, Auburn University
Muldoon, James	Rutgers University
Musto, David F.	Yale University
Overmann, Ronald J.	San Francisco, formerly program officer National Science Foundation
Petigny, Alan	University of Florida
Robert, Joseph C. (deceased)	University of Richmond
Sauer, John E.	Ohio State University
Smith, George D.	Winthrop Group and NYU Stern
Sobel, Robert N. (deceased)	Hofstra University
Sosna, Morton	Cornell, formerly Stanford University
Talley, Colin	Emory University
Unger, Irwin	New York University

people continue to buy and die from cigarettes. Historians are paid to immortalize tobacco, to make it seem natural that people should smoke. Indeed, much of modern tobacco historiography has a nicotine taint.

Here I want to explore how historians have worked for the industry, focusing on contract history, consulting, and (especially) expert witnessing for the industry in court. I also want to suggest that while historians who service the industry may not realize it, their labors have the indirect effect of keeping the price of cigarettes low, by saving the companies from having to pay out costly legal awards. Which means that when historians testify for the industry in court, they are effectively helping the industry to avoid a kind of tax. Saving the industry money in this manner keeps prices low, meaning more cigarettes smoked and more people dying from the habit. The chain of causation is indirect but nonetheless real: witnessing for the industry causes death.

CONTRACT HISTORY

Historians who have worked for the tobacco industry fall into three main categories: scholars who have been paid to write for the industry, sometimes as official corporate historians; scholars who have done more secretive consulting for the industry, usually in preparation for litigation; and scholars who have testified as expert witnesses for the industry in court, exculpating the industry's conduct by placing blame on the individual smoker.

Readers should keep in mind, though, that even this covers only a small fraction of industry-friendly tobacco historiography. There is a vast unpublished body of historical writing in the archives of the industry, covering everything from the rise and fall of specific brands to the origins of certain kinds of processing equipment. There are chronicles of marketing campaigns and tobacco paraphernalia, along with histories of tobacco-growing regions and of particular cigarette additives. There are unpublished histories of specific firms but also of specific departments and top brass within those firms. Some of this was prepared for use in litigation, though most seems to be just part of the companies' efforts to create institutional memories for themselves in the form of commemorations, time lines, literature reviews, or internal honorifics. Judging purely from the number of pages, there may be more historical writing in the industry's archives than has ever been printed in scholarly books. Some of this has been written by professional historians, but the authors are more often corporate staff assigned to prepare chronologies or literature or brand reviews of one sort or another. Hundreds of chronologies are preserved in the industry's archives; nearly twenty thousand documents contain the word *chronology*.[2]

The industry also, though, generates published histories for popular consumption. The "story" of Camels, Winstons, Marlboros, and other popular brands has been told in countless popular magazines, along with tales of how tobacco was once a medicine or barred from consumption in one part of the world or another.[3] Narratives along these lines are sometimes conveyed through museums and historical exhibits—such as that maintained by the Duke Homestead Education and History Corporation in Durham, North Carolina, or any of the dozen-odd other tobacco museums funded by the industry in different parts of the world. Tobacco museums are not as numerous as they once were—SEITA has closed its French museum, as has Austria Tabak in Vienna—but those that remain are de facto ads for the habit, displaying the golden weed as a venerable luxury and economic powerhouse. Museums are sometimes created to coincide with the penetration of a new market: Philip Morris established a museum at its Kutna Hora plant in the Czech Republic in 1995, for example, when it took over production from the former state monopoly. Some of these are sizable: the China Tobacco Museum in Shanghai (opened in 2004) cost an estimated $22 million to build; the edifice houses 150,000 historical artifacts and presents a predictable whitewash of health effects ("there is no need to object to cigarette smoking"). There has never really been an honest tobacco museum; all are essentially conflicts of interest masquerading as educational institutions.

The practice of paying historians to write for the companies dates back at least to the nineteenth century, but a historiographic watershed of sorts was 1937, when Jerome E. Brooks published the first of five volumes of a sumptuous *Tobacco: Its History Illustrated by the Books, Manuscripts and Engravings in the Library of George Arents, Jr.*, cataloging the rare books and smoking ephemera that, until recently, occupied an entire hall on the top floor of the New York Public Library.[4] Brooks went on to a stellar career as the industry's premier historian, publishing widely read books on the glories of tobacco lore, along with folksy brochures and pamphlets for the Tobacco Institute. His 1952 book, *The Mighty Leaf: Tobacco through the Centuries,* is textbook triumphalist hagiography, celebrating smoking as a "treasured necessity" and "natural right" of humankind.

Medical historians were also engaged early on. One of the first in the United States was Morris Fishbein, the iron-fisted editor of *JAMA,* who in the early 1950s was paid (by Lorillard) tens of thousands of dollars to write a comprehensive book on smoking and health. Fishbein to his credit did a pretty good job—too good in fact, which is probably why the book was suppressed. Lorillard reneged on its offer to buy several thousand copies, and Doubleday canceled his contract.

One reason for the funding of historical writing has been to be able to recommend a set of right-minded books to people inquiring about the history of tobacco. In 1975, for example, when an Arizona scholar wrote to Reynolds asking for information along these lines, the company's public relations department could recommend four "comprehensive histories": Robert K. Heimann's *Tobacco and Americans* (1960); Jerome E. Brooks's *The Mighty Leaf* (1952); Joseph C. Robert's *The Story of Tobacco in America* (1949); and Nannie M. Tilley's *The Bright-Tobacco Industry* (1948).[5] All interesting and well-written books but all activist histories dishing up slavish praise for tobacco—with virtually no acknowledgment of health harms. And all written by scholars with close ties to the industry. Robert Heimann at the time was executive assistant to the president of American Tobacco (and an NYU-trained sociologist); Jerome Brooks was a lifelong writer for the industry on Hill & Knowlton's payroll; Joseph Robert worked for Reynolds; and Nannie Tilley had served as R. J. Reynolds's official corporate historian, a position she held from 1959 through 1964.

Industry-funded historiography continued into the 1960s and 1970s. Robert Sobel's 1978 book, *They Satisfy: The Cigarette in American Life,* was financed by the industry, as was Mark Edward Lender's *A New Prohibition? An Essay on Drinking and Smoking in America,* published by Brown & Williamson in 1995. Sobel was a professor of history at Hofstra University; Lender was (and is) chair of the history department at Kean University in New Jersey. Lender acknowledged tobacco industry support for his book—a cigarette manufacturer published it, after all—but histories with cigarette links have often been published without any such acknowledgment. Francis Robicsek in his lavishly illustrated history of tobacco in Maya art and religion, *The Smoking Gods,* thanks the Tobacco Institute for its "cooperation," for example, but nowhere lets the reader know that the book was made possible by a $55,000 subsidy from that lobby body.[6]

More serious is Milton Rosenblatt's failure to disclose his tobacco industry ties in his 1964 history of lung cancer for the *Bulletin of the History of Medicine.* Rosenblatt here made the by-then preposterous argument that lung cancer rates were not in fact on the rise; the increase was only apparent, a consequence of the fact that cancers were being diagnosed more often from the growing use of X-rays. So the pandemic was really just "a tribute to progress in diagnostic acumen." Rosenblatt had been working for the industry since the 1950s and by 1961 was taking TIRC "Special Services" money. He repeated his denial of any real rise in lung cancer throughout the 1960s, testifying to this effect before Congress and on CBS Television's *Calendar Show with Harry Reasoner.* Rosenblatt also shows up in the Tobacco Institute's 1972 propaganda film, *Smoking and Health: The Need to Know,* claiming once again that the observed rise in lung cancer was illusory. The Tobacco Institute loved his dismissal of the idea of smoking causing cancer as "a colossal blunder"—and featured this prominently in its brochures and videos. Tobacco enthusiasts clearly valued his assistance: a 1962 memo from J. Morrison Brady, associate scientific director of the TIRC, to Clarence Cook Little described the industry's public relations woes, created by cancer research of the 1950s, as "like the early symptoms of diabetes—certain dietary controls kept public opinion reasonably healthy. When some new symptom appeared, a shot of insulin in the way of a news release, a Berkson antidote, a Rosenblatt television rebuttal, etc., kept the patient going."[7] The "patient" in this case was the cigarette cartel, threatened by the revelation of cigarettes causing death and disease. Rosenblatt had helped cigarette makers handle the 1954 "emergency," along with subsequent public relations problems "that must be solved for the self-preservation of the industry." CTR officers as late as the 1980s were regurgitating his denialist theory in testimony before Congress, with the man held forth as "an outstanding medical historian."[8]

Some historians who have worked for the industry do so unabashedly, and out in the open. Joseph C. Robert, a member of the history faculty of Duke and later Richmond University, for many years worked as a contract historian for R. J. Reynolds; he was also a frequent speaker at cigarette industry conferences, where he would celebrate the lore and lure of *Nicotiana* in an opening or after-dinner lecture. I've mentioned Nannie Tilley's position as official historian at Reynolds: Tilley was sometimes asked to field questions for the firm—on the composition of Estron, for example (answer: cellulose acetate, used as a filter material)—and her books include subtle and accomplished accounts of early tobacco technology, tobacco economics, and the corporate history of Reynolds itself, always with the "health issue" conspicuously overlooked. We also find unpublished histories by such authors in the industry's archives. Jerome E. Brooks in the 1970s, for example, was commissioned to write an "authorized unpublished history" of Philip Morris for the company, which we now know about only from documents submitted in response to subpoenas. Tobacco manufacturers throughout the world have commissioned such histories: British American's unpublished "History Project" from 1972 surveyed the growth of the company's trade in Australia, Brazil, China, the Congo, and more than a dozen other countries, citing thirty-six books on tobacco history and a larger number of pamphlets and magazine articles, many published by the companies or corporate agents.[9]

Some of this literature written for internal corporate use is now online, thanks to the subpoena power granted to litigators. The notorious 460-page "Corporate Activity Project" produced by Jones Day for Reynolds is now available online, for example, but there are histories of this sort we cannot access: Patrick O'Neil-Dunne's prodigious twenty-one-volume *History of U.S. Cigarette Advertising*, for example, compiled at the request of Carreras Ltd. in Britain, makers of Craven "A" and Black Cat cigarettes. That text was put together for internal use ("published on a restricted basis for distribution among the Rothmans group affiliates"), and we know of its existence only because of one single mention in *Brandstand*, the official publication of the Cigarette Pack Collectors Association, an amateur group with friendly connections to the industry.[10]

Another oft-encountered genre is the company-sanctioned corporate history, which typically treats the rise of a particular firm in the form of a business history. Howard Cox's *The Global Cigarette: Origins and Evolution of British American Tobacco, 1880–1945*, is a good example. The book is both a substantial piece of scholarship and a celebration of one of the world's largest tobacco transnationals; it is also, though, based on a detailed study of (hard-paper) BAT archives not accessible without permission from the company.[11]

What are the ethics of a historian using sources to which only he or she has access? Cox's book relies on a series of unpublished "corporate histories" prepared by BAT's legal department; how are we to evaluate such scholarship, if no one apart from the author has access to the archives? What is left out of such accounts, and what kinds of bias have been written into the story? Cox's book is dedicated to R. Glyn Davies, former editor of *BAT News* and the company's marketing information officer. Does this cozy connection have anything to do with the fact that the dangers of smoking are almost entirely ignored in this book? Or that the chronology stops just about when the lung cancer hazard is nailed down? Similar questions can be raised about most of these contract histories: B. W. E. Alford's history of W. D. & H. O. Wills, for example, or Brian Du Toit's history of Ecusta, or W. Twiston Davies's *Account of the African Organisation of the Imperial Tobacco Company, 1907–1957*, or Sue V. Dickinson's history *The First Sixty Years of Imperial's American Leaf Organization*, and so forth.[12]

PROJECT COSMIC AND THE POLITICS OF TRANSPARENCY

A more secretive prompt for contract history was Philip Morris's Project Cosmic, an effort launched in 1987 to establish "an extensive network of scientists and historians from all over the world" to produce tobacco-friendly scholarship. An Oxford historian by the name of David Harley was appointed one of six Project Cosmic "directors" and wrote several articles for this purpose: a 1987 letter in Philip Morris's files describes his plans "to start work immediately" on the history of "tobacco use in England, producing papers suitable for publication in learned journals." A 1990 progress report describes his plan to lecture at the Columbus quincentenary in Madrid and meetings of the American Society of Eighteenth Century Studies and the American Association for the History of Medicine and to publish a book-length history of tobacco. His article on "The Beginnings of the Tobacco Controversy" in the 1993 *Bulletin of the History of Medicine* failed to disclose his industry funding; there is also no mention of the fact that "creating controversy" was a central pillar in the industry's ongoing denialist campaign. Harley thanks Daniel Ennis for "encouraging" his interest in the topic, but Ennis's position as Project Cosmic coordinator for Philip Morris goes unmentioned, as does the fact that the article itself was a Cosmic project. Harley was paid handsomely for his services: $17,415 in 1988, $21,000 in 1989, $46,706 in 1990, and $31,074 in 1991.[13]

David F. Musto, a professor of psychiatry (at the Child Study Center) and the history of medicine at Yale, was another Project Cosmic director highly valued by the industry. Musto in January of 1990 was awarded $300,000 from Philip Morris to document "the history of social response to mood-altering substances." Project Cosmic directors all produced industry-friendly research and in some instances went on to help the companies with legal challenges. Ohio State's John Burnham, for example, was disclosed as an expert witness for the defense in *Cipollone v. Liggett*, where he was expected to testify that scientists were "strongly skeptical of any link between cigarette smoking and lung cancer prior to the 1950s" and that the industry's response to the discovery of tobacco mortality "was both timely and appropriate and constituted a respectable/commendable scientific effort."[14] Burnham also recruited other historians for use as experts—more on which in a moment.

Philip Morris's Project Cosmic lasted about five years, with hundreds of thousands of dollars paid to its principals, including the above-mentioned historians but also David Warburton from the psychology department of Reading University and the psychologist, eugenicist, and tobacco-phile Hans Eysenck of the University of London. Funding resulted in a number of publications, none of which acknowledged support from Philip Morris. David Musto in 1991, for example, published an article titled "Opium, Cocaine and Marijuana in American History" in *Scientific American,* with no disclosure of his ongoing work for Philip Morris. Nor was there any mention of his tobacco ties in 1992, when he hosted a *NOVA* television series on the history of drug use; indeed the show's writer and director, Eric Stange, was quite surprised when I told him that his host had been taking tobacco money throughout their filming and indeed for some years previously. The industry for its part was clearly pleased with Musto's work, judging from the praise we find in Philip Morris's archives, which commends his role in popularizing a "moderate view of substance use in the media." The tobacco giant especially liked his theory of a seventy-year cycle of tolerance and intolerance toward psychoactive substances, which could be used to naturalize the present "phase" we were going through. Musto's industry-friendly thesis was even reported on by Gina Kolata of the *New York Times,* who probably had no idea it was tobacco-tinged.[15] Yale administrators were also happy to have him bringing in these funds: Leon E. Rosenberg, dean of Yale's School of Medicine at the time, thanked Philip Morris profusely for its support, adding that Dr. Musto's research would "bring us closer to the time when our society will have a healthy relationship with substances that affect our moods."[16]

Harley's and Musto's failure to disclose financing from the industry is not unusual: other historians working for the industry have failed in similar fashion. Some have even employed assistants without letting them know whom they were really working for. Ernest Hook, a professor of public health at UC Berkeley, apparently did not tell his assistants which side they were working for, for example, and John G. Snetsinger at California Polytechnic State University in San Luis Obispo is known to have hired graduate students to help him prepare for litigation without telling them they were working for the industry. As one of his assistants later reported:

> I would not have done the work if I had known what it was for. I'm relieved that the jury rejected the tobacco industry's argument and I wish Ms. Bullock's attorneys had contacted me to a) learn about the rather selective research I was supposed to do and b) that Snetsinger was using grad students to do the work without fully disclosing who and what it was for.[17]

Historians have not yet come to grips with when and how to require disclosure of potential conflicts of interest, though confessions have begun to appear in some academic journals, mainly in response to peer reviewers raising questions about the origins of a particular piece of scholarship.[18] We should also realize, though, that disclosure and transparency can be double-edged swords. In recent years the tobacco colossus in concert with other polluting industries has sought to manipulate science by this means, using and even creating "data access" laws to deconstruct science they see as a regulatory threat. A remarkable example is the industry's work to help draft and pass the Data Access Act of 1998 and the Data Quality Act of 2000. These new federal laws allow the industry (or anyone else with sufficient resources) to obtain and reprocess the raw data from anyone publishing any kind of scientific or medical study using federal funds. The tobacco industry pushed for legislation of this sort to make it easier to reanalyze and reinterpret (i.e., look for flaws in) research critical of the industry. Philip Morris employed Multinational Business Services and other front organizations to help push through these laws—over objections from both the National Academy of Sciences and the American Association for the Advancement of Science. The new laws create a deep and disturbing asymmetry in the scrutiny applied to different kinds of science, with publicly funded research subject to a much higher level of interrogation than research conducted by the industry. The laws make it possible for corporate actors to sit as if behind a one-way mirror, directing the dissection of whatever body of data they regard as a threat to business as usual. Which is why some environmental experts have called such laws "a tool to clobber every effort to regulate" and an instrument to promote "censorship and harassment."[19]

DELUGE MATERIALS AND
THE CHICKEN SOUP DEFENSE

The industry's exploitation of historians increased dramatically in the 1980s in response to a new level of threat from lawsuits such as *Cipollone v. Liggett,* filed in 1983. Rose Cipollone was a fifty-eight-year-old New Jersey woman who had smoked Chesterfield, L&M, Virginia Slims, and True cigarettes before contracting lung cancer and then dying from the disease. Lawsuits had been filed much earlier—several hundred since 1954, in fact—but the industry had always been able to win by claiming that tobacco, while dangerous, was not *unreasonably* dangerous. And that people knew about and therefore knowingly assumed the risk when they purchased the product. Tobacco attorneys had also usually been able to outspend their opponents on trial preparations—often by an order of magnitude or more—making every case a mismatch. Industry lawyers used to brag about this:

> the aggressive posture we have taken regarding depositions and discovery in general continues to make these cases extremely burdensome and expensive for plaintiffs'

lawyers, particularly sole practitioners. To paraphrase General Patton, the way we won these cases was not by spending all of Reynolds' money, but by making that other son of a bitch spend all his.[20]

Several key elements in this landscape had changed by the 1980s, however. For one thing, a number of legal teams had become quite wealthy working for the defense in *asbestos* litigation—often by blaming cigarettes for the lung maladies suffered by shipyard workers. Attorneys working for Big Asbestos had become practiced in the art of attacking tobacco and used this to their advantage in this new wave of tobacco trials. (The asbestos companies blame everything on tobacco; the tobacco companies blame everything on asbestos.) Trial lawyers were further emboldened by new doctrines of *comparative fault* and *split liability,* allowing claims for compensation even when the plaintiffs were partly to blame for whatever harms they may have suffered. Juries have been more willing to rule in favor of plaintiffs under such circumstances, which is one reason *Cipollone v. Liggett* returned a verdict favoring the plaintiffs—the first such victory in an American court of law.[21]

Big Tobacco recognized the gravity of this confluence of events and sought to develop new weapons for its defense—which is where the historians came in. In October of 1984, acting on the request of Reynolds's chief counsel, Max Crohn, attorneys from the companies' powerful Policy Committee of Lawyers formed the Special Trial Issues Committee (STIC) "for the purpose of identifying and preparing potential nonmedical witnesses for pending tobacco liability litigation." Outside counsel were tapped to coordinate this effort, with the lead being taken by Arnold & Porter; Chadbourne & Parke; Jones, Day, Reavis & Pogue; Shook, Hardy and Bacon; Webster & Sheffield; and King & Spalding. The goal was to locate scholars who could testify to (a) the "high level of public awareness" of tobacco hazards and (b) the industry's "lack of deception." This is explained in a 1992 memo reviewing the accomplishments of the Committee:

> STIC has developed social, business and medical historians as witnesses to attest to the high level of public awareness regarding tobacco hazards and the absence of any deception by the tobacco industry. These experts will also explain more broadly the evolution of tobacco in America as a result of natural social forces, wholly unrelated to industry coercion or promotion.[22]

In a nutshell: people knew what they were doing when they decided to smoke, and the companies were never involved in any kind of deception. And however tobacco "evolved" in the United States, this was purely the result of "natural social forces."

Historians were needed to buttress these claims and so were hired—in droves. Robert Sobel from Hofstra University was hired to prepare a series of papers on the history of the cigarette (for Jones Day) under the guidance of Allen R. Purvis from Shook, Hardy and Bacon. Articles from the *San Francisco Chronicle* were assembled by a team of historians hired by PHR Associates, a Florida-based "Human Resource and Risk Management" firm guided by Janet L. Johnson of Arnold & Porter. Professor James Muldoon from Rutgers was assigned the task of combing through New Jersey newspapers, with a lawyer—John B. Kearney of Kenney & Kearney—working along similar lines under Bruce Sheffler, an attorney from Chadbourne & Parke. West Virginia newspapers were handled by Shook, Hardy and Bacon's Allen Purvis, who also supervised similar work by Professors Fred Carstensen at the University of Connecticut, Irwin Unger at NYU, and Muldoon at Rutgers. PHR Associates reviewed California's Vallejo *Times* and the Mare Island *Grapevine*, collaborating with the law firm of Rogers, Joseph, O'Donnell & Quinn. Articles assembled from Mare Island papers were supposed to provide a "test run of the materials that we can generate for plaintiff-specific cases."[23]

The plan in each instance—as in most subsequent trials—was to assemble huge files of cautionary statements on smoking and health from local newspapers, magazines, schoolbooks, and whatever else might have influenced a plaintiff's "information environment"—all cast as evidence of "fair warning." Novels and plays and short stories were canvassed, along with film scripts, editorial cartoons, and comic strips. Historians were paid to look for examples of humor revealing common knowledge, as when Mark Twain commented on how easy it was to quit, having done so hundreds of times. The point was to show that anyone with even half a brain would have been "aware" that smoking was bad for you, or at least that authorities had conveyed such warnings: plaintiffs were "deluged" by such materials. "Deluge materials" from the *New York Times* and other nationally distributed newspapers were collected, with the point being again that no one could have escaped such a flood. The Winthrop Group helped assemble "deluge materials," with Shook Hardy's Allen Purvis in many cases serving as the supervising attorney. PHR Associates were assigned Texas and Kansas newspapers, Fred Carstensen reviewed *Time* and *Newsweek,* and Shook Hardy surveyed *Reader's Digest.* Texts from such publications were copied, coded, and entered into a computerized "awareness" database maintained by Jones, Day, Reavis & Pogue, with each item indexed according to an elaborate system encompassing not just author, date, and title but also type, scope, and place of publication and several hundred other categories (type of hazard, "who was spreading the word," the role of religion or the particular slang or rhetoric used, etc.).[24] Dozens of historians and student assistants were hired to help construct this database, and it could well be that the cigarette industry by this means becomes the largest industrial employer of historians in post–World War II America.

Striking in all of this "research"—which is perhaps better described as a kind of factory-scale clerical performance—is how circumscribed (and shoddy) these investigations have been. Defense historians have rarely been asked to investigate how tobacco manufacturers influenced the "information environment"; there is no exploration of the role of Hill & Knowlton or the Tobacco Institute or any of the other PR arms of the industry. Little consideration is given to the impact of cigarette ads or the industry's "white papers" or other means by which the companies denied hazards, scoffed at medical authority, and reassured smokers. Entirely ignored is the *disinformation environment*, the deliberate effort to confuse and befuddle. The industry's historians have been led to produce testimony that is phantasmagoric from the point of view of basic human psychology: there is no effort to understand the *feelings* created by visually seductive tobacco ads, for example, or the impact of sponsoring sports, music, and the arts. Or how warnings are made invisible by "wear-out," or how impressions of "corporate social responsibility" are created by conspicuous displays of sheltering the homeless and caring for battered women. A slanted, ahistorical account of popular tobacco culture is deployed in court, with the industry virtually absent as a historical actor. Louis Kyriakoudes in his review of the industry's use of historians hits this nail on the head, concluding that the historians present "a skewed history of the cigarette in which the tobacco industry all but ceases to exist."[25]

Of course it doesn't take a great deal of talent to dig up "awareness" or "deluge" materials and to code these for storage in the industry's computers. Much of the spade work is actually done by lawyers, or by researchers contracted by defense legal teams. I've mentioned PHR Associates and the Winthrop Group, but many other firms have been hired to gather such materials. A company called Texas Energy Research was hired to read through the *Beaumont Enterprise,* the *Beaumont Journal,* and Houston's three biggest newspapers for use in *Grinnell v. American,* with Chadbourne & Parke supervising. Private research corporations such as History Associates in Rockville, Maryland, or Morgan, Angel and Associates in Washington, D.C., were engaged. Boston newspapers were reviewed by Steve Nachman, an attorney with Webster & Sheffield (for use in *Palmer v. Liggett*), and Baton Rouge newspapers were cataloged by Bill Bradner of Chadbourne & Parke for use in local trials. The Tobacco Institute had maintained a newspaper clipping service since 1959, which was pilfered for examples of "awareness," as were the collections of the Tobacco Merchants Association.

The end goal in all of this was the industry's so-called universal awareness or common knowledge defense, the point being that since everyone has always known about the hazards people have only themselves to blame for whatever illnesses they contract. Everyone has always known that tobacco is bad for you, though no one has ever been able to prove it.[26] The legal implications are obvious: people voluntarily assumed risks when they began smoking, and the companies acted responsibly in refusing to admit any proof of a danger. This has also been dubbed the "chicken soup defense," as in, people have always known that chicken soup is good for you, but medical scholars have only recently proved it. The idea is that popular knowledge often precedes expert knowledge, so ordinary people knew about tobacco harms long before they were proven by scientists.

It is important to realize that while historians who work for the industry may be well known for their scholarship, their litigation-related work is typically not widely known—even to their colleagues. In some instances the industry actually *requires* a certain measure of confidentiality. Consultants are told that their work falls under a kind of attorney work product privilege (John Burnham makes this claim, for example),[27] and some scholars sign a contract *requiring* that they not publish using the sources under investigation. James H. Jones, for example, signed a non-publication agreement when he went to work for the industry in the late 1980s, about five years after publishing his book, *Bad Blood,* on the Tuskegee syphilis experiments. Jones was being groomed as an expert witness, but after about a year and a half of work in Library of Congress archives and Arents's famous collection at the New York Public Library he was dropped, perhaps because (as he now suspects) the lawyers were unhappy with his recognition of the reality of addiction. That is how the industry works: it has enough money to hire large numbers of scholars, giving them nominally free rein to investigate certain (narrow) topics, and then promotes a select few to the status of expert witness who can be counted on to stick to the requisite script. Jones, incidentally, is the only historian with whom I have spoken who regrets having worked for the industry, though perhaps there are others.[28]

The industry was more pleased with John C. Burnham, who had gone to work for the industry a few years prior to this time, in 1986. Burnham is one of the few industry experts ever to have published on tobacco prior to his work for the companies, though it should also be noted that his book, *Bad Habits: Drinking, Smoking, Taking Drugs, Gambling, Sexual Misbehavior and Swearing in American History* (1993) was published five years *after* he began working for Philip Morris's Project Cosmic. Burnham was one of three Project Cosmic directors with a history of medicine background, along with David Harley, then at Oxford, and Yale psychiatry professor David Musto who, according to his website, should be considered "the leading historian of drug policy in the United States."[29] More than a dozen medical historians would eventually work for the industry, tainting the articles and editorial boards of the world's leading medical history journals (see Figure 33).

WITNESSING FOR THE INDUSTRY IN COURT

Among the various services rendered by historians to Big Tobacco, the most disturbing—and consequential—is their provision of testimony in court. Expert witnesses are most often recruited from the larger body of consultants already working for the companies, sometimes for months or even years. Jon Harkness, for example, was chosen to help defend the industry as an expert witness in *Boerner v. Brown & Williamson* (in 2003) after having worked for the industry for about eight years, part of which overlapped with his editorship of *Isis,* the official journal of the History of Science Society. For his tobacco work Harkness was paid about $500,000: $300,000 as salary and another $200,000 for research expenses. I analyzed the substance of his testimony in a recent article for *Tobacco Control*,[30] raising this question of disclosure: should authors be required to disclose such relationships? What about members of an editorial board or peer reviewers: should they be required to disclose? And if so, how and how often and to whom? And is disclosure always enough? When does scholarship become too tainted to publish? This last-mentioned item may sound outlandish, but the fact is that several medical journals already bar publication of any and all research funded by the tobacco industry,[31] and perhaps it is time for historians to consider doing the same.

The network of historians who have testified as expert witnesses for the industry is large, including at least forty-eight professors of history in the United States alone. (Non-historians have presented historical testimony,[32] but those persons listed in the box on pages 460–63 are all professional historians.) One particularly disturbing aspect of this business is the deep involvement of *medical* historians. Kenneth Ludmerer, M.D., a Washington University professor of medicine and medical history, was actually the first academic historian to testify on the stand for the industry—in *Kotler v. American Tobacco*, an individual plaintiff's case tried in Boston in 1990. Ludmerer had begun working for the industry in August of 1988, when Arnold & Porter hired him to prepare a response to Jeffrey E. Harris, an MIT economist who, in 1985, had written a chronicle of the recognition of tobacco health hazards for the plaintiffs in *Cipollone v. Liggett*.[33] It is not entirely clear how Ludmerer first came to the attention of tobacco attorneys, but it may have been through the recruitment efforts of John Burnham at Ohio State, who had earlier been listed as a witness for the defense in *Cipollone*. Ludmerer says he agreed to work for the industry after seeing the poor quality of historical testimony introduced by the plaintiffs, but what is remarkable is how truncated his own investigations have been—especially in light of his own self-praise.

In 2002 in *USA v. Philip Morris*, for example, Ludmerer claimed to have studied the history of tobacco and health "more thoroughly, more comprehensively, more representatively, more systematically than anyone in the world had ever done." He admitted that the Surgeon General's report of 1964 "helped erase any residual doubt" about the lung cancer hazard, but nowhere did he acknowledge the industry's refusal to admit the reality of such hazards. Remarkably, he also never consulted the industry's internal documents. In *Harvey v. Lummus* he admitted to having never asked anyone at Philip Morris what the company knew about the hazards of smoking; nor did he review any internal industry documents:

Q: Would it be correct to say that you have not reviewed a single internal Philip Morris company document?
A: That is correct.[34]

Ludmerer seems not to have been embarrassed by this; he just didn't consider it part of his assignment. That is where much of the bias in such testimony can be found: in delimitation of expertise, in the framing of questions posed and questions neglected—producing a kind of strategic myopia or tunnel vision. Asked about his neglect of such documents, Ludmerer says this had to do with the historian's unavoidable "setting boundaries" to research. Queried about the TIRC, he says only, "I have heard the term. . . . I really don't know much about it. I have not studied it, I have no intention to study it. It is again out of my area." Delimitation of expertise seems to be a deliberate industry strategy: they hire and train a scholar in only one particular area and then can be assured that when he or she is asked a potentially embarrassing question, this will be beyond their scope of competence. Ludmerer in *Cipollone* claimed not even to know whether smoking posed a public health threat:

> Q: Sir, would you agree that there is reliable evidence today to suggest that cigarette smoking is a major threat to the smoking public? . . .
>
> A: I do not have an opinion on that subject, an expert opinion.

Again, in the same deposition:

> Q: Doctor, is it your opinion that cigarette smoking contributes to the development of lung cancer in human beings?
>
> A: I have no opinion on that.
>
> Q: Do you have an opinion as a physician?
>
> A: No, I have no expert opinion.[35]

How could such a distinguished medical scholar have no opinion on what is arguably the most important medical fact of modernity? We don't have to speculate; the fact is that Ludmerer was simply following the script drafted for him by his handlers. In 1988, in a memo titled "Witness Development," Arnold & Porter's Janet L. Johnson explained to STIC's State-of-the-Art Subcommittee their need to develop a "storyteller" to tell "our version" of the history of the recognition of tobacco hazards. Jeffrey Harris's expert report for *Cipollone* had presented a detailed chronicle of the discovery of the lung cancer hazard, identifying evidence from the 1930s and the strong case for a proof by 1957. The industry wanted to counter this testimony, without having to address when a link had actually been established: "Instead of trying to defend the issue of whether and when a link between cigarette smoking and lung cancer was established, we should consider focusing our testimony on defending 1954, attacking Harris' 1957 date on which a link was 'proven,' and demonstrate that it was not 'proven' in 1957 with post-57 statements by medical experts about the existence of a controversy."[36] The industry's claim would be that controversy persisted after 1957 and that the relationship between lung cancer and cigarettes "was not even a legitimate scientific question until 1954." Johnson realized there was little to be gained by extending the state-of-the-art story into more recent times; indeed there were advantages to limiting the time span covered by their expert, insofar as this would free them from having to answer questions about when in fact the controversy was resolved. Johnson acknowledged the tightrope any such expert would have to walk when distinguishing his personal opinion from his expert testimony:

> This witness could probably testify credibly that it is his *personal* opinion that cigarette smoking is only a "risk factor" in the etiology of lung cancer. It would be less credible, however, for this witness to give expert testimony that the *community* of scientific and medical experts believe today that smoking is only a risk factor.[37]

That is why Ludmerer could make this delicate point, that he had no "expert" opinion on causality whatever his personal views might be. Recall that the conspiracy to deny *all* evidence of hazards was still in force; it would not be abandoned until the end of the 1990s, when legal settlements with the states forced a (partial) retreat. The industry's lawyers realized they were going to have to deal with certain "tensions" in the testimony of any medical history expert: "What will this witness say about general causation? What will this witness say about the current state-of-the-art? Is the 'controversy' still alive? If not, when did it end? If it's still alive, who believes it? Only tobacco interests? Who else?"[38]

Defense attorneys had earlier tried to resolve these tensions by developing a medical history witness who was not a physician—and could therefore get away with having no expert opinion on causation. This witness would be hired to focus exclusively on pre-1960 events—absolving them of having to talk about the industry's conduct after that time. As expressed in 1988, this was one of the industry's "original mandates" for developing a state-of-the-art witness:

> One of the original mandates for developing a witness to address "state-of-the-art" issues was to find a witness (a) who could not have an expert opinion on general causation, and (b) who could not address the current state-of-the-art on general causation. Following this mandate, we developed a non-M.D./medical historian [John Burnham] who, because he was not a medical doctor, could not have an expert opinion on general causation and who, because his research and expertise focused on the pre-1960 period of history, did not have an expert opinion on the current state-of-the-art. On the other hand, this witness was not qualified to evaluate specific research issues because he was not a medical doctor or a scientist. By contrast, however, a state-of-the-art expert with medical credentials will have to face squarely issues on general causation.[39]

Notice how carefully crafted this search for an expert witness was. The witness had to be ignorant on the crucial issue of causation, since the industry's denialist enterprise was still in force. Nor could the expert safely address state-of-the-art issues after 1964, because that would expose the bankruptcy of the industry's denial of causation. Ludmerer solved the latter problem: he was a medical historian but was asked to investigate only the limited time frame from 1930 to 1964, keeping the spotlight off those several decades thereafter, when the conspiracy of denial was still in full force. And the problem of causation was solved by having him separate whatever "personal" views he might have from those based on his professional expertise.

The testimony offered by defense historians in American tobacco litigation is not difficult to grasp. Indeed it can be summarized in a single sentence: "Everyone knew, but no one had proof." People have only themselves to blame for whatever suffering is caused by cigarettes, and the industry did nothing wrong in questioning statistics or stalling for more research or marketing "light" cigarettes. Of course there are sub-strategies and nuances in such testimony: Ludmerer, for example, argues that statements must be situated in the context of their times, that history is complex and messy, and that we must guard against the 20–20 vision of hindsight— "Monday morning quarterbacking." All fine truisms, but in the industry's hands all gamed as exculpatory stratagems. Ludmerer's stress on context, for example, allows him to situate, to exculpate, to make the abnormal seem normal. Admonishing against hindsight allows him to say that events back in the day were not as they appear to us now; we need to cut the past some slack and not judge too harshly. Messiness also suggests a fog of uncertainty about the past, with neither black nor white but only shades of gray. Countless variants on such arguments have been introduced to deny addiction or enfeeble advertising or otherwise exculpate the industry. The defenses are elaborate, hackneyed, and sometimes formulaic to the point of exhibiting plagiarism;[40] they are also put forward in court by such distinguished professors as Peter English of Duke (a pediatrician and medical historian), Michael Schaller at the University of Arizona, Elizabeth Cobbs-Hoffman at San Diego State, Lacy Ford at the University of South Carolina, Michael E. Parrish of UC San Diego, and dozens of others (see again the box on pages 460–63).

THE HUMAN COST

I've highlighted several different ethical breaches in the tobacco–history encounter. These ethical issues are weighty enough, but more than ethics is at stake. Let me conclude this chapter by recalling that there is a human cost to expertise and that every time a historian steps into a courtroom human lives hang in the balance. What is the human cost of expertise, when historians work for the tobacco industry in court?

According to a *Wall Street Journal* report from 2000, the U.S. tobacco industry spends about $900 million per year on legal expenses.[41] Let's call it a billion. The value of such efforts to the industry could be quite a bit higher, but let's assume this is a justifiable expense and one of their many costs of doing business. If we regard this as a normal business investment, and one for which the companies expect a reward on a par with other investments, we can calculate its impact on tobacco pricing and therefore on tobacco consumption and therefore on human health.

Let us assume the industry cannot win its cases without experts and that historians provide the industry with, say, 10 percent of its litigation expertise. Let us assume, for the sake of argument, that historians contribute $100 million a year to the industry's survival.[42] The figure could well be higher than this, since the billion or so spent on litigation may be worth many times this amount. It could be lower if you think that historians don't contribute much to the winning of such cases. Let us further assume that this $100 million is a savings passed on to consumers in a form that basically keeps the price of cigarettes low.

What would this mean for the impact of historical expertise on human health?

The cost of litigation can be considered a kind of tax on cigarettes. If the cost is passed on to consumers in the form of higher prices and higher prices means fewer cigarettes smoked, then we can calculate how many deaths are caused by the provision of historical expertise. That is because there is a close and predictable relationship between the number of cigarettes smoked in a society and the number of tobacco-induced deaths in that society twenty-five years later. The delay stems from the long but predictable "time lag" between exposure and death: Philip Morris talks about this as "not unlike a glacier," to which new smokers are "added" at one end and eventually melt away at the other, "slowly, steadily over time."[43] This relationship is consistent and predictable and basically runs as follows.

For every million cigarettes smoked in a society there will be one excess death caused by those cigarettes. And for every three million cigarettes smoked there will be one extra death from lung cancer. Both have this time lag of about twenty-five years. These are approximations of course but seem to hold pretty much true for anywhere in the world. Divide the number of cigarettes smoked in any given year by three million, and you will have the number of lung cancer deaths per annum twenty-five years later.

So what does this say about the impact of our experts? The first thing to recall is that the price elasticity of tobacco is about .4—which means that for every 10 percent increase in price, consumption will fall by about 4 percent. A $100 million increase in cost therefore causes about $40 million worth of cigarettes not to be consumed. If cigarettes cost $5 per pack with twenty cigarettes per pack, this means that an increase in the price of cigarettes by $100 million will cause a reduction in the number of packs smoked by $40 million divided by $5/pack = 8 million packs, or 160 million cigarettes. If cigarettes cause one death for every million smoked, this means that the industry's deployment of historical expertise in litigation causes about 160 deaths per year.

Of course the true figure, if there is such a thing, could be higher or lower. Maybe it's not 160 but 16 or 1,600. The point is not to calculate an exact or even an approximate figure but rather simply to emphasize that the provision of aid to polluting industries costs human lives. It's not just a question of moral or social responsibility; it's also a question of life and death.[44]

Do historians realize that lives hang in the balance when they step into the witness stand? I don't know what they are thinking, or if they really are thinking. Maybe they are dazzled by the money or the attention, or just trying to do "a good job." Some may see in the defense of smoking a higher cause of some sort, perhaps liberty or personal responsibility; many are clearly led to focus on some narrow body of historical facts and may not even know or care they are missing the forest for the trees. Some may think they are working not for Big Tobacco but for some higher truth that is supposed to come from the clash of warring experts. Most seem to take comfort in the belief that their handlers don't seem to be "influencing" their findings. Historians employed for such purposes may well be (kept) ignorant of the consequences of their actions, perhaps by the elaborate parceling up of tasks that is often entailed in such assignments. Perhaps they feel they are just following facts, if not just following orders.

PART FOUR

Radiant Filth and Redemption

What we have thus far seen of the rise of lung cancer, that is surely just the beginning of the catastrophe.
FRITZ LICKINT, 1953

If the exit gate from our market should suddenly open, we could be out of business overnight.
CLAUDE E. TEAGUE, 1982

ON MAY 26, 1995, Philip Morris made a startling announcement. The world's largest cigarette company admitted that a sizable number of its cigarettes had been "tainted" by improper mixing of a plasticizing agent ordinarily used in making filters and announced the beginning of a recall. Eight billion "smelly, bad-tasting cigarettes" were eventually pulled from the shelves, after smokers had started noticing an odor akin to certain kinds of plastics or pesticides. The recall cost the company over $100 million, but the public was assured no harm was done, and business continued as usual. A batch of improperly mixed "plasticizer" was blamed for the foul-up, though details were never released on precisely how this had gotten into the tobacco.[1] It eventually turned out that the contaminant—methyl isocyanate, a close relative of the compound that killed thousands when released from a chemical plant at Bhopal, India—was not from a plasticizer but from the paperboard used to make hard-pack cartons of Marlboros, Virginia Slims, and Benson & Hedges.

This recall is odd, though, on several levels. One of the largest consumer product recalls in history was absorbed with little more than a hiccup in the company's stock price, which had risen nearly seventy-fold since the mid-1970s, outperforming the Dow Jones Industrial Average by an order of magnitude. (FYI: $10,000 invested in Philip Morris stock in 1958 would now be worth about $50 million.) The move is also odd, though, because it must have saved many lives—albeit not for reasons one might imagine. The recall saved lives not because it prevented exposure to a defective plasticizer but rather because these were cigarettes no one ended up smoking. Since one person dies for every million cigarettes smoked, in theory at least this recall saved about eight thousand lives.

Of course if Philip Morris had had its way the cigarettes would never have been contaminated and would have been sold and smoked in the usual deadly sort of way, killing those eight thousand people. The company didn't recall the cigarettes to save lives; the recall was issued simply to protect the company's image—fouled by whatever PR mess might have come from people throwing away their stinking fags, fearing Bhopal.

The tobacco industry spends a great deal of time—and money—making cigarettes look good. The paper is bleached to a pleasing ivory white, the rod evenly shaped and uniform, the package sparkly clean and attractive. Even the color of the ash is not left to chance: the companies have learned that smokers prefer a light-colored ash, and chemicals are added to achieve this effect. Billions of dollars have gone into cigarette design, much of which involves manipulation of physical image and symbolic effluents. The modern cigarette is a work of art (or piece of work), fêted via billions in ad and promotional revenues as a handy, handsome, white, svelte, smooth, and easily fondled consumer "good."

Image and reality, however, are as night and day in this realm. We've already seen how Kents were sold with "micronite" filters containing crocidolite asbestos: billions of asbestos-laden cigarettes were smoked from 1952 through 1956, causing some number of smokers to contract asbestosis, lung cancer, or mesothelioma after inhaling the mineral needles of this Lorillard brand. Scholars have gone back to dissect old cigarettes from such packs, which reveal (via electron microscopy) asbestos fibers protruding from the business ends of these vintage cigarettes. And by smoking them on machines designed to replicate the human lung, scholars have calculated how many fibers were likely to have been inhaled. Smokers of Kents in the mid-1950s on average inhaled over a hundred million particles of asbestos every year, more than enough to cause tumors. Lawsuits against Lorillard have been filed by people suffering from mesothelioma or lung cancer, and some such cases have been won.[2]

Asbestos, though, has been only one of many "extra" ingredients in cigarettes. Smokers inhale fibers of cellulose acetate, the chemical standard for virtually all modern filters, but smokers are also known to have inhaled charcoal particles, sand, the combustion products of various machine greases, worm and insect body parts and excrement, asbestos filaments from ceiling insulation in tobacco plants, and other kinds of filth. Cigarette manufacturing is not, in fact, a very clean business. A 1958 study by British tobacco manufacturers found bits of steel from the knives used to cut tobacco, along with sand from the carborundum wheels used to sharpen those knives. Food inspectors routinely examine food for flies, vermin and rot, and various forms of adulteration, but who watches over the cigarette factories?[3]

One way to learn about such contaminants is from the many letters of complaint written to the companies. Smokers have often contacted the companies to protest finding filth or defects of one sort or another in cigarettes, and in 1983 the American Tobacco Company divided these complaints into twenty-five separate categories, as part of an effort to compare its different manufacturing plants. Most of those who complained drew attention to cigarettes broken or torn by rough handling, but stems, worms, rubber, plastic, metal shards, and other "foreign matter" were also noted. The Reynolds company preserved many such letters, containing similar complaints. A sailor stationed at Pearl Harbor in 1998 wrote about a carton he had bought containing three cigarettes with bug holes in them, including one with "at least one bug alive!"[4] A man from Alton, New York, complained about an odd taste in several of the Doral Menthol Lights he had recently purchased, prompting him to dissect one: "I decided to take one of the cigarettes apart. I found this meal worm or whatever type it is in with the cigarette tobacco."[5] A woman from Shoreline, Washington, complained about a different problem: "Today I was about halfway done with my cigarette when it suddenly flamed up! The flame was high enough that it burnt my nose and singed my hair!"[6]

The companies must have received hundreds of thousands of such complaints over the years. A man from Newcastle, Texas, complained that his Doral cigarettes tasted "so much like bug spray I couldn't smoke them." A woman from Gurnee, Illinois, reported that her Salem Lights "not only taste funny," but gave her "a blinding headache." A woman from East Baldwin, Maine, wrote after finding worms: "I know that smoking isn't good for you, but I don't enjoy smoking worms." Others wrote to complain about filters detaching or air bubbles in the wrap or a "terrible aftertaste . . . tinny or metal of some sort"; others complained about cigarettes being "as old as dirt" or full of holes or exploding into the smoker's face. A man from Tampico, Illinois, wrote that his wife had been driving when the front end of her cigarette fell off, burning her hand. A Florida man wrote, "I found a stick inside the cigarette! What is it? Tobacco? Wood? Please explain!" A Madera, California, woman wrote, "My husband thinks that because of all the law suits and attorney fees that your letting the quality of your product go down." R. J. Reynolds carefully tabulated each of these letters and categorized them by nature of complaint. In one three-month period from 1995 the company logged thirty-eight pages of complaints for the single category "Fire Falls Out" (causing burns).[7] Product complaints were traced by elaborate tracking mechanisms to specific factories and even to specific making machines; complaints about "insufficient glue," for example, were traced back to the specific machines that had produced those cigarettes.[8]

The archives also preserve examples of the companies' responses. In 1999, when a man from Martinsburg, West Virginia, wrote to Reynolds about feeling sick from smoking a cigarette with some kind of metal in it, Reynolds Consumer Response Specialist Ginger Coe wrote to reassure that the company had examined the metal and found it to be "a piece of wire composed of iron and copper." This was no cause for alarm, Coe wrote, because

> Copper is a metal with a low order of toxicity. It is also an essential trace element required for good health. The temperature encountered in a cigarette and the duration of contact is not sufficient to volatilize metallic copper (MP = 1083°C). Iron also has

a low order of toxicity and is also an essential trace element required for good health. The temperature encountered in a cigarette and the duration of contact is not sufficient to volatilize metallic iron (MP = 1535°C). Based on a thorough review of all available information, our scientists have concluded any health risk associated with the one-time smoking of this material is minimal and would not be responsible for the health effects you described.[9]

We also know there were differences from factory to factory in the particular kinds of screw-ups. "Odor" was a more common complaint for cigarettes made at American's Durham plant than at its Reidsville facility, whereas Durham was more likely to generate complaints about worms. Similar records were kept for cigarettes stained, missing, or defective in some physical aspect. In 1988 American Tobacco received thirty-nine written complaints of cigarettes being "wormy," with the highest number coming from Florida.[10] This was an improvement over previous years: in 1983, for example, eighty complaints of worms were received within the space of a single month. Perhaps you were a smoker back then and smoked some of these worms? Or their excreted feces?

Of course it is strange to think about contaminants in smoke when even pure, pristine, natural tobacco is already toxic. If even the cleanest cigarette smoke will kill you, does it really matter if there is extra filth in the form of metal shards or insect excrement? Perhaps this is different from, say, fecal pellets in your cereal or hair in your hot dog. We don't really have much of a common cultural perception of the filth in cigarettes, nothing we can compare to the rot and stench of the stockyards Upton Sinclair exposed in *The Jungle*. Which is odd, because far more people die from cigarettes than ever perished from the maggots and microbes that once tainted our meat.

The moral of this story is not that tobacco should be clean but rather that its makers cannot be trusted. To find out more about what is really in a cigarette we need to return to the archives, where we find the companies well aware of the presence in cigarettes of lead and arsenic, along with pesticides and polonium and a witches' brew of chemicals added for various purposes. Topics rarely broached in the consumer letters—because most people really have no idea what they are smoking.

What's Actually in Your Cigarette?

The belief that cigarettes contain only pure, unadulterated tobacco is almost universal among smokers . . . they are blissfully ignorant of the ungodly messes of which they are composed.

HERMAN SHARLIT, "CIGARETTE SMOKING AS A HEALTH HAZARD," 1935

There's an old saying in the food business, that people will eat almost anything if you grind it up fine enough. With food of course there is a certain amount of over-sight, and acute poisonings attract attention. But with tobacco the situation is different. Cigarette makers have had virtually unlimited freedom to add whatever they want to cigarettes—whether to elevate sales or reduce costs or kill mold or prolong shelf life or make handling by machinery easier. Or to supercharge the nicotine or to appeal to the youthful sweet tooth. And given the fertility of the tobacco man's mind, some remarkable things have been added. Tobacco chemists put a breath-taking variety of additives into tobacco leaf, cigarette paper, and packaging foils: flavorants and moisturizers, of course, but also impact boosters, burn accelerants, fire retardants, bronchodilators, smoke particle size reducers, and a broad palette of coloring and bleaching agents.

And that's just what is there by design. Smokers may think they are smoking cured tobacco leaf, but there is actually quite a bit of other stuff in cigarettes—some of which enters just by chance. The industry doesn't like to admit it, but we know from their internal archives that unwanted filth sometimes makes its way into cigarettes. This includes shards of metal or glass but also substances that enter through rough handling in the growing stage—dirt, sand, and pesticides, for example, but also grease from the machines and even chemicals that gas off from the cellophane.[1] The list of contaminants is long.

Before diving in, though, we should appreciate that additives and contaminants have never been high on the list of things that tobacco's critics worry about,[2] given that the "pure" cured leaf by itself is so toxic. What difference does it really make that a company is adding dangerous chemicals if "natural" tobacco is already super-deadly? American Spirit's much-hyped "natural" cigarettes are no less deadly than any other kind, despite having a Native American on the pack. The same with China's popular "herbal" brands. Worrying about whether your tobacco is natural or organic is like worrying about whether the fecal pellet in your cereal was excreted by a caged or free-range rat.

There is another oddity we must keep in mind. The industry has long maintained that it uses only "approved" food additives, which makes about as much sense as the rat pellet point. For many years this additives list was a closely guarded secret, and even today we know more about the constituents of cat food—which should give smokers pause. But think for a moment about this "approved food additive" point. A fruit salad eaten is quite different from a fruit salad burned and inhaled. Almost any complex organic mixture will be toxic when pyrolyzed and drawn into the lungs, and you can be sure that a fresh fruit salad dried, burned, and inhaled will not do you any good. And the same is true for many of the additives forced into tobacco. Sugar may be relatively safe when consumed in moderation (apart from cavities and the like) but when burned in a cigarette will produce acetaldehyde, a carcinogen. Glycerine is likewise innocuous when eaten but when combusted produces acetaldehyde and acrolein, carcinogens both. Protein is also of course an essential nutrient—in food—but quite toxic when burned and inhaled. Burning protein produces nitrosamines, among the deadliest of all carcinogens. (Philip Morris scientists in 1963 characterized nitrosamines as "the most potent carcinogens known," with the dosage needed to produce cancer being "exceedingly low.") So it is ridiculous to say that some specific cigarette ingredient is "generally regarded as safe" (GRAS)—as we so often hear from the industry.[3] The entire concept of GRAS is intended solely for foods, not for substances burned and inhaled. The confusion is bizarre and a typical tobacco subterfuge of the facts.

So let us ask again: What is in your cigarette? Here are a few of the choicer items, with some of the history behind how they got there.

ARSENIC AND LEAD

Arsenic and lead became a hot potato in the 1930s and 1940s, when lead arsenates and arsenites were widely used as pesticides—on tobacco but also on many kinds of food crops. Catastrophic poisonings in the 1930s inflamed the press, as when dozens of laborers in the Moselle Valley (near Germany's border with Luxembourg) died after spraying the compound on grapes. Some died from drinking wine made from the grapes, and autopsies showed that many of these victims had tumors.[4] No one knows how many people perished from handling the pesticide—or from the arsenic that lingers even today in cigarettes.

By the early 1930s the tobacco industry had already started hiding what it knew about arsenic. A letter of 1932 to Lorillard's vice president detailing the arsenic content in "Plain Havana Blossom" chewing tobacco, for example, began by noting, "Since we understand that considerable secrecy has been maintained relative to the subject, we are taking the liberty of writing you this report in long-hand, and trust that you will be able to make it out." Lorillard measured an average of 2.8 parts per million (ppm) arsenic in its tobacco, though other investigators had been finding up to 30 ppm in the actual smoke. Pesticides were one principal source, but Henry Ford—the carmaker and cigarette critic—as early as 1914 had reported arsenic being used (along with lime and lead) to toughen cigarette paper and that solutions made from paper treated in this manner had enough poison in them to kill mice.[5]

Lead got into cigarettes the same way as arsenic—mainly from lead arsenate pesticides—but there were other sources. The metal was commonly used in the *foil* used to wrap cigarettes, for example, a practice not banned in the United States until the 1940s—by the War Production Board, interestingly, which implemented the ban not to protect human health but rather to safeguard the nation's supply of metals for making ammunition. Leaded gas was also sometimes used as a fuel for cigarette lighters, which must have caused some inhalation. Pesticides, though, were clearly the predominant source, with the *Consumers' Research Bulletin* already by 1936 proposing as a cynical cigarette slogan: "Have you inhaled your lead and arsenic today?"[6]

Agricultural spraying of arsenic was drastically cut back after the Second World War, causing measured levels of both arsenic and lead in cigarettes to decline. Unpublished studies done by the Imperial Tobacco Company had documented a gradual increase in As_2O_3 in unburned leaf throughout the 1930s and 1940s, with the highest values (51 ppm) recorded in 1947. Many scholars at this time—Richard Doll, for example—thought arsenic might well be the principal carcinogenic agent in cigarettes, and speculations were sometimes voiced that eliminating the element from smoke might make cigarettes less deadly.[7] Arsenic levels in smoke have fallen ever since, with smokers today inhaling only hundreds of kilograms per year, compared with the hundreds of thousands of kilograms from previous decades. With the phasing out of arsenic insecticides, however, one ogre was simply replaced by another with just as many warts—which brings us to the synthetic pesticides of the postwar era.

PETROCHEMICAL PESTICIDES

People in the tobacco trade apply a wide variety of chemicals while growing the plant, weeding the fields, curing and aging the leaf, and rolling and packing the final product. Chemicals are used to save on time or human labor but also to keep the plant from being attacked by pathogens of one sort or another. Much of what the industry worries about in terms of "tobacco and health" is actually damage to the tobacco plant—from microbes like the tobacco mosaic virus or a bacterium of some sort but also molds, fungi, and myriad insect pests. Treatments generally involve spraying the soil, plant, or stored leaf, often with chemicals that end up as residues in groundwater or the cigarettes people smoke.[8] The threats are diverse, as are the compounds used to combat them.

Blue mold and black shank, for example, are prevented by sprayings with fungicides such as mancozeb, a carbamate nerve toxin also known to cross the placental barrier. Metalaxyl is often applied, though this benzenoid fungicide is feared for creating resistant strains in other crops. (Farmers consult the online Blue Mold Forecast System, which identifies outbreaks.) Powdery mildew is thwarted by sprayings of dinocap and benomyl, black root rot with methyl bromide and soil sterilants such as chloropicrin. Bacteria also attack the plant, causing black leg, hollow stalk, and barn rot, treated by methods similar to those used to control nematodes. Nematodes—tiny subterranean roundworms—attack the tobacco plant by roosting in the roots, where they form galls and promote the growth of fungi, causing black shank, fusarium wilt, and black root rot. Nematodes are beaten back with fumigants such as ethylene dibromide, Aldicarb, 1,3-dichloropropene, and methyl isothiocyanate.

Integrated pest management has become the fashion here as elsewhere, but chemical insecticides remain a big part of the tobacco world. Cutworms are controlled by sprayings around the base of the plant, and white grubs and false wireworms are countered by soil fumigants. Similar chemicals are used to combat aphids, flea beetles, grasshoppers, hornworms, loopers, stinkbugs, thrips, leaf miners, tobacco slugs, stem borers, and whiteflies. Predators attack the tobacco as it is stored, so dimethyl dichlorvinyl phosphate is used to control the cigarette beetle and tobacco moth, two predators that alone chew up hundreds of millions of dollars worth of tobacco stocks every year—and that's just in the United States. Cigarette beetles are found at all stages of manufacturing, presenting the specter not just of economic loss but also of cigarettes contaminated by "insect corpses or byproducts" such as feces and body oils.[9]

So even though pheromone traps and the like are sometimes used to catch cigarette moths, a great deal of poison is still sprayed on or around the leaf at one stage or another. Many such chemicals are hard to handle safely but can also be hazardous for smokers who inhale the residues and for wildlife wherever tobacco is grown. Many tobacco pesticides harm birds or cause soil depletion; some, like methyl bromide, are notorious ozone depleters. Applications tend to be quite heavy, with some tobacco crops receiving as many as sixteen different treatments. One of the most widely used is maleic hydrazide, a "suckering" agent that deserves some special remarks.

MALEIC HYDRAZIDE: PESTICIDE FOR SUCKERS

Plants often do things farmers don't like, and one of these is to sprout where they shouldn't be sprouting, depriving already established leaves of energy for growth. To prevent this, tobacco farmers apply suckering agents, the most popular of which is maleic hydrazide (MH-30), a growth retardant used to remove new shoots from the stalk of the plant after topping. (Topping involves removing flower tops to concentrate growth in the leaves.) The compound has been recognized since the 1960s—even by the industry—as a carcinogen, but farmers have been reluctant to give it up. In Rhodesia, present-day Zimbabwe, the compound was actually banned for use on tobacco in the early 1960s. Today, though, it is still widely used, and residues can be found in most cigarettes. Philip Morris in 1987 launched Project Moon to monitor contamination and found the following levels in European brands, measured in parts per million.[10]

Brand	Company	Maleic Hydrazide Levels (ppm)	
		June	December
Marlboro	Philip Morris	43.7	43.7
HB	British American	36.3	31.1
Camel	R. J. Reynolds	28.4	35.8
Lord Extra	Reemtsma	9.5	33.7
P. Stuyvesant	Reemtsma	23.2	20.0
West	Reemtsma	22.6	21.0
Ernte 23	Reemtsma	18.9	20.0
Reva1, plain	Reemtsma	44.7	35.8
R6	Reemtsma	14.2	23.7
Roth Händle, plain	BTM (Reemtsma)	<2.0	7.9
Lux	MB	13.2	10.5
Krone	British American	22.1	23.7

Cigarettes weigh about a gram, which means that if a trillion were being smoked in any given year (which is about right for Europe at that time) and residues averaged 20 micrograms per cigarette, then the total mass of just this one herbicide in cigarettes smoked by Europeans was about 20,000 kilograms per year. MH-30 residues have been recorded even higher—up to 115 ppm in some samples—with 5 to 7 percent being transferred into the smoke.[11]

Of course while exposures from any one cigarette may be small, the aggregate over a lifetime can add up—which is significant when it comes to pesticides, given how many thousands of tons are sprayed on tobacco. In the United States alone, according to the General Accounting Office, an estimated 27 million pounds of pesticides are sprayed onto tobacco fields every year. Indeed for non-agricultural workers, inhaled tobacco smoke will likely be the principal means by which smokers are exposed to pesticides—with the mode of delivery being about as dangerous as it gets. Farmworkers are exposed via several different routes, but smokers burn it right into their lungs. Environmentalists have been sounding this alarm for quite some time: Rachel Carson in her 1962 *Silent Spring* pointed to the cumulative nature of sprayings, causing the arsenic content of American cigarettes to rise more than 300 percent from 1932 to 1952.[12]

Government agencies have long been granted authority to control such compounds in foods but have never had much power to limit pesticides in cigarettes. Most countries have been apathetic: German authorities in 1988, for example, confirmed their "lack of concern" with residues of methoprene (Kabat Tobacco Protector) on imported leaf so long as it was kept below 10 ppm. And a Philip Morris document from 1991 talks about how Malaysia was being pressured—by the tobacco giant—to increase its tolerance from 1 to 15 ppm.[13] Apathy stems in part from the fact that for tobacco control advocates it doesn't really matter how tobacco kills you; the brute fact is that it does, and the details are, in a sense, a distraction. Another source of neglect stems from the fact that manufacturers rarely alert smokers to the presence of pesticides in cigarettes. Some companies have recently tried to play the "pesticide-free" card: American Spirit cigarettes, for example, are advertised as made from "100% additive-free natural tobacco" and have managed to capture much of this eco-granola market. Reynolds saw this as a growth area in the 1980s and 1990s and set out to buy the rights to this brand (from the Santa Fe Natural Tobacco Co.)—which it did for a whopping $340 million in 2002. Health-conscious smokers in the San Francisco Bay Area are enthusiastic consumers of this naturo-bunkum brand—which makes about as much sense as hoping that the car crashing into you is a fuel-efficient Prius rather than a gas-guzzling Ford.

Pesticides have also been ignored because of regulatory or administrative impotence. Cigarettes have not until recently been regulated by the FDA, so there never has been any full disclosure of what is actually in a cigarette, or virtually any limit on either contaminants or additives. And no requirement to study the health impact of an additive, prior to adding it. So regulatory myopia has encouraged industrial nonchalance. The companies have long fought to keep pesticide residues from being classed as foods (or drugs) and to keep tolerances high in those few countries where pesticides in tobacco are regulated.[14] The industry has been largely self-regulating in this realm, which is more like saying anything goes. So when specific additives are discussed, this is most often done under the irrelevant rubric "ingestion," as if eating a dried leaf soaked in licorice was the same as burning and inhaling it. With the irony that whatever pesticides end up in a smoker's lungs, even if deadly, might be no worse than the "natural" fumes from gimmicks like American Spirit.

FLAVORANTS AND ADDITIVES

Tobacco manufacturers add flavorants to cigarettes for many different reasons: to enhance pack aroma or "cool" the smoke, to attract the young or beginning smoker, or just to mask the nasty stank of nicotine. Many of these were already in use in the nineteenth century, with old-time stalwarts like cocoa, licorice, and molasses joined more recently by exotics like rose of latakia, imperial prune, and a parade of synthetics from German or Japanese labs. Many of these are described in the industry's archives, but some take detective work to decipher, as they're listed only under code names. AMSPIN, CROTAN, and MADMART, for example, turn out to be licorice, cocoa powder, and St. John's bread. (British American Tobacco began using five to seven-letter code names for additives prior even to the Second World War, continuing a practice from the trade secret–sensitive flavorants industry.)[15] Flavorants are often added not for taste at all but rather just to improve the smell of the cigarette prior to combustion—upon opening the pack, for example ("pack aroma" appears in five thousand company documents). The industry has devoted enormous resources to researching the sensory qualities of tobacco and the impact of various additives and has developed an elaborate vocabulary to talk about aroma, impact, flavor, and the like.

Oriental (Turkish) tobacco, for example, is said to have a "cheesy-sweaty-butter odor reminiscent of isovaleric acid," while other varieties are said to have aromatic notes of wood, leather, dirt, or various animal scents. Flavors are described as bitter, sour, or metallic, or as having a peppery bite or sting. Tobacco researchers developed the science of *hedonics* to distinguish such sensations, with some industry documents listing more than a hundred different ways to characterize a particular sensory impact or impression, from "putrid" or "fecal" to "malty" or "molasses."[16] Coumarin is used to impart a vanilla-like aroma, and ylang ylang provides a floral scent with notes of jasmine and custard (it's also used in motion sickness medicines). Balsam of Tolu is added to provide hints of cinnamon, and patchouli oil is added for "earthy notes." Flavorants include oil extracts from cardamom, cedar, and coriander, juice extracts from prunes and figs, and oddities like Otto of Rose or *castoreum,* an aromatic oil extracted from the anal glands of Canadian and Siberian beavers. Most of the world's herbal chests have been probed for this purpose—and scrutinized through "taste tests" in the transnationals' laboratories.

Some classes of additives have been more successful than others. Lots of fruity and chocolaty flavorants have been tried, along with extracts intended to provide "a good bourbon or whiskey flavor." In one series of Brown & Williamson tests menthol and cinnamon got good marks, but perfumes and florals didn't pass. And neither did many spices, which were often judged too sharp or hot. Perfume or floral flavors such as mimosa, jasmine, frangipani, and musk were explored to pretty up secondhand smoke and to intensify the smoking experience. Philip Morris invented its New Leaf brand using wintergreen and a Breeze menthol sauced up with cloves. Saratoga had extra licorice and chocolate; American's oddly named Mayo brand was tinctured with spearmint. And Brown & Williamson sold a fruity cigarette called Lyme, prior to the rise of the tick-borne disease. None of the companies ever fared very well with raspberry, peach, or banana, though Brown & Williamson apparently used small amounts of each in its cigarettes. Better luck was had with lemon, orange, apple, and cherry, as with brandy, rum, and bourbon—though Winston's "winey" and "raisiny" notes were thought to have been achieved with flavors of sage. Less successful were efforts to simulate scotch, cognac, or vermouth. For a time great hopes were held out for coffee flavors, with the obstacle being that most such signatures are unstable.[17]

One reason for many of these intrigues was to replace flavors lost from the rush to "low-tar" cigarettes, but tobacco chemists also hoped that low-delivery products would offer "ideal vehicles for high levels of added flavors." There was also the hope that new fruity flavors would attract young smokers. Some wild and crazy ideas were explored—like adding opposite-sex-attracting pheromones to cigarettes. Philip Morris researchers in 1978 urged the company to register trademarks such as "Male" and "Female" for this purpose.[18]

Natural flavorings can be expensive or unstable, which is why the industry has often turned to synthetics. Grape, for example, is approximated by a methyl anthranilate, peach by a complex carbon aldehyde, and banana by an amyl acetate. Many such compounds have code names: AMBROX is an ambergris odor substitute, for example, with the more technical name tetra-methyl-dodeca-hydro-naphtho-furan. Coumarin, used to impart vanilla-like aromas, has at least seven different code names and numerous synthetic counterparts. Green apple is achieved with 3-hexenyl propionate, and a "meaty smell" is obtained from hexyl 2 furcate. Hundreds of synthetic flavorants are routinely used in cigarettes, with many being obtained by the ton from chemical manufacturers. Brown & Williamson in the 1970s was using about a dozen suppliers, including Norda (for oil of lime and orange), Firmenich (imitation chocolate), Glidden (peppermint), Gentry (cherry), Givaudan (apple and cinnamon), Fritzsche (mace and bourbon), and Dragoco (coffee). These suppliers obviously knew what their products were being used for,[19] so did they ever worry about them being burned and inhaled? Did any such firm ever refuse business from a cigarette company? And what safety tests were ever done prior to shipment? Recall that if *only one percent* of all cigarette deaths have been caused by burning and inhaling such additives, this would still be a million deaths worldwide during the twentieth century—and a toll growing higher every year.

Tobacco additives have been almost entirely unregulated, which means virtually unlimited freedom to add whatever manufacturers might fancy. If plutonium were not a controlled substance, there would apparently be no obstacle to tossing it into a cigarette. What could be the objection? That it raised the likelihood of death from "high" to "extreme"? The reality is that many known carcinogens have been added to tobacco products. Angelica root extract is sometimes used in cigarettes: the compound appears in more than 1,700 internal industry documents. Safrole was apparently being used in Kent cigarettes in 1990, years after it was banned (as a carcinogen) from soft drinks.[20] One document prepared for Brown & Williamson lists over a hundred cigarette additives, from star anise oil to smokanilla, with more than forty designated by the company as "potentially hazardous." Compounds in this category range from tonka bean and saccharine to diethylene glycol and Dragoco tangerine.[21] Additives have included the food dye known as butter yellow ("found to cause liver cancer in animals"), calamus or sweet flag ("banned in 1968 because it caused malignant tumors"), cobalt and its salts ("chest pains resembling heart attacks"), ammoniated glycyrrhizin ("severe hypertension and cardiac arrhythmia"), juniper berries ("nervous system toxins which can cause hallucinations"), lithium chloride ("several human fatalities"), mannitol ("diarrhea, nausea, and vomiting"), and pennyroyal ("can induce abortion").[22]

Many of these compounds are used in substantial quantities. Licorice, for example, has been widely used—on a gargantuan scale—as a sweetener in cigarettes. Tobacco manufacturers in the 1980s in the United States alone were putting 12 *million* pounds of licorice into cigarettes every year, with an estimated 90 percent of *all* licorice in the country going into tobacco products.[23] Along with 35 million pounds of glycerol, millions of pounds of cocoa, and millions of pounds of synthetics of various sorts. These are huge investments: the U.S. tobacco industry spent $76 million on flavorings in 1977 and $113 million two years later. The U.S. Surgeon General in 1981 cautioned that additives might pose "increased or new and different disease risks"; the industry was asked to stop adding new ingredients, a request apparently ignored. The industry likes to be able to say (in effect) that "everything we use can be sprinkled on corn flakes," but how many people really want to smoke corn flakes? Widespread smoking of corn flakes would no doubt cause lung cancers.

A 1992 Covington & Burling document gives a revealing look into the quantities of hundreds of different ingredients used in American cigarette manufacturing. Here is a (small) sampling from that list:[24]

Cigarette Ingredient	Pounds Used in:		
	1989	1990	1991
Glycerol	27,310,466	28,803,951	24,910,166
Propylene glycol	26,956,893	29,732,869	22,803,628
Ethyl alcohol	8,744,830	9,925,381	8,965,715
Licorice	7,859,104	8,954,944	8,140,074
Ammonium diphosphate	5,164,491	5,203,918	6,0655,11
Menthol	1,512,984	1,742,077	1,564,759
Urea	1,900,800	1,944,000	2,376,000
Chocolate	827,697	942,664	841,405
Citric acid	374,927	315,793	184,163
Honey	271,026	523,589	139,475
Potassium sorbate	245,727	282,203	296,984
Lactic acid	31,495	38,300	32,714
Prune juice and concentrate	15,445	333,162	156,093

Levulinic acid	8,939	11,816	13,413
Peppermint oil	3,129	· 3,373	1,888
Nutmeg powder and oil	2,743	6,895	2,359
Coriander extract and oil	2,032	2,015	1,903
Dandelion root solid extract	1,601	2,026	2,044
Benzylideneacetone	1,096	2,499	2,559
Dimethylhydroquinone	30	28	19

I have selected twenty ingredients, but the document from which this is taken includes some 614 distinct compounds. Readers may be surprised to learn that American cigarettes in 1989 contained 9,725 pounds of kola nut extract, 863 pounds of monosodium glutamate (MSG), 34 pounds of myrrh oil, and just over a pound of horehound extract. Or that in 1990 manufacturers were adding 35,324 pounds of maple syrup, half a million pounds of honey, and nearly nine million pounds of licorice.

Many of these are either carcinogens by themselves or produce carcinogens upon burning. A swamp plant known as deer tongue (so named for the shape of its leaves) contains coumarin, a compound with vanilla-like flavors and aromas. Coumarin was originally extracted from deer tongue or tonka beans, with Reynolds alone by 1930 using 1,200 pounds per month in its cigarettes. The FDA banned all use of coumarin in foods in the 1950s, following research showing it causes liver damage. Some cigarette manufacturers may well have cut back, but a 1983 Mother Jones investigation found the compound still being used—and on a fairly large scale. The leaves are gathered from Georgia swamps and pine forests and sold to middlemen, who then turn the herb ("wild vanilla") over to tobacco factories. American manufacturers in the early 1980s were still buying one to three million pounds per annum, despite its broad recognition as a carcinogen. Reynolds rationalized (to itself) its continued use by claiming that the amounts added were small: a 1981 research department memo (marked "Secret") noted that "All domestic companies except PM add coumarin to one or more of their cigarette products." Philip Morris brands contained less than one microgram per gram, but Reynolds's own Now brand showed 67 micrograms and Carlton 85s a whopping 140 micrograms per gram of tobacco.[25] Do smokers know that the cigarette industry has a history of adding known carcinogens to its products?

MAKING THE POISON GO DOWN EASIER

Menthol was first added to cigarettes in the 1920s, when Axton-Fisher unrolled its "menthol cooled" Spud cigarette containing the peppermint extract. Menthol was already regarded as a medicinal cough suppressant, which is why smokers were advised (in ads) to switch to Spuds "when you have a cold." Manufacturers used mice to test for toxicity: a 1935 report for Brown & Williamson claimed that the amounts added to Kool, Polar, and Spud cigarettes (from 1.33 to 2.08 mg per cigarette) were below levels thought to be toxic—though here again we find a failure to reflect on the fact that smokers were not *ingesting* but rather *inhaling* the compound after combustion—with all the chemical shape-shifting that implied. Brown & Williamson's research at this point was preemptive: there was not yet any real opposition; the research was undertaken "simply to have it ready in case somebody starts something about mentholated cigarettes being harmful." It is already here, though, in these 1930s reports, that we find some of the first arguments of the form "There is no more menthol in 60 cigarettes than in 10 to 20 cough drops": trivialization by creative (and inappropriate) comparison. Yale University scholars working for the makers of Kool cigarettes noted that you would have to smoke twelve thousand a day to "absorb" the same amount of menthol given to patients as internal medication[26]—which, again, is like ignoring the difference between eating a pistachio nut and inhaling its carbonized remnants.

Synthetics have long been used to achieve the menthol sensation, even though BAT knew by the 1960s that some of these at least were carcinogenic. Brown & Williamson had patented monomenthyl maleate for use in cigarettes, for example, but BAT's Additives Panel in 1967 expressed their wariness of using such a compound, given that some of its by-products—maleic anhydride, for example—"had been shown to be mildly carcinogenic." Researchers at BAT raised this issue with the company's legal counsel, who advised the firm to be "extremely cautious" using such a substance "since it involved a direct allegation of carcinogenicity in a probable pyrolytic product." Worries of this sort led the firm to explore other menthyl esters: menthyl succinate and triborate, for example.[27]

Menthol is added to "cool" cigarette smoke and to make it less harsh, which means that mentholation makes a cigarette easier to smoke. Menthol is an anesthetic: it soothes or even numbs the linings of the mouth and throat and suppresses the body's natural cough reflex. And by making it easier to smoke, it also makes cigarettes more attractive to young or beginning smokers. Brown & Williamson in the late 1980s reflected on how menthol brands were "good starter products," since new smokers "already know what menthol tastes like vis-à-vis candy." Menthol today is much beloved by the industry—and few cigarettes nowadays aren't treated with at least subliminal levels. Which is also why the industry fought so hard to exclude it from the list of sweeteners barred from cigarettes by the Family Smoking Prevention and Tobacco Control Act of 2009. Strawberry, banana, vanilla, and ten other fruity/sweet additives were banned, but the industry won at least a temporary stay on menthol. The banned flavorings affected less than one percent of the American cigarette market, whereas menthol—the "ultimate candy flavoring" according to Phillip Gardiner of California's Tobacco-Related Disease Research Program—is the characterizing flavor of more than a quarter of all cigarettes sold.[28]

Menthols have long been smoked disproportionately by African Americans, which is why cigarette makers were accused of racism in fighting to keep menthols on the market. That charge is not entirely unfounded, given Lorillard's archival record of explaining menthol's appeal as part of a purported desire (by "negroes") to mask a "genetic body odor." William S. Robinson, executive director of the National African American Tobacco Prevention Network based in Durham, North Carolina, withdrew his support for the FDA bill when negotiators agreed to exempt menthols from the initial ban.[29]

The FDA in 2010 began hearings on whether to disallow menthol in cigarettes, with a recommendation due on this topic in 2011. The agency is likely to consider not just the incremental hazard but also the fact that menthols are disproportionately smoked by African Americans and other racial minorities. Regardless of whether menthol is found to confer added physical harms from a purely biochemical point of view, the question will be whether this peppermint flavoring poses a hazard by making it easier or more attractive to smoke, or harder to quit. Phillip Gardiner has urged the FDA to consider that by sweetening cigarettes, menthol makes the poison go down easier.

Menthol will be a crucial test case for the FDA's new authority to regulate cigarettes. If the FDA can ban flavorants that make the poison go down easier, it can presumably also reduce the alkaloid that keeps smokers coming back for more. (Currently it is barred from eliminating nicotine altogether, but nothing prevents it from requiring that it be reduced to, say, 3 percent of current levels, which is certainly technically feasible.) The fact is that *anything* that makes smoking more attractive will make people more likely to smoke and therefore causes harm. Menthol on these grounds is clearly a threat to public health, as is virtually everything else about cigarettes. There is certainly legal precedent for requiring that cigarettes be made less attractive: tobacco manufacturers cannot advertise on television, for example, which limits their ability to attract customers. Lives will be saved if cigarettes are made less attractive, and eliminating menthol will do just that. Lives will be saved if cigarettes are made less addictive, and reducing the nicotine will do that as well. The FDA has this power, the world is watching, and it remains only to be seen whether the government has the courage to exercise that power *pro bono publico*.

Postscript: The FDA's Tobacco Products Scientific Advisory Committee in March of 2011 issued its report on menthol cigarettes, concluding that the minty additive was not just a flavoring agent but had druglike effects, including "cooling and anesthetic effects that reduce the harshness of cigarette smoke." The report found that while menthols were no more harmful than regulars on a per-cigarette basis, mentholation could make it easier to start and harder to quit: "by reducing the harshness of tobacco smoke menthol could facilitate initiation or early persistence of smoking by youth." Menthol could also "facilitate deeper and more prolonged inhalation," resulting in "greater smoke intake per cigarette." And for those who quit, reminders of menthol from candy or even toothpaste could prompt a relapse.[30] No policy recommendations were made, and it remains to be seen what action will be taken by the FDA, if any.

BRONCHIAL DILATORS, PAPER ADDITIVES, AND PARTICULATE FILTH

Bronchial dilators have been added to "smoothen" smoke and to facilitate deep inhalation. The industry has tried many different ways to make smoke milder or easier to inhale; menthol is part of this, but so is cocoa and myriad other additives. Cocoa contains a chemical known as *theobromine,* for example, which acts to expand the airway passages of the lungs. Cocoa has been added to tobacco since the nineteenth century, but it was really only in the 1960s that manufacturers began appreciating its pharmacologic effects. The quantities used are impressive: British American Tobacco in 1978, for example, was adding 1,250 metric *tons* of cocoa butter to its cigarettes every year, and most other companies were following suit. Synthetics have also been developed. A "proprietary fat" known as Coberine (made by Unilever) has been used as a substitute for cocoa butter, and cocoa aldehyde was in use as a cocoa substitute by the 1950s. Sugar seems to have allied effects, since sugar upon burning produces acetaldehyde, which interacts with nicotine to intensify psychopharmacologic effects. Licorice also seems to have a bronchodilation effect, which is important given the enormous quantities added to tobacco. Tobacco manufacturers talk about reducing irritation by means of "quenchers," meaning agents with "anesthetic properties such as menthol, terpenoids and other pharmacoactive additives." Achieving "mildness" has long been a priority of the companies, with researchers investigating "sugar amination during toasting" and "possible effects of antioxidants as scavengers of free radicals."[31] Efforts along these lines reveal how intensively smoke chemistry has been manipulated, once cigarettes came to be regarded as drug delivery devices.

Additives to cigarette paper.   We tend to forget that you cannot smoke a cigarette without smoking cigarette paper, which means that whatever goes into the paper also gets smoked. Cigarettes often have brand names inked onto the rod, for example, which means that a bit of ink gets smoked along with each cigarette. Colorants and/or bleachings are often added, and these, too, get smoked—which is not as trivial as it sounds. Cigarette paper has many different chemicals added, from bleachings to make it white to burn accelerants to keep it lit. None of these are present in large amounts, but in the aggregate we are talking about quite a lot of stuff. Even if there is only a microgram of ink on any given cigarette, for example, this still means six million grams of ink smoked worldwide in any given year. That's more than ten thousand pounds of ink, burned and smoked along with 300,000 tons of cigarette paper. Comparable figures could be given for bleaching and whitening agents. Some of these additives are anything but innocent: in the 1980s, for example, with worries about asbestos in the news, tobacco manufacturers started wondering whether the talc used by cigarette paper makers contained asbestos, the notorious carcinogen. The Ecusta company quietly conducted an investigation, and its suppliers assured the company that no asbestos was in the talc it was supplying—at least not in "detectable" levels.[32]

The most important paper additives from a health point of view are the burn accelerants—oxidizing agents—added to keep a cigarette lit or to decrease machine-measured deliveries (because the cigarette burns up faster). The most widely used in recent decades have been sodium or potassium citrates, though many other oxidizing agents have been added (nitrates, tartrates, etc.). Additives of this sort complicate the chemicals emitted in the smoke, but their most important impact is on fire safety, since burn accelerants also keep a cigarette lit when tossed or dropped onto the ground—or onto paper or fabric—which can then cause fires. Some large fraction of the world's thousands of annual fire deaths are made possible by the industry's use of burn accelerants in cigarettes.

Particulate filth.   Particulate filth is one thing the industry tends to take quite seriously, since this poses a threat to the integrity of the machinery used to manufacture cigarettes. Smokers often complain about finding "foreign matter" in their cigarettes, and this has led to further concerns at the level of public relations. British American Tobacco in the early 1990s began working with the Chilworth Technology Centre to develop "experimental systems for separating clean tobacco from contaminates such as paper, carbon particles, filter material and silica." Techniques explored involved charging the particles by exposing them to some kind of a static electricity, following which they could be removed by exploiting the differential charge imposed.[33] It is not clear whether this particular method was ever employed, but the fact that such ideas were entertained shows that contamination was taking place.

TOBACCO SUBSTITUTES

Cigarette manufacturers have often used non-tobacco plant materials in cigarettes, and for various reasons. People in times of war, for example, have turned to substitutes when tobacco became scarce. Germans in World War II tried dozens of different alternatives, from dried lettuce and chicory to corn silk and cherry leaves, and the French even before the war were fond of cigarettes and cigars made from cocoa leaves and pods. Kids from the American South used to smoke whatever leafy weeds they could find, calling this "rabbit tobacco." Tobacco substitutes have been used to save on manufacturing costs, but there has also been a hope that inert substances might lower machine-measured tar and nicotine and provide "health reassurance." Researchers at the Roswell Park Memorial Institute in Buffalo, New York, conducted an elaborate experiment with cabbage cigarettes in 1964 and found after testing 110,000 such cigarettes that smokers "lost their desire to smoke tobacco cigarets for several hours," suggesting this as one possible way to cut down. The *Wall Street Journal* reported that cigarettes of this sort produced "an odor akin to cabbage burning in a pan."[34]

In the United States, commercial cigarettes have sometimes been made from plant derivatives judged unfit for human consumption—corn silk, for example— or inexpensive edible materials. The first factory for lettuce cigarettes was built in Hereford, Texas, in 1966 to sell Bravo cigarettes; sales by March of that year reached $50,000 but never went much further, apart from a couple of isolated markets. (In 1967 two of every hundred cigarettes smoked by students in Amarillo, Texas, the company's test market, were made from lettuce.) Triumph cigarettes—another lettuce brand—were no more successful when introduced in 1969.

Interest in tobacco substitutes remained high throughout the 1960s and 1970s, however. Fred G. Bock at Roswell Park studied several different kinds of plants to find out which, when smoked, would produce the fewest carcinogenic tars. Beets, petunias, cabbage, dandelions, maple leaves, lettuce, and catalpa all came under scrutiny. One researcher attached to the French tobacco monopoly in the 1960s described a patent for a tobacco-free cigarette—the "Santab"—made from coltsfoot, lobelia, rose petals, and cinnamon. Cocoa cigars were smoked in France in the decades prior to the First World War, and this same researcher described these as "very much appreciated by children, who would procure them from the bakery or from the grocers." Cigarettes were sometimes made from eucalyptus leaves, and chocolate cigarettes (for smoking!) for a time were made in a Marseille factory. Lots of other substitutes have been proposed: dried menthol, pulverized pine needles, coffee hulls, citrus pulp or pulp from sugar beets, algae in various forms, gum and pectin fillers of various sorts, a Celanese product known as Cytrel, and substances more generically characterized as "designed" or "low tar filler" (LTF).[35]

Tobacco makers of course have long used substitutes simply to save on costs. Laws against adulterating tobacco have been around since the nineteenth century, though many seem to have been poorly enforced. One common fad from the 1970s was to introduce nonburnable materials into the cigarette rod, much as you might reduce the calories in a certain volume of ice cream by pumping it full of air or some other inert filler. Materials added to cigarettes have included volcanic glass, ceramics, and various synthetic fibers and claylike materials. A number of British firms played this game: Peter Taylor in his *Smoke Ring* reports that some British cigarettes in 1977 contained 25 percent "new smoking material" (NSM), a tobacco substitute produced through a 20-million-pound cooperative venture between Imperial Tobacco and Imperial Chemical Industries. Millions of kilograms of NSM went into about a dozen new brands in 1977, none of which proved successful over the long haul, despite huge fanfares of publicity. As Taylor puts it, nonburnable tobacco substitutes were "a monumental flop." Cigarette manufacturers had hoped that NSM would be welcomed as helping to make a "safer" cigarette, but Britain's Health Education Council ridiculed the gimmick, comparing it to jumping from the thirty-sixth floor of a building instead of the thirty-ninth.[36]

ELEPHANT JUICE AND IMPRUDENCE

The additives considered here are only a tiny fraction of those utilized by the industry—and a much smaller part of the universe of those considered for use. The archives reveal some ideas that, to anyone outside the tobacco labs, sound quite sinister. In the 1970s, for example, when many people thought marijuana might become legalized, the industry started exploring the possible use of "super-addictors" in tobacco (and perhaps in marijuana): scientists at British American Tobacco in 1977 pondered spiking its cigarettes with etorphine, a narcotic "10,000 times more addictive than morphine"—also known as "elephant juice" for its use in immobilizing elephants.[37] The idea today sounds outlandish but is perhaps unsurprising given the industry's long history of adding substances to influence a cigarette's burn rate, smoke particle size, or nicotine potency—or even the whiteness of the paper or the color or integrity of the ash. Some companies have even added appetite suppressants, mindful of the fact that many women smoke to control their weight.

The archives also reveal tobacco manufacturers sometimes blindly adding substances about which they had no clue as to composition. BAT in the 1960s pressed one supplier, Sandoz, to reveal the composition of YOMARON, used by the company since 1950 as a bleach for cigarette paper. Sandoz eventually reported toxicity data to the company, but what is remarkable is that BAT didn't even know its chemical composition during the first ten years it was being used in cigarettes. (Sandoz in 1960 revealed it to be a "diamino stilbene derivative containing triazine groupings.") BAT regarded the Sandoz report as "clearing" the compound, even though the data were exclusively for ingestion and, according to BAT, "we still don't know what happens on burning." The company continued using this bleaching agent for several years thereafter, prior to deciding (in 1967) that it would be better to use "more desirable additives" serving this purpose.[38]

Safety has always been the odd man out in the cigarette business, and one thing we find in the archives is the presumption that a long history of use is justification enough for a compound's continued use. BAT in 1967, for example, okayed the continued use of cocoa butter (code named CELMOE) on the grounds that cocoa enjoyed "a very long history of use at quite considerable levels." Dosage was sometimes a consideration, as when BAT justified (to itself) its adding of ZAMPAR, an aldehyde supplied by International Flavours and Fragrances: "There is no reason why ZAMPAR should not be used on tobacco at an application rate of 1 oz. per 1,000 lb. cut tobacco," given that it took 18.5 grams of the stuff per kilogram to kill half the rats exposed. (The British–metric mishmash is in the original.) More cautious, perhaps, was the suggestion that a compound known as Ketonarome (1-methyl-cyclopenta-2,3-dione) was to be added to cigarettes "at the lowest level necessary," given evidence of ciliatoxicity for similar dicarbonyl structures. Formalin was likewise to be used (in starch pastes, to kill mold) "only as a last resort" because it was "physiologically active." The philosophy in most instances seems to have been: assume safety unless you can prove otherwise. That was the approach in 1967, when Australian manufacturers asked about using two different flavorants for which BAT had recommended an upper safety limit. The question was whether one should worry about synergistic effects, and Sydney J. Green's response at BAT was basically: in the absence of other information, assume no interactions.[39] I'm not sure what name to give to this violation of "the precautionary principle" (reckless endangerment?), but in the cigarette world it seems to have been business as usual.

Some additives have been banned by national legislative bodies. Diethylene glycol is prohibited in cigarettes sold in Australia, for example, and coumarin has been banned in Germany. Maleic hydrazide was banned in Rhodesia in the 1960s, as already noted. British cigarette makers in the 1950s were barred from adding either sweeteners or humectants to tobacco, though they were permitted to add spices dissolved in rum (to improve the smell) and acetic acid (to reduce mold). A number of countries have banned the use of ammoniated tobacco sheet for purposes of freebasing, and there are bans on many types of tobacco products in different parts of the world.

In most parts of the globe, however, there are few restrictions on what can or cannot be put into cigarettes. The United States has historically been lenient in this regard—one could say profoundly negligent. Prior to 2009 the country had no rules governing what could be legally added to tobacco—apart from controlled substances such as opiates or barbiturates. The tobacco industry has a stated policy of using only additives approved for use in foods and "generally recognized as safe,"[40] but that has been a purely voluntary code with no legal teeth and suffers from the already mentioned conflation of ingestion and combusted inhalation. Manufacturers of dog food are more careful—and humane—and if cigarette makers decided to make human feces or rodent hair an ingredient, there would seem to be no law stopping them. Smokers are not likely to know much about what goes into cigarettes and might well be surprised to find out the truth.

Radioactivity in Cigarette Smoke

"Three Mile Marlboro" and the Sleeping Giant

[Publishing our research on polonium] has the potential of waking a sleeping giant. The subject is rumbling . . . and I doubt we should provide facts.
PAUL A. EICHORN, MANAGER OF TECHNICAL PLANNING, TO ROBERT B.
SELIGMAN, VICE PRESIDENT OF R&D, PHILIP MORRIS, 1978

Some cigarette constituents are astonishingly little known—or rather transiently known, publicized, and then forgotten in cycles of media attention and forgetfulness. Radioactivity is a perfect example: few people today realize there are deadly radioactive isotopes in cigarettes, but the fact is that smoking is one of the principal means by which people are exposed to cancer-causing radiation. The story is a remarkable one, and little known to the world outside the companies' private laboratories.[1]

The reality is that radioactive isotopes were identified in smoke as early as 1953. D. K. Mulvany that year presented the first such evidence in a letter published in the British journal *Lancet,* raising the possibility that radioactive potassium 40 in cigarette smoke might be responsible for the upsurge in lung cancer. Mulvany reported finding twice the potassium in cigarette smoke as in ordinary air and reasoned that even though the dosage was minute, this was nonetheless "the only naturally occurring radioactive element that gains entrance not merely to the cytoplasm of a cell but to its very nucleus," where cancers were thought to begin. Richard Doll picked up on this shortly thereafter and hypothesized that radioactive potassium might be responsible for the cigarette–cancer epidemic. V. C. Runeckles from Imperial Tobacco of Canada reviewed this question in a 1961 article for *Nature,* concluding that the amounts inhaled were far lower than those ingested in ordinary foods and that whatever made its way into the lungs would be quickly expelled. The idea was of sufficient interest to others in the industry, however, that by 1959 librarians working for British tobacco manufacturers were listing radioactivity as one of the "Physical Properties of Tobacco & Tobacco Smoke." The TIRC in the United States also had a program exploring "trace metals and radioactivity" in smoke—or such at least was the claim of its executive director, Willson T. Hoyt, responding to a University of Tennessee scholar who had wondered whether the radioactive thorium used in cigarette lighter flints might be making its way into the lungs of smokers.[2]

The floodgates didn't really open until 1964, however, when two scholars from Harvard's School of Public Health identified polonium 210, a powerful alpha emitter, in cigarette smoke. The quantities measured were small—roughly .04 picocuries per cigarette—but the element was known to be energetic, releasing tens of thousands of times more radiant energy, gram for gram, than the plutonium used in the atom bomb dropped on Nagasaki. So the obvious question was: could this be why smoking was causing cancer? Timing enlivened the question, as Radford and Hunt's paper appeared in *Science* magazine on January 17, 1964, only six days after the press conference accompanying the release of the Surgeon General's report.[3]

HOT SPOTS

Radford and Hunt's paper caused a flurry of scientific activity over the next few years, as scholars outside the industry confirmed the findings while cigarette makers watched with nervous apprehension—and quietly conducted their own research. The pattern by then was familiar and well rehearsed. *Publicly* the industry dismissed any such hazard, calling it just the latest "scare tactics" used against the industry.[4] *Privately,* however, the companies also launched a series of efforts to measure radioactivity in cigarettes, while trying also to develop filters and other methods to keep the carcinogen from reaching smokers' lungs. While this part of the story should not be surprising, what *is* remarkable are some of the tricks used to trivialize the hazard—and the fact that the companies ultimately abandoned any effort to reduce the polonium threat. Because they judged it not worth the expense, given the lack of public worries.

Brianna Rego in her history of this episode has shown that while Radford and Hunt's measurements were quickly verified, industry researchers did so using methods that produced conveniently lower values. Radford and Hunt, after all, had stressed that while *total* exposure to the lungs averaged only about 36 rems (over a lifetime of smoking), the more alarming fact was that radiation could accumulate in *particular parts* of the lungs—notably the deciliated branching points, or "segmental bifurcations"—creating "hot spots" with far greater potential for causing harm. Radford and Hunt measured the radioactivity in these hot spots and found that tissues at pulmonary branching points could be receiving upward of 1,000 rems over a period of twenty-five years—a substantially higher dose than revealed by looking only at averages over the lungs as a whole. (The *rem* is a unit of exposure *per mass of tissue exposed,* so radioactivity concentrated unevenly in tiny areas can have disproportionately high exposures—"hot spots.") The industry was clearly trying to minimize the measured effect by calculating only total-lung exposures.[5] Both methods were technically correct, but the industry's was deceptive, as if to say, "Hey, it's not so bad getting shot, since the force of any one bullet is trivial when spread over your whole body." Alpha radiation is like a real-world bullet in this sense, impacting only one small part of the body—but with whole-body consequences. The isotope lodges in some particular spot in your lungs, from where it starts mutating tissues. Calculating exposures in terms of whole-lung dosages while ignoring hot spots was deceptive and failed to capture the deadly force of smoking.

More disturbing even than this dosage deception, however, is the fact that the industry researched polonium in cigarettes for many years, without ever warning the public of a possible danger. For decades, too, the industry worked hard to find out how polonium came to be in cigarette smoke, exploring the path by which it entered the tobacco plant, its chemistry in the burning cigarette, its mode of deposition in the body, and what methods might be used to eliminate it.

One early discovery was that tobaccos grown in different parts of the world harbor different levels of radioactivity. North Carolina leaf, for example, had about three times the polonium as tobacco grown in Maryland, and tobacco grown in the United States was more than twice as radioactive as tobacco grown in New Zealand. These differences were explained as coming from the soil or method of culture or something about the environment or curing process; fallout from nuclear tests was one early suspect, for example, but experiments exposing tobacco plants to high levels of radon in greenhouses showed this was unlikely. T. C. Tso and his colleagues at the USDA realized soon thereafter that polonium was probably coming from the "superphosphate" fertilizers routinely applied to tobacco plants (superphosphates contain high levels of natural uranium).[6] Phosphates had been attractive to tobacco farmers, to lower the nitrogen concentrations in the leaf. Nitrogen affected taste, but it also increased nitrate concentrations in the leaves, which produced nitrosamines and other poisons upon burning. Scholars would later claim that tobacco grown in countries such as India, Indonesia, and Turkey had lower concentrations of radioactive polonium because tobacco farmers there used organic fertilizers rather than the high-uranium phosphates favored in the Americas.[7]

The tobacco industry's reaction to all of this was interestingly different from how they had reacted to Wynder's 1953 mouse-painting experiments or the 1964 Surgeon General's report. These two previous challenges had been accompanied by broad publicity, but the public response to polonium was muted, relatively speaking. Philip Morris assigned a staff radiochemist to look into the question, which resulted in a report by Gonzalo Segura, since 1959 head of the company's Isotope Committee, that polonium could indeed cause cancer if dosages were sufficiently high. Segura in 1964 advised the company to stay "ahead of adverse publicity and be in a position to counter it quickly whenever necessary"; he also suggested that since it was apparently through the decay of lead 210 that polonium got into tobacco, one solution might involve "loading the soil with non-radioactive lead-206" to cut down on the uptake of lead 210.[8]

The industry also tried to keep embarrassing research at bay. John E. Noakes from Oak Ridge Associated Universities in 1967 applied to the CTR for funds to study polonium, for example, and despite impressing the industry as "knowing what he was talking about" and having a well-thought-out plan and "a relatively simple and inexpensive means of reducing" polonium in cigarettes (by switching to low-uranium fertilizers), Noakes's proposal was rejected. The CTR was not in the business of exploring potentially embarrassing facts, and polonium was clearly too hot to handle—publicly.[9]

Privately, though, the companies developed a number of different methods to monitor and to manipulate radioactivity in cigarette smoke. Changing fertilizer was an obvious intervention, but American Tobacco also tried to develop *filters* to take out some of the polonium (Project PTT-A-68-A), while Philip Morris explored the possibility of *washing* tobacco leaves to render them less radioactive. Edward Martell, a radiochemist from the National Center for Atmospheric Research in Boulder, Colorado, in 1974 had published a new proposed route by which polonium entered cigarettes: Martell agreed that phosphate fertilizers were the ultimate source of the contamination but disagreed that polonium was absorbed through the roots. His proposal: radioactive lead 210 (from the fertilizer) lands as "fallout" on the leaf via a decay chain from uranium 238 through radium 222; lead 210 is then inhaled when the cigarette is burned. And only then, after lodging in the lungs of a smoker, does the lead decay into polonium.[10]

Crucial also to Martell's view was that the lead 210 formed through decay of radium sticks to the tobacco leaf by attaching to the small sticky hairs known as *trichomes* coating the surface of the leaf; cigarettes rolled from these leaves incorporate these radioactive trichomes. Martell's theory opened up the possibility of *washing* the tobacco leaves prior to processing, which would prevent the radioactive trichomes from ever reaching the finished cigarette. A number of tobacco companies explored such a possibility, and in 1980 Stauffer Chemical obtained a patent on a washing process. The tobacco companies were quite taken with this prospect—experiments seemed to lower polonium counts significantly—and the hope was to be able to use such methods in the event of negative publicity. America had suffered its worst nuclear accident in March 1979—a partial core meltdown of a reactor at Three Mile Island Nuclear Generating Station in Pennsylvania—and the tobacco industry didn't want to have to deal with talk of "Three Mile Marlboro."[11]

NO COMMERCIAL ADVANTAGE

By the 1980s a number of different methods had been developed to keep polonium out of tobacco:

- Polonium could be reduced by *changing fertilizers*. T. C. Tso at the USDA had shown that fertilizer choice influenced polonium content and that polonium in finished tobacco could be dramatically reduced by applying fertilizers low in natural uranium.
- Polonium could also be reduced *by including only low-polonium tobacco varieties* in tobacco blends. As early as 1965 Philip Morris was pondering whether to select tobaccos for use in manufacturing "to be sure these are not high in polonium content."[12]
- Polonium could be reduced by *breeding tobacco plants without the sticky trichomes* to which radiolead and polonium were sticking. Tso had bred a "glandless" variety of tobacco at the USDA's Tobacco Research Station at Oxford, North Carolina, and found that glandless yielded whole smoke condensate "with a 20% reduction in soluble 210 Po . . . indicative of lower leaf retention of radioactivity by airborne deposition due to the less sticky nature of the glandless leaf."[13]
- Polonium could also be reduced by *washing the tobacco leaves* prior to processing. A patent was obtained for this process in 1980, involving washing of tobacco leaves with a dilute solution of acid and hydrogen peroxide.

None of these methods was apparently ever put into commercial practice. R. J. Reynolds's "resident expert on polonium," Charles W. Nystrom, rejected the trichome washing procedure on the grounds that it would have "no commercial advantage." Philip Morris regarded washing as too expensive—and at one point actually worried about the "proper disposal" of the resulting radioactive waste. (Better just to let smokers smoke it, apparently.) Other methods were rejected as ineffective—the use of ion-exchange resin filters, for example. The companies may even have feared that acid washing might alter the acid-base balance of cigarette smoke, affecting nicotine pharmacology. All of this was discussed behind closed doors; indeed, as Rego shows, the principal character of the industry's public response was silence. Alan Rodgman at Reynolds in 1982 noted that since the polonium question had already "appeared and disappeared" several times, the company should not worry about taking it too seriously. The public had forgotten before and would presumably forget again.[14]

The industry eventually made a conscious decision not to even measure polonium, consistent with Wakeham's dictum that "you couldn't be criticized for not knowing something." And here it does seem that by artful divisions of labor and keeping silent, knowledge of the polonium "problem" began to disappear, even within the companies. In 1982, when Thomas Winters and Joseph Difranza from the University of Massachusetts revived the issue with a letter in the *New England Journal of Medicine*—equating pack-and-a-half per day smoking with three hundred annual chest X-rays—Brown & Williamson's senior field manager was shocked: "Our R&D

Dept. will just love to hear this!"[15] As if they didn't already know. Researchers inside the companies had been keeping tabs on polonium for years, but little effort seems to have been given to instructing employees in other departments. In 1985, when Miriam Adams in Reynolds's PR department received an inquiry on this topic, she had to report she had "no information in file" to give to her correspondent.[16]

Radioactivity in smoke was clearly not something the companies wanted people to know about. Winters and Difranza commented on receiving hundreds of letters from smokers who had quit after learning about radioactivity in cigarettes, and the companies feared they could "lose many customers" if attention were to be drawn to the topic. They didn't want to say it was safe, but they also didn't want to draw attention to the problem by criticizing the science. The smoking gun memo is from 1978, when Philip Morris debated whether to go public with a critique of Martell's work prepared by company researchers. Paul A. Eichorn, Philip Morris's manager of technical planning and information, decided the risk was not worth any possible benefit and penned a handwritten note to his vice president of R&D, Robert Seligman, warning of the danger of "waking a sleeping giant." The industry's critique, originally intended for publication in *Science,* was filed and forgotten.[17]

CYCLES OF ATTENTION AND FORGETTING

It is hard, and perhaps impossible, to say how many fewer people would have died from smoking if the polonium had been removed; we don't really know what fraction of all cigarette cancers are caused by radioactivity. It could be 10 percent; it could be one percent. In the United States alone 10 percent would be 16,000 lives per year, counting only those lost to lung cancer. And even one percent would be 1,600 deaths. The fact is that the industry really didn't care one way or another, or at least not enough to threaten business as usual. They appear to not care even today, if actions are any measure of intentions. Cigarettes on the market today are all still radioactive.

What is also remarkable, though, are the perennial cycles of attention and forgetting in this sphere. Polonium seems to be rediscovered—and republicized and then quickly forgotten—every decade or so. Why this cycling of discovery and forgetfulness?

The principal reason, I believe, is that cigarette nuclearity falls into a kind of "ideological gap" or "disinterest pit." The story never really gets political legs, because no one has been able to attach it to more familiar agendas. For the industry of course the whole topic is anathema, so their silence is hardly surprising. Antinuclear groups have always been happy to propagandize against radioactivity, but natural radiation in tobacco or anywhere else (think of radon or the natural radioactivity in Brazil nuts) appears to have been regarded as a distraction from man-made nuclearity—notably atomic weapons and atomic plants but also X-rays and exposures suffered by miners. The dangers of smoking have often been used to trivialize workplace hazards or environmental pollutants, and this may well have fostered a lack of interest in tobacco mortality from experts in occupational health.

And public health activists have additional blinders. Anti-tobacco activists have never been terribly interested in precisely *how* smoking kills you; indeed they've tended to regard inquiries into carcinogenic mechanisms as *distractions* from the brute fact of tobacco mortality. Which is why the polonium story has never received more than passing attention from any of the professional groups one might expect to have focused on this issue. The radioactivity of cigarettes is periodically exposed but quickly falls back thereafter into silent slumber. Knowledge evaporates; ignorance recovers.

RUSSIAN SPIES AND RADIATION WARNINGS

I was recently involved in one of these perennial cycles of discovery and forgetfulness, when polonium hit the news from a rather different direction. In November 2006 I was intrigued to read in the press about Alexander V. Litvinenko, the former KGB agent, being fatally poisoned using this same polonium 210 isotope that had swung in and out of the news since the 1960s. This time, though, I was surprised to see no reference to tobacco. I published an opinion piece about this in the *New York Times,* which caused yet another flurry of attention, followed by yet another quick loss of memory. British health authorities responding to the poisoning commented that the isotope posed "no threat to the general population," which of course was wrong. Smokers inhale it every day—as does anyone who breathes other people's smoke. The oversight is perhaps understandable: if tobacco is killing six million people every year, does it really matter which of these many constituent poisons is to blame? Tobacco manufacturers have never been under any obligation to make cigarettes any less deadly—which hopefully will change some day. Monique Muggli and her colleagues have proposed requiring radiation warnings on all cigarette packs[18]—an excellent suggestion—but the fact is that far more dramatic action is needed.

The Odd Business of Butts—
and the Global Warming Wildcard

The slopes on the sides of the Kunati Valley, near Mount Kenya, are now completely bare . . . their former covering of trees has been cut down to be used as fuel for curing tobacco.
"TOBACCO DEPLETES FOOD-CROP LAND," *SMOKE SIGNALS*, 1982

The final scene of the 1950 sci-fi flick *Destination Moon* shows a team of American astronauts faced with a life-or-death crisis. The spacecraft has successfully landed on the moon, but faulty navigation has forced the voyagers to use up more fuel than expected, and they realize they cannot make it back to earth without shedding some weight. The crew starts looking everywhere to lose some pounds: a ladder is jettisoned, along with wrenches, clothing, and pretty much everything else not absolutely essential. Self-sacrifice is the leitmotiv, and only some clever and drastic pruning prevents them from having to leave one of their own behind.

For us here on earth, too, there may come a time—if it is not already upon us—when we will be forced to think about what parts of our consumptive lifestyle we can do without. The wealthy of the globe now live in an unsustainable world of wanton excess, where a newspaper may have a hundred pages of colored-ink ads, lawns grow useless crops of chemicalized grass, and water is drunk from throwaway plastic cups and bottles. The talk is all of energy efficiency and alternative fuels, but surprisingly little has been done to cut effectively into excess and waste, or even to slow the rate of exhausting unrenewable fuels.

Where does tobacco figure in this equation? How sustainable is the cigarette, and what contribution does it make to global pollution, global resource use, and global climate change?

A BILLION KILOGRAMS OF TOXIC TRASH

We tend to take it for granted, but cigarettes are actually among the world's biggest sources of toxic trash. Six trillion are rolled and smoked every year, and since most have filters this means nearly six trillion butts discarded every year. If each cigarette weighs a gram and the butt is one-sixth of that, that's a *billion kilograms* of plasticized, nicotine-soaked, cellulose acetate refuse, much of which gets tossed onto the ground. This is a nontrivial body of litter; it is also a substantial mass of toxic waste. Cigarette butts contain benzene, nicotine, cadmium, and dozens of other poisons, not the kind of thing you want in your environment.

Not all butts remain unconsumed. Especially in poorer parts of the world and more miserable moments of history, discarded butts are often gathered, re-rolled, and re-smoked. Germans in the early years after World War II would collect discarded butts and twist them into cigarettes—five or six would usually do the trick. The practice has even been commercialized. In Indonesia, butts are sometimes gathered up off the ground and sent back to the factory, where they are recycled into "new" cigarettes. The more common fate, though, is for them to remain where they have been thrown—until they are washed downstream or eaten by birds or picked up by litter patrols. The quantity is such that these are often the single most common form of litter—gauged by number of pieces. In the United States alone an estimated 68,000 *tons* of cigarette waste are discarded every year—and that's not counting the paper/cellophane packs. Even the Cigarette Litter Prevention Program financed by Philip Morris admits that cigarette butts account for about a third of all litter in the United States, measured by number of individual pieces. And whereas in the pre-filter era these were fairly quickly degraded—or re-smoked—the use of plasticizers in recent designs has made them more durable. The net result: poison-laced filters are a ubiquitous feature in modern civilization, fouling sidewalks and sewers and urinals—and virtually every other place smokers frequent. Butts end up on beaches and in waterways, releasing toxins as they degrade.

How toxic, though, is a cigarette butt?

Environmental scientists have developed techniques to measure the extent to which a body of water has been fouled, using organisms with predictable responses to pollutants. One standard method uses a freshwater flea, *Daphnia magna*, a tiny crustacean sensitive to a broad range of toxins and a vital link in aquatic food chains. *Daphnia* eat algae and are eaten in turn by a wide variety of fish. So the extent to which a lake or stream has been polluted can be assessed by asking, how dirty does a body of water have to be to kill half the *Daphnia* in it? "Whole effluent" tests of this sort provide useful assessments of how badly a body of water has been polluted, without having to go through costly and time-consuming assays of individual contaminants.

Cigarette butts don't fare very well in such tests. Smoke of course is toxic and kills people, so it is hardly surprising that the used butt ends of cigarettes can toxify water. Experiments have shown that a single used "filter" placed in eight liters of water will kill half the *Daphnia* living therein. And cigarette butts can even kill fish. Richard Gersberg of San Diego State University has shown that one used butt

dropped into a liter of water will kill half of all exposed freshwater fish (fathead min-
nows) or marine fish (topsmelt). More surprising is his demonstration that filters
even from *unsmoked* cigarettes can kill. One might think that filters fresh from the
pack would be inert, but even these are often infused with humectants, flavorants,
plasticizers, and other compounds that can leach into groundwater (not to mention your lips and lungs). Gersberg has shown that sixteen unsmoked filters placed
into a liter of water release enough toxins to kill fish.[1]

There is a certain irony in all this, insofar as the growth of outdoor cigarette waste
is partly the result of successful efforts to abolish indoor smoking. Bans on indoor
smoking have pushed smokers onto the streets, which is one reason butts get tossed
onto the ground. And one reason even non-smokers who live in places like New
York have so much *cotinine*—a nicotine metabolite—in their blood. Cotinine is the
most easily accessed nicotine biomarker, and the fact that New Yorkers show elevated blood cotinine is due in part to their exposure to secondhand smoke outdoors.
The same is no doubt true in many other parts of the world. In European cities such
as Vienna, where outdoor smoking is nearly ubiquitous, non-smokers partaking of
café culture must have high levels of tobacco toxins in their blood.

A number of communities have started organizing to prevent cigarette butt waste.
In California, Tom Novotny at San Diego State University has formed the Cigarette
Butt Advisory Committee and Cigarette Butt Pollution Project with the goal of reducing toxic waste from discarded butts (see Cigwaste.org). A number of countries
have taken aggressive steps along these lines: in Singapore, for example, tossing a
butt on the ground can earn you a $300 fine, and convicted litterbugs are required
to help clean city streets. The anti-butt movement was also strong early on in Sydney, Australia, where in 1996 cigarette butts were declared "a compact concentrate
of hazardous waste" and the city's "number-one environmental problem." An estimated 6.7 billion butts were being discarded annually on the city's streets, clogging
drains and polluting Sydney Harbor. The problem had become more acute in the
1980s, when the city's 800,000 smoking workers were barred from smoking indoors
and flooded onto the streets. The city's "Please Bin That Butt" campaign posted a
fine of A$200 for anyone found littering, and though the ordinance became the butt
of many jokes, the city did manage to solve much of its litter problem.[2]

Other solutions have been proposed. In 2009 San Francisco Mayor Gavin New-
som sought a 33-cent-per-pack fee to cover the $11 million cost of cigarette litter
removal (the enacted version was 20 cents). Others have suggested a deposit tax,
like the bottle bills from the 1960s that dramatically reduced glass and plastic waste
from American roads and parks. Bottle deposits aided both in cleanup and recycling, and there is no reason to think this would not work for cigarette butts. Thomas
Frieden in New York and Kelly Brownell in Connecticut have proposed taxing sug-
ary soft drinks to curb obesity ("a penny per ounce tax is a public health home-
run"),[3] and similar measures could help reduce both smoking and cigarette waste.

The tobacco industry has proposed its own solutions—like making cigarettes more biodegradable.[4] Biodegradability usually involves making a substance more vulnerable to moisture and heat, however, which does not bode well for a product that is essentially a conduit for moist hot gases. We should not expect to see anything useful from the industry on this score, apart from minor tinkering and showy displays. The industry will continue to support placement of ashtrays (yet more trash, one might say) and use of portable ashtrays, but the simpler and more intelligent solution will be to bar smoking from parks, urban streets, and other outdoor places where people congregate. Smoking is already barred along 140 miles of the California coast, and we are likely to see more smoke-free zones in the future.

ARE CIGARETTES SUSTAINABLE?

We don't often hear about tobacco as a cause of global climate change, but that is because we tend to ignore the entirety of the cigarette economy: the cutting of forests to make new land for planting or charcoal for flue-curing; the spraying of pesticides on the soil and finished leaf; the heat curing and chemicalization of the product and its transport to factories; the chopping and rolling of the leaf; the paper and plastics used in the affixing of "filters"; the cellophane and foil consumed in packaging; the fuel used for transport and the waste involved in advertising; the ignition and burning of the final product by a billion smokers; the resources used in the manufacture of ashtrays, matches, and plastic or metal lighters; the energies squandered cleaning up cigarette waste; the fires caused by careless disposal; the heaters used to warm smokers taking outdoor breaks; and the costly medical services used to treat diseases caused by cigarettes—all of which exact a toll on the environment. Ten trillion packs of cigarettes have been smoked over the past century, and if each of these (empty) weighs about five grams we are talking about 50 billion kilograms of packaging waste—including paper, ink, cellophane, foil, and glue. Piled into a heap, that would be enough to make a mountain 2.5 kilometers wide and 2.5 kilometers high, or enough to cover the island of Manhattan with a layer about 25 meters thick. Trillions of pages of color-inked ads have been printed in newspapers and magazines, billions of square feet of billboard space occupied, billions of coupons and mail offers mailed, and so forth and so on.

Tobacco manufacturers used to brag about how central cigarettes were to the modern economy, employing three million people in the United States alone, where cigarettes consumed

> over 40 million pounds of moisture-proof cellophane, more than 70 million pounds of aluminum foil, nearly 27 billion cartons, all of which contribute greatly to the economies of these industries and in turn the economy of the nation. Altogether about 1,500,000 businesses share in the tobacco trade, supplying equipment, materials, transportation, advertising, distributing and merchandising services in every part of the country.[5]

Of course in a world where "the economy" is measured by the sheer volume of "goods" consumed, such facts might be impressive. But cigarettes are, in fact, a drag on modern economies, a productive sink, a cause of poverty and of labor incapacity, inter alia. A waste and not a good. For the tobacco man reciting these facts, however, this was obviously a point of pride—which helps explain why this exact passage was plagiarized by at least four other tobacco industry advocates, following its first appearance in 1968 in an article by Frank B. Snodgrass in the *United States Tobacco Journal*.[6] Snodgrass was talking only about the United States, but the global toll is now larger by more than an order of magnitude. Six *billion* kilograms of cigarettes are smoked worldwide every year, which doesn't count the packaging, cartons, or cases in which they are housed and transported.

So it should hardly come as a surprise that cigarettes are leaving a sizable carbon footprint on the planet. Global climate change has stimulated a great deal of interest in what are known as "life cycle" comparisons, meaning comparisons of how different industries contribute to greenhouse warming. And sophisticated models have been developed to calculate impacts for different kinds of industry. In 2002, for example, according to the Economic Input–Output Lifecycle Assessment (EIOLCA) models developed by Carnegie Mellon University's Green Design Institute, the $47 billion tobacco industry in the United States was responsible for generating about 16 million metric tons of carbon dioxide equivalents. American automobiles emit an average of about 4.4 tons of carbon per year (driving 12,000 miles), which means that if cigarettes were to disappear from the United States the country would see a carbon benefit equivalent to taking nearly 4 million cars off the road.[7]

The benefit would actually be significantly higher than this, however, since EIOLCA modelers measure the carbon footprint of an industry (or product) only as far as the factory gate. Ignored are whatever emissions may stem from transporting cigarettes to retail outlets, or from smokers driving to the store to get their fix. More important, though, are the carbon costs of the medical care required to treat illnesses caused by smoking. Health care in the United States is estimated to have a total carbon footprint of about 550 million metric tons of carbon dioxide,[8] and since about 5 percent of all U.S. health care costs stem from tobacco—about $100 billion per year—we can assume that about 5 percent of this health care carbon burden could be avoided by eliminating smoking. That adds another 28 million tons of carbon to our cigarette greenhouse gas burden. But there is more.

Tobacco manufacturing is a significant cause of deforestation.[9] A 1991 estimate put the amount of land under cultivation for tobacco at 5.3 million hectares, making it the world's leading non-food crop. Tobacco at that time displaced land that could feed an estimated 10 million to 20 million people.[10]

Cigarettes are also a major cause of fires, including forest fires, and a substantial contributor to industrial disasters. The largest single industrial accident in the United States was directly caused by smoking: in 1947 careless handling of cigarettes was blamed for igniting 2,600 tons of ammonium nitrate on a ship in the harbor of Texas City, Texas, killing six hundred people and causing an explosion so powerful it knocked planes from the sky. Smoking caused the crash of a Russian-made Ilyushin-18 plane on Christmas Eve 1987 at Canton, killing twenty-three passengers. And cigarettes caused the infamous Triangle Shirtwaist Factory fire in 1911, killing 146 New York City garment workers.

Tobacco fires don't get a lot of attention, but in the United States alone from 1970 through 2000, fires killed about four thousand people per year, with about a quarter of these being traceable to cigarettes.[11] The tragedy is magnified by the fact that it is not that hard to make (relatively) fire-safe cigarettes: all you have to do is wrap a few tiny bands of thickened paper around the rod; these bands extinguish the cigarette unless a smoker is actively pulling on it, preventing a dropped cigarette from kindling a fire. Designs of this sort were patented in the 1920s, and the negligence of the industry is such that cigarettes were not made fire-safe until the new millennium. (Manufacturers actually exacerbated the danger by adding burn accelerants to help keep cigarettes lit—and even organized fire marshals to oppose fire-safety standards.) New York was the first state to mandate fire-safe cigarettes—in 2004—and other states have since followed this lead. The shocking fact is that tens of thousands of people have died needlessly from tobacco fires—including people who fell asleep with a cigarette lit. Fire deaths would surely merit a greater public outcry, were it not for the fact that cigarette deaths from heart disease and cancer dwarf those caused by fires by a couple orders of magnitude.

A WIN-WIN-WIN SITUATION

Cigarettes contribute substantially to the global climate crisis. In the United States alone, eliminating cigarettes would yield carbon savings equivalent to raising the fuel efficiency of all cars and trucks by several miles per gallon—or to converting the entire electrical grid of a state like Massachusetts to solar power. Eliminating cigarettes would probably make a bigger dent in the country's total carbon footprint than is presently made by all of the nation's wind and solar energy combined. We tend of think of saving the planet as involving painful sacrifices or breakthroughs in science and technology, but in this case global environmental health could be boosted by eliminating the world's leading cause of preventable death. This is a win-win-win situation, given that most smokers don't even enjoy their cigarettes—and wish they didn't smoke. The only real loss, apart from profits for the racketeers extruding the product, will be to governments hooked on cigarette taxes. When the real costs in terms of human health are factored in, however—including lost productivity and the costs of treating smoking illnesses—we return to our triple or even quadruple win: environmental health, medical savings, smokers' hopes, and the end of the world's biggest killer.

"Safer" Cigarettes?

Philip Morris is committed to domestic violence.
PHILIP MORRIS COMPANIES INC., "DOMESTIC VIOLENCE
FACT SHEET," 1998

Tobacco companies have sometimes claimed it is not possible to make a "safe" or even a "safer" cigarette, though the basis for that argument has shifted somewhat in recent years. The claim used to be there was *no point* to making cigarettes "safer," since they had never been shown to be unsafe. In the late 1990s this argument was given a bizarre twist, as the companies began characterizing cigarettes as *inherently* risky. The hope was to glide safely through the collapse of the denialist project, using the reassuring rhetoric of "risk": Isn't life, after all, inherently risky? So isn't the cigarette very much like life in this respect?

Smoking, then, entails certain "risks." We are also reassured, though, that the companies are trying to reduce those risks through research. That is one reason Philip Morris built a new $350 million research facility in downtown Richmond, Virginia. One of the main goals of this high-tech "Life Sciences Park," staffed by three-hundred-odd research scientists, is to explore "reduced harm" tobacco products, using nanotechnology and metagenomics and other state-of-the-art science fashions. "Harm reduction" has become the industry's new mantra; the companies now want us to believe that less hazardous products can be and are being made and marketed—in the form of cigarettes, of course, but also chewing tobacco, oral snuff, and that sexy spittle-soaked item known as Swedish "snus," which causes mainly tooth loss and mouth tumors.

Unquestioned in all of this is the ideology of consumer sovereignty: the presumption is that consumers should have unlimited *choices* when it comes to what kinds of products they might consume. It is the myopia that leads us to encourage *cessation of consumption* while ignoring opportunities in the realm of *cessation of production*. Consumers are encouraged to stop consuming, but producers are never discouraged from producing. Applied to harm reduction, the presumption is that we should only think of "safer" cigarettes in terms of products added to those already on the market. Harm reduction is envisioned in terms of *inventing new products* rather than *restricting or banning* those already being sold.

But first: Can cigarettes be made less lethal? Of course they can! Cigarettes are highly engineered artifacts and can be made in a thousand different ways—and some will obviously be less deadly than others, depending (partly) on how they are used. Tobacco control advocates have often been leery of making this point, not wanting to seem to be helping the industry find ways to "improve" cigarettes—which might well discourage people from quitting (or never starting). Health advocates are, in fact, divided over whether it is good for cigarettes to be made "more safe," and for interesting reasons.

On the one hand, there are those who ask: How could anyone *not* want cigarettes to be less hazardous? If people are going to smoke, shouldn't they be able to smoke in ways that are less likely to kill them? Comparisons are made to the use of drugs such as heroin: so long as people are going to shoot junk into their veins, shouldn't they at least be able to use clean needles? Such has been the basis for needle-exchange programs in various parts of the world, and the tobacco industry has worked hard to piggy-pack onto at least part of this rhetoric—the "harm reduction" part. People are always going to smoke, so shouldn't we at least make cigarettes as safe as possible?

There are good reasons to be skeptical of harm reduction, however. I tend to agree with those who sense that as most commonly imagined "harm reduction" may end up causing even greater harm, by dangling false or even true hopes in the market. Quitting (or never starting) is really the only way to prevent harm, and if products touted as "safer" make smokers less likely to quit, then harm reduction could do more harm than good. There is the added legal twist that a tobacco manufacturer might have trouble obtaining approval for a novelty that might provide, say, only a 10 percent chance of killing you—compared with the 50 percent of traditional cigarettes (over a lifetime of smoking). Cigarettes made in the conventional (= superdeadly) way have been "grandfathered in" by the health and safety myopia of times gone by, but imagine a world in which cigarettes had never been invented, and the question were posed de novo: is the cigarette an acceptable drug or consumer product? Patent offices would presumably refuse it; regulators would bar it. That is why new tobacco products, even those that are marginally less lethal, may not be welcomed with open arms. A California law (Proposition 65) defines a "significant risk level" as anything that would result in more than one excess cancer in 100,000 individuals exposed over a seventy-year lifetime; cigarettes are thousands of times more deadly, so even a thousandfold improvement wouldn't pass the Golden State's test of "significant risk." Hence the difficulty. Of course given how low the bar is for cigarette safety, almost anything will appear "safer" by comparison. Talk of "safer cigarettes" is rather like talking about safer terrorism, or safer smallpox, or safer forms of drowning: it's oxymoronic.

AN UGLY IRONY

Again, it would not be hard to make a "safer cigarette" or even one that is *perfectly* safe, so long as we are willing to stretch our definitions. A cigarette made entirely of solid wood or stone could not be smoked, for example, and therefore would be quite safe. The same would presumably be true for any cigarette that does not deliver toxins into the body. Cigarettes of this sort are not made, of course, because no one would buy them. People buy cigarettes because they have a craving for nicotine, and if cigarettes don't deliver "the goodies" they won't get bought.

The law also has a say in this matter. Cigarettes are regulated for purposes of taxation—and now in the United States by the FDA—which means we have legal definitions of a cigarette. In the United States a cigarette has traditionally been a smokable tobacco product wrapped in paper. How important, though, is the paper to this definition, or the smokability, or the tobacco? What if we are talking about a nicotine delivery device that emits no smoke, or is not wrapped in paper, or contains no tobacco, or is not burned but rather heated—is that still a cigarette? The question is not an academic one, since regulators have to decide whether a particular device is or is not a cigarette, in order to know how or even whether to regulate it. This was one problem encountered by Premier and Accord in the 1980s and 1990s: the devices were introduced as cigarettes but didn't so much burn as warm and release a kind of flavored nicotine steam. The industry called these "cigarettes" and included tobacco to have them grandfathered into the FDA's regulatory neglect (since the agency was barred from regulating cigarettes), but not everyone agreed they were enough like cigarettes to ignore.

There is an ugly irony here: cigarettes that are not deadly enough may not be classified for regulatory purposes as cigarettes—especially if they don't contain (and burn) tobacco. Electronic cigarette manufacturers often include some small amount of tobacco in their products, just to guarantee these will be classed as cigarettes and not as inhalers or some other kind of drug device. Nicotine inhalers have to be approved by the FDA, whereas cigarettes generally speaking do not (though that is now beginning to change). And drug delivery designs that stray too far from traditional cigarettes may not be approved even if—and in a sense *because*—they are less deadly. Designs that well might kill fewer people may not be classed as cigarettes and might not obtain regulatory approval. Cigarettes get grandfathered in as sacrosanct, while devices that might kill fewer people get barred as unsafe.

From the industry's point of view, of course, it would be great to be able to make less deadly cigarettes, so long as profits could be kept high. The companies are not in the business to kill people; that is more of a side effect and one they would surely rather avoid, everything else being equal ("unattractive side effects," is how Brown & Williamson once described lung cancer and heart disease from smoking.)[1] The companies have tried from time to time to make cigarettes less deadly, albeit always within the confines of maximizing profits and fending off lawsuits. Many of these efforts were kept quiet, since the industry didn't want to admit that cigarettes were at all unsafe.

And most such efforts involved little more than tinkering. Scientists working for Reynolds once summarized ten different ways that cigarettes had been redesigned to offer "safer smoking," following the arguments of Gio Gori, their ally at the National Cancer Institute. These included use of high-porosity cigarette paper; air-dilution filters; use of reconstituted tobacco and stems, along with inert fillers ("tobacco extenders") such as clay or dolomite; novel methods of cultivation and curing; and reductions in machine-measured tar, nicotine, nitrogen oxides, carbon monoxide, and hydrogen cyanide to "appropriate" levels.[2]

The industry now likes to display such efforts as proof of good-faith efforts to make cigarettes safer, but the fact is that none of these are anything but minor tinkerings. High-porosity paper helps the companies control the oxygen flow to the burning rod, affecting the temperature and rate of burn. Tar and nicotine look lower to smoking robots because the cigarettes burn up faster. Air dilution is just ventilation, a trick overcome by compensation and "lipping behavior." Recon is primarily a way to save on factory costs and to fine-tune composition, and inert fillers make smoking safer if you believe that a few glass marbles in a bottle of soda will lower its calorie count. The industry's principal stabs at creating "safer" cigarettes ignore—or sometimes even capitalize on—the reality of compensation and can even cause *more* harm by delaying quitting. Untold millions of smokers have continued to smoke, imagining that by switching to extra longs, filters, menthols, low tars, or lights they were smoking safer.

There are two chief problems in this "safer cigarette" business. The first is that no matter how you modify the product, repeated inhalation of smoke is going to cause disease. The second is more of a legal nature, having to do with the fact that so long as cigarettes in their super-deadly form are legal, there really is no incentive for a manufacturer to make less deadly cigarettes. Think about it from a (rather misanthropic) marketing point of view: why bother selling a "safer" cigarette when no one is stopping you from selling your unsafe brands? That was the problem with Lorillard's "little cigars," launched with the brand name Madison in 1958. These were basically cork-tipped cigarettes made with brown instead of white paper and a smoke pH so high—on a par with cigars—they would not be inhaled ("You Need Not Inhale to Enjoy Them"), which would have been a genuinely less deadly tobacco product. A few people even outside the industry realized this and grasped the underlying rationale: as *Consumer Reports* put it in 1959, "cigar smoke is too strong and irritating for most people to want to inhale it, and smoke which merely is taken into the mouth does not, so far as is now known, cause or aggravate lung cancer."[3] "Little cigars" never met with much commercial success, however, despite a burst of popularity following the 1964 Surgeon General's report. The companies never made any serious effort to advertise these as less lethal and never withdrew cigarettes with more easily inhalable smoke.

The lawyerly complications stem from the fact that once you start saying your new version of Luckies, Marlboros, or Virginia Slims will kill fewer people, this would seem to be an admission that your old-school brands have not been on the up and up. Lots of "safer" cigarettes marketed or proposed for marketing have bitten the dust on these grounds—Liggett's palladium cigarette, for example.

LIGGETT'S PALLADIUM FIASCO

In Liggett's case the company had launched this effort jointly with the Arthur D. Little company in the 1950s, spraying palladium nitrate onto cured tobacco leaves to achieve a more complete combustion.[4] The idea was that the metal would act as a catalyst, helping to burn up some of those nasty polycyclic aromatic hydrocarbons thought responsible for causing cancer. Catalytic converters were known to have done something similar for cars: automobile exhaust is basically forced past a reactive catalyst at a high temperature, which breaks up some of the uglier complex molecules into softies like carbon dioxide and water. The afterburners attached to jet engines work on a similar principle, albeit with the goal being not to reduce emissions but rather to extract more energy from the fuel. Catalytic conversion might well have "worked" in cigarettes—preliminary tests showed a lessening of carcinogenic potency—but the idea seems to have foundered on legal shoals.

Everything else being equal, it could well be that switching from, say, Marlboro Reds to a cigarette with a palladium nitrate catalyst might make you less likely to die from smoking. Liggett in the 1960s and 1970s put quite a few eggs into this basket, spending $15 million over about twenty years on projects with code names like Project Tame and Project XA. Smoke from such cigarettes caused fewer tumors when condensed and smeared on the backs of experimental animals, and the company purchased 200,000 ounces of the precious metal—at $52.50 per ounce—from Engelhard Minerals. But legal fears eventually caught up with and snagged the cigarette, which was never sold commercially. This was a great disappointment to the program's chief architect, the chemist James D. Mold, who wanted very much to see this "safer cigarette" marketed. Liggett's attorneys realized this would be difficult without admitting that cigarettes cause cancer; there was also the worry that the Federal Trade Commission might not even allow any mention of such additives in advertising. Mold has testified that the company hoped for help from the White

House; Jimmy Carter was president when the cigarette was being readied and was friendly enough to promise North Carolina growers help with making smoking "even more safe than it is today."[5]

Liggett would later claim that its palladium cigarette was dropped because it had a "metallic taste" and failed marketing tests. Testimony from the project's researchers, however, reveal that the company came under pressure from some of the larger manufacturers, who didn't want to hear anyone in the business conceding that smoking caused cancer. According to Mold, the company worried that the sale of palladium cigarettes "would seriously indict them for having sold other types of cigarettes"; he also recalls Liggett's president and CEO, Kinsley Van R. Dey, talking about a threat from Philip Morris that the Marlboro men would "clobber" Liggett if it were to market such a product. Shortly after announcing the new cigarette, Liggett researchers got word from the company's lawyers that the device could put them in legal jeopardy.[6]

Liggett's low-cancer palladium cigarette was announced in the fall of 1978, with a press release by Arthur D. Little identifying Liggett as "the first cigarette maker to acknowledge tobacco produces cancer in laboratory animals." A Liggett spokesman immediately rejected this conclusion, stating that the admission pertained only to certain animal experiments using smoke condensate—which were flawed by virtue of using "the wrong substance on the wrong tissue, on the wrong species in the wrong amounts." A Liggett press release of September 26, 1978, reaffirmed that the company and the cigarette industry as a whole "continue to deny . . . that any conclusions can be drawn relating such test results on mice in laboratories to cancer in human beings." The company's acquisition of a patent on the palladium process was not to be considered an admission of a cancer link:

> Liggett has made no such admission; the fact is that for more than two decades scientific researchers have produced tumors on mouse skin by the application of enormous dosages of smoke condensate. Neither the industry nor Liggett has denied these results. Liggett and the cigarette industry continue to deny, as they have consistently, that any conclusions can be drawn relating such test results on mice in laboratories to cancer in human beings. It has never been established that smoking is a cause of human cancer.[7]

Plaintiffs' attorneys later had a field day with the confusion, after learning that Liggett had spent $15 million over twenty-four years to research a project whose relevance to human smoking they now repudiated. Had Liggett really spent so much money just to save the lives of a few shaved mice?[8]

SUPPRESSING NICORETTE

The palladium cigarette is remarkable as a case of product suppression, regardless of whether it would have actually saved lives. It was suppressed for legal and PR reasons, but it is certainly not the only instance of tobacco-related product suppression. Another example took place in the 1980s, when Philip Morris pressured Merrell Dow Pharmaceuticals to rein in its marketing of Nicorette chewing gum. Nicorette was a nicotine replacement therapy developed by the Swedes in the 1960s and approved for use in Switzerland in 1978 and in the United Kingdom in 1980, by which time Merrell Dow was readying it for sale in the United States. FDA approval didn't come until 1984, but in 1981 the company had launched the *Smoking Cessation Newsletter* to publicize the virtues of nicotine replacement therapy. Philip Morris was furious at Merrell Dow for publishing "anti-smoking propaganda" and called a meeting with the company to demand that it "cease further publication." Philip Morris also threatened to stop buying humectants from the company's parent, Dow Chemical, which by 1982 was doing $8 million in business with the cigarette manufacturer. Merrell Dow bent under the pressure, and the *Smoking Cessation Newsletter* was canceled after only one issue.[9]

Philip Morris continued to pressure Merrell Dow on other matters, including the pharmaceutical manufacturer's support for the National Interagency Council on Smoking and Health, a distinguished group of representatives from the American Heart Association, the American Public Health Association, the American Cancer Society, and other public health agencies. Philip Morris didn't like the council's support for scholars who refused tobacco industry money, its urging of athletes to renounce tobacco sponsorship, or its call for "a Smoke-Free Society by the year 2000." Merrell Dow also continued to promote Nicorette gum, prompting Philip Morris to honor its threat to halt all purchases of glycerine, glycol, and other humectants from Dow Chemical (in May 1984). Philip Morris explained in internal correspondence that Dow had apparently decided that Nicorette was "more important" than its trade with tobacco manufacturers; indeed Dow was engaged in an audacious program "to motivate Philip Morris customers to stop smoking." Philip Morris expressed its disappointment that a loyal customer (itself) would spend millions of dollars purchasing materials from a company (Dow Chemical) whose profits would then be used "to attack that customer's product and perhaps reduce the customer's sales." Dow protested that it was not in fact trying to combat smoking, but the cigarette maker was rightly skeptical. Philip Morris warned that future relations between the two companies would be "predicated" on "the course of the Nicorette program."[10]

Philip Morris continued with its effort "to eliminate, or at least tone down," Dow's marketing of Nicorette but eventually realized that the cigarette maker was as dependent on Dow as vice versa. Philip Morris resumed purchasing from Dow but only after the chemical company had withdrawn its support for the Interagency Council.[11] By pressuring Dow in this manner and by helping to quash the *Smoking Cessation Newsletter*, Philip Morris may well have delayed the spread of effective methods of smoking cessation in the United States. Which of course was precisely its intent.

. Bhavna Shamasunder and Lisa Bero at UCSF have shown that tobacco manufacturers have pressured pharmaceutical manufacturers in other ways—to limit the marketing of nicotine transdermal patches made by Merrell Dow and CIBA-Geigy (Nicoderm and Habitrol), for example. Philip Morris here again was worried about patches cutting into its cigarette business and actually calculated a loss of sales to the industry on the order of 11.2 billion cigarettes per year by 1996, based on a market for patches predicted to reach $1 billion per year by 1995. Philip Morris "took offense" at CIBA-Geigy's marketing of Habitrol and used its position as a major buyer of pesticides to pressure the company to rein in its "anti-tobacco" advertising. Intimidation of this sort resulted in CIBA-Geigy revising its marketing of Habitrol, with a "Groundrules" agreement between the company's agricultural and pharmaceutical divisions requiring that the drug maker target only those people already "committed to quitting." Habitrol was not to be considered "a substitute for smoking" or to violate "the freedom of choice for smokers." Philip Morris was apprised of all these changes and appeared satisfied that CIBA-Geigy would "remain sensitive to the concerns of the tobacco grower organizations and the rest of the tobacco industry."[12]

There are many other examples of the industry flexing its muscles to suppress products, policies, or programs perceived as obstacles to the continued sale of cigarettes. In an earlier chapter we saw how dependence on tobacco advertising revenue made it hard for popular magazines to criticize cigarettes; this same influence worked to encumber cessation advertising. *Consumer Reports* as early as 1959 noted how hard it was for the manufacturers of Bantron, a prescription pill designed to help smokers cut down on smoking, to get magazines to take their ads, given the risk of offending cigarette makers. The *New York Times* cautioned that magazines wanting to publish such ads would have to "think twice" before risking their lucrative cigarette accounts. Shamasunder and Bero compare this to the industry's use of its considerable financial might to pressure airlines not to enact smoking bans.[13]

These are only tiny slivers from the industry's larger history of political machinations, much of which has been designed to keep radical tobacco exceptionalism alive. Tobacco managed to have itself excluded from regulation by the FDA for more than a century, just as it was excluded from regulation by the Consumer Product Safety Commission when that body was founded in 1973. The commission has always had the power to rein in dangerous cigarette *lighters*, for example, but has never had any authority over tobacco products. It has the power to require furniture makers to design upholstery to withstand ignition from cigarettes but no power to demand a reduction in the ignition propensity of cigarettes themselves.[14] A medievalist colleague once remarked on how the government of the United States is byzantine with political fiefdoms and legal exceptions, and I cannot think of a better example than the parochial exceptionalism granted to Lord Tobacco.

ILLUSIONS OF SAFETY

"Safer" cigarette designs number in the hundreds if not the thousands. What we've mainly seen from manufacturers, however, are *illusions of safety,* conveyed by intimations of health via branding categories like "lights," "low tars" and "milds," along with healthy-seeming additives such as menthol, with its medico-bogus implication of sanitation. (For the tuxedoed "Dr. Kool," complete with black bag and stethoscope, see Figure 34). *King-sized* cigarettes (Pall Mall, introduced in 1939) were also supposed to offer protection by virtue of "traveling the smoke" farther, and even "toasting" (Lucky Strike) was heralded as removing poisons. *Filters* were all the rage in the 1950s, forcing smokers to pull somewhat harder on their cigarettes but doing little to change the quantity inhaled or its carcinogenic character. *Selective filtration* was supposed to be the next big hope, though here, too, the difficulty was that while one kind of compound might be partially trapped (say, hydrogen cyanide or phenols), others were as likely to be augmented (carbon monoxide or nitrosamines, for example). Cigarette makers found themselves faced with a chemical hydra, with new poisons cropping up when old ones were vanquished. Smokers were then urged to switch to "low tar" and eventually "light" cigarettes—concocted by blending tricks and ventilation and hand waving—though here, too, the benefits were illusory. Smokers tended to adjust their smoking behavior, drawing harder to maintain their accustomed level of "satisfaction." "Lights" became the main new branding concept in the 1970s, formalizing this low-tar subterfuge. With Lights this suggestion of a benefit from "stepping down" in tar was built into the very brand name, a novelty in the history of marketing. Competition for the "worrier" or "concerned segment" prompted brand extensions into ever lower tar regimes, with the late 1970s seeing the invention of "Ultra Light" and "Lowest Tar" brandings—all bogus.

Additives were another great hope. Dozens if not hundreds of substances were tested to see whether specific poisons might be destroyed: to eliminate benzpyrene, for example, companies tried adding metal nitrates of various sorts, hoping these would act as catalysts to break down carcinogenic polycyclics. Absorbents were added, along with chemicals to lower the burning temperature (to reduce polycyclics), or even hemoglobin to gobble up carbon monoxide.[15] Carbon was added to filters to capture ciliastats, and while American companies were toying with Parmesan cheese and kitty litter, the Japanese were patenting a bovine milk protein that was supposed to adsorb onto a carbon surface.

The problem with almost all such manipulations is that tobacco smoke is a complex and chemodynamic brew, with many interacting components. David Townsend, director of product development at R. J. Reynolds, saw a certain amount of humor in the situation:

You know, we—we joke a lot in the laboratory about it, all the heads are tied to all the tails. If you change one thing, in fact, everything changes because it's such an interactive system . . . it's technically very difficult to go into something complex—complex like cigarette smoke with a scalpel and carve out one compound or one group of compounds.[16]

Which is also why so few of these manipulations offered anything in the way of genuine safety. All were essentially gimmicks, as was revealed to the outside world when cancer rates failed to fall as many scholars had hoped. Per-cigarette cancer rates today remain about what they were in the 1950s and 1960s, with no real benefit from the shift to lights and low tars. Indeed since there is significantly less tobacco in cigarettes, on a per-gram basis cigarettes are actually more deadly now than ever before—as we have seen.

One new and radical step taken in the 1980s and 1990s was to try to make a *nonburning cigarette*—basically a smoke-free nicotine delivery device that would release some kind of warm nicotine steam with flavors. The idea here again was that smokers should be able to obtain their requisite nicotine fix without all that nasty admixed tar. Reynolds spent hundreds of millions of dollars along these lines: the goal of Projects Spa, Q, and Y, for example—which eventually yielded the Premier cigarette—was to develop a device heated by a battery or chemical reaction of some sort that would emit no secondhand smoke and near-zero tar while still delivering nicotine "satisfaction."

TEXAS BABOONS ON CRACK

Reynolds announced its Premier cigarette in the summer of 1988, but the brand was a flop from the get-go. The new cigarette never sold, despite a massive marketing campaign encompassing one-on-one briefings with university presidents, medical school deans, science writers, and medical organizations, along with politicians and "opinion leaders" throughout the world. The plan included cultivation of academics as spokespersons and witnesses—including Stanford's Nathan Rosenberg, who was hired to testify on "technology policy" for the company—along with more traditional use of hot lines, sampling vans and kiosks, and "very elegant cigarette girls to sample product in trendy restaurants and clubs." And contacts with key friendlies in the House and the Senate. The new device—basically a nicotine steam dispenser with a hollow, pellet-filled, metal heating element running through the center—was clumsy to light, hard to dispose of, and had a pretty wretched taste. Test panels reported flavors reminiscent of "burnt biscuits" and "glue made from fish or horses," with the remnant heating element left after smoking looking rather like "the heating rods in nuclear reactors—very industrial." One user described the smell as redolent of "a grave opened on a warm day."[17] And while tar deliveries were lower, "gas" yields were actually higher, including classic nasties like carbon monoxide and hydrogen cyanide, released by the smoldering of the charcoal tip (which you lit to get the thing fired up). So it was never even clear that a shift to such a cigarette would be an overall plus, even if it didn't stink (which it did). Smokers found the thing disgusting, but there was also the legal/PR rub that devices such as this could not be advertised as "safer," so long as no one was willing to admit that ordinary cigarettes were dangerous. Critics charged that the only reason it contained tobacco at all was to exempt it from regulation as a new kind of drug delivery device— to which Reynolds responded by launching a series of investigations forcing baboons to smoke crack cocaine.

The stimulus here was the complaint that Reynolds's Premier cigarette could be used to deliver other kinds of drugs—like cocaine. Jack Henningfield and Edward Cone from the National Institute of Drug Abuse had replaced the nicotine in Premier with 200 milligrams of crack cocaine and found that the contraption functioned tolerably well as a crack pipe. Reynolds ridiculed the suggestion ("They call Premier a 'drug delivery device': well, so is a spoon") but was forced to respond, prompting a series of Reynolds-financed experiments in which baboons were taught to smoke cigarettes laced with crack cocaine. The goal was to see whether this new "smokeless" cigarette could be used "as an efficient system for the delivery of 'crack' or free-base cocaine." Reynolds in January 1989 had at least nine baboons smoking crack (or controls), with laboratory analyses farmed out to the University of North Carolina in Chapel Hill and the crack-addicted baboons lodged at the Southwest Research Institute in San Antonio, Texas—which at that time had the world's largest baboonery. A psychiatrist by the name of Mario Perez-Reyes was the company's point man at UNC, with Walter R. Rogers doing the dirty work in San Antonio. The cocaine was provided by the Georgia Bureau of Investigation. The experiments went on for several months, with mixed results. Perez-Reyes for a time was worried that the baboons had not been properly trained and might only be "puffing" without inhaling. Researchers did find evidence of compensation: "As in humans, baboons are very sensitive to draw resistance. They can learn to modify their puffing to compensate."[18]

There is much we cannot know about such experiments: the document just cited, for example, begins with a redacted section censored as "Privileged material." We do know, though, that Southwest Research by the mid-1970s already had thirty-five baboons hooked on cigarettes: Walter Rogers had trained them to smoke by depriving them of water and then allowing them to drink only through a tube through which smoke was also introduced. Helmut Wakeham led a Philip Morris team to San Antonio to observe the creatures, several of whom by 1975 had already been addicted for more than two years. Operant conditioning had turned them into precision instruments for the study of smoking behavior, with their carefully timed puffs resulting in "the buildup of a heavy pall of smoke about the animal's head."[19]

As for the baboons: we don't yet have a good study of experimental animal abuse in the tobacco industry. Tens and probably hundreds of thousands of animals have been sacrificed for no good purpose. We also need further study of *human* experimentation in the industry. Philip Morris in 1969, for example, launched a series of experiments titled "Smoking under Conditions of Shock Produced Anxiety" to see whether college students would become more or less interested in smoking after exposure to electric shock. Virginia Commonwealth University students were jolted with electric current to show that smoking "is more probable in stress situations than in nonstress situations." Shock intensity was to be adjusted for each subject "according to the subject's pain threshold," and the protocol explained that "the shock will be painful." This particular series was abandoned in October of 1972, when Philip Morris psychologists realized that "fear of shock" was "scaring away some of our more valuable subjects." Industry employees have also been subject to human experiments, testing experimental cigarettes or even experimental pesticides with little or no regulatory oversight.[20]

CIGARETTE DOUBLESPEAK

Premier's failure was, in a sense, both pre- and overdetermined. Quite apart from being awkward, unpleasant, and a bigger emitter of carbon monoxide even than ordinary cigarettes, protests were also voiced that this was just another effort by the industry to keep people hooked on nicotine. Trenchant criticism also came from those who realized that the "safety" offered was trivial at best: Arnold M. Katz, head of cardiology at the University of Connecticut Health Center, noted that to market such a product as preventing disease would be like urging us to sleep with rattlesnakes because they are less toxic than cobras.[21]

Criticism of this sort seems not to have been much of a deterrent, however. Philip Morris's Project Advance (from 1984) was yet another effort to investigate "nonburning pleasure articles," quasi-cigarettes that would deliver an aerosol of "nicotine, flavors and other satisfying components" with "very low biological activity" and little or no sidestream smoke. The goal was to avoid combustion, with alternate heat sources ranging from electric batteries to chemical power (photoflash or thermite). The same company's Project Vanguard expanded this to include cold unpowered vapor devices, flashbulb heating mechanisms, piezoelectrics, and mechanical devices for atomization, along with devices incorporating whistles, capillaries, and something called "packed beds-pulsed power." A common idea behind the "electric cigarette" was that a battery of some sort would heat a nichrome wire, warming and vaporizing the nicotine (developed under the company's Project Leap). Philip Morris also worked with General Electric "to provide additional expertise in developing the electric cigarette concept."[22] Efforts along these lines—supported by $200 million in development costs—culminated (in 1997) in the debut of Accord, an "ultra low tar" cigarette that could be smoked only while inserted into a large, handheld, battery-powered Puff Activated Lighter™, complete with a micro-processor to indicate how many puffs remained. This, too, was an instant flop: the electronic lighter alone cost $50 and required a recharge of batteries after every pack smoked. Richard Daynard called it a "weird contraption," and the *New York Times* likened it to smoking a kazoo. The device also failed when test marketed in Germany as the "Heatbar."[23]

Other companies developed similar designs. Brown & Williamson in 1991 filed for a patent on a cigarette that would generate a warm tobacco-flavored liquid, and Imperial Tobacco patented a cigarette that would burn only while the smoker was inhaling. But most projects of this nature during the development phase at least were kept quite confidential. The companies usually didn't want it known that they were trying to make (some) cigarettes less dangerous, and the dilemma continued even after new products were announced. It was hard to advertise such innovations: the companies couldn't really say they were "safer," without admitting their other brands were less than safe. The solution was a kind of doublespeak, in which Premier and the like were offered only as reducing "many of the controversial compounds" in cigarette smoke. And smokers just didn't buy it. Why should they, when the manufacturers were not even admitting any harms from plain old regular smokes?

Reynolds in the 1990s retreated to a less radical redesign with Eclipse, which was more like a traditional cigarette with reduced (visible) secondhand smoke emissions. Eclipse was introduced in the United States in 1996 but also simultaneously in Germany as Hi.Q and in Sweden as Inside. None of these were popular, however. The cigarette was supposed to yield fewer smoke solids and to be "safer" from the point of view of starting fires (since it wasn't really burning the tobacco so much as just heating it to produce a flavored nicotine aerosol). But the taste again was foul: not as "sweet and sickly" as Premier but still unpleasant with "fungal" and "metallic/toxic" taste overtones. And hard to light and hard to tell how far down you'd smoked, since the tubular outer casing never went away. Test panels judged it overall "a good cigarette to smoke if you want to quit"—mainly because it was so disgusting.

The hard lesson learned through such misadventures was that while cigarettes could be made that might well be less likely to kill you, they weren't likely to attract much of a following. And in a smug sort of way the companies must have welcomed this, since it could be used to blame the victim—that is, the consumer. The companies could basically say, "Look how hard we tried to make safer cigarettes, but people don't want to smoke them! What more can we do? If smokers don't want safety, then it's not our fault."

Recent years have seen renewed efforts to produce "less hazardous" cigarettes, most of which use batteries to provide some kind of flavored nicotine steam. Electric or "electronic" cigarettes, for example, warm a soup of nicotine fluid, which then vaporizes and can be sucked into the lungs. Many such devices are now being produced in China—the Ruyan cigarette, for example, which can be bought on various Internet sites or through eBay, or competitors like the Ploom (a pipe) or Njoy. The idea is for these to be used ("vaped") in places where traditional cigarettes cannot—on airplanes, for example, or in bars where smoking is banned. None of these devices have been tested for safety, however, and since all deliver nicotine, sometimes accompanied by a propylene or diethylene glycol mist, we can assume they will all cause addiction. Electronic cigarettes have been banned in Australia and in Hong Kong and are restricted in many other countries. Regulatory oversight is likely to depend on whether they are imagined for use as cigarettes, cigarette substitutes, or smoking cessation instruments. Some are being promoted as quasi-therapeutic—like Vapir One, a "revolutionary" vaporizer designed to "intoxicate your senses" by inhaling "the essence" from various herbs, spices, or tobacco. Vapir's inhaler is advertised as useful in the treatment of asthma, congestion, or anxiety, eliminating "all of the discomfort" associated with traditional cigarettes. Users are invited to "inhale the future."[24]

Most such devices have been greeted with skepticism from the medical community, since the long-term consequences of inhaling nicotine or glycol steam or herbal "essences" are not at all clear. There is also the worry that such devices will be used in combination with smoking or to avoid quitting. The U.S. Food and Drug Administration in 2009 barred the import of electronic cigarettes into the United States, though a federal court shortly thereafter lifted this ban, classifying the devices as cigarettes and therefore subject to the new regulatory authority of the FDA. Electronic cigarettes have been banned in many countries—Brazil, Australia and Canada, for example—where cigarettes themselves (for now) remain legal.

IGNORED OPTIONS

There is no such thing as a "safe" or even a "safer" cigarette, judging purely from the intrinsic physical properties of some smoking article. Cigarettes are more or less lethal, depending on how they are used. The tarriest Lucky Strike from the 1950s wouldn't be so bad if you just puffed once on it lightly without inhaling and then tossed it (fireless) into the trash. And the "healthiest" ultralight is a tumor tube if you suck on it like a vacuum pump to the bitter end. All those numbers printed on packs for so many years were virtually meaningless—and highly deceptive—and the fact is that a cigarette advertised as delivering 20 milligrams of tar could be smoked to deliver 2 milligrams and vice versa. The only really safe cigarettes are those you never smoke.

That being said, it is important to realize that the industry easily could have designed and manufactured cigarettes that would have been *inherently* less deadly—

by virtue of being difficult to inhale. Cigars, for example, cause far less damage to the lungs than cigarettes, because they are harder to inhale. They are harder to inhale because the tobacco is cured in such a way as to make the resulting smoke quite alkaline. Alkaline smoke (anything above pH 7) is harsh and if pushed higher than about pH 8 becomes almost impossible to inhale without coughing. Tobacco manufacturers have been manipulating the pH of cigarette smoke for more than a century, and it would be easy for them to redesign cigarettes—back to the uninhalable form that existed prior to that time and still exists today in most pipe and cigar tobaccos. Cigarettes would once again become little cigars and lose part of their deadly force. Cigarettes would still cause mouth and throat cancer and heart attacks and just as many deaths from secondhand smoke, but the total burden of death would still be significantly less than we have at present. The FDA's new Center for Tobacco Products—charged with regulating cigarettes—should consider this fact: if cigarette manufacturers were barred from making products with a smoke pH less than 8, there would be significantly less inhaling and significantly less lung cancer. It's a no-brainer.

Tobacco manufacturers have realized this for quite some time, and some have even tried to capitalize on it. In the 1970s, for example, the Consolidated Cigar Corporation marketed "little cigars" delivering nicotine with a sufficiently high pH that they did not have to be inhaled. (Recall that high-pH nicotine easily penetrates the mucosal membranes of the mouth and so needn't reach the lungs to deliver "satisfaction.") In testimony before the U.S. Congress in 1973, Consolidated's president defended his company's Dutch Treat cigars by claiming that their goal had been to develop "a little cigar that would be acceptable to the consumer and to the authorities as a safer alternative to cigarette smoking." The claim was that cigar smoking presented "reduced, if not negligible health risks." This is one of the few concessions at this time by a tobacco manufacturer of the reality of "health risks." Consolidated kept the pH of its cigar smoke around 7—but if it had been elevated to 8 or above and smokers had no access to "milder" smokes of the more traditional sort, this would have dramatically reduced the lung cancer risk.[25]

Cigarettes could easily be redesigned to be difficult to inhale. There is no iron law saying that cigarette smoke must be inhalable; indeed as late as the 1930s it was fairly common for cigarette smoke *not* to be taken into the lungs. Inhalation was promoted to facilitate nicotine delivery; there is no more effective way to administer such a drug. (Recall also that we are not talking here about "taste"; there are no taste organs in the lungs.) The modern inhalable cigarette is the product of decisions that could have been reversed at any time during the past century—or today for that matter. Had a decision of this sort been taken in the 1950s, cigarettes would not be causing the 160,000 annual lung cancer deaths we now have in the United States. Millions of lives could have been saved.

Tobacco companies could also have produced cigarettes that were not addictive, simply by reducing the amount of nicotine in the rod to less than about 1 milligram per cigarette. Manufacturers like to keep the nicotine up around the 10-milligram mark—even in cigarettes marketed as "light" or "low tar"—and reducing the absolute (rather than machine-measured) nicotine in the rod by a factor of ten or more would make it virtually impossible for smokers to sustain their addiction. Manufacturers have sometimes made such cigarettes—Merit Free or Next, for example—but they have never been commercially successful. The companies realize that people smoke for the nicotine and that without nicotine people will not smoke. Not tobacco at any rate.

ATLAS VERSUS HERCULES:
A DIGRESSION ON DIVERSIFICATION

Safety has never been a high priority for the industry—except when it comes to their own self-preservation. An immense amount of money is spent by the companies to defend themselves in court—close to a billion dollars per year in the United States. Yet another strategy has been to diversify into products such as candy, food, and alcohol, to secure for themselves a future in a post-tobacco, or at least a post-cigarette, world.

This was shrewd, given that it has never been clear when the bottom might drop out of the cigarette market—as a result of consumer revolt, litigation, or regulation. Liggett & Myers began the trend in 1964 by acquiring the Allen Products Company, makers of Alpo dog and cat food, for $15 million. American Tobacco shortly thereafter bought Sunshine Biscuits and Sara Lee, and Lorillard in 1965 acquired the Golden Nugget Candy Company. Reynolds that same year bought My-T-Fine Desserts and Vermont Maid Syrup by acquiring Pennick and Ford. Philip Morris bought Miller Beer in 1969, prompting a move into the liquor business by Liggett, which by the 1970s was making not just cigarettes but also Bombay gin and vermouth, Grand Marnier liqueur, and J&B scotch. And popcorn and vacuum cleaners. Imperial Tobacco did something similar in England and by the end of the 1960s was supplying 10 percent of the country's turkeys and a quarter of its chickens. Reynolds then bought Nabisco (in 1985, for $4.9 billion), forming RJR Nabisco, a conglomerate cranking out Camel cigarettes alongside Oreo Cookies, Fig Newtons, Saltine Crackers, and Planters Nuts.

The biggest deal of this sort was Philip Morris's purchase of Kraft Foods in 1988. The company had earlier bought Miller Beer and a Canadian brewery, and by the 1970s was holding American Safety Razor (makers of Personna razors) and Clark Gum (makers of chewing gum). The Kraft acquisition launched Philip Morris big time into the food business, which continued in 2000 with its acquisition of Nabisco

Holdings, a spin-off from RJR Nabisco, for $18.9 billion. This turned Philip Morris into the largest food producer in the United States, controlling products such as Altoids, Maxwell House Coffee, Lifesavers, Planters peanuts, Oscar Mayer wieners, Jell-O, Boca Burgers, Kool-Aid, and all Nabisco and Post cereals. The thinking was that if tobacco ever went down the tubes, then the people who brought you the Marlboro cowboy and millions of deaths from cardiac arrest could fall back on quality foods like Velveeta Cheese, Cool Whip, and Oreo Cookies. Ordinary consumers who bought such products probably had no idea they were enriching the coffers of the tobacco magnates.

Nor, I suspect, did they realize they were helping the world's largest cigarette maker mobilize support for the industry. Philip Morris on a number of occasions used its subsidiaries to do its political dirty work, to protect its core cigarette market. In 1994, for example, the tobacco maker sent Corporate Affairs reps to its food divisions to urge employees to write to their congressmen to oppose an increase in federal cigarette taxes. The "Talking Points" prepared for these agents offered samples of what kinds of resistance might be encountered and how best to deal with it:

Anti: "You people should pay for health care. Your cigarettes kill hundreds of thousands of people a year."

You: "We could debate tobacco issues all day. But that's not why I'm here. I'm here to tell you that if it's tobacco today, it will be pickles tomorrow. Did you know they tried a snack tax in California a couple of years ago?"

The company had earlier organized focus groups to find out what kinds of arguments would be most persuasive, identifying "slippery slope," "fairness," and "jobs" as the "most involving." So the argument to these makers of hot dogs and cookies was to go something like this: "Look, if they get cigarettes this year, they're going after beer and gasoline next, and then it will be everything else—baked goods, fast food, sports equipment, boats, anything they think you like enough that you'll keep using it, even if you have to pay an increased tax." The company also organized a "Beat Federal Excise Tax Week" (starting March 21, 1994), with letters mailed to each of Philip Morris's 150,000 employees urging them to act to defeat the tax. The company also shut down its Richmond plant to bus its entire staff to Washington, D.C., to meet with a congressional delegation and rally at the Capitol. Philip Morris used similar tactics to fight FDA regulation: in 1995, when the Clinton administration began making noises along these lines, Philip Morris mobilized its Oscar Mayer employees to write letters opposing any such move. Philip Morris's venture into foods thus had a political value over and above its economic worth.[26]

Marlboro's diversification was not achieved without a struggle, however. When William Farone was hired by the company in 1976 he had two principal duties: to develop "safer" cigarettes and to ease the company away from tobacco and into foods. As he tells the story, this was a time of titanic struggle within the firm, with two chief factions: "Hercules" versus "Atlas." Farone was on the Hercules side, believing cigarette making to be a kind of labor the company had to endure before emerging as a producer of some more socially acceptable product, like food. The Atlas faction, by contrast, held that cigarettes were a burden the company must bear forever, just as Atlas shouldered the earth. The Atlas faction had triumphed by the time Geoffrey C. Bible was named president and CEO in 1994; Bible retrenched the company and continued to deny all health effects from smoking, even as late as 1998. Altria—the friendly-sounding new name for Philip Morris as of 2003—spun off its Kraft shares in 2007, becoming once again a pure tobacco play.

SMOKELESS HOPES

Smokeless tobacco is another direction in which the industry has recently diversified, part of its ongoing hope for "reduced harm" products. Oral snuff, snus, and chewing tobacco have all been revived, principally because the companies now see this as one solution to the problem of secondhand smoke. The hope is also to co-brand with cigarettes, helping thereby to keep people smoking. (That may be one reason Marlboro Snus has been designed to deliver so little nicotine: the hope may be to supplement rather than supplant cigarette use.)[27] Global tobacco manufacturers have invested heavily in smokeless products, imagining these as a "safer" business bet given current threats to the cigarette enterprise. Reynolds in 2006 bought Conwood Sales, maker of Kodiak and Grizzly smokeless, for $3.5 billion. Philip Morris in 2007 test-marketed Marlboro Snus, a tobacco pouch that you basically suck on as you might a tea bag, swallowing whatever juices mix with your saliva. This so-called Swedish experience has become a bright hope for several of the transnationals, imagining that snus will prove more socially acceptable than cigarettes. And while it is probably true that gram per gram oral snuff won't kill as many people, this is by no means a benign indulgence.

Chewing tobacco has long been associated with cancers of the mouth and jaw. Baseball players are notoriously vulnerable, given their historic preference for a salivated plug bulging from inside the cheek. Chewing tobacco was banned from American collegiate sports in 1994, but the practice quietly continues, and Major League Baseball to this day has refused to take a stand against the drug. So in summer 2007, when Barry Bonds was creeping up on Hank Aaron's home run record, television cameras revealed the telltale circle in his back right pocket, the signature impression of the tobacco tin. It is unclear whether Bonds was paid for such a display, but it wouldn't be the first time an athlete has taken money to promote tobacco. Thousands of athletes have contracted cancers of the mouth, lips, and throat—Baseball Hall of Famer Tony Gwynn is one recent victim, following in the footsteps of Babe Ruth and numerous other baseball greats—and vivid pictures of such tumors can now be found on tobacco products in many parts of the world. And will appear in the United States before very long.

Some cigarette critics hope that smokeless will "reduce harm," but we don't really know what the long-term consequences might be. Sweden is held up as an example, but there is actually a huge variability in the constituents of chewing tobacco. In some parts of Africa, where oral snuff is widely used, smokeless tobacco is quite high in deadly nitrosamines. And in Sweden itself many health professionals are horrified that the "Swedish experience" is being used to promote this new form of drug use. Margaretha Haglund, head of tobacco prevention at Sweden's National Institute of Public Health, debunks the "myth" of using smokeless to quit smoking and notes that few of Sweden's former smokers—only about 5 percent—quit with the help of snus. While snus use itself has skyrocketed. Twenty-two percent of Swedish men use snus on a daily basis, up from about 9 percent in the mid-1970s. Swedish Match sells 250 million cans per year, and nearly 40 percent of Swedish users still smoke cigarettes. Only about a quarter of these are former smokers. Snus may well help some smokers quit, but it also seems to be promoting a kind of "dual use"—allowing cigarette users to get a nicotine fix where they are no longer allowed to smoke (on long airplane flights, for example). Snus and other new forms of "spitless" tobacco are perhaps best regarded as the flailing grasp of an industry thrown off-balance by successful campaigns to make offices, restaurants, bars, and an increasing variety of outdoor spaces smoke-free.[28]

The industry's overarching goal, of course, is to create and sustain addiction, which is also why other kinds of smokeless articles have been introduced in recent years—including flavored "dissolvable tobacco" in the form of Camel Strips, Sticks, and Orbs, which are meant to be sucked or chewed while still delivering a nicotine punch. Greg Connolly has commented on how the new cinnamon- and mint-flavored Camel Orbs look like Tic Tac candy and contain about a milligram of nicotine in a highly freebased form (pH 7.9). The danger of appealing to kids is not far-fetched, given the 13,705 reported cases of poisonings from tobacco products from 2006 to 2008, most of which (90 percent) involve children. Connolly in a recent interview with the *New York Times* described making nicotine look like candy as "recklessly playing with the health of children."[29] Of course the real purpose of Reynolds et al. may be just to tie up the new FDA with trivial pursuits while business goes on as usual in the big-killer cigarette market.

A LICENSE TO KILL?

Talk about "safer" cigarettes is often misinformed. We might as well talk about safer ways to inhale asbestos, or safer forms of drowning. The word *safer* itself is mischievous in this context, since talk of making something "safer" implies it is already "safe." (Think "safe," "safer," "safest.") Cigarettes could certainly be made less lethal, but there is always the chance that in doing so we end up causing more harm by delaying quitting—and encouraging starting. A *safe* cigarette is one that cannot be smoked, or one you leave unsmoked in the pack. Cigarettes are less deadly when fewer of them are smoked, however they are made. The industry has tried to make cigarettes that yield less smoke, and while some of these might well cause less death per cigarette—*ceteris paribus*—they have never been introduced coincident with any kind of plan to withdraw the more obviously deadly. Smokers are often given a "choice," but the industry's own choices remain invisible, as if sacrosanct. Which is why still today you can go out and buy Camels, Marlboros, 555s, Mild Sevens, or Panda or Chunghwa cigarettes that if smoked as intended by the manufacturers will increase your chances of contracting cancer by several thousand percent. Half of all regular smokers will die from the habit, and all will show evidence of pathology at autopsy. The industry seems never to have removed a product because of evidence it was killing people. It is hard to name another business with so little regard for its customers. Viewed from afar, one would almost think that cigarette makers have been granted a license to kill.

Globalizing Death

Tobacco exports should be expanded aggressively because Americans are smoking less.

DAN QUAYLE, VICE PRESIDENT OF THE UNITED STATES, 1990

We stand on the threshold of a global pandemic of tobacco-related diseases that is nothing short of colossal.

ALLAN BRANDT, HARVARD UNIVERSITY, 2007

Humans are naturally inquisitive, and it would probably be hard to find an animal, vegetable, or mineral that has not, at some time or another, been put to the inhalation or ingestion test. Tobacco has been helped along, however, by certain properties of the plant itself. The plant is weedily easy to grow, with a range now extending from the tropics into places like Germany or even Sweden and Canada. Also, the seeds are astonishingly small: thousands fit into a tablespoon, which helps explain how easily the herb was transported from South America and (later) Mesoamerica and North America. Francisco Hernández de Toledo brought living plants back to Spain in 1559, and it was not long before enterprising agriculturalists were growing it in North Africa. Tobacco arrived in the Philippines in 1575, in Russia in 1585, and in China in the late 1500s. India first saw tobacco in 1605, which is also about when Japan took up the habit. Tobacco was most often smoked in pipes and later in roll-your-own versions, flavored with lime (calcium oxide), cloves (especially in Indonesia), and sweeteners of various sorts.

The tobacco industry likes to dredge up such facts, to make of smoking a kind of venerable tradition. As if smokers today are doing what Americans and Europeans have been doing for centuries, or Native Americans for millennia. The fact, however, is that today's use of cigarettes is on an entirely different *scale* from anything in former times. Scale here is everything, and the long reach of the leaf in modern times is largely due to mechanization and, more recently, globalization. The net effect is the spread of tobacco death across the planet on a scale nearly unimaginable, a process hastened by the penetration of transnational corporations into markets previously inaccessible.

Consider that in the early years of the cigarette epidemic, circa 1900, Buck Duke's American Tobacco conglomerate produced more than 90 percent of the world's cigarettes, which at that time was only about four *billion* sticks. Consider also that today's global consumption is higher by a factor of more than a thousand: about six *trillion*. State-of-the-art cigarette-making machines have been installed in factories throughout the world, transforming a rich man's fashion into a poor man's addiction, albeit increasingly dual-gendered. Smoking has become an impoverishing luxury, the companion of benighted affluence. Decolonialism and economic progress following the Second World War are partly to blame, as are tax-thirsty governments, but global tobacco also represents a new kind of cardiopulmonary colonialism wreaking havoc on the world's vital organs. Americans and Europeans as recently as the 1940s were smoking nearly half the world's cigarettes, whereas today that fraction is down to around 10 percent. The big growth has come from places like India and China and nations formed from the breakup of the former Soviet empire, where affluence and aggressive free trade have opened the door to *laisser-fumer* carcinogenic consumerism.

CHINA AND INDIA

Smoking has grown especially fast in China, where about a third of the world's cigarettes are now smoked. The Communist Party leadership for many years encouraged smoking—the pragmatic pro-Western Deng Xiaoping was key here, with his stress on cigarettes as part of China's push for "modernity with Chinese characteristics." Tax revenues fuel the attraction: the Chinese government in 2008 received $31 billion from tobacco taxes, though cynics might wonder whether the Middle Kingdom has not just found a brutal way to end its time-honored tradition of filial piety. Tobacco kills mainly the elderly, and the government may even welcome this as a way to unburden itself of the unproductive aged and infirm. (Milos Zeman, prime minister of the Czech Republic, offered this callous calculus in 2001, claiming that tobacco use actually saved the state money by killing off the elderly.)[1] Health professionals have been largely powerless to stop the onslaught, and in the first decade of the new millennium nearly half of all Chinese physicians still smoke. And millions of farmers and traders make their living from the habit. Cigarette consumption peaked in the United States in 1981 but may not even yet have peaked in China.

The Chinese are used to smoking domestically produced cigarettes and as recently as the 1990s had nearly a thousand different brands available for purchase. That number is being consolidated, as the China National Tobacco Corporation prepares to compete with imports such as Marlboro, Camel, and BAT's 555 and JTI's Mild Seven. Prices range from under 50 cents for a pack of cheap peasant smokes to more than $18 for the classiest kowtow-to-your-boss Panda brand. Super luxury brands can go even higher—up to $35 for a pack. The Chinese state and economy depend on tobacco both for revenue and for agricultural stability, which is why we should not be surprised to find a doubt-mongering apparatus similar to our notorious "Tobacco Institutes" of Australia, New Zealand, Hong Kong, Taiwan, and the United States. The Yunnan Tobacco Institute in Yuxi, south of Kunming, is the nerve center of Chinese tobacco propaganda, where vested interests combine with cowardice to keep the horrors of smoking hidden.

Foreign manufacturers, though, have long been trying hard to gain a foothold in the Middle Kingdom. Prior even to the twentieth century James "Buck" Duke opened a world map and tapped his finger on China to announce, as the story is told, "Here is where we'll build our kingdom." Multinationals have salivated over the prospects ever since: Robert Fletcher of Rothmans in 1992 likened the Chinese market to thinking about "the limits of space," while Philip Morris characterized China as "the most important feature on the landscape." Yet another Philip Morris Asia official has gushed, "In every respect, China confounds the imagination."[2] There is no mystery here, though. The global transnationals are busily having their way with poorer parts of the world as they once did with the rich. Philip Morris has recently struck a deal with China, acquiring rights to market Marlboros in the country in exchange for help with popularizing Chinese brands in other parts of the world. China could well become a global cigarette superpower, even as foreign brands gain entry.

India's tobaccosis has risen almost as fast as China's. This is all the more remarkable since it was not so long ago that few manufactured cigarettes were smoked on the subcontinent. Smoking has been encouraged both by economic growth and transnational penetration, with the film industry lending a hand as well. Bollywood films were chock full of cigarette implants until 2005, when a policy was adopted barring depictions of smoking on films (and television). According to a WHO-financed study released just prior to the ban, 89 percent of Hindi-language films depicted smoking, with two-thirds showing the lead character in the act and nearly half showing specific brands. A surprisingly large percentage of Indian films—more than a quarter—belittled or mocked people worrying about tobacco harms. India's ban was reversed by the Delhi High Court in 2009, following protests about limitations on artistic freedom. One director, Mahesh Bhatt, complained early on that the problem was not so much films as reality and that "if the government has the courage, it should ban smoking in real life."[3]

Tobacco kills nearly a million Indians every year, a number that will grow as exposures from the 1980s, 1990s, and 2000s take their toll. Cigarette consumption has probably not yet peaked in South Asia, however, since more people still smoke hand-rolled "bidis" than manufactured "white" cigarettes. Bidis are cheaper and more often made by hand—though even that is changing. Significant also is that while bidis account for about 80 percent of Indian smokes, "white" cigarettes account for 90 percent of the country's total tobacco tax revenue.[4] Unusual also in the Indian situation is the fact that tobacco here kills far more people via *tuberculosis* than via lung cancer. Epidemiologists have shown that about three quarters of all people dying from tuberculosis in India would not have died from that disease if they had not smoked. The lung irritation seems to create a fertile ground for infection by the tubercle bacillus and may weaken the body in other ways, making it more vulnerable.[5] (Smoke is known to disable macrophages and weaken the immune system, for example.) Tobacco is a "communicable" disease, in more ways than one.

India is also unusual in the diversity of ways in which tobacco is consumed. Cigarettes and bidis have been mentioned, but Indians also use a toxic cigarlike smoke known as a *cheroot* and a variety of local oral chews such as *paan* and *gutka,* which are typically betel leaf wrapped around a mixture of tobacco, the alkaloid-rich areca nut, and spices of various sorts with slaked lime added as a freebasing agent (to promote nicotine absorption). Pound for pound "white cigarettes" are still a minor part of total tobacco consumption, but that is changing, as wealth generates Western imitations. Three quarters of the cigarette market is controlled by the Indian Tobacco Company, a subsidiary of BAT, with the most popular brands being Bristol, Scissors, Gold Flake, and Capstan. A Philip Morris subsidiary is the second largest manufacturer, with Vazir Sultan Tobacco third in the rankings.

Indonesia doesn't get a lot of attention in the global tobacco wars, but the island chain nation has become a virtual playground for the cigarette transnationals. A third of the country's 250 million people are regular smokers, especially of clove-flavored cigarettes known as *kreteks,* so called for the crackling sound they make when the stems inside are smoked. The country is heavily dependent on cigarettes, with an estimated 8 million to 10 million people making a living bringing them to market, including farmers who grow the leaf and/or the cloves. Advertising is technically prohibited, but the ban is widely ignored, and visitors to Jakarta will find virtually every lamppost plastered with tobacco ads. Modernization of production is ongoing, with manufacturers claiming even to be using "carbon capture" to produce the dry ice used in making expanded tobacco—via the so-called DIET process.[6]

GLOBAL CONSPIRACIES

There are of course parts of the world where tobacco has never penetrated. Smoking is extremely rare in the Nevis half of the island nation of St. Kitts-Nevis, for example, and is not very common in the landlocked mountain redoubt of Bhutan, where public smoking and the sale of tobacco has been banned since 2004. Smoking has also been rare in some of the poorer parts of Africa and South America. Nigeria in 2007 had one of the world's lowest smoking rates: according to a recent

Gallup poll only 6 percent of Nigerians answered yes when asked, "Did you smoke yesterday, or not?" Highest was Cuba, where 40 percent of the population answered yes to the same question. Other surveys show smoking rates even higher among certain subpopulations: more than three quarters of all Yemeni men smoke, for example, as do 71 percent of all women in the Cook Islands and nearly two-thirds of all male Albanian third-year medical students.[7]

Part of the problem is that the industry has been organizing as a global force far longer—and with much deeper pockets—than public health advocates. Buck Duke had already hoped for a global monopoly in the nineteenth century, and his British American offshoot quickly captured much of the world market. I've mentioned the denialist efforts of Germany's Academia Nicotiana Internationalis and Bremen's International Association for Scientific Tobacco Research—plus of course the doubt-mongering apparatus of Hill & Knowlton and the American tobacco magnates—but similar efforts have been launched in other parts of the world. Denialist science has been purveyed by many different organs, from Germany's Verband der Cigarettenindustrie to the Paris-based Center for Cooperation in Scientific Research Relative to Tobacco (CORESTA), Britain's Tobacco Manufacturers' Standing Committee (today the Tobacco Manufacturers' Association),[8] and the myriad "Tobacco Institutes" established throughout the world. Plus of course the many corporate law firms paid extraordinary sums to defend the industry in court. Tobacco has paid more for its legal defense than any other industry in history, with the possible exception of asbestos.

Global tobacco collaborations date from early in the twentieth century, but formal ties were strengthened in the 1970s, principally to deal with the new threat from evidence that secondhand smoke was causing death and disease. Evidence along these lines had been building since the 1960s, when steps began to be taken to eliminate smoking from airlines, hospitals, restaurants, and the "clean rooms" where computers were expected to operate. Smoke fouled magnetic tapes, prompting operators to ask, if smoke can harm computers, might it not also be harming people? Most such measures were mild or even laughable by today's standards: separate smoking sections in restaurants did little to reduce exposures, for example, and in some instances made a mockery of physics (see Figure 35). I'll never forget riding in buses with one side reserved for smoking while the other was supposed to be smoke-free.

The tobacco industry saw what was coming and recognized a potential catastrophe (for profits) if the problem was not deftly managed. In the summer of 1976 the Philip Morris Chairman's Conference in Hot Springs, Virginia, came to the "unanimous agreement" that limitations on public smoking posed "a more serious threat to the Industry's future than any other." In Australia that same year W. D. & H. O. Wills listed two "serious threats" to the industry: (1) "the threat that smoking could become anti-social and unfashionable" and (2) "passive smoking." For cigarette makers in Australia, as in other parts of the world, the question now became, "what positive action should be taken to change the smoking and health question from one that already has been decided, to one that is open to debate?"[9]

Secondhand smoke denialism grew from these concerns over social acceptability, with the companies realizing that the scale of the problem demanded new kinds of collaboration. Efforts along these lines were quickly globalized; groups such as the International ETS Management Committee (IEMC), the Confederation of European Community Cigarette Manufacturers (CECCM), Britain's Tobacco Advisory Council (TAC), and the International Committee on Smoking Issues (ICOSI) all had a hand in the action. Different groups were assigned different tasks, so whereas the CECCM coordinated the European response, the IEMC was supposed to handle the rest of the world. As one ICOSI agent put it in 1979, the goal was to "unite with common targets and common approaches" against threats from international cancer agencies and movements to restrict indoor smoking. Coordination with the United States was typically through the Tobacco Institute, though law firms were also hired to craft strategy and to sanitize documents. One key concern was to ensure that decisions taken abroad wouldn't jeopardize the American legal situation. The fear was also of a domino effect—that legal setbacks in the United States could harm the global industry—which is why Lovell, White & Durrant in London and Chadbourne & Parke in New York were hired to make sure documents produced by the industry's trade associations would not create legal embarrassments. Shook, Hardy and Bacon had long been doing similar work. A great deal of consideration was given to "the legal position in the United States," with the fear again being that actions taken abroad could weaken the American litigation front.[10]

Operation Berkshire was the code name given to one such collaboration, launched on December 3, 1976, when Tony Garrett, chairman of Imperial Tobacco of London, asked Hugh Cullman at Philip Morris International for help in crafting a "defensive smoking and health strategy." The goal, among other things, was to ensure that "no concessions beyond a certain point" would be made on smoking and health by the industry, by which was meant not just Philip Morris and BAT but also Reynolds, Reemtsma, and Rothmans International, all of whom had already signed on to the plan. Garrett was worried that uncoordinated action would allow the companies in different parts of the world to be "picked off one by one"—meaning effective public health controls on smoking—with the resulting "domino effect" having an impact on "all of us." Cullman agreed, and the group began meeting at Shockerwick House, a training center owned by W. D. & H. O. Wills near Bath, England, in summer 1977. The premise for these meetings had been outlined in a precirculated "Position Paper," wherein we find the companies refusing to accept "a causal relationship between smoking and various diseases." The Position Paper—also referred to as the "charter" for a new International Committee on Smoking Issues (ICOSI)—postulated that "the issue of causation remains controversial and unresolved" and that further research was needed. Crucial also was the need for the industry to speak "with one voice." The goal was to mount a "Smoker Reassurance" program to counter "the increasing social unacceptability of smoking."[11]

Berkshire's principal outcome was the formation of ICOSI, a body later reorganized as the International Tobacco Information Center (INFOTAB) and then again (in 1992) as the International Tobacco Documentation Center (TDC). ICOSI members in these early years included Philip Morris, BATCo, Imperial Tobacco, Gallaher, Reynolds, Reemtsma, and Carreras Rothmans but by 1984 would encompass sixty-nine members operating in fifty-seven countries. Separate working groups were established, with Reynolds taking the lead for "Social Acceptability," BAT for "Smoking Behavior," and Imperial for "Medical Research." The overarching goal was to meet "discreetly to develop a defensive smoking and health strategy," gathering information to assess threats but also taking steps to develop countermeasures. The focus was to be transnational and proactive, with "action kits" distributed to help members challenge regional health initiatives. As BATCo put it, the goal was to conduct "defensive research aimed at throwing up a smoke screen and to throw doubts on smoking research findings which show smoke causes deceases [sic]." Initiatives along these lines were made possible by the enormous political power of the companies: W. D. & H. O. Wills in 1976, for example, bragged about the Australian industry having achieved "a high degree of access to government on the relevant issues and a considerable ability to delay and/or amend proposed restrictive legislation and regulation."[12]

Power of this sort was made possible by elaborate and well-funded alliances in academia, the media, and government—but also by well-heeled corporate lawyers, who in many respects acted as an arm of the industry itself. In 1978, for example, representatives from Britain's Tobacco Advisory Council met with Philip Morris, Reynolds, Shook, Hardy, and Covington & Burling to coordinate denialist efforts, especially in the secondhand smoke realm. Covington & Burling was also key to the success of Operation Whitecoat, a Philip Morris–led effort to restore social acceptability by developing European networks of experts—"whitecoats"—to help produce industry-friendly science and policy. Covington & Burling's London office helped coordinate this effort, with the goal being to "resist and roll back smoking restrictions" and "restore smoker confidence." Whitecoat operatives collaborated with the Center for Indoor Air Research in the United States and INFOTAB in Europe, working to insinuate doubt and misinformation globally, including in Latin America. In the Latin Project, for example, Covington & Burling organized a team of medical experts to publicize doubts about secondhand smoke hazards, drawing up and vetting lists of Argentine experts for this purpose. The country's Tobacco Industry Chamber established an entire department titled "The Controversy," distributing leaflets and reports for the press to challenge evidence of hazards.[13]

A NEW OPIUM WAR?

Much of the industry's global muscle in recent years has gone into making sure that tobacco companies have free access to markets in poorer parts of the world, seen as the last great opportunity for expansion now that smoking rates are falling in virtually all of the richer parts of the globe. The goal has been to guarantee that tobacco remains a freely traded "good," supported by governments desperate for the revenue and citizens eager to emulate the West.

One method used by the transnationals has been to weaken state monopolies. Tobacco has long been an enterprise of the state in many parts of the world and still today is monopolized in Thailand, Vietnam, China, Iran, Romania, and a dozen other nations. Many of these monopolies have come under pressure to open their markets to foreign competition, and global trade treaties such as the General Agreement on Tariffs and Trade (GATT) and its successor, the World Trade Organization, have made it easier for the transnationals to gain access. Allan Brandt in his *Cigarette Century* shows how the White House under Ronald Reagan launched a formidable campaign to force Japan, South Korean, Taiwan, and Thailand to open their markets, using the office of the U.S. Trade Representative. Tobacco companies managed to convince the head of that office, Clayton Yeutter, that they were victims of unfair trade practices and in need of assistance; heavy political artillery was then brought to the negotiations, with no consideration given to how breaking into such markets might affect public health. Free trade carried a big stick, and Japan, South Korea, Thailand, and Taiwan were all quickly forced to eliminate their import tariffs, causing cigarette consumption in those countries to skyrocket. U.S. cigarette exports climbed by over 600 percent in the years following these agreements, and in Japan alone the proportion of women smoking more than doubled from 1987 to 1991. Clayton Yeutter himself characterized this as "a marvelous success" and was promoted to secretary of agriculture in the first Bush administration (in 1989) and joined the board of British American Tobacco (in 1991).[14]

Hundreds of thousands of deaths can be blamed on this bullied liberalization of trade. Judith Mackay in Hong Kong as early as 1987 was talking in terms of "neo-imperialism" and "a new opium war,"[15] and even the normally restrained British journal *Lancet* decried a "new slave trade." Transnational tobacco giants ever since have sold cigarettes in poorer parts of the world using a double standard, employing tactics no longer allowed elsewhere. Attractive young females are employed to offer free samples, for example, and marketing to the young is often blatant, via pop music and sports and the other tricks from decades of experience in the "developed" world. Cigarettes are sometimes even sold without warning labels. The only positive outcome has been the outrage of health authorities, notably those in the countries victimized by the forcible liberalization of trade. In Thailand, for example, which had put up some of the strongest resistance, health authorities responded by banning advertising, increasing education on health risks, and placing graphic warnings on cigarette packs. And the World Health Organization began a series of moves that would culminate in the passage of the Framework Convention on Tobacco Control, the world's first public health treaty, in 2003.

The Framework Convention is no panacea, but it does call for graphic warnings along with increased taxation, bans on print and media advertising (including sponsorships), bans on vending machines, exclusion of industry participation in the making of tobacco policy, and bans on representing cigarettes as "light," "mild," or otherwise healthful. As of 2011 a total of 169 nations had signed the treaty, with more even than this ratifying it. (Ratification designates a stronger level of commitment, implying that the party is bound under international law to the provisions of the treaty.) Russia ratified in 2008, leaving only the United States among the major powers not to have done so. The Bush administration was never friendly toward global efforts to limit tobacco use; indeed American hostility to the FCTC was so vehement that the country was asked at one point to remove itself from deliberations. Governments from Britain, Germany, Japan, and China also worked to water down the treaty, which is one reason its ratification is sometimes regarded as a victory of the developing world over the richer tobacco-manufacturing nations.

It remains to be seen how effective the FCTC will be in curbing global tobacco use. There are no real provisions for enforcement, and some nations may implement only the bare minimum of recommended policies or give only lip service to the treaty. There is also the problem that tobacco control is viewed principally in terms of *curtailing demand,* ignoring opportunities in the form of mandating changes in the production process. The FCTC has tended to emphasize demand-side solutions, assuming free and unimpeded access to cigarettes. Protocols are being drafted for product regulation, but there is a risk that these may be limited to adjustments in the balance of specific smoke constituents rather than more effective—and simpler—interventions that could dramatically reduce the harm or addictiveness of smoking (mandating the removal of nicotine from tobacco products, for example). The treaty has built-in mechanisms for improvement, however, and we are likely to see its importance grow as new protocols are added and pressures increase to strengthen global public health and environmental sustainability.

Policy-wise, we can also see a more hopeful future emerging as individual countries or parts of countries push the envelope in specific directions—as Canada, Brazil, and Thailand have done with graphic warnings, or India did with its (short-lived) ban on smoking in films, or Australia has recently done with its plain package mandate. Bhutan has a ban on cigarette sales, and in parts of the United States we now have bans on smoking on beaches and in parks and multi-unit housing. Californians, New Yorkers, and residents of Massachusetts have made some quite remarkable strides in this area, but we shouldn't be fooled: Americans still smoke more than 300 billion cigarettes per year, and even Californians smoke nearly the same as the global average—and only slightly less than the French on a per capita basis.

Europeans have surprised many Americans by their willingness to take strong action: Ireland, France, and Italy have all banned smoking in all restaurants, workplaces, and public buildings—though outdoor urban air remains quite smoky in many of those countries. Cigarette smoke remains the deadliest form of pollution in most European cities, where outdoor cafés are routinely bathed in radioactive, toxin-laden smoke—thanks to blind-eyed ignorance, smokers' indifference, and the industry's political powers. The European Union is seeking to establish EU-wide tobacco policies, though we have also seen clever efforts to circumvent the bans that already exist—as in Bavaria, where smokers at one point started a "church" with "parishioners" allowed to smoke while in "services" (i.e., a pub, bar, or restaurant). Minnesotans were equally creative when an attempt was made to evade smoking bans by turning bars into "theaters" and all patrons into "actors"—since actors in a play were exempt. These are comical sideshows, of course, but we can certainly expect such shenanigans in the future—and far more serious resistance from the industry—given the grip of addiction and the global financial empires at stake.

. . .

So where does the ethical circle close? How far can we extend blame for these many millions of deaths? Of course the cigarette makers, but what about the companies making the paper or flavorings or freebasing agents for cigarettes? What about the public relations and marketing firms or those tattoo artists who help with pack design? What about the agricultural research experts helping to grow the leaf, or the farmers planting the seeds, or the journalists dropping the ball? Or those many scholars who provide cover for the industry? What about the law firms that protect Big Tobacco in court, or the filmmakers who write smoking into scripts, or governments that turn a blind eye, or the libertarians who justify it in the name of personal freedom? Or the smokers who keep the companies in business with their cash? Where does the ethical circle close, and what can and must be done?

What Must Be Done

In searching for the obscure, do not overlook the obvious.
HIPPOCRATES

Our goal should be to *prevent* tobacco death. Smoking already kills more people than all the world's infectious diseases combined: the number has now reached six million per year and will stay high for decades even if everyone stops smoking tomorrow. The industry wants us to think about tobacco as a "solved problem" or an issue from the distant past, but the reality is that most tobacco death lies in the future. Only about 100 million people died from smoking in the twentieth century, whereas we in our century can expect a billion tobacco deaths if we continue on our present course. A public health catastrophe is unfolding, and even keeping the final death toll under 300 or 400 million—which is certainly possible—would be a great success. None of these deaths are necessary: tobacco mortality is easily preventable. And the solutions are actually fairly simple.

It is no longer fashionable to talk about "magic bullets" in medicine, but here we really do have a magic bullet, requiring (in theory) nothing more than the stroke of a pen. Ninety-plus percent of all tobacco death can be prevented *by banning the sale and manufacture of cigarettes.* Even short of a clean sweep, however, there are many smaller steps that could help reduce tobacco mortality. Which is not to say that the political obstacles are not formidable; we live in a world of powerful vested interests. So it is useful to have short-term goals as well as higher aspirations.

IMPERATIVES

Here first are ten relatively obvious solutions, followed by ten that are somewhat less obvious, including proposals for redesigning the cigarette itself.

1. *Ban smoking in all indoor public places and in outdoor spaces where people congregate.* Public parks and beaches should be completely smoke-free, and smoking should not be allowed on streets or sidewalks of densely populated urban areas. Smoking should also be barred from apartment complexes and any other form of housing where fumes can move from one domestic unit to another. People don't seem to realize that in crowded urban spaces—outdoor restaurants, for example—smoke from other people's cigarettes can generate toxic exposures comparable to those from indoor smoking.

2. *Increase cigarette taxes.* Tobacco has a price elasticity of about .4, which means that for every 10 percent rise in the price of a pack we can expect a 4 percent fall in consumption. Some will say this unfairly taxes the poor, which is why taxes should be combined with subsidies for smoking cessation services, including nicotine replacement therapies and non-drug services (such as hypnotherapy) made available free of charge. Taxes are already high in many parts of Europe, and in some places we have $12 and even $15 minimum-price packs. But twice this amount is not impossible. Americans can still buy cigarettes for only $4 or $5 per pack, and in tax-free zones (military commissaries or duty-free shops, for example) they can be even cheaper. All loopholes of this sort should be closed, and taxes should be collected *at the point of production*—not at the retail counter—to prevent smuggling and illegal sales via the Internet. New tax revenues should be used for tobacco control and cessation, to break the dependence of governments on the continued sale of cigarettes. Pressure should also be exerted on countries with low tax rates to raise those rates to prevent buttlegging and organized crime more generally.

3. *Ban all cigarette marketing, including all advertising and promotion.* Bans in certain media (magazines, billboards, television, etc.) are already in place in many countries; these should be extended to cover *all* marketing and promotion, including direct mail, movie plugs, viral marketing, brand stretching ("Marlboro gear"), cultural sponsorships, coupons, Internet offers, and advertising at retail point of sale. Package design is an effective and ubiquitous form of advertising, and no cigarettes should be sold in anything but a plain white wrapper accompanied by a graphic warning. Advertising bans should cover not just the product but also the name of the company making that product, and manufacturers should be barred from sponsoring sports, music, or any other cultural event, including philanthropy designed to create an illusion of "corporate social responsibility."

4. *Make warning labels on cigarette packs large, graphic, and disgusting.* Tobacco packs are miniature mobile ads and the most common way smokers encounter their cigarettes. Psychologists have studied warning labels and found that certain kinds are more effective than others; some of the most graphic are power-

ful enough to make people return their cigarettes, and different images will of course resonate differently in different cultures. In Canada, for example, the most provocative have been images of a diseased mouth and teeth, whereas in Brazil the images of premature babies have been quite off-putting. Research should also continue to determine which images are most likely to discourage smoking.

5. *Bar the sale of cigarettes everywhere except for special state-licensed outlets.* In the United States, as in most other parts of the world, it is far too easy to find and purchase cigarettes. Several states allow hard liquor be sold only in state-sanctioned stores, and the same should be true for cigarettes. In the meantime, cigarettes should be removed from "impulse" purchase areas at checkout counters and made available only by request from a sequestered source. And to help prevent youth access, cigarettes should be sold only by the carton and not within one thousand feet of a school. Vending machines should also be banned, along with distribution of free samples and brand-themed merchandise.

6. *Place an R rating on all feature films depicting smoking.* Exposure to smoking in movies causes young people to take up the habit; indeed there is no more effective form of advertising. Smoking in Hollywood films grew substantially in the 1990s, and by 2002 three quarters of all American films portrayed cigarette use. An R rating for all films showing smoking would help reduce tobacco use, since most of the profits in this business come from youth-audience films. Hollywood movies have a global reach, which means that the impact of such a rating would extend beyond the United States. It would help to denormalize smoking, which in most parts of the world is still regarded as rather like drinking coffee or eating a bar of chocolate. Present-day tobacco brands should never be shown in general-audience feature films, and producers of films displaying cigarette use should certify that they have not accepted money or goods from a tobacco company or its agents. Directors would still be free to include smoking, just as they are free to include nudity or foul language; they would just have to accept a restricted audience.

7. *Stop all tobacco subsidies and supports.* Governments throughout the world encourage the planting and cultivation of tobacco, treating it as an ordinary agricultural commodity like corn, beans, or rice. Why should farmers be encouraged to grow the world's deadliest crop? Tobacco has benefited from state-sanctioned protectionism, and what is needed are incentives for crop substitution. Global free-trade agreements should also not treat tobacco as an ordinary commodity but rather as the product of a rogue agricultural enterprise—an economic "bad" and not an economic "good." Trade in tobacco should be treated more like the trade in weapons, which is tightly controlled and falls outside the governance of global trade agreements.

8. *Increase funding for tobacco prevention and cessation* to a level commensurate with the harms caused. Nowhere in the world is tobacco prevention—including smoking cessation—funded on a scale appropriate to the magnitude of its medical cost. In Sweden tobacco prevention receives only a mere 0.003 percent of the health care budget, even though treatment of diseases caused by tobacco consumes more than 8 percent of the nation's health care costs. In China there are perhaps fifteen people working full-time on tobacco prevention while more than 15 *million* work to get people to smoke as much as possible. The allocation is off by several orders of magnitude. Tobacco mortality is easily preventable, and tobacco control can save a nation money by reducing medical costs. Tobacco prevention also brings with it side benefits in the form of reduced harm to the environment, savings on costs from fires, and savings for individuals freed from the financial burdens of lifelong addiction. Private philanthropists (notably Mayor Michael Bloomberg of New York and Bill and Melinda Gates) are funding creative work, but governments also need to take more responsibility. Cessation promotion should be part of this: toll-free numbers (e.g., 800-QUIT NOW) should be established to direct people to cessation services, and research into creative new means of cessation should be funded.

9. *Teach tobacco prevention early, graphically, and creatively.* The lesson is not just that cigarettes kill but also that the industry uses devious means to hook you. Crucial is to instill a sense of informed discontent: children should begin learning about tobacco mendacity ("Look how they are trying to trick you!") in their third or fourth year in school, which is also about when they should learn that humans share a common ancestor with apes and have duties to safeguard biodiversity. Megafacts of this sort are empowering and must be taught to help boost civic literacy and environmental responsibility. Children should be taught that cigarettes contain a menagerie of poisons, and contests should be sponsored to encourage kids to develop their own ideas on how tobacco impacts life and our ecosphere—and what should be done about it. Prizes should be large and numerous, with rewards going to imaginative insights and creative presentation. The rhetoric in any successful campaign must avoid paternalism and should strive to recapture high ground values of life, liberty, and the pursuit of happiness. The struggle, after all, is not about health versus choice, or purity versus freedom, or parents versus teens, or the righteous versus the weak, but rather *a useless polluter versus the rest of us.*

10. *Listen to the voices of smokers.* Half of all smokers will die from their habit, and we need to know more about what *they* think should be done, especially those who have contracted diseases from smoking. What do they advise? They are on the front lines, and their voices must be heard.

LESS OBVIOUS IMPERATIVES

And now for a series of less obvious imperatives, most of which involve imaginative cigarette redesign or governance of production.

11. *Make cigarettes uninhalable by raising smoke pH.* Cigarettes have been
    designed to create and sustain addiction, but they could easily be redesigned
    to be far less deadly—and not at all addictive. Cigarettes would be far less
    lethal, for example, if the pH of cigarette smoke were restored to levels
    prevailing prior to the invention of flue-curing. Flue-curing lowered the pH
    of cigarette smoke, allowing it to be inhaled; this fatal design flaw has spread
    throughout the world, part of efforts to make cigarettes ever "milder." Ciga-
    rette smoke pH is easily manipulated, and no cigarette should be sold that
    delivers smoke with a pH less than 8. By returning smoke pH back to where it
    was prior to the nineteenth century cigarettes would no longer be inhaled, and
    most of the lung cancer hazard would vanish. Much of the appeal of smoking
    would also disappear, especially for "starters." A century of morbid cigarette
    engineering would be reversed and millions of lives saved. Care must also be
    taken, however, to ensure that *cigars* are not redesigned to become low-pH
    inhalable "big cigarettes." FDA authority should therefore be extended to
    cover *all* tobacco products, to make sure that new design mandates for
    cigarettes are not circumvented by some other form of nicotine delivery.

12. *Reduce the nicotine content of cigarettes.* Nicotine is the sine qua non of all
    tobacco addiction. And if we can take safrole out of root beer and lead out
    of paint and asbestos out of insulation, then surely we can take nicotine out
    of cigarettes. This is not hard from a manufacturing point of view—nicotine-
    free cigarettes have been available since the nineteenth century—and few
    people will continue to smoke without this deadly hooker. The new FDA in
    the U.S. is barred from eliminating nicotine entirely, but nothing prevents it
    from establishing a maximum of, say, 0.5 or even 0.4 milligrams per ciga-
    rette, reduced from present values of about 10 mg. (Here again we are talking
    about total nicotine in the cigarette, *not* smoke delivery; see the box on page
    380.) This would still allow people to smoke for "taste" and whatever pleasure
    comes from fondling the cigarette or gazing at its smoke; cigarettes with
    dramatically reduced nicotine in the rod, however, would no longer have
    the power to create and sustain addiction.

13. *Tax or ban the machines.* We often hear about the importance of *cessation
    of consumption* but rarely about the value of *cessation of production.* Three
    or four companies dominate the world's cigarette-making-machine business,
    and high taxes should be levied on any factory wanting to make or sell such
    machines, or any company wanting to import them. Global cigarette-
    machine manufacturing is dominated by the Hauni corporation in Ham-

burg, Arenco-Decouflé in Paris, G.D (Generate Differences) in Bologna, and Molins in London. The Hauni company is the largest, but Italy's G.D offers stiff competition. Hauni's and G.D's machines are the deadliest in all of human history, cranking out twenty thousand cigarettes per minute, nearly 10 million per eight-hour shift. And since one person dies for every million cigarettes smoked, this means each of these machines causes the death of ten people per eight-hour shift. Taxing or banning these machines would be an excellent way to lower tobacco mortality. Manufacturers would pass these higher production costs on to consumers, but taxation would also create an incentive to switch to less deadly products. Tobacco control advocates have ignored this crucial link in the chain of causes leading to cigarette death, but the fact is that manufacturers also have choices, much as they would like us to think they do not. Caveat emptor is not enough; we should not place all the burden of fateful "choice" on smokers. We have to go to the root of the problem and stop the machines: *caveat fabricator!*

14. *Put an end to research sponsored by the tobacco industry at all colleges and universities.* The companies have long sponsored research to boost their credibility, using the good name of Stanford, Harvard, or the University of California to claim, in essence, "How can we be so bad if such fine institutions are willing to work with us?" The companies use these sponsorships to cultivate experts and to twist the substance of science in their favor. Ending such collaborations would improve research integrity and help scholars who hold unpopular opinions repudiate charges of being "hacks" for the industry. If you really think nicotine-coated stents might help prevent heart attacks, then stop taking tobacco money, and people might actually believe you! If you really want to show that pilots fly better under the influence of nicotine, then do this research with untainted funds, and you won't be accused of selling your soul. Barring cigarette sponsorship is crucial for both academic freedom and scholarly integrity.

15. *Sue the racketeers!* Litigation can be an effective means to limit the power of the industry, and the cost of successful suits will be passed on to consumers in the form of higher prices—which means that litigation functions more or less as a (rather inefficient) cigarette tax. Few countries take advantage of this opportunity; most of the world's litigation has taken place in the Americas and, to a lesser extent, Australia and Great Britain. Japan has had only one small trial, and there are a scattered few elsewhere. Litigation can help force documents into the open, revealing the scope of the industry's chicanery. This can then be used as a springboard to further health advocacy and disease prevention.

16. *Establish a single-payer national health care system offering universal coverage.* Some countries won't need this advice, since they already have such systems in place. The United States is virtually alone among the richer nations of the

world in having no single-payer medical system. The only good to have come from this is that some powerful insurance companies and governments have been led to sue the industry, hoping to recover some of the financial costs of smoking. Establishing a national health service would force governments to shoulder some of this burden and help bring to light the social and human costs of cigarette complacency. Governments are more likely to take serious steps against tobacco when they realize that the cost of treating cigarette maladies exceeds the benefits generated through cigarette taxes.

17. *Recognize tobacco as a significant source of toxic pollution and environmental destruction.* Tobacco manufacturing is costly from an environmental point of view: 23 million pounds of pesticides are applied to tobacco every year in the United States alone, for example, and far more globally. This has environmental consequences but is also a waste from the point of view of scarce global resources. Millions of people make their living growing and selling the golden leaf, and substantial planetary resources are squandered in the process. Tobacco cultivation is also a significant cause of deforestation. Old growth forests continue to be razed to establish fields for planting tobacco and wood for fuel for curing. Every year, an old growth forest the size of twenty Manhattans is cleared to bring new tobacco fields into cultivation. Massive quantities of fossil fuels are consumed during the growing, manufacture, and transport of tobacco, all of which contributes to greenhouse emissions and the global climate crisis.

18. *Be creative in the language we use.* We hear lots of talk about "tobacco control" but not enough about "tobacco prevention" and "prevention of tobacco death." And suffering. Control talk is a bit defensive and has a regulatory ring out of synch with the magnitude of the catastrophe. Control talk implies a certain accommodation or collaborative tolerance, which is why we don't talk about "asbestos control" or control of lead in children's toys. We can't stop floods, which is why we have "flood control." And it is an oxymoron to talk about socially responsible cigarette manufacturing; we might as well talk about socially responsible traffic accidents or the proper way to drive while drunk. The industry has captured much of the rhetorical high ground here, denigrating talk of "bans" or "prohibition" as beyond the pale. We need to recapture this rhetorical advantage and broaden how we envision smoke-free futures. The industry presents itself as the natural ally of liberty, romance, and the good life lived to its fullest—values most of us would hold higher even than health or longevity.[1] The public health community needs to learn that these "higher values" must be embraced if we are to stop cigarette suffering. We also need to learn to call a spade a spade, even if that means talk of killer machines, toxic polluters, world-class liars, cancer mongers, drug lords, child abusers, pulmonary criminals, death dealers, RICO

racketeers, and so forth. The so-called vilification clause of the Master Settlement Agreement's Public Education Fund (administered by the American Legacy Foundation) bars any use of such monies "for any personal attack on, or vilification of, any person," but the rest of us should resist the industry's rhetorical bullying and sleight of hand.

19. *Expose cigarettes through film and fine arts.* The California State Tobacco Control Program and the American Legacy Foundation's Truth Campaign have done a great deal to dramatize the duplicity of the industry and the ravages of smoking. Filmmakers and journalists as a whole, however, have done little to capture and dramatize this catastrophe. We need movies on the killer machines of Hamburg and Bologna and on how Big Tobacco's denialist tricks were adopted and used by deniers of global warming. We need animated renderings of how tobacco attacks the heart and nicotine rewires the brain; and we need hard-hitting exposés of how transnationals penetrate local cultures. We need graphic public art treating the corruption of science and tobacco's threat to the environment—including contributions to global warming. And Hollywood needs to switch sides.

20. *Expand our imagination of what is possible!* This is the imperative from which all others should follow. Nothing that is good, true, or beautiful is ever achieved without a measure of creative fantasy. If phasing out tobacco seems out of reach, this is only because our imaginations are impoverished. Recall that people once found it hard to imagine courtrooms without spittoons, or television without tobacco ads, or smoke-free restaurants, but who now regrets those decisions? The industry fought hard to keep smoking on planes and in elevators, but who now feels this as a loss of human freedom? The industry fought hard against warning labels and bans on vending machines and sports sponsorships; all were denounced as the death of liberty, but who now would bring those back? Who now misses being able to light up on a crowded bus or train? Surveys show that even smokers appreciate smoke-free settings, since it gives them an incentive to quit.

THE SPECTER OF PROHIBITION

There is one last recommendation I shall make, which in the final analysis trumps all the others: *The sale and manufacture of cigarettes must be banned.* This is the simplest way to approach disease prevention and would obviate the need for most other solutions commonly proposed. It is remarkable how seldom this simple solution is entertained. How and why did the idea of a comprehensive ban come to be so far outside our ordinary imagination? Why does the end of cigarettes appear so unthinkable? Why do we assume that cigarettes, like the poor of biblical lore, will always be with us?

The short answer of course is the power of the industry, which acts as a virtual state within a state to influence policy and what we imagine to be possible. (Global revenues for Altria in 2009 were $25 billion, which makes the makers of Marlboro cigarettes richer than half the nations of the world.) Governments also fear losing the tax revenues that flow from cigarettes, and there are fears that smokers will revolt or smugglers run rampant. There is also, though, the myopia that looks for solutions only in the realm of "consumer choice" and "free markets." Our bizarre starting point is the well-stocked shelf of cigarettes, to which we respond by begging people not to purchase them. Nothing impedes the trucks that deliver the cigarettes or the factories that churn them out by the billions. We are led to believe that "information" and "choice" are the answers—however compromised by the grip of addiction. We are told that banning cigarettes would be tantamount to Prohibition, which we all know has been tried and failed.

This specter of 1920s-style prohibition is commonly invoked, as if the prohibition of alcohol were an appropriate comparison. It is not. Alcohol and tobacco are very different. The most important difference is that alcohol, unlike nicotine, is a recreational drug. Many people like to drink, and most do so responsibly with little or no harm to their health. Only about 3 percent of all people who drink are alcoholics; the overwhelming majority of "drinkers" do so without compromising their freedom. They are not addicts, which means that apart from that tiny minority of abusers, they choose to drink. That is the main reason Prohibition failed: *people like to drink* and can usually do so responsibly and in moderation.

Tobacco presents us with a very different situation. Nicotine is not a recreational drug. Most people who smoke wish they didn't, and most smokers (90 percent) regret ever having started.[2] That is because *most smokers are addicted*—80 to 90 percent, compared with the 3 percent among consumers of alcohol. Few people who drink regret their indulgence; few will say, "Gee, I wish I wasn't going to have this glass of wine tonight." Smokers are quite different; most smokers do not enjoy it; they smoke because it relieves their cravings, and they don't feel they can endure the pain required to quit. Alcohol and nicotine are very different in this respect, which is crucial to keep in mind when considering what must be done.

One thing I have noticed after many years of exploring this question is that there are really only two groups who take seriously the prospect of a total cigarette ban: smokers and tobacco industry executives. Smokers are open to the prospect, because they usually know they have a problem and need help. They want this monkey off their backs. They are often not the wealthiest people in the world and are acutely aware of the money they are wasting. They don't like the idea of higher taxes, because they know they will probably end up just paying more to scratch the diabolic itch. They regret having started and realize that "strong medicine" is needed to help them stop.

The archives make it clear that the industry has been anticipating the end of cigarettes for quite some time. Tobacco companies have no special love for cigarettes; they make them only because they know they can profit from doing so. And they would just as soon shift to something else, if their stockholders could be satisfied. Recall that William Farone, director of applied research at Philip Morris from 1976 to 1984, was hired to help guide the firm into a post-tobacco era; the company had bought Miller Beer and 7-Up as part of this effort and for a time considered getting entirely out of cigarettes. (Farone recommended the company buy Genentech—which would have been a smart move.) Recall also how hard the companies have worked to make a world without cigarettes seem unimaginable. Prohibiting cigarettes is cast as a grave threat to the liberties we hold dear.

If banning cigarettes seems like a drastic act, that is partly because we have been led to believe that prohibition *as a general policy* is impractical—or insufferable. The reality is that there is much in life that we prohibit, and for very good reasons. We prohibit slavery and child labor and a thousand varieties of crime, from murder to mayhem. Most laws are prohibitions, as is a great deal of morality (think of the Ten Commandments). We ban foods that contain poisons and drugs with deadly side effects. We've banned leaded gas and asbestos insulation, and we don't allow ordinary citizens to possess (most) military-grade weapons. Some bans are site- or age-specific: you cannot carry knives with you onto an airplane or into a school—and lots of things allowed for adults are off-limits to children. In a sense we live in a world awash in bans, a world radically delimited by constraints that most of us take for granted and would not want to see disappear. Many such prohibitions we think of more as protections, which we unthinkingly accept as crucial for the full expression of human liberties.

California bars the import of certain kinds of plants and animals, for example, to prevent pathogens from hitchhiking into the state. Do California farmers mind such prohibitions? How free would California farmers feel, having to cope with a ravenous new fruit parasite or an unstoppable nematode? Addictive psychoactive drugs are banned throughout the world, because of fears of potential abuse (heroin and cocaine, for example). Would we feel ourselves freer by allowing the sale of heroin on every street corner?

And what about hazardous materials, or extra-powerful poisons or weapons? Handguns are banned in many parts of the world, but even in America a private citizen is not supposed to own a sidewinder missile or armor-piercing ammunition. Are we happy to have such prohibitions? And how about the United Nations' prohibition of the use of dumdum bullets or chemical and biological weapons? Would we be freer with such items in broad circulation? Are we unduly hamstrung by the Geneva Convention, or international rules governing how prisoners must be treated, or treaties prohibiting the proliferation of nuclear technology?

Safety is perhaps the most common rationale for modern prohibitions. Employers are barred from exposing workers to hazardous substances, and restaurants cannot serve food from filthy kitchens. Aren't those good prohibitions? And what about laws punishing the fouling of public air or water, or laws barring products that threaten the health or safety of children? Childhood safety is protected by many different kinds of laws, including consumer product regulations. Toys cannot be sold with small pieces that can detach, posing a swallowing hazard. You cannot sell a baby crib with the bars so far apart that a child might squeeze through, risking strangulation. You cannot sell toys coated with lead paint, or pills in bottles without safety caps. Should we be free to market such products?

Food and drug laws include prohibitions that few of us would want to see relaxed. Food manufacturers are barred from using additives known to cause cancer; they are not supposed to include filth or misrepresent contents on packaging. Safrole (from sassafras) is now banned (in the United States) for use in root beer but also for use in perfumes and soaps by the International Fragrance Association. Six different food dyes used to color artificial butter were banned in the United States in the 1950s, when experiments revealed these could cause cancer.

Of course not all industries are equal in their power to resist such bans: recall the American Cancer Society's observation from 1956 that if the same evidence indicting cigarettes had been found against spinach, the leafy green would not be legal for very long. Most consumer products suffer far greater scrutiny. For pharmaceuticals in the United States, the burden of proof now lies with the manufacturer, which cannot market a drug until it has passed strict safety tests. Mandatory testing of drugs is surprisingly recent, and largely a response to widely publicized abuses. I've mentioned the sensational case of diethylene glycol, which killed over a hundred people in the 1930s, but there are many other instances where harms have come from untested medications. Thalidomide was commonly used (in Europe) as a painkiller and an anti-emetic against morning sickness, prior to its recognition (in the 1950s) as a cause of birth defects. The drug caused more than ten thousand malformations worldwide prior to its removal from the market. In the United States the scandal led to a ruling that drugs must be tested prior to release—which means that untested drugs are, in effect, prohibited, banned.

Automakers are barred from selling vehicles that do not meet safety standards. We may not think much about it, but every automobile on the road today is a rolling embodiment of hundreds if not thousands of mandatory performance standards. You cannot make a car without headlamps of a certain brightness or brakes and tires that pass strict tests. Windshield and window glass must not shatter into deadly shards, airbags must inflate, and seatbelts have to be a certain strength. New car designs have to pass impact and rollover tests, fuel economy tests, visibility tests, crash tests, crush tests, and dozens of others. Even the stick shift knob must be large enough not to penetrate the human optical orbit, a lesson learned after some number of brains got skewered. All of which helps explain why traffic fatalities are lower now than at any time since 1950: only 35,000 Americans died on the road that year—

the same as in 2009. (Contrast this with the growth of smoking deaths from about 100,000 to more than 400,000 during this same time frame.) Every stretch of highway, like every car, is a physical expression of hundreds of safety and performance standards, which don't strike us as prohibitions only because we don't generally see what is not, and indeed by law cannot, be built. Vehicles, roads, and signs not up to snuff are effectively banned.

Otherwise put: we live in a world of ubiquitous prohibitions. Government-financed institutions establish standards for air, food, and water quality, along with the health and safety of work, the safety of transportation, standards at schools and hospitals, and limits on how, when, or what we hunt or fish. And how we hire or fire workers or trade stock or treat children. These all involve prohibitions, safeguards against threats to one or another aspect of human life and freedom.

My point is not that these are perfect institutions or even that they are doing a satisfactory job; there is always room for improvement. The point is rather that many of our freedoms depend on limits on takings, along with punishments for the negligent. We also live in a world where loud libertarian ideologues try to make it sound as if regulation is inherently a bad thing, the enemy of freedom, when the fact is that every family vacation completed safely on a highway, every airbag inflated properly during a crash, every airplane landed safely with the aid of an air traffic controller, every life saved by a shear-bolt breakaway sign post, every antibiotic not fouled by a charlatan, every doctor with a medical license, every house built in compliance with an electrical code, is proof of the value of standards properly enforced. I would also suggest that anyone with a knee-jerk objection to "prohibition" can-vas some of the 500,000 hits returned from a Google search of "laws prohibiting"; I suspect that most of these are things that few people would like to see overturned.[3]

Safety of course is not the only rationale for prohibitions. Performance-enhancing drugs and gear are barred from many sports, to ensure fairness and the integrity of competition. Many environmental laws entail prohibitions—on hunting certain animals or improper discharge of wastes, for example—often with the goal of protecting air or water quality but also to preserve our ability to appreciate nature's untamed splendor. Pesticides are sometimes banned to protect endangered wildlife, and heritage laws prohibit destruction of natural monuments or historical artifacts. Sustainability is sometimes the goal, as when Irish fishermen organized to prohibit mechanized trawling in Northern Ireland's Lough Neagh, home to the tastiest eels in all of Europe. Trawling in the 1950s and 1960s had led to a dramatic fall in the catch, so a decision was made to allow only line fishing and draft nets—no trawling. Eel populations have rebounded as a result, and local fisher folk have preserved their livelihood based on this prohibition—along with a host of other sustainable management practices.[4]

So we already live in a world of routine if invisible prohibitions, established to protect the weak from the powerful, the innocent from the abuser, the prudent from the greedy, the public from the polluter. Prohibitions of this sort may often go unnoticed, rendered invisible by the absence of the barred artifact from consumption or circulation. Further clouding our perception is the rancor of libertarians, who denounce all "intrusions" by "the government" as onerous. This man-alone-on-an-island myopia makes it hard to keep in mind the myriad bans from which most of us benefit every day. Insofar as we live in a world of freedoms preserved through laws, prudent prohibitions are a crucial part of this.

EYES ON THE PRIZE

The cigarette is the deadliest artifact in the history of human civilization. It is also a defective product. The cigarette is the seatbeltless car, the lead-painted crib, the car with faulty brakes, the open unguarded manhole, the rickety ladder, the fouled maggoty meat, the Dalkon shield, the smokestack spewing fumes. It is lead paint and asbestos and arsenic and worse, since it kills so many more and so slowly and seductively. And it is still, apparently, the only consumer product that kills when used as directed. Half its users, in fact.

There will come a time, I am convinced, when tobacco will no longer be widely smoked, and people will marvel at this odd obsession of the past. And historians will puzzle over how and why nicotine captured as many people as it did, and for so long. The change won't come about overnight, and for a time we can expect the industry to continue bullying and buying off its critics. Change in some parts of the world will come from grassroots movements, with local policies quilting into ever larger policies. Elsewhere change will come from the reasoned actions of elected officials, acting under pressure from an informed and outraged public. Smoking will persist in parts of the world for many years, but tobacco will one day become part of a closed chapter of history. Cigarettes will join lead paint and ubiquitous asbestos and other abandoned artifacts—like the spittoon or buggy whip—and this chapter of history will come to an end.

To bring this about, though, we need to keep our eyes on the prize. Cigarettes are the world's most widely abused drug and the world's largest preventable cause of death and suffering. We are talking about the bane of a billion living smokers and an unparalleled corruption of science and the human lung. A destroyer of forests and the world's leading cause of fires. A cause of global impoverishment and global disease—and a burden abhorred even by smokers. To reclaim clean air for the commons, and to prevent needless suffering, including millions of those not yet born, the manufacture and sale of cigarettes must be abolished.

INTRODUCTION

1. The Ecusta company's website, http://www.ecusta.com/products.htm, accessed January 2006, has since been taken down. For background on the company, see *The Echo— Anniversary Edition—1939–1949* (Pisgah Forest, NC: Ecusta Paper Corp., 1949).

2. Richard Doll and A. Bradford Hill suspected arsenic; see their "Smoking and Carcinoma of the Lung: Preliminary Report," *British Medical Journal* 2 (1950): 739–48. Franz Hermann Müller suspected the increasing use of stems; see his "Tabakmissbrauch und Lungencarcinom," *Zeitschrift für Krebsforschung* 49 (1939): 57–85. J. J. Durrett of the Federal Trade Commission suspected the humectant diethylene glycol; see Hiram R. Hanmer to Paul M. Hahn, "Memorandum on Alleged Causative Relation between Cigarette Smoke and Bronchiogenic Carcinoma," Sept. 15, 1950, Bates 950218815–8825, p. 7.

The "Bates numbers" I shall be citing are used to identify documents prepared for release in the discovery phase of litigation. These numbers have been stamped onto documents by handheld automatic stamping machines, such as those patented by the Bates Manufacturing Company of Orange, New Jersey, in the 1890s. Bates numbers allow large sets of documents to be uniquely sequenced, though in practice, when archives from multiple trials are combined, more than one document may end up with the same Bates number. Readers can retrieve documents from the online Legacy Tobacco Documents Library by entering the first part of the Bates number (preceding the hyphen) in the search field at http://legacy.library .ucsf.edu.

3. See Louis Kyriakoudes, "Historians' Testimony on 'Common Knowledge' of the Risks of Tobacco Use: A Review and Analysis of Experts Testifying on Behalf of Cigarette Manufacturers in Civil Litigation," *Tobacco Control* 15 (2006): iv107–16; also my "Should Medical Historians Be Working for the Tobacco Industry?" *Lancet* 383 (2004): 1174–75.

4. U.S. liability laws generally do not require proof that parties guilty of negligence *knew*

they were doing harm; it is enough that they failed to act in accord with the "state of the art." For legal purposes, then, the question is not so much when the industry "knew" but rather when they "should have known."

5. Testimony of the "Seven Dwarfs" before Henry Waxman's congressional committee can be found at http://www.pbs.org/wgbh/pages/frontline/shows/settlement/timelines/april942.html#nope. For the testimony of Geoffrey Bible, see *Minnesota v. Philip Morris,* March 2, 1998, Bates BIBLEG030298, p. 5782.

6. Richard Kluger, *Ashes to Ashes: America's Hundred-Year Cigarette War, the Public Health, and the Unabashed Triumph of Philip Morris* (New York: Knopf, 1996).

7. The Plaza Hotel meeting is described in "Tobacco Industry Meeting, New York, December 14, 1953," Bates 680262226–2228.

8. On January 26, 2006, the Air Resources Board of California's Environmental Protection Agency recognized secondhand smoke as a significant cause of breast cancer, based on a five-year review of epidemiology. The report also concluded that secondhand smoke constitutes a "toxic air contaminant" responsible for more than fifty thousand American deaths per annum. For documentation, see http://www.arb.ca.gov/regact/ets2006/ets2006.htm; and for an updated assessment, Canadian Expert Panel on Tobacco Smoke and Breast Cancer Risk report of April 2009, http://www.otru.org/pdf/special/expert_panel_tobacco_breast_cancer.pdf.

9. Industry executives were privately admitting the reality of cigarette addiction more than a quarter-century prior to the Surgeon General's report of 1988, the first to arrive at this conclusion. British American Tobacco (BAT) Chief Scientist Sir Charles Ellis in 1961 characterized smokers as "nicotine addicts," for example, and two years later Brown & Williamson's chief counsel and executive vice president confessed (privately) that "nicotine is addictive" and that the company was "in the business of selling nicotine, an addictive drug." See Ellis, "Meeting in London with Dr. Haselbach," Nov. 15, 1961, Bates 301083862–3865; Addison Yeaman, "Implications of Battelle Hippo I & II and the Griffith Filter," July 17, 1963, Bates 435.

10. Louis Kyriakoudes notes that American etiquette guides as late as the 1970s (Amy Vanderbilt's, for example) were still recommending that a good hostess provide cigarettes and ashtrays for her guests after a dinner party; he cites this as evidence that many people were not yet ready to talk about smoking as a deadly addiction. See his testimony in *Boerner v. Brown & Williamson,* May 9, 2003, Bates Kyriakoudeslo50903.

11. On baldness: J. G. Mosley and A. C. C. Gibbs, "Premature Grey Hair and Hair Loss among Smokers: A New Opportunity for Health Education?" *BMJ* 313 (1996): 1616. On premature menopause: E. R. te Velde, P. L. Pearson, and F. J. Broekmans, eds., *Female Reproductive Aging* (London: Parthenon, 2000), p. 255. On Hollywood films: M. A. Dalton et al., "Effect of Viewing Smoking in Movies on Adolescent Smoking Initiation: A Cohort Study," *Lancet* 362 (2003): 281–85; also James D. Sargent, "Effect of Seeing Tobacco Use in Films on Trying Smoking among Adolescents," *BMJ* 323 (2001): 1394–97. On plasticizers released into the lungs: D. E. Mathis (Eastman Kodak Co.), "Factors Affecting Filter Firmness," n.d., Bates 599006814–6819. On hookah: Wasim Maziak, "The Waterpipe: Time for Action," *Addiction* 103 (2008): 1763–67; also Erika Dugas et al., "Water-Pipe Smoking among North American Youths," *Pediatrics* 125 (2010): 1184–89.

12. U.S. Department of Health and Human Services, *Reducing the Health Consequences of Smoking: 25 Years of Progress: A Report of the Surgeon General* (Washington, DC: U.S. Government Printing Office, 1989), chap. 4, tables 6, 15, and 16 and figs. 1 and 2.

13. Steven A. Schroeder, "Tobacco Control in the Wake of the 1998 Master Settlement Agreement," *New England Journal of Medicine* 350 (2004): 293–301; J. R. Hughes et al., "Prevalence of Smoking among Psychiatric Outpatients," *American Journal of Psychiatry* 143 (1986): 993–97; R. J. Reynolds, "Project Scum," Dec. 12, 1995, Bates 518021121–1129. Simon Chapman, Mark Ragg, and Kevin McGeechan have published a fascinating account of how scholars tend to exaggerate the fraction of mentally ill who are smokers; see their "Citation Bias in Reported Smoking Prevalence in People with Schizophrenia," *Australian and New Zealand Journal of Psychiatry* 43 (2009): 277–82.

14. *Eavescasting* is a word I asked the linguist Iain Boal to craft to designate this hidden intent to broadcast; the word is formed from a truncated amalgam of "eavesdropping" and "broadcasting."

15. See my " 'Everyone Knew but No One Had Proof': Tobacco Industry Use of Medical History Expertise in US Courts, 1990–2002," *Tobacco Control* 15 (2006): iv117–25.

16. Lorillard in 1963 launched a newspaper—*Science Fortnightly*—to cloak its popular Kent brand in the authority of science. The publication was designed for doctors' offices, with careful attention given to the quality of paper used and even the font and format of the typeface, all to catch the doctor's eye and the attention of patients. Published from 1963 through 1964, the paper actually makes quite a good read, with articles on cosmology and dinosaurs and the achievements of racial minorities in science. The hope was to use top-notch popular science reporting to burnish the image of Kent as a "safer" cigarette, which is why every issue had at least two prominent ads for that brand and for no other product. *Science Fortnightly* was good popular science, but it was also an effort to convince doctors of the superiority of Kent, with its "Micronite" (formerly asbestos) filter. Doctors were always a group the industry wanted to influence and for obvious reasons: a 1950s industry document noted that for every physician "reached," a thousand patients were also being reached. Lorillard in 1994 ordered the destruction of its collection of *Science Fortnightly* along with associated documentation; see "Record Transfer List," May 5, 1994, Bates 87929836–9837.

17. My Stanford colleague Matthew Kohrman has recently mapped over three hundred of the world's tobacco factories—"cigarette citadels"—which can now be viewed interactively at https://www.stanford.edu/group/tobaccoprv/cgi-bin/wordpress/.

PART I

1. Francis Robicsek, *The Smoking Gods: Tobacco in Maya Art, History, and Religion* (Norman: University of Oklahoma Press, 1978).

2. Robert K. Heimann, *Tobacco and Americans* (New York: McGraw-Hill, 1960), p. 203. Heimann was an NYU-trained sociologist who skyrocketed into the executive ranks of the American Tobacco Company (AT) in the early 1950s. His book was actually a collaboration between AT, Hill & Knowlton, the Tobacco Institute, and Philip Morris. Details of the publication history can be found in J. S. Fones and E. P. Quinby to George Weissman, "Notes and Suggestions on 'Americans and Tobacco,' " May 4, 1959, Bates 1005038147–8155.

3. Harris Lewine, *Good-Bye to All That* (New York: McGraw Hill, 1970), pp. 11–12. Several other versions of this story circulate: the Rizla rolling paper company in France, for example, talks about soldiers in the Napoleonic wars using pages from books to wrap tobacco; see http://www.rizla.co.uk/riztory/riztory.php. Accounts of the origin of the cigarette differ according to whether one is talking about "small cigars," the word *cigarette*, or paper wrapping.

CHAPTER 1

1. There are three principal ways to classify tobacco: by breed, place of growth, and method of curing. The categories blend into one another, since the varieties grown in specific regions tend also to be cured in specific ways, and the quality of the smoke produced is strongly influenced by the soil in which it is grown. Flue-cured, or "bright," tobacco is also known as *Virginia* tobacco, because that is where it was originally cultivated. Seeds taken from Virginia tobacco and planted in Cuba, however, will produce leaves best suited for Cuban cigars. American Tobacco's Robert K. Heimann commented on this in 1960, noting that the tobacco plant was "more true to the earth in which it grows than the seed from which it springs"; see his *Tobacco and Americans*, pp. 146–85.

2. Direct heating by means of propane gas, begun after World War II, has been suspected of increasing the production of carcinogenic nitrosamines in tobacco and cigarette smoke; see Dietrich Hoffmann and Ilse Hoffmann, "The Changing Cigarette: Chemical Studies and Bioassays," in *Risks Associated with Smoking Cigarettes with Low Machine-Measured Yields of Tar and Nicotine* (Bethesda, MD: National Cancer Institute, 2001), pp. 159–91.

3. Laurence Brockliss and Colin Jones in their *The Medical World of Early Modern France* (Oxford: Clarendon Press, 1997) note that eighteenth-century methods for reviving bodies fished from the Seine included "rubbing eau-de-vie and ammoniac on various parts of the body and blowing tobacco smoke up the anus" (p. 744).

4. Heimann, *Tobacco and Americans*, p. 244.

5. A good review is G. F. Peedin, "Flue-Cured Tobacco," in *Tobacco: Production, Chemistry and Technology*, ed. D. Layten Davis and Mark T. Nielsen (Oxford: Blackwell, 1999), pp. 104–42.

6. Turkish leaf also produces a low-alkaline smoke, which is why it has often been used in cigarettes. American's Pall Mall brand, introduced in 1913, originally used Oriental (= Turkish) tobacco and didn't shift over to flue-cured until 1936. *Chambers' Edinburgh Journal* in 1868 reported on the popularity of cigarette smoking following the Crimean War of 1853–56, advising that "for full benefit" smoke from Turkish-leaf cigarettes should be inhaled into the lungs; see Richard B. Tennant, *The American Cigarette Industry: A Study in Economic Analysis and Public Policy* (New Haven: Yale University Press, 1950), p. 130.

7. Francis J. Weiss (Sugar Research Foundation, for R. J. Reynolds), "Tobacco and Sugar," Oct. 1950, Bates 502477793–7881. An excellent review of the role of sugars in tobacco chemistry is Reinskje Talhout, Antoon Opperhuizen, and Jan G. C. van Amsterdam, "Sugars as Tobacco Ingredient: Effects on Mainstream Smoke Composition," *Food and Chemical Toxicology* 44 (2006): 1789–98.

8. Fritz Lickint, *Ätiologie und Prophylaxe des Lungenkrebses* (Dresden: Steinkopff, 1953), pp. 68, 134–35.

9. See Prabhat Jha and Frank J. Chaloupka, eds., *Tobacco Control in Developing Countries* (New York: Oxford University Press, 2000); also my "Tobacco and the Global Lung Cancer Epidemic," *Nature Reviews Cancer* 1 (2001): 82–86. For the hypodermic needle comparison: Henner Hess, *Rauchen: Geschichte, Geschäfte, Gefahren* (Frankfurt: Campus, 1987), p. 49.

CHAPTER 2

1. Thomas H. Steele et al., *Close Cover before Striking: The Golden Age of Matchbook Art* (New York: Abbeville Press, 1987).

2. "Camel Is Still Going Strong after 60 Historic Years," *RJR World* (Jan.–Feb. 1974): 4, Bates 507849712–9729.

3. "George W. Hill: Pioneer Dynamo," *Newsleaf*, Nov. 1984, Bates 950213874–3877, p. 8.

4. James A. Bonsack, "Cigarette-Machine," U.S. Patent No. 238,640, awarded March 8, 1881; B. W. C. Roberts and R. F. Knapp, "Paving the Way for the Tobacco Trust: From Hand Rolling to Mechanized Cigarette Production," *North Carolina Historical Review* 69 (1992): 257–81.

5. An excellent source on the history of tobacco mechanization is the Philip Morris document by Pat Walford: "The Development of Cigarette Technology," Feb. 28, 1979, Bates 1000774237–4245; compare also "Cigarette Manufacture: A Backward Glance," *Molinismo* (London: Molins Machine Co., Ltd., 1971).

6. Richard Hall, *The Making of Molins: The Growth and Transformation of a Family Business, 1874–1977* (London: Molins Ltd., 1978), p. 2. Bernhard Baron, an American inventor, began manufacturing cigarette-making machines in London's East End in the 1880s and in 1896 incorporated his Baron Cigarette Machine Company. John Player & Sons started using the Baron in Nottingham in 1893 and by the end of the century had installed eighteen such machines in its factories. The Glasgow firm of Stephen Mitchell & Son also bought sixteen Barons; see Howard Cox, *The Global Cigarette: Origins and Evolution of British American Tobacco, 1880–1945* (Oxford: Oxford University Press, 2000), p. 53.

7. Cited in Allan M. Brandt, *The Cigarette Century: The Rise, Fall, and Deadly Persistence of the Product That Defined America* (New York: Basic Books, 2007), p. 510 n. 49.

8. Cox, *Global Cigarette*, p. 53.

9. On Italy's machines, see Giuseppe Cavallini, "La machina italiana per la confezione delle sigarette," *Il Tabacco*, no. 548 (1942); and for Germany's: M. Richard Creuzburg, "Die Tabakmaschinenindustrie," *Chronica Nicotiana* 1, no. 2 (1940): 30–53.

10. BATCo, "Report on Visit to U.S.A., May 1973," 1973, Bates 100226995–7033, p. 2; "Administration January-March, 1971" (BATCo), Bates 105360706–0735, p. 1; J. H. Simpson and I. W. Tucker, "The Technical Research Department of Brown & Williamson Tobacco Corporation: A Comprehensive Report of Its History, Current Status and Recommendations," Dec. 1953, Bates 650032904–2943, p. 29. For Reynolds's machines: "QA Production Division," July 25, 1986, Bates 509908904–8948. The Molins Machine Company of London for many years was an innovator in cigarette machine design; Desmond Walter Molins was running the company in the early 1970s, when rumors swirled that the Russians had bought 150 of his Mark VIII machines. Molins was also a pioneer of packing (vs. rolling) machines: its Mark I machine from 1919 fit ten cigarettes into a soft pack, eliminating hand-packing; see

Walford, "Development of Cigarette Technology," pp. 4–5. Liggett in 1974 patented an "automatic feed device" linking makers with packing machines, allowing them to pack upwards of 3,600 cigarettes per minute; see Philip Morris's *Technical Newsletter,* April 1974, p. 2. An excellent analysis of machine speeds is BAT's "Technological Forecasting: A Brief Survey of Trends," 1976, Bates 526022434–2566. For Hauni: "Status of Manufacturing Department Projects and Activities," May 13, 1981, Bates 500253245–3255. In 2008 the Hamburg-based Hauni company, with a staff of 3,700, claimed to be "by far the largest and most successful provider of technologies and solutions for tobacco processing" and "the global market and technology leader in machine building" for the industry; see http://www.hauni.com/about_uso .html?&L = 0.

11. Bryan Burrough and John Helyar, *Barbarians at the Gate: The Fall of RJR Nabisco* (New York: Harper and Row, 1990), p. 218.

CHAPTER 3

1. Philip Morris, Public Affairs Department, "Tobacco Action Program Manual," 1980, Bates 2053630242–0341, pp. 1-1–8.

2. Puffing on cigarettes could give away one's position, which is why Sassanian soldiers developed the habit of smoking *from the lit end* of the cigarette, to hide the coal. In more recent wars smoking has become more dangerous from the use of night-vision goggles, which can easily spot the heat from a cigarette.

3. Ted Bates and Co., "Copy of a Study of Cigarette Advertising Made by J. W. Burgard: 1953" (Lorillard), n.d., Bates 04238374–8433.

4. "Tobacco Boosts Defense Morale," *News* (Paris, TX), Nov. 29, 1959, Bates 1003543302–3654.

5. See my *The Nazi War on Cancer* (Princeton: Princeton University Press, 1999), pp. 258–347.

6. George Seldes, "US to Force Europe to Take $911,100,000 in Tobacco, Only 2 Billions in Food in ERP Plan," *In Fact,* March 22, 1948, pp. 1–3. The Marshall Plan was designed to send goods rather than cash to Europe, with the goal of keeping Europe's "farm and factory production machine humming." The goal was also, though, to help keep U.S. farm prices high; see "How to Do Business under the Marshall Plan," *Kiplinger Magazine,* May 1948, p. 6.

7. In September 1947 the Committee for European Economic Cooperation (CEEC) drew up a plan for European reconstruction and presented it to the U.S. government. Tobacco, significantly, was not included in this. Compare also the list in "First official meeting of the OEEC in Paris to determine national needs prior to passage of appropriations bill by U.S. Congress," April 15, 1948, in the U.S. National Archives.

8. George Seldes, *Lords of the Press* (New York: Julian Messner, 1938); also his "Tobacco Shortens Life," *In Fact,* Jan. 13, 1941, pp. 1–5; and Jan. 27, 1941, 3–4.

9. Hill & Knowlton, "Confidential Memorandum," 1954, Bates 501941222–1229.

10. "To Smoke or Not: The Issue Involves Personal Choice, Not the Public Health," *Barron's,* Jan. 20, 1964, p. 2. The U.S. government by 1970 was paying $31 million per year for

tobacco for the Food for Peace program, plus another $28 million for tobacco export subsidies and $240,000 for promotion of cigarettes in places such as Japan, which used some American tobacco.

CHAPTER 4

1. Francisco Comin and Pablo Martin Acena, *Tabacalera y el estanco del tabaco en España: 1636–1998* (Madrid: Fundación Tabacalera, 1999); Jacob M. Price, *France and the Chesapeake: A History of the French Tobacco Monopoly: 1674–1791*, 2 vols. (Ann Arbor: University of Michigan Press, 1973).

2. For 1935 data: C. F. Bailey and A. W. Petre, "The Modern Cigaret Industry," *Industrial and Engineering Chemistry* 29 (1937): 11–10, where we hear that "generally, the world over, tobacco revenues rank first or second in importance as a source of governmental income of this class." For France, Italy and Formosa: "Tobacco's Taxing Dilemma," *Time*, May 7, 1965, http://www.time.com/time/magazine/article/0,9171,898779,00.html. Many Eastern European nations have (or formerly had) state-owned tobacco companies. Bulgartabac, for example, remains a state-owned enterprise despite numerous recent efforts at privatization. TEKEL is Turkey's state-owned alcohol and tobacco monopoly; other monopolies combine tobacco and salt (Japan, the Vatican), wine (Taiwan), ginseng (Korea), etc.

3. See my *Nazi War on Cancer* for details.

4. See Yali Peng, "Smoke and Power: The Political Economy of Chinese Tobacco" (Ph.D. diss., University of Oregon, 1997). The World Health Organization has published a bibliography on smoking in China; see Joy de Beyer et al., *Research on Tobacco in China: An Annotated Bibliography* (New York: WHO, 2004). For China's earlier history, see Cox, *Global Cigarette*; and Sherman Cochran, *Big Business in China: Sino-Foreign Rivalry in the Cigarette Industry, 1890–1930* (Cambridge, MA: Harvard University Press, 1990).

5. Tobacco taxes in the latter part of the nineteenth century—prior to the establishment of a national income tax—provided the U.S. government with nearly a third of its total revenue. As recently as 1992 Philip Morris was still the largest single taxpayer in the United States, coughing up $4.5 billion in income taxes.

6. According to a study by the Center for Public Integrity in Washington, D.C., BAT, Philip Morris, and Reynolds have all "worked closely with companies and individuals directly connected to organized crime in Hong Kong, Canada, Colombia, Italy, and the United States." The Center also comments on an Italian government report, according to which Philip Morris and Reynolds agents in Switzerland were "high-level criminals who ran a vast smuggling operation into Italy in the 1980s that was directly linked to the Sicilian Mafia"; see International Consortium of Investigative Journalists, "Tobacco Companies Linked to Criminal Organizations in Lucrative Cigarette Smuggling," CPI Special Report, March 3, 2001 (online).

7. Canada's remarkable story is told in Rob Cunningham's excellent *Smoke and Mirrors: The Canadian Tobacco War* (Ottawa: IDRC, 1996), pp. 125–35. For Sweden: AFP, "Sweden Scraps Its Heavy New Tobacco Tax Due to Booming Smuggling," July 29, 1998, Bates 106012256. For Colombia: Mark Schapiro, "Big Tobacco," *The Nation*, May 6, 2002 (online).

8. "North-East Argentina" (BATCo), 1992, Bates 503918336–8348.

9. Brown & Williamson, "Tobacco in Italy," 1982, Bates 501016079–6083. Luk Joossens in 2007 estimated that 11 percent of the world's cigarette transactions were "illicit," including smuggling, illicit manufacture (by legitimate companies), and counterfeiting. In 2007 this amounted to about 600 billion cigarettes. BAT in 1992 predicted how many cigarettes would be smuggled into Hong Kong as a result of the island's duty increases; see Graham Burgess, "Company Plan 1993—1997," Oct. 16, 1992, Bates 304010203–0231 at 0216.

10. For the Ukraine: F. Delman, "Taxation & Smuggling," *TMA Executive Summary,* Jan. 29, 1999, Bates 519977898–7901. For BAT: Jennie Matthew, "Company Denies Cigarette Smuggling Allegations," *Cyprus Mail,* Dec. 18, 2001. For Chinatown: Angelica Medaglia, "Cigarettes Are Costly, but Often Less So in Chinatown," *New York Times,* Sept. 18, 2007.

11. Susie Mesure, "Imperial Director Charged after German Customs Swoop," *The Independent* (London), Jan. 15, 2003.

12. Luk Joossens and Martin Raw, "Cigarette Smuggling in Europe, Who Really Benefits?" *Tobacco Control* 7 (1998): 66–71. BAT Nigeria's Richard Hodgson on Jan. 16, 2005, in the Lagos journal *This Day* opined, "Tobacco use is risky but counterfeit cigarettes are lethal."

13. See Brandt, *Cigarette Century,* pp. 431–38.

CHAPTER 5

1. Nannie M. Tilley, *The R.J. Reynolds Tobacco Company* (Chapel Hill: University of North Carolina Press, 1985).

2. A fine history of trademarks and brand names is Susan Strasser, *Satisfaction Guaranteed: The Making of the American Mass Market* (New York: Pantheon, 1989).

3. For thirty thousand brands: Mark W. Rien and Gustaf N. Dorén, *Das neue Tabago Buch* (Hamburg: Reemtsma, 1985), p. 119. For Susini and Sons: Tony Hyman, "Louis Susini's *La Honradez:* Cuban Cigarettes & the 1st Collectible," National Cigar Museum Exhibit, www.cigarhistory.info/Cuba/Honradez.html. For Police Club: Jerome E. Brooks, "The Philip Morris Century," ca. 1978, Bates 96746624–6648.

4. Philip S. Gardiner, "The African Americanization of Menthol Cigarette Use in the United States," *Nicotine & Tobacco Research* 6 (2004): S55–65; also "The Black Menthol Cigarette Market, February, 1979," prepared by William Esty for Reynolds, Bates 501071047–1122.

5. Susan Wagner, *Cigarette Country: Tobacco in American History and Politics* (New York: Praeger, 1971), pp. 56–60.

6. "Call for Philip Morris," *PM People,* Jan. 1992, Bates 2054407245–7249.

7. See Rizla's website, http://www.rizla.co.uk/riztory/riztory.php, where you can also play various video games.

8. David E. Rudd, *Illustrated History of Baseball Cards: The 1800s,* http://www.cycleback.com/1800s/tobacco1.htm.

9. Brandt, *Cigarette Century,* p. 7. For skycasting: "Voice from the Sky Resounds over the City," *New York Times,* Sept. 18, 1928.

10. S. Clay Williams to W.R. Hearst, Sept. 10, 1935, Bates 501771783–1787; Hearst to Berkowitz, n.d., Bates 501771781–1782.

11. "Radio Continuity, Lucky Strike, 1928–29," 1929, Bates 945263197–3552.

12. For other shows developed by the industry, see Louis M. Kyriakoudes, "The Grand Ole Opry and Big Tobacco: Radio Scripts from the Files of the R. J. Reynolds Tobacco Company, 1948 to 1959," *Southern Cultures* 12 (2006): 76–89.

13. http://www.youtube.com/watch?v = yNuQ6G1G_KQ#.

14. "A New Advertising Medium for KOOL Cigarettes," *Information* (BAT), July 1948, 17–18, Bates 400566440–6490.

15. Kyriakoudes, "Historians' Testimony," p. iv112.

16. Kim Chong-wan documents these events in his book, *One Hundred Years of Korean Film* (in Korean), noting that the first screening of "moving pictures" in Korea was in October 1897 (personal communication, Yumi Moon).

17. "PM's Mobile Cinema," *Tobacco Control* 17 (2008): 147–50.

18. Kristen L. Lum, Jonathan R. Polansky, Robert K. Jackler, and Stanton A. Glantz, "Signed, Sealed, and Delivered: Big Tobacco in Hollywood, 1927–1951," *Tobacco Control* 17 (2008): 313–23; also http://www.smokefreemovies.ucsf.edu/problem/earlyhollywood.html.

19. R. A. Rechholtz, "1971 Management Plan," Sept. 28, 1970, Bates 501706277–6278.

20. Sylvester Stallone to Bob Kovoloff, Associated Film Promotion, April 28, 1983, Bates 690132319; and for details, J. F. Ripslinger to Stallone, June 14, 1983, Bates 2295; and more generally: Randall Poe, "Invasion of the Movie Product-Pushers," *Across the Board,* Jan. 1984, 36–45; and C. Mekemson and S. A. Glantz, "How the Tobacco Industry Built Its Relationship with Hollywood," *Tobacco Control* 11 (2002): 181–91.

21. Gene Tunney, "Nicotine Knockout, or the Slow Count," *Reader's Digest,* Dec. 1941, pp. 21–24. The irony is that even Joe Louis allowed his image to be used in ads for Chesterfields.

22. See the American Tobacco file labeled "Tuxedo, 1913–17," Bates 945164313–4423. The "King" appellation is from the back of Cobb's 1910 T206 tobacco card.

23. For Newman, Connery, and Eastwood: "AFP Payments," 1983, Bates 682154636–4641. For Lark: Michael G. Wilson to Thomas A. Luken, July 19, 1989, Bates TIMN0305044–5045 and 685086478. For *Superman II:* Pierre Spengler (Dovemead Ltd.) to P. McNally (Philip Morris Europe), Oct. 18, 1979, Bates 2046788819–8821. For props in fifty-six films: "Tobacco Issues, Hearings before the Subcommittee on Transportation and Hazardous Materials, House of Representatives," July 25, 1989, Bates 2406.01. For "no shortage": John A. Kochevar (Philip Morris) to Thomas A. Luken, Feb. 2, 1989, Bates 87703545–3547. For merchandising: Frank A. Saunders to James C. Bowling, Jan. 9, 1984, Bates 2021280500.

24. Gary Messatesta to Bill Degenhardt (American Tobacco), "Movie Memorandum," Nov. 10, 1989, Bates 980345339–5750. Charlton Heston also smokes in at least one *Planet of the Apes.*

25. Warren Cowan to Gerald Long (Reynolds), May 4, 1981, Bates 503579240–9244.

26. A. R. Hazan, H. L. Lipton, and S. A. Glantz, "Popular Films Do Not Reflect Current Tobacco Use," *American Journal of Public Health* 84 (1994): 998–1000.

27. Robert F. Kennedy's words are from Sept. 12, 1967, and online at smokefreemovies.ucsf.

28. A. Charlesworth and S. Glantz, "Smoking in the Movies Increases Adolescent Smoking: A Review," *Pediatrics* 116 (2006): 1516–28.

29. Sarah Jessica Parker flashes a pack of Marlboro Lights in *Smart People* (2008) in a

scene clearly crafted to highlight the brand. British films may be using product placements, judging from the prominent role played by BAT's Senior Service in the *The Bank Job* (2008), for example. Filmmakers sometimes use fictional brand "prop" cigarettes: Quentin Tarantino used a Red Dog brand in *Pulp Fiction,* for example, and the 1994 film *The Shadow,* with Alec Baldwin, features a fictional Llama brand made to look like Camels.

30. Kelly, Weedon and Shute, "Philip Morris Cigarette Marketing—A New Perspective," Nov. 1989, Bates 2501057693–7719, p. 11. James Cameron's *Aliens* (1986), also starring Sigourney Weaver, is full of extraterrestrial smoking.

31. American Tobacco Co., "Lucky Strike, 1922–23" (Advertisements), 1922–23, Bates 945196562–6665.

32. Reynolds, *Magicians Handy Book of Cigarette Tricks* (Winston-Salem, 1930s).

33. *Arthur Selwyn Brown v. R. J. Reynolds Tobacco Co.*, "Transcript—Vol. II. Defendants' Evidence," May 1938, Bates 501820114–0257.

34. Martha N. Gardner and Allan M. Brandt, " 'The Doctors' Choice Is America's Choice': The Physician in US Cigarette Advertisements, 1930–1953," *American Journal of Public Health* 96 (2006): 222–32. For more ads, see http://lane.stanford.edu/tobacco/index.html.

35. See the collection of ads in "Philip Morris Newspapers," 1940–42, Bates 1003071050–1338.

36. Brown & Williamson in 1948 invited six thousand leading U.S. nose and throat specialists to send in a postcard to obtain twenty-five complimentary packs of Kool cigarettes to hand out to their patients "suffering from colds and kindred disorders." An astonishing 56 percent "readily and cheerfully accepted" the free cigarettes. The offer was soon thereafter extended to all practicing physicians in the United States; see "Unique Kool Campaign Has Warm Reception," *Information* (BAT), July 1948, pp. 9–10, Bates 400566440–6490. Nose and throat specialists were also sent Dr. Kool penguin paperweights as "goodwill builders," with the hope that these could be placed on the desks of "practically every physician in the United States." See also Fig. 34.

37. See the schedule for Tareyton cigarettes prepared for American Tobacco by the Lawrence C. Gumbinner Advertising Agency, updated from 1966, Bates 990042857–3531, p. 442.

38. Emerson Foote is cited in L. Heise, "Unhealthy Alliance," *World Watch,* Oct. 1988, p. 20; compare John H. Crowley and James Pokrywczynski, "Advertising Practitioners Look at Ban on Tobacco Advertising," *Journalism Quarterly* 68 (1991): 329–37. For the impact of advertising: R. W. Pollay et al., "The Last Straw? Cigarette Advertising and Realized Market Shares among Youth and Adults, 1979–1993," *Journal of Marketing* 60 (1996): 1–16; J. P. Pierce et al., "Does Tobacco Advertising Target Young People to Start Smoking? Evidence from California," *JAMA* 266 (1991): 3154–58; Michael Klitzner, Paul J. Gruenewald, and Elizabeth Bamberger, "Cigarette Advertising and Adolescent Experimentation with Smoking," *British Journal of Addiction* 86 (1991): 287–98. For examples of the industry admitting advertising's impact, see Bates 506768775, 507632657, and 501928462.

39. For "get more triers": "Resume of Sales Meeting Held in New York Office on December 5, 6, 7, and 9, 1966" Bates 990146737–6773, p. 7. For patches, see Art Padoan (Philip Morris), "Nicotine Skin Patch (NSP) Industry Fact Summary Sheet," Nov. 3, 1992, Bates

2040573155–3163, where we hear that "Advertising of the patches was halted by the companies in the late spring to cool off demand, which had quickly outstripped supplies."

40. "YAFScan: A Qualitative Overview of Values Lifestyles Brand Images among Northeast Urban Young Adult Female Smokers," Oct. 1997, Bates 2073775413–5477.

41. O. P. McComas, "Annual Report Philip Morris," 1954, Bates 2048017883–7921.

42. "Corporate Totals" (Lorillard), Jan. 16, 1961, Bates 01793607–3612.

43. "Some Reflections on Our Present Discontent—Or Why We Are Losing the Public Affairs War on Tobacco?" 1990, Bates 2500057725–7729.

44. For rivals: Liggett & Myers, "Chesterfield #25A," March 28, 1951, Bates LG0071270–1300. As of 1991 "Courtesy of Choice" had more than 8,500 participating outlets in forty-nine countries; see Wilson Jones, "Issues Book 2000," 1991, Bates 2082100111–0279A; and for Australia's participation: "ETS Activity Status," Sept. 1993, Bates 2500156096–6105. For PM's Accommodation Program, see Monique Muggli, Jean L. Forster, Richard D. Hurt, and James L. Repace, "The Smoke You Don't See: Uncovering Tobacco Industry Scientific Strategies Aimed against Environmental Tobacco Smoke Policies," *American Journal of Public Health* 91 (2001): 1419–23; J. V. Dearlove, S. A. Bialous, and S. A. Glantz, "Tobacco Industry Manipulation of the Hospitality Industry to Maintain Smoking in Public Places," *Tobacco Control* 11 (2002): 94–104.

45. For "not too bad an advertisement": Addison Yeaman (Brown & Williamson) to W. E. McCabe, Dec. 3, 1946, Bates 682349456. For "create Philip Morris": Jack Porterfield to J. E. Gallagher, "Johnny, Jr. Operation," Dec. 19, 1953, Bates 2010019434. The Tobacco Institute's William Kloepfer on Nov. 24, 1976, asked Arthur Stevens, general counsel of Lorillard, "why, if the cigarette companies do not want to promote smoking among young people, [do] they allow candy cigarette manufacturers to use their brand names"? (Bates 00487616–7617). Much of my discussion of candy cigarettes is from an unpublished paper coauthored by Julia Powell and myself in 2006–7.

46. "American Tobacco Co., Fiscal Statement," Dec. 31, 1928, Bates 945284363–4810; W. T. Woodson, "*Lorillard v. Glick*," Sept. 9, 1929, Bates 88106915.

47. Addison Yeaman to P. J. Trantham, March 18, 1949, Bates 682349439.

48. Robert B. Meyner to Addison Yeaman, Feb. 20, 1967, Bates 682349375; Addison Yeaman to Meyner, March 7, 1967, Bates 682349373.

49. Addison Yeaman to Tell Chocolate Novelties, March 16, 1948, Bates 682349453; also his letters to Victoria Sweets, Oct. 14, 1948, Bates 682349448; to Stephen Szilagyi of the Smiley Candy Co., Jan. 17, 1950, Bates 682349433; and to Sylvan Sweets, April 7, 1950, Bates 682349428. The Lorillard document cited is Anna F. Woessner to Fujio Inoue (Hakuhoda Inc.), Jan. 31, 1961, Bates 00487966.

50. Gus Wayne to J. E. Gallagher, "Sales Promotion," Dec. 6, 1953, Bates 2010019425–9427, with punctuation corrected. Gallagher considered this notion of giving kids Philip Morris chocolate cigarettes "an excellent suggestion"; see his letter to Ray Jones, Dec. 24, 1953, Bates 2010019424. Gus Wayne, Buddy Douglas, Al Altieri, and Leon Polinsky were the four "Johnny Juniors" used to market Philip Morris cigarettes when the original "Johnny" (Roventini) wasn't available. Philip Morris valued the "Johnny Junior" trademark at $300 per month in 1949, though the "Johnnys" themselves weren't paid very well and were regarded as more

perishable than the usual trademark: advertising executive Seymour Ellis pondered "the comparatively short life" of a Johnny—"they are not much good to us after 40, or even before"—and so urged a salary of about $70 per month for their services. See Seymour Ellis to Allan Thurman, July 27, 1949, Bates 2010017043–7044.

51. Alan Blum, "Candy Cigarettes," *New England Journal of Medicine* 302 (1980): 972; Jonathan Klein et al., "Candy Cigarettes: Do They Encourage Children's Smoking?" *Pediatrics* 99 (1992): 27-31.

52. Margaret E. Hilton, "Teaching them Young," *Medical Officer,* Feb. 22, 1963, p. 111; Robert C. Conlon (Lorillard) to World Candies, Inc., Jan. 31, 1969, Bates 88682607; Guy M. Blynn (Reynolds) to World Candies, Inc., Jan. 15, 1980, Bates 515864270–4271.

53. J. S. Speer III to E. W. O'Toole, "Kent Trade Mark," Feb. 5, 1969, Bates 00487906.

54. For "ugly heads": R. E. Scanlan to New York State TAN Advisory Committee, "New York Activities," Feb. 15, 1983, Bates 680532741–2742. For Tootsie Roll: Henry F. Mohler to T. J. Kelly (Kelly Candy and Tobacco), May 29, 1971, Bates 1005098971–8975. For ban defeated: "Committee against Unjust Cigarette Taxes Reactivated," *Tobacco Reporter,* Feb. 1968, p. 66.

55. For leaflets: William Kloepfer (Tobacco Institute) to J. Kendrick Wells, May 26, 1978, Bates 680546989–6999. For lobbying: Michael F. Brozek to William P. Buckley, "Legislative Update—Minnesota," May 10, 1985, Bates LG0304982–4986. For friends: Philip Morris, "Tobacco-Related Web Addresses," 1995, Bates 2078863603–3617.

56. J. Kendrick Wells to Samuel Cohen (World Candies), May 9, 1985, Bates 640516197–6198; J. Kendrick Wells to Counsel for World Candies, May 22, 1985, Bates 521002266.

57. D. M. Antonellis (Stark Candy) to C. G. Lamb (Brown & Williamson), Oct. 23, 1990, Bates 486100575.

58. For "BIG TOBACCO BUSINESS": R. J. Reynolds, "School Days Are Here," Sept. 9, 1927, Bates 502399083–9085. For "most cigaret experts": George Seldes, "Cigarets for Children," *In Fact,* July 28, 1947, p. 1.

59. For Japan: Yoshihiro Nagai to Yutaka Suzuki (Philip Morris), "Book Cover Advertising Report," Feb. 18, 1987, Bates 2504042177–2178. For Argentina: G. Irman (Brown & Williamson), "Notes on Project 'Bristol,' " April 1980, Bates 661122258–2277.

60. For "new starters": D. V. Cantrell (Brown & Williamson) to I. D. Macdonald et al., "Kool Isn't Getting the Starters," Feb. 17, 1987, Bates 621079918. For "replacement smokers": Diane S. Burrows (Reynolds), "Younger Adult Smokers: Strategies and Opportunities," Feb. 29, 1984, Bates 505458067–8160. For "young adult market aged 14–21": Charles A. Tucker, "1975 Marketing Plans Presentation, Hilton Head" (presented to RJRI Board of Directors), Sept. 30, 1974, Bates 501421310–1335. For "initiation": "Smoking-Cigarettes and Advertising" (Brown & Williamson), 1975, Bates 680561705–1712. The Roper report is at Shirley Wilkins and Bud Roper to Steve Fountaine, "Suggestions for Research," June 12, 1970, Bates 2078100038–0042. For "today's teenager": Myron E. Johnston to Robert B. Seligman, "Young Smokers," March 31, 1981, Bates 1003636640–6688. For "aggressive monkeys": Frank J. Ryan, "Hyperkinetic Child as a Prospective Smoker," July 18, 1975, Bates 680903115–3143, p. 22.

61. For "Marlboro's leadership": "Philip Morris EEC Region Three Year Plan 1992–1994," Bates 2500064227, p. 30. For "prime target group": A. G. Buzzi (Leo Burnett Advertising for Philip Morris Holland), "Marketing Plans 1982," Jan. 14, 1982, Bates 2501026818–6952, p.

18. For YAMS: "Soccer Sponsorship," Feb. 9, 1994, Bates 2504051405–1451. For "starters" and "switchers", see Imperial Tobacco Ltd., "Fiscal '80 Media Plans: Phase 1," March 1, 1979, Bates 202345172–5352, pp. 19–22. The "young skew" of the marketing plan for du Maurier reflected, according to company marketing experts, the "large amount of starters duMaurier receives."

62. Roper Research Associates (for Philip Morris), "A Study of Cigarette Smokers' Habits and Attitudes in 1970," May 1970, Bates 1002650000–0392, pp. 3–4.

63. T. L. Achey to Curtis Judge (Lorillard), "Product Information," Aug. 10, 1978, Bates 94684934–5122 at 5039.

64. Lorillard, "Replies to 5-Year Plan Questionnaire," 1981, Bates 85525469–5510, p. 27.

65. Claude E. Teague Jr., "Some Thoughts about New Brands of Cigarettes for the Youth Market," Feb. 2, 1973, Bates 502987357–7368, pp. 10–11.

66. For Teague's 1973 memo, see note 65 above. For the 1975 update: Jim F. Hind to C. A. Tucker, Jan. 23, 1975, Bates 505775557. Hind states that Reynolds's "Meet the Turk" campaign was designed "to shift the brand's age profile to the younger age group." Compare the same company's secret "Planning Assumptions and Forecast for the Period 1977–1986," March 15, 1976, Bates 503327127–7146. For "perfect Camel demographics": Stadium Motorsports, "Camel Point of Sale and Increased Exposure Opportunities 1983," Aug. 24, 1982, Bates 504054574–4576. For Sweden: Marie Friefeldt (IMU-Testologen), "Changes in Smoking Habits and Attitudes towards Marlboro Red," Oct. 18, 1990, Bates 2501173074–3134.

67. For "youthful eye": Philip Gaberman (Creative Director, Brian Associates) to Charles Seide, Aug. 13, 1970, Bates 92352889–2890; also the exposé in *Consumer Reports,* Jan. 1971, p. 5, Bates 504823488. For "video game craze": M. A. Sudholt to S. T. Jones (Lorillard), "New Idea Sessions in the Research Department, July 1982," Aug. 13, 1982, Bates 96509462–9472. In *Minnesota v. Philip Morris* (1998), when evidence was presented that the industry had marketed to twelve-year-olds, the defense argued that this was "a typo and they meant 21 year-olds"; see Devarati Mitra (quoting Channing Robertson), "Tobacco: Behind the Smokes and Mirrors," *Stanford Scientific* (Spring 2003): 26.

68. Marketing and Research Counselors, Inc., "What Have We Learned from People? A Conceptual Summarization of 18 Focus Group Interviews on the Subject of Smoking" (for Ted Bates Advertising for Brown & Williamson), May 26, 1975, Bates 680559454–9490; original emphasis.

69. Lev L. Mandel, Stella A. Bialous, and Stanton A. Glantz, "Avoiding 'Truth': Tobacco Industry Promotion of Life Skills Training," *Journal of Adolescent Health* 39 (2006): 868–79; Melanie Wakefield, Kim McLeod and Cheryl L Perry, "'Stay Away from Them Until You're Old Enough to Make a Decision': Tobacco Company Testimony about Youth Smoking Initiation," *Tobacco Control* 15 (2006): iv44–53. For "alarmingly like a colorful pack": "Blown Cover," *Advertising Age,* Sept. 11, 2000, 34–35.

70. http://tobaccoanalysis.blogspot.com/2006/03/harvard-medical-school-professors .html. Produced by Sunshine Communications with the help of PM's Youth Smoking Prevention Department. For "Raising Kids Who Don't Smoke": http://www2.pmusa.com/en/prc/ activities/downloadresources.asp. And for the impact of such ads: M. C. Farrelly et al., "Getting to the Truth: Evaluating National Tobacco Countermarketing Campaigns," *American Journal of Public Health* 92 (2002): 901–7.

71. R. Dunn, "Camel and the Hollywood Maverick," 1986, Bates 515606728–6729.

72. Teague, "Some Thoughts about New Brands of Cigarettes for the Youth Market," pp. 10–11, with thanks to Geoffrey Schiebinger for this insightful analysis of dual rhetoric.

73. Paul M. Fischer et al., "Brand Logo Recognition by Children Aged 3 to 6 Years: Mickey Mouse and Old Joe the Camel," *JAMA* 266 (1991): 3145–48; Henry A. Waxman, "Tobacco Marketing Profiteering from Children," *JAMA* 266 (1991): 3185–86; Kathleen Deveny, "Joe Camel Is Also Pied Piper, Research Finds," *Wall Street Journal*, Dec. 11, 1991, pp. B1–B4; and for the whitewash: David Smith, *A Camel Called JOE: The Illustrated Story of an American Pop Icon* (Boston: duCap Books, 1998).

74. Bruce Eckman and Shelly Goldberg (for Philip Morris), "The Viability of the Marlboro Man among the 18–24 Segment," March 1992, Bates 2040178502–8519, p. 13.

75. For Jews: Gehrmann Holland (Reynolds), "A Study of Ethnic Markets," Sept. 1969, Bates 501989230–9469; also the ninety-seven-page listing of Reynolds slogans in Bates 514029640–9736. For the military market: Action Marketing Ltd., "Brown & Williamson Military Marketing Plan," April 1978, Bates 660048045–8308. For gays and lesbians and pets and gold jewelry: Leo Burnett Agency (for Philip Morris), "1995 Media Recommendation for Benson & Hedges 100's," Dec. 8, 1994, Bates 2060370113–0175, p. 14; also Joanne Lipman, "Philip Morris to Push Brand in Gay Media," *Wall Street Journal*, Aug. 13, 1992, Bates 2045995474–5475. For "breath conscious": J. W. Carson and B. W. McCarthy, "Report of the Final Days of the SCIMITAR Campaign for B.A.T.," July 1990, Bates 400211403–1465, pp. 4–8; also Bates 506254897. For "virile segment": D. W. Shouse to J. A. Herberger, "Project LF," Feb. 3, 1987, Bates 507371356. For "work is a job": Tobacco Merchants Association, "A Cigarette for You," *TMA Tobacco Weekly*, Feb. 22, 1990, Bates 2501285534–5535. For "burnouts": R. J. Reynolds, "Differentiating within the FUBYAS Group," 1984, Bates 503897087–7101. For "They got lips": Hilts's interview from May 20, 1996, Bates 2070090240–0259.

76. "Benefits—Brand Family Segments" (Reynolds marketing document), Bates 503046115 –6123; Reynolds, "Segment Summary" (Reynolds), 1981, Bates 501984818–4823.

77. For Arabs: Yankelovich, "Marlboro Qualitative Research Presentation, Saudi Arabia," June 1993, Bates 2501084045–4103. For Poland: Philip Morris International, "Poland Marketing Plan," 1993, Bates 2501261059–1171. For Virginia Slims in Korea: "Brand History: Virginia Slims," Sept. 1993, Bates 2057095264–5322 at 5291. For "highly focused attack": Flemming Morgan (BAT Nederland) to T. M. Wilson, Nov. 2, 1993, Bates 500012270–2272. For "hedonic rating": Brown & Williamson, "Total Competitive Smokers," n.d., Bates 465710875–0982. For "Camel Loyal Segments": GRD et al. to D. H. Murphy, "Camel/Winston Significant Activities," July 20, 1994, Bates 514211259–1260. For "on the verge": Gerald H. Long, "Remarks . . . to the Tobacco Seminar," June 8, 1983, Bates 85173427–3654, p. 6.

78. "Cigarette Promotion at Sri Lanka's Major Religious Festival," *Marketing News* (BAT), Dec. 1974, 11–15, Bates 400953289–3319.

79. For "Negroes read": Moss H. Kendrix to J. W. Glenn (Reynolds), March 16, 1948, Bates 500322204; and the marginal note by EHD on Kendrix to W. T. Smither, June 8, 1948, Bates 500322201. For communist agitators: Tilley, *Reynolds Tobacco Company*, 373–414. For Nigger Hair: "The American Tobacco Co.," *Fortune*, Dec. 1936, pp. 96–102, 154–60, in "Publicity Articles," Bates 945359792–0452. *Niggerhead* was a term widely used outside the to-

bacco context, describing specific varieties of coal, termites, oyster tins, and a species of New Zealand sage. Kansas Niggerhead was a flower in the American Midwest, niggerhead coal was a variety that comes in large roundish lumps, and so forth.

80. "'Sold American': Basic Plan," 1944, Bates 945246830–7157, p. 5.

81. For "Negro dollar": A. Bernstein (American Tobacco) to J. F. McDermott, "Pall Mall Sales in Southern Negro Market," Dec. 30, 1958, Bates 990066086–6090. For "negro cigarette": "Philip Morris Campaigns for Negro Market," White Sentinel, ca. July 1956, Bates 2045990400. For 27 percent: G. Weissman (Philip Morris), Oct. 7, 1953, Bates 1001750585–0590. For boycott of "nigger lovers": "Klan Chief Urges Boycott of 3 Firms for NAACP Aid," New York Post, June 24, 1956, Bates 2041942549.

82. J. F. Craft, "Winston Negro Problem Markets," June 21, 1966, Bates 501106692–6701; James Spector to R. Fitzmaurice, "Marlboro Menthol Analysis—Grand Rapids," Sept. 12, 1974, Bates 2040321326–1330.

83. Lorillard, "Why Menthols? A Meandering Rationale Relating Certain Phenomena about Menthol Smokers to an Interesting Opportunity for Newport," 1970, Bates 00486171–6175; original emphasis. This document is not signed, but it appears in Lorillard's files in close proximity to documents to and from Arthur J. Stevens, chief counsel for the company in its New York office. The surrounding documents include correspondence from Stevens to Lennen & Newell, the advertising agency handling the company's Newport account, on how additives such as menthol influence "mouth taste" and "breath freshening." Much of this correspondence is unavailable, having been sequestered as "privileged."

84. For Big Boy: Brown & Williamson, "Project Big Boy," Nov. 14, 1988, Bates 621708903–8929. For military markets: "Special Markets," Pipeline (May 1983): 3, Bates 670118791–8811. For "plums": G. R. Telford to R. D. Hammer et al., "Newport Planning," Jan. 26, 1983, Bates 85172803–2806.

85. For Hispanics operating on a "fantasy level": J. Pericas to C. L. Sharp, "Analysis of the MDD Segmentation Study among Hispanic Smokers," Feb. 18, 1982, Bates 503522931. For Doris Day vs. Clint Eastwood: "Cigarette Market Segmentation Study" (Reynolds), Aug. 12, 1974, Bates 03537963–8000.

86. For "high Jewish populations": Nancy S. Kaufman to J. W. Goss, "1983 Jewish Market Pantry Survey," Feb. 13, 1984, Bates 503490299–0302. For Yiddeshen taam: Joseph Jacobs, "The Sounds of Tel Aviv—Winston Filter Cigarettes," Feb. 20, 1962, Bates 500110339–0344. Reynolds's 1986 "Strategic Summary" talks about Vantage, Salem, and Now as "priority brands in the Jewish market" and notes that Vantage cigarettes were sampled "through the Joseph Jacobs organization that reaches major gatherings of Jewish people in the New York Metropolitan market" ("Jewish Market," Oct. 15, 1985, Bates 504952070–2072).

87. For "short in length": R. . Reynolds, "Segment Summary," 1981, Bates 501984818–4823. For "worrier segment": Ron Beasley et al., "R. J. Reynolds Tobacco Company, Philadelphia Metro," July 23, 1976, Bates 501792034–2077. For "Blatant Lesbians": F. B. Satterthwaite (Lorillard) to R. Smith et al., "Segmenting the Women's Market by Women's Role, Women's Lib and Other Social Forces," June 18, 1973, Bates 84277013–7022. The goal of this latter study was to explore ways to harness "social forces for the cigarette market," including "Women's Lib, Ecology, Homosexuality, Consumerism, Anti-Materialism, Self-Fulfillment, etc."

88. Richard Klein, Cigarettes Are Sublime (Durham: Duke University Press, 1995).

CHAPTER 6

1. Alexis Smith, " 'Satisfiers,' Smokes, and Sports: The Unholy Marriage between Major League Baseball and Big Tobacco," *Sport History Review* 38 (2007): 121–33.

2. Liggett & Myers, "Minutes of Annual Meeting," March 8, 1948, Bates LG0155486–5497; "Statement of Chairman," March 14, 1949, Bates LG0154785–4790; "Statement of Chairman," March 13, 1950, Bates LG0154791–4795.

3. Liggett & Myers, "The Perry Como Show," Jan. 1, 1950, Bates LG0368276–8500; Oct. 11, 1950, Bates LG0084016–4021; Liggett & Myers, "Chesterfield Contract Advertising," Dec. 15, 1950, Bates LG0282755–2756. A swell photo of the Chesterfield Star Team can be found in the *Sporting News* of October 4, 1950.

4. Liggett & Myers, "The Perry Como Show," Oct. 10, 1951, Bates LG0084444–4450; Liggett & Myers, "Personal #5 Philadelphia Only," May 5, 1953, Bates LG0392119; "Young America," Aug. 21, 1953, Bates LG0392167; "Factory Visit #2" (Liggett & Myers), Aug. 21, 1953, Bates LG0392158; "The Chesterfield Supper Club," Jan. 1, 1944, Bates LG0374195–4293; "The Chesterfield Supper Club," Jan. 1, 1945, Bates LG0374294–4816; James E. Kleid to Larry Bruff, Dec. 20, 1957, Bates LG0301956–1959.

5. Alan Blum, "Tobacco Industry Sponsorship of Sports: A Growing Dependency," paper presented to the Surgeon General and Interagency Committee on Smoking and Health, Oct. 27, 1988, Bates 980171240–1336.

6. "Sponsorship: List of Activities Currently and Previously Sponsored by T.A.C. Member Companies," Dec. 18, 1978, Bates 2024928572–8573.

7. Philip Morris, "Why Tobacco Sponsorship?" July 1980, Bates 2025015678–5681.

8. Motorsports Merchandising, "R. J. Reynolds and Automobile Racing," March 23, 1970, Bates 505579294–9314. An excellent early review is BAT's "Motor Sport Sponsorship . . . A Review," *Marketing News,* Feb. 1972, pp. 1–15, Bates 400952490–2781.

9. R. A. Rechholtz, "1971 Management Plan," Sept. 28, 1970, Bates 501706277–6278.

10. "Action on Smoking and Health," *Social Audit* 2 (Autumn 1974): 5–7. John Player & Sons sponsored auto racing in Canada beginning in 1961, and the company's Gold Leaf logo was on Lotus cars at Australia's Grand Prix in Melbourne by 1968. Rothmans took over South Africa's famous Durban July Handicap in 1964 and for thirty-seven years the country's premier horse race was known as the "Rothmans July."

11. "Blum—Tobacco and Sports," 1988, Bates 2025867484–7485.

12. Lisa Greene (Sports Marketing Enterprises) to Seth Moskowitz, Oct. 18, 1989, Bates 507760716–0718; and "1990 Fact Sheet: Sports Marketing," Bates 512574950–4954.

13. N. W. Glover to W. H. Melton (Reynolds), "Doral Skiing Program," Dec. 29, 1970, Bates 500743623–3624; "Proposed United States Ski Association Doral Citizens Racing Program," Oct. 12, 1972, Bates 500767255–7258; also Bates 500743927–3938 and 500079297–9302.

14. "1995 Motorsport Conversion Efforts," March 22, 1995, Bates 514179190–9204; "Camel Conversion Programs," Nov. 1, 1996, Bates 516459420–9430; "Winston Select Expert Panel #1: Conversion Program," 1995, Bates 513254093–4110.

15. For cost per convert: "Conversion #'s: 1995 Camel Character Conversion," July 15, 1996, Bates 515125113–5118. For "conversion specialists": "Motorsports Conversion,"

March 31, 1994, Bates 509239981–9984. For "cost per smoker": "Camel Event Marketing," 1996, Bates 515125133–5138. For personal "intercepts": "Camel Cash Conversion Results," July 20, 1992, Bates 513827243. For strippers as "Camel ambassadors": Cultural Initiator Task Force, "Requirements," July 17, 1997, Bates 520399812–9815.

16. David Fell to P. Turner et al., "1996 World Cup Cricket," July 12, 1993, Bates 303564376–4377.

17. Alan Turner to Peter Turner (W. D. & H. O. Wills), "Potential International Sponsorship for Benson & Hedges World Cup of Cricket 1996," May 19, 1993, Bates 303564380–4388.

18. "Virginia Slims Tennis Sponsorship," June 21, 1994, Bates 2047527761–7763.

19. WTA, "Program Overview," Dec. 1993, Bates 2043686293–6304; ad text is from a 1987 Virginia Slims ad in "Marketing Intelligence Report," Bates 505894926–4954 at 4945.

20. For the MCBF: Mrs. Frank A. Jeffett (Nancy), Chairman, Virginia Slims of Dallas, and President, Maureen Connolly Brinker Tennis Foundation, to Ellen Merlo, Philip Morris, Nov. 7, 1986, Bates 2049403232–03233. For players as young as eleven: "Virginia Slims of Dallas," 1989, Bates 2043631397–1587. For the Ginny, see Bates 2058503716.

21. Canada's tobacco–tennis tryst is nicely sketched in Robert Boughton, "Canadian Open Tennis Hall of Shame," April 23, 2003, http://airspace.bc.ca//content/view/25/53/.

22. Arthur Ashe in his autobiography notes that while tobacco sponsorships troubled some of his colleagues, many were willing collaborators—players such as Roy Emerson of Australia, Manuel Santana of Spain, Rafael Osuna of Mexico, and Ashe himself, all of whom served as consultants for Philip Morris in the 1960s. Ashe also befriended Philip Morris President Joseph F. Cullman III, who, he said, became "a second father to me, an invaluable mentor"; see Ashe's *Days of Grace* (New York: Random House, 1993), p. 207.

23. The "Ginny" insignia first appears as the "coveted 'silver Ginny' trophy" awarded to the player who had accumulated the most points on the Virginia Slims Circuit at the 1973 Virginia Slims Championship in Boca Raton, Florida.

24. "New Virginia Slims Circuit Bows," *Philip Morris Call News*, May 1982, Bates 5001 59505–9520.

25. For under age eighteen: William Esty Co., "Salem Cigarettes: Professional Male Tennis as New Special Event," June 1973, Bates 500726538–6553. For "brand activity": F. Saunders, "Corporate Relations Report," March 30, 1971, Bates 2010027749–7752. For "hypocrite": "Why We Accept Cigarette Ads," *Business and Society Review*, Oct. 1, 1977, Bates TIMN 0066734–6737.

26. Leo Burnett U.S.A., "Philip Morris, U.S.A. Magazine Ad Position Report," 1977, Bates 2040670554–0574.

27. The sarcastic query is Kluger's in his *Ashes to Ashes*, p. 390.

28. Tip Nunn's Events, "Virginia Slims Opinion Poll 2000: Publicity Proposal," March 29, 1999, Bates 2070648649–8660; compare Ellen Merlo to T. Keim et al., Oct. 17, 1983, Bates 2049404778–4779.

29. "Attachment 3—1975 Bowling Program," n.d., Bates 503994403–4404; "Winston-Salem Bowling," n.d., Bates 501316467–6472, p. 57. Bowling was the third most heavily sponsored sport for Reynolds, behind racing and rodeo. For Negro bowlers: C. B. Malcolm to J. O. Watson (Reynolds), "Information Sheet on Bowling," Oct. 24, 1973, Bates 501163466–3467.

30. "Accommodation Program," Nov. 1, 1994, Bates 2045518816 and 8817; "Accommodation Program: 1995 Plan," Bates 2045518949–8981.

31. "Raleigh Cigarettes to Sponsor Professional Purse for Bowling Spectacular" (B&W Press Release), Feb. 27, 1976, Bates 699009908–9909.

32. An excellent overview is J. F. Torroella (Brown & Williamson) to K. Daily, "Lucky Strike Sponsorships and Parallel Communications," May 10, 1983, Bates 660921173–1182.

33. National Cancer Institute, *The Role of the Media in Promoting and Reducing Tobacco Use—Monograph 19* (Bethesda, MD: USDHHS, 2008). In 2000 Nottingham University accepted £3.8 million from British American Tobacco to create an International Centre for Corporate Social Responsibility; see Derek Yach and Stella Aguinaga Bialous, "Junking Science to Promote Tobacco," *American Journal of Public Health* 91 (2001): 1745–48.

34. Rogers & Cowan, "Final Report on Research for the RJR Social Responsibility Program," Jan. 1984, Bates 502658739–8805. For "small business": World Health Organization, "Tobacco Industry and Corporate Responsibility . . . An Inherent Contradiction," Feb. 2003, WHO.

35. One goal of Philip Morris's Virginia Slims Legends tour was to generate names for the company's computerized database and to extend "brand visibility . . . through advertising and public relations"; see "Virginia Slims Creative Brief," 1998, Bates 2071664865–4866. For Merit: Philip Morris, "Merit Bowling Key Talking Points," Aug. 17, 1994, Bates 2024253002. For useful allies: International Bowling Industry, "Smoking: Neutral Stance Sought," Jan. 1, 1996, Bates 2070109386. For Steve Podborski: "Most Feel Tobacco, Booze Firms Should Sponsor Sports, Poll Says," *Toronto Star*, June 4, 1984, Bates TIMN452658.

36. For Palmer: "Bay Hill Classic 1981," Feb. 23, 1981, Bates 680409736–9826. For Bunn: Tobacco Advisory Council, "Sports Sponsorship by Tobacco Companies," April 1985, Bates 2501214107–4118. For Mancuso: Camel Mud & Monster Series press release, Nov. 20, 1989, Bates 507443942–3944. NASCAR driver Richard Lee Petty in 1983 claimed that being able to sell oneself to a well-heeled sponsor was "about as important in racing today as driving ability" (Bates 2172326–2929). Grand National Champion Bobby Isaac, holder of the world record for a closed speedway, hailed Winston sponsorship as "a terrific boost" for stock car racing; see "Company to Sponsor 'Winston 500' Stock Car Race," *Intercom*, Dec. 16, 1970, Bates 503139801–9802.

37. Lacy Lee Rose (Stanford) to Clifford H. Goldsmith (Philip Morris), July 19, 1982, Bates 2040941149, with thanks to Josh Wong. For sponsorship requests, see the letters from Meg Meurer, Manager of Event Promotions, Philip Morris, April 9, 1990, Bates 2048481264 through 2048481277.

38. Frank Saunders "Report of Meeting," *Corporate Relations Report,* March 30, 1971, Bates 2010027749–7752.

39. Ron Scherer, "Tobacco Sponsorships Disputed," *Christian Science Monitor,* Jan. 16, 1991, Bates TIMN 371435; A. Charlton et al., "Boys' Smoking and Cigarette-Brand-Sponsored Motor Racing," *Lancet* 350 (1997): 1474.

40. R. J. Reynolds, "Corporate Public Relations and Public Affairs Monthly Events Calendar, Sept. 1985," Aug. 22, 1985, Bates 505466959–6964; also Bates 661200261.

41. BAT Central Africa by 1966 was sponsoring golf and motor racing but also "soccer,

rugby, cricket, horse racing and show jumping"; see the company's "Annual Report and Accounts," Nov. 10, 1966, Bates 300076922–6936.

42. For $77 million: Barry Meier, "A Controversy on Tobacco Road," *New York Times,* Dec. 4, 1997. For "world's leading corporate sponsor": "A Day in the Life: This Is Philip Morris," 1994, Bates 2050272003.

43. "Soccer Sponsorship," Feb. 9, 1994, Bates 2504051405–1451.

44. "Some Non-Tobacco Trademarks Owned by US Tobacco Companies," 1994, Bates 2041221080–1084. Skoal also sponsored the U.S. ski team and NASCAR and by the 1990s was broadcasting a daily "Skoal Motorsports Report" on more than a hundred radio stations; see "Corporate Sponsors Drive the Right Messages Home," *U.S. Tobacco and Candy Journal,* July 27–Aug. 24, 1987, pp. 46, 84. For Louis Bantle: Mike Knepper, "Speed Merchants: Why are American Companies Spending $5 Million at the Track?" *Continental,* Feb. 1983, pp. 58–61 and 78–79, Bates 990750922–1020.

45. Chris Hastings and Patrick Hennessy, "Revealed: The Truth about Tony Blair's Role in the Ecclestone Affair," *Sunday Telegraph,* Oct. 11, 2008.

46. For BAT's Kent: Samuel Abt, "Take a Puff, It's the Tour of China!" *International Herald Tribune,* Nov. 3, 1995. BAT sponsored the 555 Hong Kong–Beijing Rally annually from 1990. For television: "Marketing Conference PRC Presentation," Dec. 10, 1992, Bates 2504017237–7257. For Beckham: Geoffrey A. Fowler, "Treaty May Stub out Cigarette Ads in China," *Wall Street Journal,* Dec. 2, 2003, http://www.mindfully.org/WTO/2003/China-Cigarette-Ads2dec03.htm.

47. "Soviet Union: Low Nicotine Novelty," *World Tobacco* (Sept.–Oct. 1973): 35, Bates 1000271932; Anastasia Osipova, "Smoke of the Motherland," *Russian Life* (Jan.–Feb. 2007): 51–54.

48. J. T. McCarthy (Reynolds), "Winston Rodeo Series," Oct. 1, 1979, Bates 500138938–8944.

49. "Benson & Hedges Series Night Cricket in South Africa," *Marketing News* (BAT), Aug. 1983, pp. 4–7, Bates 400981948–2247.

50. For Kim logo: "Promotional Activity Report: BAT Pleads Not Guilty to TV Loophole Charge," June 14, 1983, Bates 660938618–8619. For Winston 500: "Sponsoring a Major GN NASCAR Race," July 9, 1970, Bates 500728566–8575. For "under ten years of age": *Trees Newsletter,* March 1986, Bates 107342173–2206, p. 12. Philip Morris ended its Marlboro Trail racing sponsorship in 1972, when Brown & Williamson started entering powerful Viceroy cars. Philip Morris didn't relish the idea of seeing "Viceroy entries carrying off Marlboro prize money"; see "In the U.S.A. Viceroy Takes to the Track," BAT's *Marketing News,* Feb. 1972, Bates 400952490–2781.

51. B. L. Murtaugh to T. B. Owen, "Winston Championship Auto Shows," Jan. 15, 1982, Bates 503897257–7269.

52. Peter Chapman to Monty Kiernan, "Kent Sports Business," Sept. 16, 1983, Bates 87277428–7429.

53. For African American reps: B. M. Bruner and R. N. Gladding to H. R. Hanmer and W. R. Harlan, Aug. 23, 1961, Bates 966003997–3999. For Newport giveaways, see the deposition of Marie R. Evans for *Evans v. Lorillard,* May 29, 2002.

54. KNT Plusmark, "Camel: Project Big Idea Concept Development," June 21, 1988, Bates 506888749–8801.

55. "1981 Winston Pro Series: Motorcycle Racing Program," 1981, Bates 503777627–7637.

56. Lauren Lazinsk to Ina Broeman, "Virginia Slims Fashion Spree Markets," Feb. 28, 1992, Bates 2043524905–4908.

57. For press clippings: Cohn & Wolfe, "Virginia Slims Championships, 1993 Wrap-Up," Jan. 24, 1994, Bates, 2040233876–4240. For readership: "Event Marketing Publicity Results," 1998, Bates 2071664878. For protests: "1997 Spring Results," 1997, Bates 2071664874.

58. "Conference Addresses Domestic Violence," *PM Globe,* Oct. 1998, Bates 2076281639–1642.

59. See the NCI's *Monograph 19,* esp. Lisa Henricksen's chapter 6, "Tobacco Companies' Public Relations Efforts," pp. 184–85.

60. "Philip Morris Companies Inc. and the Virginia Slims Legends Salute Pittsburgh AIDS Task Force," in "The Virginia Slims Legends Tour," Oct. 17, 1998, Bates 2070897424–7470 at 7429.

61. Philip Morris America Latina, "Por un mundo mejor: Protegemos nuestros recursos naturales," 1998, Bates 2074086560–6575; Cathy L. Leiber to William Webb, Jan. 9, 1998, Bates 2074086559.

62. Bob Herbert, "Tobacco Dollars," *New York Times,* Nov. 28, 1993, Bates 20246012635; Steve Herman, "Cartoons, Cotton-Candy, and the Marlboro Man: The Targeting of Children for Addiction by the Tobacco Industry," Dec. 23, 1995, Bates 2075792203–2243.

63. *BAT Marketing News,* July 1983, Bates 690133902–3929, pp. 1–7.

64. J. DeParle, "Warning: Sports Stars May Be Hazardous to Your Health," *Washington Monthly,* Sept. 1989, pp. 34–49.

65. BAT, "Note to the Chief Executive's Committee: Formula One Sponsorship Proposal," 1997, Bates 800414168–4181.

CHAPTER 7

1. Charles E. Lewis (president of Charlie's) to Ina Broeman (PM's director of marketing), Oct. 26, 1989, Bates 2048669807–9808; compare Vicki Berner to Brian Cury, Dec. 14, 1989, Bates 2047987689–7690. Philip Morris's sampling procedures are detailed in its "Marlboro Sampling Manual," 1980, Bates TIMN0064405–4417.

2. "PM USA Sponsorship," 1999, Bates 2064977096.

3. For Gold Club: "Gold Club Surveillance in Kitchener-Waterloo Region March-June 2003," in *Filter-Tips: A Review of Cigarette Marketing in Canada,* 4th ed., Winter 2003. For viral advertising: Yogi Hendlin, Stacey J. Anderson, and Stanton Glantz, "'Acceptable Rebellion': Marketing Hipster Aesthetics to Sell Camel Cigarettes in the US," *Tobacco Control* 19 (2010): 213–22.

4. An excellent overview is Reynolds's "Special Promotions," Sept. 28, 1982, Bates 504021512–1546—which also has a précis of sponsorships by the alcohol industry. For Spanish language media: Mary Munkenbeck to Jack McAuley, Oct. 18, 1982, Bates 2045086452–6453. For Marlboro Menthol: C. Cohen, "Marlboro Menthol Inner City Bar Night Program," May 11, 1988, Bates 2048479521.

5. R. W. A. Hermans (Philip Morris Europe) to R. W. Murray, "Sponsorship of the Arts," July 14, 1978, Bates 2024258179–8181, where we also hear that support for the arts "enhances the image of the sponsor because it has the tendency to be aimed at the top end of the social scale. In that sense it certainly has commercial value."

6. Alisa Solomon, "The Other Nicotine Addiction," *Village Voice,* Oct. 18, 1994, Bates 2041128423–8548.

7. For examples in the United States, see "Miscellaneous Anti-Smoking Subjects," 1995, Bates 2072914997–5005, also at http://www.tobacco.org/Misc/collaborators.html#aa1.

8. For "innocence by association": http://www.tobacco.org/Misc/collaborators.html#aa1. For "Elgar and Tchaikovsky": Peter R. Taylor, *The Smoke Ring: Tobacco, Money, and Multinational Politics* (New York: Pantheon, 1984), p. 28.

9. Solomon, "The Other Nicotine Addiction."

10. Philip Morris, "Marlboro Music Stage: Bringing the Best Latin Talent to the Marlboro Music Stage," 1995, Bates 2040591382.

11. "Kool Strategic Brand Plan—Executive Summary," 1980, Bates 661081684–1713.

12. " 'Kool Jazz Festivals' Promotion Study," Sept. 21, 1979, Bates 670548387–8438. Other manufacturers established music labels: Silk Cut in the mid-1990s produced a CD titled *Silk Cut Classics,* for example, and Reynolds had earlier reissued Benny Goodman and his Orchestra through its Camel Caravan Label, decked out in full cigarette regalia.

13. For "half a million Blacks": "To: All Field Personnel: Kool Jazz Festivals General Information," June 18, 1981, Bates 670138027–8028. For "great bonanza" and "dream come true": "George Wein Presents the Kool Jazz Festival," 1982, Bates 685053242–3302.

14. Louanna O. Heuhsen to Martha W. Verscaj, May 14, 1990, Bates 2065055750.

15. Reynolds, "Field Marketing Presentation Draft," Dec. 15, 1982, Bates 504072296–2304.

16. Brandt, *Cigarette Century,* p. 94.

17. Reynolds, "Camel Expeditions Presentation," March 1, 1981, Bates 501482619–2629.

18. "Tobacco: External Communications" (for Reynolds), 1982, Bates 500657677–7683.

19. For Green Fashion Fall: Brandt, *Cigarette Century,* pp. 84–86. For Ebony Fashion fairs: M. G. McAllister to C. W. Fitzgerald, "Ebony Fashion Fair," May 7, 1975, Bates 501139280–9281, and Reynolds's "Field Marketing Presentation," Dec. 15, 1982, Bates 504072296–2304. For Newport tattoos: Apres Events, "Proposal to Lorillard for Newport Special Events and Sampling Program for Long Island," May 7, 1994, Bates 93114296–4299. And for wilder ideas: "Virginia Slims Idea Generation," March 2000, Bates 2078801860–1863.

20. Guy L. Smith IV to R. William Murray, Oct. 9, 1989, Bates 2023277090–7091. For a film festival, see " 'Benson & Hedges 100 Movie Classics' Booking Schedule," June 1976, Bates 2042016629.

21. BAT, "Guidelines on Communication Restrictions and New Opportunities in Marketing," June 14, 1979, Bates 670828367–8381.

22. "Salem Business Review," July 27, 1998, Bates 522879546–9548.

23. Kathryn Mulvey, Mary Assunta, and Konstantin Krasovsky et al. for INFACT, *Global Aggression: The Case for World Standards and Bold US Action Challenging Philip Morris and RJR Nabisco* (New York: Apex Press, 1998), pp. 57–58.

24. C. A. Tucker, "1975 Marketing Plans," Bates 501421310–1335 at 1320.

25. Mulvey et al., *Global Aggression,* 86.

26. Paul Nuki, "Tobacco Firms Brew up Coffee to Beat Ad Ban," *Sunday Times,* Jan. 18, 1998, Bates 2074783874.

27. HotNews.ro, "Multinationals in Breach of Romanian Tobacco Ads Law," *Romanian-Newsy,* Oct. 3, 2006.

28. "Elementary Schools Named after Tobacco Industry in China," *China Hush,* Jan. 20, 2010; "Should Tobacco Sponsorship of Education Be Banned?" *Beijing Review,* Feb. 5, 2010; "China Wrestles with Tobacco Control: An Interview with Dr. Yang Gonghuan," *Bulletin of the World Health Organization* 88 (2010): 241–320.

29. Philip Morris, "Marketing New Products in a Restrictive Environment," 1990, Bates 2044762173–2364 at 2236.

30. For an impressive list of promotional activities of one company in just one month, see Reynolds's "Competitive Promotional Activity Report," Dec. 1971, Bates 2049307194–7198. More than a hundred possible ideas for how to market the company's Dakota brand can be found in "Other Ways to Reach the Target," Oct. 2, 1989, Bates 507176999–7016.

31. See my *Cancer Wars,* 270–71.

CHAPTER 8

1. The literature here is vast; see Joe Giesenhagen, *Collector's Guide to Vintage Cigarette Packs* (Atglen, PA: Schiffer, 1999); Fernando Righini and Marco Papazonni, *International Collectors' Book of Cigarette Packs* (Atglen, PA: Schiffer, 1998); Mark F. Moran, *Warman's Tobacco Collectibles* (Iola, WI: Krause Publications, 2003).

2. More familiar is the theory that baseball's "bullpen" derives from American Tobacco's practice of giving players prizes for hitting its Bull Durham billboards at the back of the field—behind which were cages where the pitchers warmed up.

3. Charles Henry Bingham, "Vending Apparatus for Cigars, Cigarettes, &c.," U.S. Patent Office, Aug. 23, 1887, Patent No. 368,869.

4. H. A. Kent (Lorillard) to Todd Wool, March 17, 1938, Bates 80686600–6601.

5. Philip Morris Research and Development, "Vending Machine Growth," *tif Smoke Signals,* June 8, 1979, Bates 1000769885–9892.

6. J. W. Marsh (Reynolds), "Status Report—December 1982," Jan. 10, 1983, Bates 5040 90775–0780. And for the elaborate fees paid by the companies to place specific brands in specific rows, see AT's "Circular Book" for Aug. 1 to Sept. 30, 1963, Bates 947043747–4226.

7. See the Computer History Museum's "Timeline of Computer History," http://www.computerhistory.org/timeline/?category = cmptr.

8. Clara L. Gouin, "Non-Smokers and Social Action," in *Proceedings of the Third World Conference on Smoking and Health,* vol. 2 (Washington, DC: U.S. Government Printing Office, 1977), p. 356.

9. "Attachment II: General Line of Questioning," Oct. 30, 1997, Bates 466853974–3978; compare Bates 2060569570–9574.

10. Edward Sanders to Cathy Ellis, Aug. 18, 1998, Bates 2060569578–9581. Phillips poured about $600,000 into this project in the mid-1990s, prior to pulling out when the tobacco industry started having significant legal difficulties.

11. Tobacco Documentation Centre, "Directory of Internet Resources," June 1996, Bates 503921732–1764.

12. Tobacco Research Board, "Tobacco and the Internet," ca. 1995, Bates 800159973–9990.

13. Michelle Pentz, "Smoke Gets on the Net," *Convergence,* Summer 1996, Bates 50392 1783–1790.

14. http://www.tobaccofreekids.org/reports/internet/. In October 2008 the official site for Marlboro Miles listed twelve clickable sites for purchasing cigarettes online. Cigarettes bought on such sites are much cheaper than retail: $14.90 for a carton of 200 Marlboro Reds, for example, which is less than a third what one would pay in, say, New York City. See http://marlboromiles.cigarettes-online-store.com/marlboro-miles-catalog.html.

15. U.S. General Accounting Office, *Internet Cigarette Sales* (Aug. 2002), http://www.gao.gov/new.items/do2743.pdf.

16. Kurt M. Ribisl, Rebecca S. Williams, and Annice E. Kim, "Internet Sales of Cigarettes to Minors," *JAMA* 290 (2003): 1356–59.

17. Kathleen Hunter, "States Hunt Down Online Cigarette Buyers," May 3, 2005 (online).

18. "Credit Card Firms Agree Not to Enable Web Cigarette Sales," *Direct Newsline,* March 21, 2005, Bates 551804079.

19. See, for example, the Wiki CigarettePedia site, http://www.cigarette.pedia.com, where you can view tens of thousands of different kinds of cigarette packs.

20. See http://www.trinketsandtrash.org/tearsheet.asp?ItemNum = 212384.

21. http://www.smokingfetishsites.com/scores.htm; compare http://www.smokinbabe.com/free/index.php. Lorillard's Youth Smoking Prevention website in the early 2000s was www.buttoutnow.com; it has since become a pornography site.

22. http://www.oltra.org/a trade association. OLTRA itself links to a number of pro-smoking groups, such as smokinglobby.com, The Smoking Outdoorsman, etc.

23. "BlackBerry Connection," http://www.blackberry.com/newsletters/connection/it/i6–2007/sampson.shtml. And on YouTube more generally: Becky Freeman and Simon Chapman, "Is 'YouTube' Telling or Selling You Something? Tobacco Content on the YouTube Video-Sharing Website," *Tobacco Control* 16 (2007): 207–10.

24. http://whyquit.com/pr/043008.htmlQuit.

25. G. T. Fong, D. Hammond, and S. C. Hitchman, "The Impact of Pictures on the Effectiveness of Tobacco Warnings," *Bulletin of the World Health Organization* 87 (2009): 640–43.

PART II

1. Egon Lorenz et al., "The Effects of Breathing Tobacco Smoke on Strain A Mice," *Cancer Research,* 3 (1943): 123; compare also Egon Lorenz, "Experimental Studies on Tobacco Smoke," *Proceedings of the National Cancer Conference,* 1949, p. 203. Nowhere in either publication is it mentioned that major support for these projects came from the American Tobacco Company.

2. Ecusta documents were first introduced into litigation by Woody Wilner et al. in *Henry W. Boerner v. Brown & Williamson,* tried in May 2003 in Arkansas; I introduced further documents testifying in *Frankson v. American Tobacco,* Nov. 18–19, 2003.

3. Ernst L. Wynder, Evarts A. Graham and Adele B. Croninger, "Experimental Production of Carcinoma with Cigarette Tar," *Cancer Research,* 13 (1953): 855–66; and for its impact: Kluger, *Ashes to Ashes,* pp. 162–66, and Stanton Glantz et al., *The Cigarette Papers* (Berkeley: University of California Press, 1996), pp. 33–35.

CHAPTER 9

1. Glenn Sonnedecker, "Drug Standards Become Official," in *The Early Years of Federal
Food and Drug Control* (Madison, WI: American Institute of the History of Pharmacy, 1982),
pp. 28–39. Karl L. Reimann and Christian W. Posselt isolated nicotine in pure form in 1828;
see Paul Koenig, *Die Entdeckung des reinen Nikotins im Jahre 1828 an der Universität Heidelberg* (Bremen: A. Geist, 1940).

2. *United States Pharmacopoeia,* 8th rev. (Philadelphia: Lippincott, 1905), p. lxii. This new
edition still recognized belladonna, opium, cannabis, cocaine, silver cyanide, and numerous
arsenic and mercury compounds as legitimate drugs.

3. See M. V. Cornil, "Sur les greffes et inoculations de cancer," *Bulletin de l'Académie de
médecine* 25 (1891): 906–9.

4. K. Yamagiwa and K. Ichikawa, "Experimentelle Studie über die Pathogenese der Epi-
thelialgeschwülste," *Mitteilungen aus der medizinischen Fakultät der kaiserlichen Universität
zu Tokyo* 15 (1916): 295–344.

5. Wilhelm C. Hueper, *Occupational Tumors and Allied Diseases* (Springfield, IL:
Charles C. Thomas, 1942); Donner Foundation, *Index to Literature of Experimental Cancer
Research 1900 to 1935* (Philadelphia: Donner Foundation, 1948), pp. 994–95.

6. Anton Brosch, "Theoretische und experimentelle Untersuchungen zur Pathogenesis
und Histogenesis der malignen Geschwülste," *Virchows Archiv für pathologische Anatomie
und Physiologie* 162 (1900): 32–84, esp. p. 70.

7. Ulysses S. Grant's death from cancer of the throat in 1885 was widely traced to his
smoking; see James T. Patterson, *The Dread Disease: Cancer and Modern American Culture*
(Cambridge, MA: Harvard University Press, 1987), pp. 1–35. Tobacco industry chronologies prepared for internal use in the 1940s and 1950s recognized smoking as an undisputed
cause of oral and esophageal cancer; see Paul Larson and Harvey Haag, "Cancer of the Esophagus, Stomach and Intestines, Liver and Bladder," Jan. 1—Dec. 31, 1950, Bates 500508793–8794.

8. Victor E. Mertens, "Zigarettenrauch eine Ursache des Lungenkrebses? (Eine Anregung)," *Zeitschrift für Krebsforschung* 32 (1930): 82; R. G. J. P. Huismann, "Tobacco and Lung
Cancer," 1940, Bates 503244772–4792.

9. Fritz Lickint, "Tabak und Tabakrauch als ätiologischer Factor des Carcinoms," *Zeitschrift für Krebsforschung* 30 (1929): 349–65; Herbert L. Lombard and Carl R. Doering, "Cancer Studies in Massachusetts," *New England Journal of Medicine* 198 (1928): 481–86.

10. Müller, "Tabakmissbrauch," 78, emphasis in original; and for background, see my *Nazi
War on Cancer,* 173–247.

11. Eberhard Schairer and Erich Schöniger, "Lungenkrebs und Tabakverbrauch," *Zeitschrift für Krebsforschung* 54 (1943): 261–69; also my *Nazi War on Cancer,* 183–217. Ernest L.
Wynder and Evarts A. Graham, "Tobacco Smoking as a Possible Etiologic Factor in Bron-

chiogenic Carcinoma," *JAMA* 143 (1950): 329–36. Austin Smith, Fishbein's successor as editor of *JAMA*, solicited the articles by Wynder and Graham and by Morton Levin published in the May 27, 1950, issue of *JAMA;* see Hiram R. Hanmer, "Memorandum on Telephone Conversation with Mr. Hahn," June 16, 1950, Bates MNAT00733134. Wynder and Graham's research had already attracted attention; see William L. Laurence, "Cigarettes Linked to Cancer in Lungs," *New York Times,* Feb. 27, 1949. Doll and Hill's careful work includes their "Smoking and Carcinoma" and their "The Mortality of Doctors in Relation to Their Smoking Habits," *BMJ* 1 (1954): 1451–55. And for an overview: Colin White, "Research on Smoking and Lung Cancer: A Landmark in the History of Chronic Disease Epidemiology," *Yale Journal of Biology and Medicine* 63 (1990): 29–46.

12. Lorenz et al., "Effects of Breathing Tobacco Smoke." For "reassuring experiments": Hiram Hanmer to Henry S. Patricoff, March 9, 1949, Bates 950204894. And for a press report: "Smoking Mice Live Normal Span: U.S. Experiments Fail to Prove Cancer Rise," *U.S. News and World Report,* Feb. 3, 1950, pp. 22–23.

13. A. C. Hilding, "Phagocytosis, Mucous Flow, and Ciliary Action," *Archives of Environmental Health* 6 (1963): 61–73.

14. Otto Mühlbock, "Carcinogene Werking van Sigarettenrook bij Muizen," *Nederlands Tijdschrift voor Geneeskund* 99 (1955): 2276–78, Bates 2023693883–3885; Murco N. Roegholt to Sydney Negus, Sept. 5, 1955, Bates 950166932. Roegholt here also mentions the view of the pathologist H. E. Schornagel of Rotterdam affirming the link between smoking and cancer of the lung as "doubtless."

CHAPTER 10

1. Angel H. Roffo, "Was Man von dem Krebs wissen muss. Auflklärungsschrift," Buenos Aires, 1928.

2. Angel H. Roffo, "Durch Tabak beim Kaninchen entwickeltes Carcinom," *Zeitschrift für Krebsforschung* 33 (1931): 321. Roffo had earlier produced precancerous leukoplakias on the ears of rabbits using tobacco tars; see his "Leucoplasia tabáquica experimental," *Boletín del Instituto de Medicina Experimental* 7 (1930): 130–44.

3. Angel H. Roffo, "El tabaco como Cancerígeno," *Boletín del Instituto de Medicina Experimental* 42 (1936): 287–336; also his "Krebserzeugendes Benzpyren gewonnen aus Tabakteer," *Zeitschrift für Krebsforschung* 49 (1939): 588–97. Some of this work was done by Roffo's son, A. E. Roffo Jr.; see his "Espectrografía de los derivados obtenidos por destilación directa de los tabacos y su relación como agentes cancerígenos," *Boletín del Instituto de Medicina Experimental* 45 (1937): 311–99. R. J. Reynolds scientists later claimed to have "corroborated the published findings with respect to 3,4-benzpyrene, obtained this compound in crystalline form, and positively identified it as a constituent of cigarette smoke on the basis of its chemical and physical properties"; see Alan Rodgman to Kenneth H. Hoover, Nov. 2, 1959, Bates 500945942–5945, p. 1. Reynolds measured 81 micrograms of 3,4-benzpyrene in the smoke of one kilogram of Winstons; see A. Rodgman and L. C. Cook, "The Analysis of Cigarette Smoke Condensate," Dec. 1, 1958, Bates 504912197–2250. Brown & Williamson scientists in 1952 reported "a partial isolation and identification of the aromatic hydrocarbon, ben-

zopyrene, in both smoke and original tobacco from Raleigh blend cigarettes." The report refers to benzopyrene as a "carcinogenic hydrocarbon"; see "Report of Progress," Dec. 24, 1952, Bates 650200084–0095.

4. Angel H. Roffo, "Krebserzeugende Tabakwirkung," *Monatsschrift für Krebsbekämpfung*, 8 (1940): 97–102; also his "El tabaco rubio como cancerígeno," *Boletín del Instituto de Medicina Experimental* 47 (1938): 5–22; Roffo, "El tabaco como cancerígeno," p. 333.

5. For large pool, see Angel H. Roffo, "Krebserzeugende Einheit der verschiedenen Tabakteere," *Deutsche medizinische Wochenschrift* 65 (1939): 963–67. For skin cancer: Angel H. Roffo, "Cáncer y sol: Carcinomas y sarcomas producidos por la acción del sol total," *Boletín del Instituto de Medicina Experimental* 11 (1934): 353 ff. For skin pigmentation: Roffo's son authored the most elaborate study of this type; see A. E. Roffo Jr., "Reacción cutanea a las radiaciones actinicas en relación con la pigmentación congenita de la piel," *Boletín del Instituto de Medicina Experimental* 43 (1936): 287–408. For sex differences: Roffo, "Durch Tabak," p. 322. For *"fast experimentelle Wert"*: Angel H. Roffo, "Der Tabak als krebserzeugendes Agens," *Deutsche medizinische Wochenschrift* 63 (1937): 1268. This last-cited article can be found in translation in Lorillard's files; see "Selected Lorillard Chronology Materials," n.d., Bates 98919147–9546.

6. Sir Richard Doll, "Commentary: Lung Cancer and Tobacco Consumption," *International Journal of Epidemiology* 30 (2001): 30–31.

7. Schairer and Schöniger, "Lungenkrebs"; Müller, "Tabakmissbrauch"; Fritz Lickint, *Tabak und Organismus: Handbuch der gesamten medizinischen Tabakkunde* (Stuttgart: Hippokrates, 1939), pp. 869–71; Leonard Engel, "Cigarettes Cause Cancer?" *Reader's Scope* (Aug. 1946): 3–7; Edwin J. Grace, "Tobacco Smoking and Cancer of the Lung," *American Journal of Surgery* 60 (1943): 361–64.

8. For "until recently": Hanmer to Hahn, "Memorandum on Alleged Causative Relation." For "highly carcinogenic": Claude E. Teague, "Survey of Cancer Research," Feb. 2, 1953, Bates 504184873–4894. For the industry's expert witness: Lauren V. Ackerman (Expert Report), Oct. 1, 1959, Bates 2025018461–8608. For "plaintiffs may focus": Jones, Day, Reavis & Pogue, "Dr. Claude E. Teague, Jr., Deposition Preparation," Oct. 16, 1990, Bates 515873224–3304, p. 6; henceforth cited as: Jones Day, "Teague Depo. Prep." Roffo was cited in most of the cancer research bibliographies constructed by the industry: Paul S. Larson, Harvey B. Haag, and H. Silvette's massive *Tobacco: Experimental and Clinical Studies: A Comprehensive Account of the World Literature* (Baltimore: Williams and Wilkins, 1961), for example, cites forty-three Roffo articles. The Donner Foundation's 1935 *Index to Literature of Experimental Cancer Research* lists fifty-nine.

9. H. R. Hanmer to Edward Elway Free, May 11, 1939, Bates MNAT00637003. Hanmer cited a passage from the *Zeitschrift für Krebsforschung* (translated from the German) questioning the methods Roffo had used to diagnose carcinoma, showing that the industry by this time was employing translators to render foreign medical publications into English. The only known full-article translations of Roffo prior to 2006 are those done by Lorillard in the 1980s, probably for litigation; see Bates 85869514–9521 and my "Angel H. Roffo: The Forgotten Father of Experimental Tobacco Carcinogenesis," *Bulletin of the World Health Organization* 84 (2006): 494–95.

10. Ernst L. Wynder, Evarts A. Graham, and Adele B. Croninger, "Experimental Pro-

duction of Carcinoma with Cigarette Tar" *Cancer Research* 13 (1953): 855; Roffo, "Der Tabak," p. 1269.

11. Hans Reiter, "Der Stand der wissenschaftlichen Erforschungen der Tabakgefahren," *Reine Luft* 23 (1941): 97–101. On nicotine-free cigarettes and "light beer": "Vorsorge und Fürsorge am Menschen und am Arbeitsplatz—Entwöhnung—Ersatzmitttel," *Reine Luft* 23 (1941): 65–67.

12. Leonardo Conti, "Der Reichsgesundheitsführer," *Reine Luft* 23 (1941): 87–93. Smoking caused "den schwersten Schaden, der dem deutschen Volke zugefügt werden kann." Lickint by 1953 found it "inconceivable" that a serious argument could be made against the smoking–lung cancer link; see his *Ätiologie und Prophylaxe des Lungenkrebses,* translated as "Tobacco Smoke as a Cause of Lung Cancer," Bates 501902445–2559.

13. Lawrence K. Altman, "Experts Re-Examine Dr. Reiter, His Syndrome and His Nazi Past," *New York Times,* March 7, 2000.

14. The epidemiology referenced is Schairer and Schöniger's "Lungenkrebs"; see my *Nazi War on Cancer,* pp. 206–17. Karl Astel's remarks are in "Der Rektor der Friedrich-Schiller-Universität Staatsrat Prof. Dr. K. Astel," *Reine Luft* 23 (1941): 93–96.

15. Hitler's telegram of April 5, 1941, to Reichsgesundheitsführer Leonardo Conti and Gauleiter Sauckel is reproduced in *Reine Luft* 23 (1941): 81.

16. G. Becher, "Sind Wir wirklich Muradisten?" *Reine Luft* 21 (1939): 119–22; "Forschung oder Behauptung?" *Deutsche Tabakzeitung,* reprinted in *Chronica Nicotiana* 2, no. 1 (1941): 22–24.

17. "Die Entwicklung der Internationalen Tabakwissenschaftlichen Gesellschaft," *Chronica Nicotiana* 1, nos. 3–4 (1940): 25 ff. Helmuth Aschenbrenner was general secretary of the International Association, and it would be useful to have a biography of this man. On Forchheim, see *50 Jahre: Landesanstalt für Tabakbau und Tabakforschung, Forchheim* (Baden-Württemberg, 1977).

18. "Ergebnisse der Tabakforschung," *Deutsche Tabakzeitung,* Dec. 4, 1940, cited in *Reine Luft* 23 (1941): 40.

19. For a photo of the Führer's bust in the nerve center of German tobacco apologetics, see *Chronica Nicotiana* 2, no. 1 (1941): 8.

20. Friedrich Richter, *Raubstaat England* (Hamburg-Bahrenfeld: Cigaretten-Bilderdienst, 1941), 129; compare *Adolf Hitler: Bilder aus dem Leben des Führers* (Altona-Bahrenfeld: Cigaretten-Bilderdienst, 1935), 300,000 copies of which were printed.

21. For "tar" denial, see the comment on Br. Steinwallner's "Tabak und Zähne," *Chronica Nicotiana* 1, no. 2 (1940): 118–19. Regarding moderation: "If someone drinks 15–20 cups of coffee a day, that is just as bad from a health point of view as smoking 30–40 cigarettes a day, or drinking 15 or more liters of beer"; see "Einiges über die Schädlichkeit oder Unschädlichkeit von Genussmitteln," *Chronica Nicotiana* 1, no. 2 (1940): 97–100; compare Fritz Lickint, "Gegen den Missbrauch des Tabakmissbrauches: Eine Erwiderung und Richtigstellung," *Reine Luft* 21 (1939): 118–19. And for "crazy" to inhale: Adolf Wenusch commenting on Otto Schmidt, "Der Kohlenoxydgehalt des Blutes bei Raucher," *Chronica Nicotiana* 1, no. 2 (1940): 121–24.

22. Peter Schesslitz, "Tabak und Krebs," *Deutsche Tabakzeitung,* 1941, reprinted in *Reine Luft* 22 (1941): 39.

23. "Verkort de Tabak het menselijk Leven?" from *Le Cigare* via *De Tabakskoerier*, Holland's leading tobacco industry journal, reproduced in *Chronica Nicotiana* 1, nos. 3–4 (1940): 49.

24. R. G. J. P. Huismann, "Tabak und Lungenkrebs," *Chronica Nicotiana* 4 (May–June 1943): 7–19; 4 (July–Aug. 1943): 5–15. The referenced Ph.D. dissertation is by Frits Vaandrager in Utrecht. Pieter de Coninck informs me that Huismann died in January 1972 in Appeltern (Walstraat 2). We need to know more about his life and work—whether he continued to work for Big Tobacco after 1945, for example, and whether he ever accepted cigarette causation.

25. For "many questions remain open": Huismann, "Tabak und Lungenkrebs." For Helmuth Aschenbrenner's "Autoreferat": "Psyche und Krebs," *Chronica Nicotiana* 4 (April 1943): 42. For Aschenbrenner on "big fire," see my *Nazi War on Cancer*, p. 242.

26. On Raynaud's disease: L. Brigatti, "Versuche einer Therapie," *Chronica Nicotiana* 4 (May–June 1943): 29. For "prohibitionist afterlife": *Vereinigte Tabakzeitungen*, Oct. 28, 1938, cited in Fritz Lickint, "Gegen den Missbrauch des Tabakmissbrauches," *Reine Luft* 21 (1939): 119. Dr. med. H. Brückner of Berlin offered the following summary in his review of H. Lungwitz's "Tabak und Neurose," *Chronica Nicotiana* 4 (July–Aug. 1943): 30–32:

> In der Lungwitzschen metaphysikfreien Weltanschauung gibt es keine Kausalität, die irgend etwas verursacht, etwa eine Krankheit bedingen könnte; das kausale Denken ist als ein Überbleibsel der dämonischen Weltanschauung erkannt und entfällt somit als Irrtum und Fiktion. Die Meinung, dass der gesunde Mensch durch Tabakrauchen als ein wirkendes Agens krank werden könne, wird eindeutig widerlegt.

27. "Die Gefahr im Schatten: Chronica et acta phantastica," *Reine Luft* 23 (1941): 34–43.

CHAPTER 11

1. Alan Finder, "At One University, Tobacco Money Is Not Taboo; It's a Secret," *New York Times*, May 22, 2008, p. A1.

2. Asked about Trani's tobacco board membership, the university spokeswoman Pam Lepley responded: "I don't see any connection between these two. . . . And his being on the board doesn't really pertain to the university." The journalist Chris Dovi had a different interpretation, commenting, "Trani is the tobacco industry"; see his "VCU President Gets Paycheck from Tobacco Company," *Style Weekly*, May 28, 2008.

3. Upton Sinclair, *I, Candidate for Governor: And How I Got Licked* (Los Angeles: End Poverty League, 1935).

4. Charles L. Van Noppen, *Death in Cellophane* (Greensboro, NC: Charles L. Van Noppen, 1937), pp. 10–20. For "quick and virulent": E. E. Free, "Color of Tobacco Tells Who Will Get Cancer," *The Week's Science*, May 1, 1939, Bates 60359253. For Ochsner: "Sharp Rise in Lung Cancer May Be Due to Cigarettes," *Richmond News Leader*, Nov. 1940, Bates 950229634.

5. American Tobacco's clippings and abstracts from the *British Medical Journal* on Hitler's antitobacco campaign can be found in "Physiological Action of Tobacco Smoke," Bates 01055000–5005; the company's familiarity with German-language research is also evident

in its "Memorandum on A. Alleged Effects of Smoking B. Improvement of Cigarette Tobaccos with Special Reference to Irritation," Jan. 4, 1943, Bates 950291224–1339. For filter designs, see "German Patent No. 612,737," trans. Carl Demrick, May 3, 1935, Bates 950293926–3927. Demrick did contract work for American Tobacco and the TIRC from the 1930s through the 1980s, translating Otto Mühlbock from the Dutch, Fritz Lickint from the German, tobacco patents from France, Austria, and the Soviet Union, and articles from Spanish and other languages.

6. Franz H. Müller, "Abuse of Tobacco and Carcinoma of Lungs," *JAMA* 113 (1939): 1372; Raymond Pearl, "Tobacco Smoking and Longevity," *Science* 87 (1938): 216–17; Alton Ochsner and Michael DeBakey, "Primary Pulmonary Malignancy," *Surgery, Gynecology and Obstetrics* 68 (1939): 435–51. For the smoke machine: J. A. Bradford, W. R. Harlan, and H. R. Hanmer, "Nature of Cigaret Smoke: Technic of Experimental Smoking," *Industrial and Engineering Chemistry* 28 (1936): 836–39, Bates 962007682–7686; also "Evolution of the Smoking Machine," 1945, Bates 950110818–0824. B. Pfyl in Germany had earlier developed smoking machines; see his article with Ottilie Schmitt: "Zur Bestimmung von Nicotin in Tabak und Tabakrauch," *Zeitschrift für Untersuchung der Lebensmittel* 54 (1927): 60–77. Automatic smoking machines were developed principally to identify (and quantify) poisons in tobacco smoke; Hanmer as early as 1934 had reported to a confidant his plans "to attack the problem [of tobacco and health] soon from a biological angle"; see his letter to Clarence W. Lieb, Dec. 3, 1934, Bates 950160643. This letter also contains the earliest known reference to—and disparagement of—the work of Fritz Lickint by an American tobacco manufacturer. Manufacturers were already familiar with the cancer threat, however. Charles J. Kensler in 1955 reported the following conversation with Peyton Rous (1879–1970), who would later win the Nobel Prize for discovering the world's first cancer virus:

> At a cocktail party, I met Dr. Peyton Rous of the Rockfeller Institute, who is examining Dr. Wynder's histological sections of the skins of rabbits. Dr. Rous has spent about thirty years working on carcinogenesis in rabbit skin and is particularly well qualified to do this. Dr. Rous, in passing, informed me that when he was a young man one of the tobacco companies approached the National [Research] Council and offered to give them $20,000 to study the tobacco cancer problem. This was somewhere between 1910 and 1920. Dr. Rous would have liked to undertake this work but the National Research Council refused the offer.

See C. J. Kensler to R. Stevens et al., "Visit with Dr. Ernest Wynder," Oct. 25, 1955, Bates LG 0265184.

7. E. S. Harlow to H. R. Hanmer, "The Importance of Biological Research," Feb. 3, 1941, Bates 0060250848–0852, p. 1. American Tobacco's research department was founded in 1911 and by 1936 had twenty-two chemists and technicians; see "Memorandum on the Research Department of the American Tobacco Company," Aug. 3, 1936, Bates MNAT00818698–8721. The research department in 1949 had "60 trained specialists," and by the mid-1950s Hanmer had 115 people working under him. See his testimony in *Schweizer v. Internal Revenue*, June 14, 1956, Bates 950388530–8628.

8. Harlow to Hanmer, "Importance of Biological Research," p. 1.

9. Ibid., p. 2.

10. "MCV History Tidbits," http://www.medschool.vcu.edu/alumni/history.htm. The college was put on "confidential probation" by the American Medical Association Council on Medical Education in 1919, a stigma not erased until 1953; see Ricki D. Carruth, *A Medical College of Virginia Story* (Richmond: Medical College of Virginia, 1988), p. 23.

11. Carol Ballentine, "Taste of Raspberries, Taste of Death: The 1937 Elixir Sulfanilamide Incident," http://www.fda.gov/oc/history/elixir.html; James Harvey Young: "Sulfanilamide and Diethylene Glycol," in *Chemistry and Modern Society: Historical Essays in Honor of Aaron J. Ihde*, ed. John Parascandola and James C. Whorton (Washington, DC: American Chemical Society, 1983), pp. 105–25; also the 2003 film *Elixir of Death*.

12. For "unwarranted" and "not at all similar": Morris Fishbein to Willard F. Greenwald, Nov. 9, 1937, Bates 1003080094; Greenwald to Fishbein, Nov. 4, 1937, Bates 1003080095–0096. For "no evidence": "Deaths Following Elixir of Sulfanilamide-Massengill," *JAMA* 109 (1937): 1367, Bates 1003080066.

13. "Progress Report on Detection and Estimation of Acrolein in Cigarette Smoke," June 3, 1935, Bates 950109466–9470; C. F. Bailey (Mellon Institute), "Progress Report," Jan. 11, 1936, Bates 1003081919–1931.

14. See the USDA's "Report of Conference on Problems of the Tobacco Manufacturing Industry," May 14, 1942, Bates 950064215–4218.

15. See, for example, Adolf Wenusch's review of F. Hoff's book, *Über "Raucherkachexie,"* in *Chronica Nicotiana* 4, no. 2 (1943): 31.

16. Hiram Hanmer to W. E. Witzleben, Nov. 1, 1935, Bates 950202427.

17. J. H. Weatherby, H. B. Haag and R. C. Neale, "A Preliminary Report on Toxicity of Propylene Glycol," Aug. 19, 1936, Bates 950162821–2830; G. Z. Williams and H. B. Haag, "Effect on Guinea Pigs of Inhalation of Atomized Glycols," 1941, Bates 962000091–0094; "Research Work of Dr. Howard B. Hucker at the Medical College of Virginia," 1953, Bates 0060250847. For "splendid connection": H. R. Hanmer to C. F. Neiley, Jan. 14, 1937, Bates 950248520. For Sanger's gratitude: W. T. Sanger to H. R. Hanmer, May 27, 1941, Bates 9502 48459. And for Miller's work: H. R. Hanmer to C. F. Neiley, May 21, 1936, Bates 950248535. Miller may have been the author of the MCV's 1942 "Survey of Medical Schools of North America" (Bates 962007373–7374), which turned up "no investigative work having to do with tobacco" in more than sixty schools surveyed. The dean of the University of Vermont's Medical School did, however, volunteer that his faculty "smoke Luckies."

18. E. S. Harlow and P. S. Larson, "Testimony: Determination of the Effect of Nicotine on the Irritation of Cigarette Smoke," Jan. 22, 1948, Bates MNAT00399035–9040.

19. For Larson and Haag's remuneration: "American Tobacco Company Payments for Various Research and Consulting Services," May 26, 1967, Bates BBAT023713. For "sold American": Harlow to Hanmer, "Importance of Biological Research," p. 2 (the double entendre references the tobacco auctioneer's well-known slogan). Hanmer repeated Haag's being "sold American" in a letter to the company's advertising manager, S. L. Weaver, on March 20, 1946, Bates 950204841. In correspondence with the public, however, Haag was characterized as "an impartial authority"; see Hanmer to C. C. Langdon, March 30, 1946, Bates 950205030–5032.

20. For "sterilizing": American Tobacco Co., *Effect of Subjecting Tobaccos to High Temper-*

atures: An Explanation of the Phrase "It's Toasted" (New York: American Tobacco, 1928). For "proceed with all haste": H. R. Hanmer to P. M. Hahn, Dec. 16, 1935, Bates MNAT00484003.

21. John Daffron, "Something in Human Body Takes Nick out of Nicotine," *N. L.* (Roanoke), Oct. 27, 1943, Bates 950229582; compare Bates 950229583.

22. Paul S. Larson, "Obituary for Harvey Haag," ca. Oct. 14, 1961, Archives, Thompkins-McCaw Library, Virginia Commonwealth University.

23. John J. Trotter to AT, July 23, 1946, Bates 950204297. Engel later became an industry ally, as Hill & Knowlton provided him with "help" with a pro-industry assignment for *Harpers* in 1954; see Hill & Knowlton, "Report of Activities through July 31, 1954," Bates 95527373–7395; also their "Tobacco Industry Research Committee Information Activities," Oct. 7, 1954, Bates TINY0001828–1833, where we find the assessment that Engel's article will be "a defense against the cigarette attacks," lending weight to the industry's "no proof" contention.

24. Haag, "Comments on 'Cigarettes Cause Cancer' by Leonard Engel" (for Hanmer), Aug. 1946, Bates 950278708–8713; H. R. Hanmer to John J. Trotter, Aug. 5, 1946, Bates MNAT0076499–6500.

25. Alfred F. Bowden to C. Estelle Smith, Feb. 27, 1948, Bates MNAT00800321.

26. For "dangerous implications": Hanmer to Herstein, Dec. 25, 1946, Bates MNAT0075 6039. For "more satisfaction": Hiram R. Hanmer to John Holley Clark Jr., Jan. 23, 1950, Bates MNAT00648779–8780. In 1948 Harlow boasted that American Tobacco was building "undoubtedly the best library on tobacco and related subjects in the world"; see Harlow to Hanmer, July 21, 1948, p. 4, Bates MNAT00380519–0526.

27. For "highly significant": Lombard and Doering, "Cancer Studies in Massachusetts," p. 486. For "just enough evidence": H. B. Parmele to Adam Riefner, July 29, 1946, Bates 04365255–5256.

28. For "destructive distillation": Hiram R. Hanmer, "Memorandum on the Research Department of the American Tobacco Company," Aug. 3, 1936, Bates MNAT00818698–8721, p. 9. For "did not smoke tobacco": Hanmer to Karl M. Herstein, Dec. 25, 1946, Bates MNAT00756039–6040. Hanmer was also not entirely correct to say that "the life insurance companies and the National Cancer Institute disagree with Roffo." Frederick L. Hoffman, chief statistician for Prudential Insurance, was one of the first Americans to take Germany's tobacco–cancer research seriously; see his "Cancer and Smoking Habits," in *Cancer . . . Comprising International Contributions*, ed. Frank E. Adair (Philadelphia: Lippincott, 1931), pp. 62–66. Hoffman here speculated that female cancer of the lung might well stem from exposure to "air pollution" caused by "almost universal smoking habits" (p. 67; compare his *Cancer and Diet* [Baltimore: Williams & Wilkins, 1937], p. 489). For American's defense of "toasting," with explicit mention of "destructive distillation," see the "Memorandum Submitted by the American Tobacco Company" (to the Federal Trade Commission), Dec. 9, 1930, Bates 968312154–2362.

29. Harvey B. Haag, J. B. Weatherby, Doris Fordham, and P. S. Larson, "The Effect on Rats of Daily-Life Span Exposure to Cigaret Smoke," *Federation Proceedings* 5 (1946): 181.

30. Negus had handled press relations for the AAAS at its 1938 convention in Richmond, for which the science writers covering the event gave him an award for presenting "the first indisputable proof ever offered of the theory of evolution," meaning his "mutation" from "a

scientist "into a higher type of human being—a newspaper reporter." See "Accolade for Dr. Negus," *Richmond Times-Dispatch,* Jan. 1, 1963. For "approved by you": Sidney S. Negus to H. R. Hanmer, Feb. 17, 1941, Bates 950210624–0625. The industry maintained massive lists of names and addresses of science writers in many different countries; see, for example, the fifty-page "National Association of Science Writers, Inc., Membership List," July 1978, Bates 10399837–9887. For "friendly atmosphere": H. R. Hanmer to Sidney S. Negus, Jan. 27, 1942, Bates 962000277. Negus worked for American Tobacco into the 1960s, earning $ 17,000 from 1955 through 1963; see "American Tobacco Company Payments," May 26, 1967, Bates BBAT023 713. MCV scholars published dozens of articles on nicotine metabolism and toxicity in the 1930s, 1940s, and 1950s; for abstracts see Bates 950612959–2998, and for reprints, Bates CTRMN030078Y-0097. For Hanmer et al.'s flawed epidemiology, see E. S. Harlow, "Heavy Smokers with Low Mortality: A 14 1/4-Year Test of the Anti-Cigarette Hypothesis," discussed with Larson and Haag, May 8, 1961, Bates 950277196–7197.

31. For MCV publications produced under contract with American Tobacco as of 1949, see "List of Reprints of Articles by Members of MCV Staff," 1949, Bates 950210691–0692. Herbert McKennis was supported by TIRC/CTR funds continuously beginning in 1956, primarily to research nicotine metabolism. He received substantial funding for this work—$60,000 in 1972 alone, for example, plus funds from the AMA's ERF; see R. C. M. to Bing, Jacobson, and Sommers, "Herbert McKennis," Sept. 14, 1976, Bates HK2255032-5033. American Tobacco considered McKennis "the leading authority" on nicotine metabolism at this time. For witness tampering: Harlow to Harlan and Hanmer, April 2, 1958, Bates 950165636.

32. Paul S. Larson, "Comments at Formal Opening of Nutriculture Laboratory," May 10, 1956, Bates 950247795–7797. American Tobacco had earlier forced C 14–labeled smoke into the lungs of dogs to see how fast it would be cleared from the body; see "Determination of the Rate of Elimination of Tobacco Smoke from the Body," 1954, Bates 962006829–6830. For Harlow's travel: E. S. Harlow to H. R. Hanmer et al., "Visit to Argonne National Laboratory," Aug. 5, 1955, Bates 950247872–7873. For publicity spin: E. S. Harlow to W. R. Harlan, "Dr. DuPuis' Letter," Jan. 5, 1956, Bates 950139972.

33. "Conference of Tobacco Research Chemists," Oct. 1953, Bates 950264444–4445; E. S. Harlow to H. R. Hanmer and W. R. Harlan, "Preliminary Draft of Proposed Statement for Mr. Hahn," March 19, 1956, Bates 950281178–1180; R. W. Davis to E. S. Harlow, R. H. Irby, and E. C. Cogbill, "Visit to Industrial Reactor Laboratory (Highstown, N.J.) and Radiation Science Center—Rutgers University," Aug. 14, 1967, Bates 950113464–3465; R. W. Davis to E. C. Cogbill, "Progress Report," March 6, 1969, Bates 950282988–2989.

34. H. R. Hanmer to R. K. Heimann, Sept. 15, 1964, Bates 950133747–3750.

35. E. P. Richardson, "The American Tobacco Company Research Laboratory," July 1941, Bates 950133122–3178.

36. For large "NO": Hiram R. Hanmer to Preston L. Fowler, Feb. 14, 1949, Bates 95013 3824. American Tobacco researchers published only sixty-four scientific papers from 1929 through 1971; see "Papers Published by Staff Members of the Research Laboratory, The American Tobacco Company—1929–Current," n.d., Bates 966103488–3494. For "more liberal policy": J. M. Moseley to H. R. Hanmer, July 28, 1948, Bates MNAT00380513–0518, p. 6. For nicotine as "tranquilizer": Mary Grant, "Tobacco (in report) Poses as Tranquilizer," *Palo Alto Times,* Dec. 9, 1958, Bates 0000715.

37. For Philip Morris, see "Summary of the Research Program," Nov. 21, 1950, Bates 507141834–1834. Arthur D. Little, Inc., in the early 1950s had a staff of 850, about half of whom were scientists. The company conducted extensive biological tests for Liggett & Myers, including tests of the carcinogenicity of cigarette tars; see "The Biological Test Program at Arthur D. Little," n.d. (pre-1960), Bates LG0385256–5272. Charles J. Kensler directed biological research at Arthur D. Little from July 1954 to January 1957, supervising experiments in which tobacco smoke condensates were painted on the skins of mice. Kensler was called to testify in *Otto Pritchard v. Liggett & Myers* (on April 29, 1960), where he claimed that the only carcinogen isolated from tobacco smoke was benzpyrene and that even this had been found only in trace amounts. Internal company reports, however, had referenced "not one or two but probably many compounds" in cigarette smoke capable of causing cancer; see "Biological Test Program at Arthur D. Little," p. 102. For Kensler's autobiography, see his Nov. 21, 1985, deposition for *Cipollone v. Liggett,* Bates kenslerc112185.

38. H. B. Parmele to W. J. Halley, Feb. 12, 1954, Bates 89751850–1852; Fishbein to Alden James, Nov. 17, 1953, Bates 01150396. Fishbein was already working for Lorillard by 1952; see Parmele to R. M. Ganger (president of Lorillard), Nov. 21, 1952, Bates 00620708. Fishbein arranged to have an article by Morris T. Friedell placed in *JAMA;* the resulting paper, claiming that Kent cigarettes produced less vasoconstriction than other brands, failed to disclose that the author had received many thousands of dollars from Lorillard; see M. T. Friedell, "Effect of Cigarette Smoke on the Peripheral Vascular System," *JAMA* 152 (1953): 897–900. Subsequent papers by Friedell were rewritten by Lorillard prior to publication; see Parmele to Friedell, Sept. 10, 1954, Bates 01151457. Fishbein praised Friedell to Lorillard: "he has an excellent case for Kent" (Fishbein to Parmele, Feb. 2, 1953, Bates 01150446). Fishbein loved plugging Kents: "There is to be a small meeting of the board of the International Poliomyelitis Congress in New York on May 27 and I will see to it that they hear all about Kents at that time" (Fishbein to Parmele, April 28, 1953, Bates 89752346). The "only drawback" to Friedell's study, according to Parmele, writing to Lorillard's director of advertising, was that Friedell had also found that other filters filtered about as effectively—or poorly—as Kent. This inconvenient fact was fortunately "not mentioned in the report and there is no reason why it should ever be known" (Parmele to Alden James, May 7, 1953, Bates 89752349–2350). A 190-page draft of Fishbein's book, titled "Effects of Tobacco and of Cigarette Smoking on the Body," April 1954, scheduled for publication by Blakiston, can be found at Bates 01150580–0768. And for Fishbein's placement of cigarette-friendly pieces, see his letter to R. M. Ganger, March 9, 1953, Bates 00620694–0695.

39. See, for example, "Are They Harmful?" *Consumer Reports,* Feb. 1953, p. 71, where Haag's defense of diethylene glycol is cited without any mention of his work for the tobacco giant.

40. Parmele to Halley, Feb. 12, 1954.

41. Paul M. Gross (Duke) to Preston L. Fowler (AT), June 13, 1951, Bates 950153142–3143.

42. William Stepka, "Isotope Farming at Medical College of Virginia," *Commonwealth* (July 1956): 49–51, Bates 962007772–7774. Stepka directed the MCV's Nutriculture Laboratory and served as an American Tobacco Company consultant throughout the 1960s and 1970s.

43. See, for example, E. S. Harlow to C. F. Hetsko, June 21, 1966, Bates 970318304.

44. Arthur W. Burke Jr., "Oscar Auerbach: Report of a Lecture Delivered at the Medical College of Virginia," June 4, 1970, Bates 962007474–7478. Burke prepared reports for AT on other MCV visitors—Seymour Ochsner, for example, who lectured at the college on April 20, 1970 (Bates 962000214–0216).

45. For Smith's gratitude: R. Blackwell Smith, Sept. 4, 1957, Bates 950248258–8259. For MCV appointments of American Tobacco personnel: "Planned Site Visits of Candidates for Positions in the M.C.V. Biological Program," May 4, 1966, Bates 950161648. Egle obtained $52,500 in research support from American Tobacco from 1966 through 1969 (Bates 50201119–1158). For "salubrious situation": "Conference March 23, 1966 at New Products Division," April 25, 1966, Bates 962000312–0315. For legal consultations: Arthur W. Burke Jr. to Janet Brown, July 28, 1966, Bates 950219413. For other consulting: William T. Ham to E. S. Harlow, May 25, 1965, Bates 950163600; and Rodney C. Berry to Kenneth S. Rogers, May 12, 1967, Bates 950163587. For Gallaher's visit: A. W. Burke, "Report of Information Conveyed by Dr. Paul B. Larson," March 14, 1967, Bates 950163591.

46. For "safest mild stimulant": D. T. Watts to E. S. Harlow, Oct. 16, 1968, Bates 95500 4249–4251. For $200,000: "Current Research Grants to the Department of Pharmacology," Sept. 25, 1968, Bates 955004252. For "will protect people": Marvin A. Friedman, "Application for Research Grant," Jan. 31, 1974, Bates 50201119–1158. Other MCV scholars receiving TIRC/CTR funding included Ebbe C. Hoff, psychiatry; William Regelson, oncology; and Jan F. Chlobowski, biochemistry. And from pharmacology, apart from Haag, Larson, and McKennis: Mario D. Aceto, Jack Freund, John A. Rosecrans, and Ronald P. Rubin.

47. Jesse Steinfeld's remarks from Feb. 1, 1977, are cited in Bates 500270479–0866.

48. On titration: William L. Dunn, "Smoker Psychology," Nov. 11, 1977, Bates 1003287995–7996. On Suter: William L. Dunn, "Smoker Psychology," Aug. 8, 1977, Bates 1003287997–7998. On DeSimone: M. L. Reynolds to Thomas A. Pyle, Jan. 3, 1983, Bates 682320785. For Kilpatrick: S. James Kilpatrick, "To Show that the Association in the Hirayama Study between ETS and Lung Cancer Is Not Significant," Oct. 17, 1988, Bates TIBU0034471–4475. Kilpatrick was a member of the industry's ETS Advisory Group; see "Research Projects on Environmental Tobacco Smoke," July 1985, Bates TI05201794–1796.

49. On Accord: D. Ress, "Accord Device Cuts Nicotine, Eliminates Poison, Study Hints," Times Dispatch, March 23, 1999. "ETS and IAQ Consultants," Oct. 8, 1990, Bates 507778674–8690.

50. "Cast of Characters," Sept. 1992, Bates 2025884159–4213; also "People's Court," 1992, Bates 2025884135–4142.

51. See, for example, Joseph L. McClay to Barbara Zedler, "Metabolomics ms," Feb. 19, 2001, Bates 5024446083. The Legacy Library contains hundreds of emails exchanged between VCU faculty and Philip Morris; most of these can be accessed by searching "vcu.edu." This is a useful way to explore the involvement of particular universities in tobacco industry collaborations; "vcu.edu," for example, returns 1,835 separate documents; "Stanford.edu" returns 295; and "Harvard.edu" returns 1,164. VCU scholars identified by this means for 2006–10 include Daniel E. Adkins, Kellie Archer, William H. Barr, Russell M. Boyle, Eleanor D. Campbell, W. Hans Carter, John A. DeSimone, Carleton Garrett, Chris Gennings, Sunil S. Iyer, Vijay Lyall, Joseph L. McClay, Edward Lenn Murrelle, Edwin van den Oord, Misook Park, Ramesh Ramakrishnan, Domenic A. Sica, Bradley Todd Webb, and Timothy P. York.

CHAPTER 12

1. Mark Parascandola stresses the role of the germ theory in elevating the status of laboratory experimentation; Koch's postulates required laboratory experiments to isolate causative agents, and population inferences suffered in the evidentiary status hierarchy. See his "Epidemiology: Second-Rate Science?" *Public Health Reports* 113 (1998): 312–20. Epidemiology was not so much weak science as novel science, and a form of science that, by virtue of its strength, came under attack as "weak" (from the tobacco industry). For a critique of "gold standard" evidentiary exceptionalism, see Brandt, *Cigarette Century,* pp. 120–48. For "put in context": Jones Day, "Teague Depo. Prep.," pp. 16–21. On exculpation via contextualization, see again my "Should Medical Historians Be Working for the Tobacco Industry?"

2. Wynder, Graham, and Croninger, "Experimental Production of Carcinoma."

3. "Experimental Cancer in Mice Produced by Cigarette Smoke" (Press release, Memorial Center for Cancer and Allied Diseases), April 11, 1953, Bates 950167557–7559.

4. Hanmer, "Memorandum on Alleged Causative Relation," Supplement, p. 5. Wynder's November 19, 1952, letter to Rhoads was supplied clandestinely to American Tobacco by J. H. Teeter of the Damon Runyon Memorial Fund and can be found at Bates MNAT00587276.

5. For "flavoring laboratory": Jones Day, "Teague Depo. Prep.," p. 8. For "frightening": Roy Norr, "Cancer by the Carton," *Reader's Digest,* Dec. 1952, pp. 7–8; Alton Ochsner, "Lung Cancer: The Case against Smoking," *The Nation,* May 23, 1953. Norr's article was an abbreviated version of his "Smokers Are Getting Scared!" from the October 1952 *Christian Herald.*

6. Teague, "Survey," p. 5. For "Because of the possible connection": Jones Day, "Teague Depo. Prep.," p. 6. We don't know precisely when Teague was asked to prepare his review, but it was probably not long after the publication of Norr's "Cancer by the Carton" in *Reader's Digest* in December 1952. Wynder et al.'s mouse experiments—unpublished but circulating—must have provided an additional prompt. Reynolds scientists have testified that Teague's review was produced at the request of Kenneth H. Hoover (head of Reynolds's research department) and "widely disseminated" at Reynolds but also sent to the "B.G.M.C." (Bowman Gray Medical Center); see Jones Day, "Teague Depo. Prep.," p. 7.

7. Teague, "Survey," p. 8; G. M. Badger, "The Carcinogenic Hydrocarbons: Chemical Constitution and Carcinogenic Activity," *British Journal of Cancer* 2 (1948): 309–48.

8. For "firmly establish": Teague, "Survey," 10–11. For "beyond a reasonable doubt": Earl Ubell, "Cigarette–Lung Cancer Link Proved, Dr. Hammond Says," *Herald Tribune,* Oct. 20, 1954, Bates 966039727. Hiram R. Hanmer at American Tobacco also regarded Hammond's survey as "the most portentous thing in the offing . . . the crux of the whole situation. If unfavorable to cigarette smoking, it will practically clinch everything Wynder and Graham have said" ("The Situation with Respect to Cancer Research," Nov. 13, 1953, Bates 950164216–4217).

9. Teague, "Survey," p. 6.

10. Ibid., pp. 14–15.

11. Tommy Ross, counsel for American Tobacco, drafted this first "white paper"; see Bates JH000502EXHIBIT18905. For 176,800 copies: Hill & Knowlton, "Report on TIRC Booklet, 'A Scientific Perspective on the Cigarette Controversy,'" May 3, 1954, Bates 01138747–8782. For "authorities from the Damon Runyon Fund": "Cigaret Controversy: Tobacco Industry's

'White Paper' Counters Smoking-Cancer Tie-in," *Wall Street Journal,* April 14, 1954, Bates CORTI0014324. For "relatively unimportant": TIRC, *A Scientific Perspective on the Cigarette Controversy,* April 14, 1954, Bates 961008056–8076. The McNally reference is William D. McNally, "The Tar in Cigarette Smoke and Its Possible Effects," *American Journal of Cancer* 16 (1932): 1502–14. McNally's paper was used to pitch a filter device to American Tobacco; see Otto Muller to American Tobacco, Dec. 9, 1932, Bates 950190634.

12. For Senkus: Claude E. Teague Jr., Deposition for *Minnesota v. Philip Morris,* July 8, 1997, vol. 1, Bates TEAGUEC070897, p. 51. Teague's survey was "updated" by Alan Rodgman shortly after he arrived at the company in June 1954; this update—never released by Reynolds—impressed the company's top lawyer, Henry H. Ramm, enough to earn Rodgman an assignment "preparing for and defending litigation"; see Rodgman's deposition testimony for *Arch,* Aug. 4, 1997, Bates RODGMANF080497, pp. 608–9. In the 1990 document prepared to coach Teague prior to his deposition, lawyers working for Reynolds suggested that Teague's survey was merely "a review" and not an attempt to evaluate this literature critically. They also asked him not to "speculate" about the extent to which management had knowledge of hazards prior to 1953 (Jones Day, "Teague Depo. Prep.," p. 7). For Teague's interview: Jones, Day, Reavis and Pogue, "Report Containing Analyses Concerning Research Development Activities Prepared by RJR outside Legal Counsel," Dec. 31, 1985, Bates 515871651-2176, p. 14. I accessed this document prior to its removal from the archives as "Privileged Content." For "caused concern" and "recall all copies": Jones, Day, Reavis and Pogue, "RJR Research and Development Activities: Fact Team Memorandum," Dec. 31, 1985, Bates 515871651–1912, p. 8.

British tobacco researchers in the mid-1960s characterized the Policy Committee as "the main power in the smoking and health situation . . . extremely powerful; it determines the high policy of the industry on *all* smoking and health matters . . . and it reports directly to the Presidents." See Phillip J. Rogers and Geoffrey F. Todd, "Report on Policy Aspects of the Smoking and Health Situation in U.S.A.," Oct. 15, 1964, Bates 1003119099–9135, pp. 6–7.

13. Teague wrote "annual" and "long-range assumption and forecast" papers beginning in 1969; these later turned into the firm's Strategic Plans; see Jones, Day, Reavis and Pogue, "Management and Legal Supervision and Control of R&D Activities," Dec. 31, 1985, Bates 519198732–8819, p. 14. For "specialized," see Teague's "On the Nature of the Tobacco Business and the Crucial Role of Nicotine Therein," April 14, 1972, Bates 83570661–0670, p. 2; and for "pre-smokers," see his "Some Thoughts about New Brands of Cigarettes for the Youth Market," p. 1. For "most of our customers," see Teague's memo to G. R. Di Marco, "Nordine Study," Dec. 1, 1982, Bates 500898255–8257. For his job titles, see Bates TEAGUEC0 70897.

14. For pride in having found benzpyrene: Jones Day, "Teague Depo. Prep," p. 59; Alan Rodgman, "Analysis of Cigarette Smoke Condensate," Feb. 12, 1964, Bates 501008855–8928. Reynolds was the first to find cholanthrene and several other carcinogenic hydrocarbons in tobacco tars; see Rodgman to Hoover, Nov. 2, 1959, p. 1. For "strong indications": Claude Teague, "Disclosure of Invention," Nov. 18, 1955, Bates 504912040–2042. For publication bans: Ralph L. Rowland to Managers, "Management Meeting, March 22, 1971: Rewards and Recognition," April 20, 1971, Bates 515873927–3929; Alan Rodgman, "A Critical and Objective Appraisal of the Smoking and Health Problem," Sept. 12, 1962, Bates 504822823–2846.

15. For "little or no effect": Claude Teague to Kenneth Hoover, "Disclosure of Invention: Filter Tip Materials Undergoing Color Change on Contact with Tobacco Smoke," Dec. 17, 1953, Bates 511235573. Murray Senkus, Carroll S. Tompson, and Walter M. Henley also signed off on Teague's disclosure. Liggett & Myers researchers explored similar gimmicks; see Jean P. Eaves, "Stenographic Minutes of a Conference Held at the Research Laboratory," Jan. 23, 1952, Bates LG0205897–5926. For "illusion of filtration": M.E. Johnston, "Market Potential of a Health Cigarette," June 1966, Bates 1001913853–3878.

16. Claude E. Teague Jr., Deposition for *Minnesota v. Philip Morris*, vol. 1, July 8, 1997, Bates TEAGUEC070897, pp. 72–73, 77–78; compare Bates TEAGUEC070897, TEAGUEC07 0997, TEAGUEC071097, and TEAGUEC071197; and Jones Day, "Teague Depo. Prep."

CHAPTER 13

1. On Runyon's cancer, see Jimmy Breslin, *Damon Runyon* (New York: Ticknor and Fields, 1991), pp. 382–83. Walter Winchell in the 1950s supported Joe McCarthy's anticommunist witch-hunt; he also served as the announcer for *The Untouchables* for several years beginning in 1953. In the 1930s he had allowed his name to be used in advertisements for Lucky Strike cigarettes.

2. Separate letters from John H. Teeter to Paul M. Hahn, O.P. McComas, and J.C. Whitaker are all dated Sept. 28, 1950, Bates MNAT00730768, 2022238737, and 502407922.

3. Hiram R. Hanmer to John H. Teeter, Oct. 18, 1950, Bates MNAAT00901168. The reference is to "Smoking in Lung Cancer," *Science News Letter,* Oct. 7, 1950.

4. John H. Teeter to Hiram R. Hanmer, Dec. 27, 1950, Bates MNAT00730758.

5. George Weissman to R.N. DuPuis, Oct. 7, 1953, Bates 2022239142–9147.

6. Hiram R. Hanmer to Preston L. Fowler, May 16, 1951, Bates MNAT00730744–0746, copied to American Tobacco President Paul M. Hahn.

7. Hanmer to Fowler, May 16, 1951, p. 2. For "airborne infection": Lanza to Hanmer, Nov. 11, 1952, Bates 950164267–4268; John H. Teeter to W.F. Greenwald, March 25, 1952, Bates 2022238892.

8. For "petroleum industry problem": Hiram R. Hanmer, "Meeting, 9 A.M., November 5, 1953, Sloan-Kettering Institute," Nov. 17, 1953, Bates 950167411–7415, p. 2. From 1926 to 1948 Lanza was associate director of medicine for Metropolitan Life Insurance, during which time he also worked for Johns Manville, exonerating asbestos from charges of causing lung cancer. Lanza claimed that people working with the fiber died not because the mineral was scarring their lungs but rather because their lungs did a bad job of clearing out the fibers. Lanza had also vigorously defended mining companies in the Tri-State area around southwestern Missouri; see his deposition for *William Burns v. St. Joseph Lead Co.,* June 8, 1934, where he denied any hazard from breathing lead sulfide and denied any silicosis hazard from dust in mines where the rock had a free silica content less than about 30 percent. See also Barry I. Castleman, *Asbestos: Medical and Legal Aspects,* 5th ed. (New York: Aspen, 2005).

9. Hiram R. Hanmer, "Observations Concerning Individuals Participating in the Meetings" (of Nov. 5, 1953, at NYU), n.d., Bates MNAT00688881–8886, p. 2.

10. For Wynder's later funding: Nicole Fields and Simon Chapman, "Chasing Ernst L. Wynder: 40 Years of Philip Morris's Efforts to Influence a Leading Scientist," *Journal of Epi-*

demiology and Community Health 57 (2003): 571-78. For Wynder "collaborating on the N.Y.U. investigations": Marcus E. Hobbs, "Notes on Trip to New York University," Jan. 27, 1953, Bates 950164340-4343, p. 1. It is not clear how much of Wynder's 1953 work with Graham and Croninger can be traced to tobacco industry funding. His 1953 paper, "Experimental Production of Carcinoma with Cigarette Tar," credits only "a research grant from the National Cancer Institute," but we also know that at least part of his salary was being paid by American Tobacco via the Runyon Fund.

11. Hanmer to Fowler, Feb. 26, 1953, p. 5, Bates MNAT00615509-5514.

12. For Parmele's suspicions, see H. P. Parmele to John H. Teeter, May 22, 1953, Bates 01183002. For Hanmer's keeping tabs, see Hobbs, "Notes on Trip to New York University."

13. Hanmer, "Observations Concerning Individuals," p. 3; original emphasis. For "more of a fanatic," see Hanmer's Sept. 22, 1950, memo to American Tobacco's Hahn, where Wynder's father is described as "a missionary preacher who once stumped the country inveighing against the evils of tobacco." Wynder at this time (1950) was still only a fourth-year medical student at Washington University, and Hanmer suspected him of "inheriting some of his father's zeal"—all of which made Wynder's offer to direct research sponsored by the industry "inexplicable" (Bates MNAT00509599).

14. Hanmer, "Meeting, 9 A.M., November 5, 1953," p. 2.

15. Hanmer, "Observations Concerning Individuals," p. 6. Minutes from this meeting reveal a desire "to get rid of Wynder," meaning to exclude him from future industry funding; see Bates 950164205-4206. Hanmer by this time had an annual salary of $40,000, raised to $45,000 effective Jan. 1, 1954; see Bates 945324522-4823, p. 24.

16. "Cigaret Controversy: Tobacco Industry's 'White Paper' Counters Smoking-Cancer Tie-in," *Wall Street Journal*, April 14, 1954.

17. For "goldfish bowl": H. R. Hanmer to Paul M. Hahn, Nov. 17, 1953, Bates 950153110. For "not controlling": H. R. Hanmer to P. L. Fowler, Dec. 1, 1952, Bates 950152768.

18. Hanmer, "Meeting, 9 A.M., November 5, 1953," 3. Hanmer by this time was resigned to having "mouse carcinogens" found in tobacco smoke. A November 13, 1953, document titled "The Situation with Respect to Cancer Research" predicted that Wynder, Graham and Ochsner "will convert more and more doctors, directly or indirectly, to their way of thinking" (Bates 950164216-4217). Hanmer outlined a series of recommendations for the company, including an end to the use of arsenic insecticides, continued support for scientific skeptics, cooperation with Reynolds's new Bureau of Scientific Information, and the establishment of "a tobacco industrial research institute" ("Recommendations," Bates 950164218).

19. Hanmer, "Meeting, 9 A.M., November 5, 1953," pp. 3-4.

20. Ibid., p. 5.

21. Frederick R. Darkis to W. A. Blount, Feb. 4, 1954, Bates LG0090704-0708.

22. Hobbs, "Notes on Trip to New York University."

CHAPTER 14

1. Otmar Freiherr von Verschuer, the notorious Nazi racial hygienist and Mengele *Doktorvater,* was hired by British tobacco makers to verify Fisher's genotype hypothesis, using his extensive archive of identical and nonidentical twins. See "T.M.S.C. Scientific Re-

search," Feb. 9, 1959, Bates 105386966–6973. Fisher had recommended Verschuer to Geoffrey Todd as an "old scientific acquaintance"; see R. A. Fisher to Todd, Oct. 19, 1956, Bates 105409457.

2. Milton B. Rosenblatt, "Lung Cancer in the 19th Century," *Bulletin of the History of Medicine* 38 (1964): 395–425.

3. Concerns about paper continue even after the formation of the TIRC; see Tobacco Industry Research Committee, "Confidential Report, Industry Technical Committee Meeting," July 30, 1954, Bates CTR0021997–1999.

4. Edison's letter of April 26, 1914, is reproduced in Henry Ford, *The Case against the Little White Slaver* (Detroit: Henry Ford, 1916), p. 2.

5. "Sloan-Kettering Institute—Cigarette Paper Tars," n.d. (March 1952), Bates MNAT0058 7275.

6. Bruce Barton to Preston L. Fowler, Oct. 9, 1951, Bates 950166649.

7. William W. Carroll and H. J. Rand, "A Fluorospectrographic Indication of Carcinogens in Cigarette Papers," March 17, 1952, Bates 950166333–6336.

8. Carroll and Rand, "Fluorospectrographic Indication of Carcinogens," p. 4; and for the spectroscopy: E. L. Kennaway and I. Hieger, "Carcinogenic Substances and Their Fluorescence Spectra," *British Medical Journal* 1 (1930): 1044–46.

9. "Sloan-Kettering Institute—Cigarette Paper Tars." On cellophane: Richardson, "American Tobacco Company Research Laboratory," July 1941.

10. C. M. Flory, "The Production of Tumors by Tobacco Tars," *Cancer Research* 1 (1941): 262–76.

11. For "disagreeable odor": W. F. Greenwald to R. E. Matthews, March 28, 1951, Bates 1003079865. For chlorophyll-impregnated paper: Louis L. Long (Philip Morris) to L. H. Davis, Aug. 15, 1952, Bates 2000755428; W. F. Taylor Jr. (Ecusta) to W. F. Greenwald, Aug. 27, 1951, Bates 1003079871. For "closer together": Milton O. Schur to Robert N. DuPuis, Oct. 30, 1952, Bates 1001912005. On aldehydes, see H. W. Sigmon to J. C. Rickards, "Analysis of Aldehydes in Smoke," Sept. 8, 1953, Bates 1001904272–4273.

12. M. O. Schur to H. R. Hanmer, Sept. 26, 1952, Bates 969006729.

13. M. O. Schur and J. C. Rickards, "Ecusta Method for the Preparation of Cigarette Smoke Condensate," Jan. 26, 1953, Bates HK2387865–7873.

14. Minutes of meeting on Jan. 14, 1953, between Milton O. Schur (Ecusta), Lanza (NYU) and Nelson (NYU), Bates MNAT00587091–7092.

15. M. O. Schur to H. R. Hanmer, April 7, 1953, Bates 950167556.

16. American Tobacco, "'AC' Content of Cigarette Smoke," May 29, 1953, Bates 95010 9311; H. R. Hanmer to M. O. Schur, July 1, 1953, Bates 950154413–4414.

17. Joseph J. Blacknall to H. B. Parmele, July 1, 1953, Bates 00065829; "Results of Accelerated Animal Tests" (from Ecusta), June 9, 1953, Bates 00065830.

18. J. C. Rickards to H. R. Hanmer, June 24, 1953, Bates 969006724–6725. Also present at these meetings were O. L. (Chick) Hillsman, Ed Harlow, Richard C. Irby, and W. B. Wartman.

19. M. O. Schur to H. R. Hanmer, July 7, 1953, Bates 950154411–4412.

20. J. C. Rickards to P. S. Larson, July 8, 1953, Bates 950154408–4410. The methods followed were close to those of Kanematsu Sugiura, "Observations on Animals Painted with Tobacco Tar," *American Journal of Cancer* 38 (1940): 41–49.

21. M. O. Schur to H. R. Hanmer, Aug. 24, 1953, Bates 969006717.

22. J. C. Rickards to H. B. Haag, Sept. 9, 1953, Bates 969006705-6710.

23. For "rabbit will scream": Janet C. Brown, "Confidential Memorandum to Mr. Hetsko RE Conference with Messrs. Harlan and Harlow," Aug. 25, 1965, Bates 0026861-6916, p. 15. For edema "definitely greater": H. R. Hanmer to C. W. Lieb, Aug. 14, 1935, Bates 95016 0620-0621. For Philip Morris grumbling: W. F. Greenwald to Morris Fishbein, Feb. 15, 1937, Bates 1003080097-0102.

24. Schur to Larson, Sept. 24, 1953, Bates MNAT00586741.

25. See Norton Nelson to A. Grant Clarke et al., Oct. 13, 1953, Bates 950164292-4293; William E. Smith, Alvin I. Kosak, Ernest L. Wynder, and Norton Nelson, "Investigation of the Chemical Nature of Environmental Carcinogens," Sept. 15, 1953, Bates 950164294 and 950164295-4316.

26. M. O. Schur to P. S. Larson, Nov. 6, 1953, Bates 969006694 (copied to Dixon, Rickards, and Hanmer); M. O. Schur to P. S. Larson, Nov. 10, 1953, Bates 950154386; "Histological Examination of Skin Sections of Eight Mice," Nov. 6, 1953, Bates 950154387-4389.

27. P. S. Larson to M. O. Schur, Nov. 17, 1953, Bates 950154384-4385; M. O. Schur to P. S. Larson, Nov. 20, 1953, Bates MNAT00586733, original emphasis. Schur's letter, like most having to do with Ecusta's experiments, was copied to Hanmer at American Tobacco. William E. Smith was already dissatisfied with the New York group in January 1954, by which time he was discussing "the possibility of Ecusta opening a laboratory near Asheville with him to head it up" (Darkis to Blount, Feb. 4, 1954). Smith was living in Maine as recently as the 1990s and once remarked that naming a university laboratory after Lanza was like naming a synagogue after Hitler (Barry Castleman, personal communication, referring to NYU's Lanza Lab).

28. Darkis to Blount, Feb. 4, 1954.

29. Hiram R. Hanmer, "Meeting, 10:30 A.M., November 5, 1953, New York University—School of Industrial Medicine," n.d., Bates MNAT00688875-8878.

30. Ibid., p. 3.

31. "Beyond Any Doubt," Time, Nov. 30, 1953, pp. 60-63.

32. "A Vote for Acquittal," Time, Dec. 7, 1953, p. 54.

33. "Lung Cancer Rise Is Laid to Smoking," New York Times, Dec. 9, 1953.

34. "Tobacco Stocks Hit by Cancer Reports," New York Times, Dec. 10, 1953.

35. Darkis to Blount, Feb. 4, 1954.

36. Stuart D. Cowan to Ecusta, June 1, 1954, Bates 500718917. Cowan sent this invitation to Ecusta "at the suggestion of Mr. E. A. Darr, president, R. J. Reynolds Tobacco Company."

37. Gauvin to Meyer, "Monthly Development Summary," Feb. 2, 1984, Bates 2022217620-7621. Häusermann talked about a "Dial-A-Tar Cigarette with Adjustable Filter Sleeve or Holder for Varying Dilution and Tar in Cigarettes"; see Nov. 16, 1981, Bates 570312400. For "reduced visibility sidestream": N. Egilmez to J. G. Esterle, June 27, 1986, Bates 620502449-2455.

38. Jones, Day, Reavis and Pogue (for Reynolds), "Corporate Activity Project," Nov. 17, 1986, Bates 681879254-9715, p. 171.

CHAPTER 15

1. George Davey Smith, Sabine A. Ströbele, and Matthias Egger, "Smoking and Death," *BMJ* 310 (1995): 396; also their "Smoking and Health Promotion in Nazi Germany," *Journal of Epidemiology and Community Health* 48 (1994): 220–23.

2. For a collection of consensus statements in the 1950s and early 1960s, see the FTC's "Statements on Cigarette Smoking and Health by United States and Foreign Health Associations," 1964, Bates 503808686–8768.

3. Wynder and Graham, "Tobacco Smoking"; Clarence A. Mills and Marjorie M. Porter, "Tobacco Smoking Habits and Cancer of the Mouth and Respiratory System," *Cancer Research* 10 (1950): 539–42; Morton L. Levin et al., "Cancer and Tobacco Smoking: A Preliminary Report," *JAMA* 143 (1950): 336–38; Robert Schrek et al., "Tobacco Smoking as an Etiologic Factor in Disease: I. Cancer," *Cancer Research* 10 (1950): 49–58; Doll and Hill, "Smoking and Carcinoma of the Lung."

4. Doll and Hill, "Mortality of Doctors."

5. E. C. Hammond and D. Horn, "The Relationship between Human Smoking Habits and Death Rates: A Follow-up Study of 187,766 Men," *JAMA* 155 (1954): 1316–28.

6. L. C. Lewton, "Substances Present in Tobacco Smoke Which Are Irritating to the Nose and Their Removal by a New Process," Oct. 23, 1932, Bates 950192832–2838. Compare T. Umeda, "The Influence of Structural Change of Some Chemical Substances on the Movement of the Ciliated Epithelium," *Acta Dermatologica* 11 (1928): 501–4; and W. L. Mendenhall and K. Shreeve, "Effect of Tobacco Smoke on Ciliary Action," *Journal of Pharmacology and Experimental Therapeutics* 69 (1940): 295.

7. H. R. Hanmer, "Proposed Reply to Letters Suggesting Methods of Eliminating Carbon Monoxide From the Smoke of Lucky Strike Cigarettes," Feb. 16, 1933, Bates 950192864; "Suggested Reply to Inquiries Concerning Lead and Arsenic in Cigarettes," Feb. 24, 1936, Bates 950202433.

8. A. C. Hilding, "On Cigarette Smoking, Bronchial Carcinoma and Ciliary Action," *New England Journal of Medicine* 254 (1956): 1155–60.

9. Oscar Auerbach et al., "The Anatomical Approach to the Study of Smoking and Bronchogenic Carcinoma," *Cancer* 9 (1956): 76–83; also his "Changes in Bronchial Epithelium in Relation to Cigarette Smoking and in Relation to Lung Cancer," *New England Journal of Medicine* 265 (1961): 254–67. For "missing link": "Report Links Smoking to Lung Tissue Change, Possible Cancer Tie," *Wall Street Journal*, June 2, 1955. For "fully consistent": "Lung Cancer, Cigaret Link Found in Study," *New York Post*, Nov. 11, 1956; Oscar Auerbach et al., "Changes in the Bronchial Epithelium in Relation to Smoking and Cancer of the Lung," *New England Journal of Medicine* 256 (1957): 97–104.

10. See Wynder's testimony (p. 67) in *False and Misleading Advertising (Filter-Tip Cigarettes)*, Hearings before a Subcommittee of the Committee on Government Operations, House of Representatives, 85th Cong., July 18–26, 1957 (Washington, DC: U.S. Government Printing Office, 1957), referenced hereafter as *Blatnik Report*.

11. "Report of Progress—Technical Research Department" (B&W), Dec. 24, 1952, Bates 6502000084–0095, p. 8.

12. R. Guillerm, R. Badré, and B. Vignon, "Effets inhibiteurs de la fumée de tabac sur l'activité ciliare de l'épithélium respiratoire et nature des composants responsables," *Bulletin de l'Académie Nationale de Médecine* 145 (1961): 416–23.

13. Rodgman, "A Critical and Objective Appraisal," p. 7. For "cancer causing": Arthur D. Little, Inc., "L&M—A Perspective Review," March 15, 1961, Bates 2021382496–2498.

14. A. H. Roffo, "Tabak und Krebs," *Reine Luft* 21 (1939): 123–24. For the parallel between tobacco and coal tar: Johann von Leers, "Gespräche mit Rauchern," *Reine Luft* 22 (1940): 97.

15. For the argument for confluence, see Emerson Day et al., *Investigative Approaches to the Lung Cancer Problem* (New York: Sloan-Kettering Institute, 1955), Bates 502853000–3014.

16. Jerome Cornfield et al., "Smoking and Lung Cancer: Recent Evidence and a Discussion of Some Questions," *Journal of the National Cancer Institute* 22 (1959): 173–203.

17. "Seventh International Cancer Congress, 1958," Bates 966015130–5134.

18. Joseph Garland, "Cancer of the Lung," *New England Journal of Medicine* 249 (1953): 465–66; also his "Tobacco and Carcinoma of the Lungs," *New England Journal of Medicine,* 250 (1954): 125.

19. Geoffrey F. Todd, "Smoking and Health: The Present Position in the U.K. and How It Came About," 1963, Bates 1000215063–5085.

20. Iain Macleod's speech is reported in "Heavy Smoking and Cancer: Some Relationship Established," *The Times* (London), Feb. 13, 1954, Bates 01138497; Johannes Clemmesen's prediction is in his "Bronchial Carcinoma—A Pandemic," *Danish Medical Bulletin* 1 (1954): 37–46.

21. For "no question of the facts": American Cancer Society, "Lung Cancer and the Smoking Question," *Annual Report* (Atlanta: ACS, 1954), pp. 16–19, Bates TIMN0209916–9919. Dr. George V. Brindley of the University of Texas School of Medicine drafted the text of the ACS resolution, which was unanimously approved by the ACS Board of Directors at its annual meeting in October 1954. For Rhoads: "Your Chances of Lung Cancer from Cigarets," *PIC,* April 1954, pp. 20–23, Bates 502817806–7809. For "can no longer be ignored": Sloan-Kettering Institute, "Progress Report," Nov. 1954, Bates 503270356–0380, pp. 9–10. For Public Health Cancer Association: "Cancer Unit Calls Cigarettes Harmful," *New York Journal American,* Oct. 12, 1954, Bates 950299092. The PHCA resolution was adopted by a 13 to 3 vote. For patents, see Bates 108095559–6023 (filed Oct. 8, 1954) and Bates 108183492–3944 (filed 1957), the second of which states that scientists "have proved that there is a connection between smoking and lung cancer."

22. Horace Joules is cited in American Tobacco's "Report on Special Research No.11, November, 1954, Part I—U.K.," Nov. 1954, Bates 966001993–2003.

23. Carl V. Weller, *Causal Factors in Cancer of the Lung* (Springfield, IL: Charles C. Thomas, 1955), pp. 99–100, cited in Brandt, *Cigarette Century,* pp. 154–55.

24. Charles S. Cameron, "Lung Cancer and Smoking: What We Really Know," *Atlantic Monthly,* Jan. 1956, p. 75.

25. "Smoking and Cancer," *The Times* (London), May 8, 1956, Bates HT0038363.

26. For "direct cause and effect": "Tobacco Smoking and Cancer of Lung: Statement by the Medical Research Council," *British Medical Journal* 1 (1957): 1523–24. For "most rea-

sonable interpretation": Ministry of Health, Statement in the House of Commons, "Smoking and Lung Cancer," June 27, 1957, Bates 503273370.

27. For "sum total of scientific evidence": Frank M. Strong et al., "Smoking and Health: Joint Report of Study Group on Smoking and Health," *Science* 125 (1957): 1129–33. American Tobacco had agents operating inside the closed meetings of the Study Group; see H. B. Haag to E. S. Harlow, Oct. 31, 1956, Bates 950168097 and 950168095–8096. For "beyond reasonable doubt": "Statement by Surgeon General Leroy E. Burney of the Public Health Service . . . on Excessive Cigarette Smoking and Health," July 12, 1957, Bates 966016828–6833.

28. Netherlands Ministry of Social Affairs and Public Health, *Press Notice No. 1233* (The Hague: NMSAPH, 1957).

29. "Transcript of Investigation Made by the Swedish State Medical Research Council into the Biological and Medical Effects of Smoking," Aug. 13, 1958, Bates 11329502–9505.

30. Warren H. Cole, "Statement of American Cancer Society on Cigarette Smoking and Lung Cancer," *JAMA* 172 (1960): 1425.

31. P. Dorolle et al., "Epidemiology of Cancer of the Lung: Report of a Study Group," *WHO Technical Report Series* 192 (1960): 3–13.

32. For "principal causative factor": Fred Poland, "Cigarets Linked to Lung Cancer by CMA Council," *Montreal Star,* June 21, 1961, Bates 1003044717. For "beyond any reasonable doubt": Norman C. Delarue, "A Review of Some Important Problems Concerning Lung Cancer," *Journal of the Canadian Medical Association* 84 (1961): 1374–85.

33. Royal College of Physicians of London, *Smoking and Health* (London: Pitman, 1962).

34. Janet C. Brown to Cyril F. Hetsko, "AT—Lung Cancer Litigation General," Nov. 21, 1961, Bates MNATPRIV00037878–7880.

35. Janet C. Brown, "Theories for Defending Smoking and Health Litigation," Aug. 20, 1985, Bates 680712251–2260.

36. Brandt, *Cigarette Century,* pp. 211–39. Peter V. Hamill, medical coordinator for the Committee Staff of the Surgeon General's Advisory Committee, was the key player in selecting members of the Advisory Committee in 1962–63; see his deposition for *Cipollone v. Liggett,* Nov. 25, 1985, Bates 515857777–7826, beginning at 7783.

37. U.S. Department of Health and Human Services, *Nicotine Addiction: A Report of the Surgeon General* (Washington, DC: U.S. Government Printing Office, 1988), p. vi, where nicotine is identified as "addicting in the same sense as are drugs such as heroin and cocaine." For Fieser: Charles J. Kensler to L. W. Bass, "Report of Meeting between Dr. Louis Fieser and Dr. Kensler," Aug. 18, 1954, Bates LG0044505–4506.

38. P. K. Knopick to W. Kloepfer (Tobacco Institute), Sept. 9, 1980, Bates TIMN0097164–7165.

39. Kluger, *Ashes to Ashes,* p. 257.

40. Kluger, *Ashes to Ashes,* pp. 360–62, 447–48; Nicolas Rasmussen, *On Speed: The Many Lives of Amphetamine* (New York: New York University Press, 2008), and personal communication. For a massive 363-page compilation of scholarly statements on addiction, see "Tobacco, Nicotine and Dependence-Producing Drugs," May 1, 1976, Bates 681869726–0114, and supplementary updates at 681870116–0126, 681870127–0189, and 681869699–9725.

41. Rhetorical overcaution is a problem in all the Surgeon General's reports. The 1988 report on *Nicotine Addiction,* for example, is tedious nearly to the point of torture. The long

preface by C. Everett Koop doesn't even mention the tobacco industry, apart from its (purported) work to provide nicotine replacement therapies (p. vi). Smokers were supposed to shoulder all responsibility for quitting. For more on the 1964 report, including its characterization as "unimpeachable," see Brandt's *Cigarette Century*, pp. 211–39.

42. Charles Ellis, "Meeting in London with Dr. Haselbach," Nov. 15, 1961, Bates 301083 862–3865; Yeaman, "Implications of Battelle Hippo"; Charles Ellis, "The Effects of Smoking," Feb. 13, 1962, Bates 301083820–3835.

43. For "life or death": George Weissman to Joseph F. Cullman, Jan. 29, 1964, Bates 1005038559–8561. For "grave crisis": Stanton A. Glantz, John Slade, Lisa A. Bero, Peter Hanauer, and Deborah E. Barnes, *The Cigarette Papers* (Berkeley: University of California Press, 1996), pp. 50–52.

44. Joseph Califano, personal communication, Nov. 2004.

45. Johnson is cited in Naomi Oreskes and Erik M. Conway, *Merchants of Doubt* (New York: Bloomsbury Press, 2010), pp. 170–71.

46. R. L. Swaine, "Liggett & Myers Conference on March 25, 1954" (Minutes), March 29, 1954, Bates 2022969452–9459, p. 8.

47. H. R. Hanmer to Albert R. Stevens, May 13, 1952, Bates 950164500–4501. The ad can be found at Bates 950164504–4507.

48. H. R. Hanmer to Hahn, Nov. 19, 1953, Bates 950156733–6734.

49. J. M. Moseley (American Tobacco), "Second International Tobacco Congress, Brussels, Belgium and Visit to Research Institutes and Cigarette Factories in Central Europe," July 1958, Bates 950158605–8664.

50. For Moseley: Robert Heimann to Alfred F. Bowden, "Verbal Report of J. M. Moseley," July 2, 1958, Bates 966015128. For Cuzin: J. M. Moseley to Hanmer and Harlan, "15th Tobacco Chemists Research Conference," Oct. 13, 1961, Bates 950264148–4153.

51. France stopped producing its black tobacco Gauloises in 2005, by which time only about 12 percent of all cigarettes sold in France—6 billion of 55 billion—were dark tobacco.

52. British lung cancer mortality fell from 52/100,000 to 16/100,000, whereas French mortality for this same 35–54 age group (males) rose from 13/100,000 to 42/100,000; see "UK Lung Cancer Deaths Halved by Smoking Cessation," CTSU Press Release, Aug. 2, 2000, http://www.ctsu.ox.ac.uk/pressreleases/2000-08-02.

53. Data are from the WHO Mortality Database, http://www.who.int/healthinfo/morttables/en/, plus Tomomi Marugame and Itsuro Yoshimi, "Comparison of Cancer Mortality (Lung Cancer) in Five Countries: France, Italy, Japan, UK and USA," *Japanese Journal of Clinical Oncology* 35 (2005): 168–70. Thanks also to my British colleague Richard Peto for drawing this interesting French-British contrast to my attention.

54. Moseley, "Second International," p. 24. For the life of Herbert Bentley, see Martin Sherwood, "Smokers' Friend," *New Scientist* 75 (1977): 105–7. Bentley established Britain's Tobacco Research Council laboratories at Harrogate in 1963; he also played a crucial role in developing the "New Smoking Material" (NSM) British companies hoped would prove less carcinogenic.

55. For "good technique": Moseley, "Second International," p. 25. For Kennaway "greatly impressed": McKeen Cattell, "Report on Visit to Laboratories Concerned with Tobacco in Relation to Health," Aug. 24, 1956, Bates 501941142–1150. Cattell here noted that the PR

firm of Campbell-Johnson was doing for British tobacco what Hill & Knowlton were doing for the Americans. For T. D. Day's reproduction of Wynder's experiments, see "Report by Dr. T. D. Day," March 11, 1959, Bates 105386919–6932, where we learn that "liberal applications to the backs of mice of fresh condensate provided by T.M.S.C. gave rise to papillomata and presumptive carcinomata in a yield similar to that described by Wynder and his associates."

56. For "everyone should work together": Moseley, "Second International," pp. 10–12. For "true causes of this disease": "Extract from the First Report of the Scientific Research Station of the German Cigarette Industry," Oct. 1959, Bates 105615112–5114. For "hardly be subject to further doubt": H. Druckrey et al., "Vergleichende Prüfung von Tabakrauch-Kondensaten, Benzpyren und Tabak-Extrakt auf carcinogene Wirkung an Ratten," *Die Naturwissenschaften* 47 (1960): 605–6, Bates 504112821–2823, with an English translation at 504112824–2829.

57. For "tacit agreement": Robert K. Heimann to Alfred F. Bowden, "Verbal Report of J. M. Moseley," July 2, 1958, Bates 966015128. For "legal considerations": S. J. Green, "Cigarette Smoking and Causal Relationships," Oct. 27, 1976, Bates 109938433–8436. For "first reaction of the guilty": S. J. Green, "Smoking, Associated Diseases and Causality," 1980, Bates 322043191–3196.

58. Richard Doll, "Etiology of Lung Cancer," *Advances in Cancer Research* 3 (1955): 1–50. Doll's chart is also reproduced in the 1964 Surgeon General's report, p. 176.

59. See my "Tobacco and the Global Lung Cancer Epidemic." I did not know about Doll's chart when I produced my calculations in the 1990s (one death for every million cigarettes), which are nicely consistent with his work and the elegant epidemiology of Richard Peto.

60. HEW Secretary Joseph A. Califano reported in January 1978—and often throughout that year—that more than 300,000 Americans died in 1977 from cancer and heart disease for which smoking was "a major factor"; for a Tobacco Institute history and critique of the 320,000 figure from 1979, see Bates 03736412–6427.

61. Harry Dingman, *Risk Appraisal* (Cincinnati: National Underwriter Co., 1946); Frederick L. Hoffman, "Cancer and Smoking Habits," *Annals of Surgery* 93 (1931): 50–67. The earliest known actuarial report of smokers dying, on average, earlier than nonsmokers appears in the *Proceedings of the Association of Life Insurance Medical Directors* (New York: Knickerbocker Press, 1912), pp. 473–75, where Edwin Wells Dwight, chairman of the Medical Directors' Association, presented data from 180,000 New England Mutual policyholders showing that "tobacco abstainers" had a 43 percent lower mortality than expected from American Experience Tables. Ten years later, a Life Extension Institute study of Dartmouth College graduates (class of 1868) showed smokers dying about seven years earlier than nonsmokers; see Cassandra Tate, *Cigarette Wars: The Triumph of the Little White Slaver* (New York: Oxford University Press, 1999), p. 143.

62. Maurine B. Neuberger, *Smoke Screen: Tobacco and the Public Welfare* (Englewood Cliffs, NJ: Prentice-Hall, 1963), p. 6. Earl T. Opstad, assistant medical director at Northwestern National Life Insurance Co., in 1963 published a calculation of how many people must be dying prematurely as a result of smoking. Using "extremely conservative" figures so as not to be accused of "blowing up something way out of proportion," he came up with a per annum minimum of 101,646 excess deaths for American males aged thirty to sixty-four. About half of these were from coronary heart disease, with lung cancer adding another 32,000 to

34,000 and emphysema another 12,000 to 14,000. See his "Smoking and Heart Disease," *New England Journal of Medicine* 268 (1963): 903, Bates TI04703357.

63. John Ingram (Commissioner of Insurance, State of North Carolina) to Horace Kornegay, May 25, 1979, Bates TI07710818.

64. For Farmers: "NARB Okays Non-Smokers' Auto Policies Insurance Ad," *Advertising Age*, Dec. 15, 1975, Bates TI07710819. For "never been scientifically proven": Horace R. Kornegay to Robert W. Graf, March 6, 1980, Bates TIFL0537465–7466. Kornegay characterized the Allstate plan as the first example of a major advertiser using television "to carry an anti-smoking message for commercial purposes"; see his speech of Sept. 13, 1979, Bates TIMN0067878–7882. When J. C. Penny offered a similar discount, Fred Panzer wrote to Kornegay, his boss at the TI: "you might want to organize an effort similar to that used with Sears" (Dec. 1, 1980, Bates TIMN0067468).

65. James Bowling to William Kloepfer, July 12, 1979, Bates TIFL0537447; Robert S. Seiler (Allstate) to Harold B. McGuffey (Kentucky Commissioner of Insurance), Sept. 11, 1979, Bates TIMN0333248–3249; and for the science relied on by Allstate, Bates TIMN0333250–3251; Bates TI07710807; TI07710800. Bowling didn't want it to be known that Burnett had been funneling Allstate ad campaign plans to Philip Morris, which is why he insisted to Kloepfer at the TI that "Burnett's identity as a source must be protected" (July 23, 1979, Bates TIFL0537444).

66. Robert S. Seiler (Allstate) to Kirk Wayne (Tobacco Associates), Sept. 20, 1979, Bates TIMN0333241–3244.

67. For "identify and support": John Lyons to Susan M. Stuntz and Martin J. Gleason, "Anti-Smoking Practices of the Insurance Industry," Nov. 22, 1989, Bates TIMN0034730–4731; Anne Landman, "Push or Be Punished: Tobacco Industry Documents Reveal Aggression against Businesses That Discourage Tobacco Use," *Tobacco Control* 9 (2000): 339–46. For "Gays": Sparber and Associates, Inc., "Recommendations: The Anti-Smoker Practices of the Insurance Industry," Oct. 1989, Bates TIMN0034733–4742. Earle Clements in the early 1970s had assigned Marvin Kastenbaum at the TI "to the insurance watch"; see Bates TI077 10805. We need to search insurance industry archives for more examples of such pressures.

68. Bertram Harnett to Frank T. Crohn, Jan. 30, 1981, Bates 03736224–6256.

69. Michael J. Cowell and Brian L. Hirst (State Mutual), *Mortality Differences between Smokers and Non-Smokers*, Oct. 22, 1979, Bates TI47381555–1562; "Surgeon General's Statement," Oct. 22, 1979, Bates TIFL0537439. State Mutual's paper appeared in the *Transactions of the Society of Actuaries*; see Michael J. Cowell and Brian L. Hirst, "Mortality Differences between Smokers and Non-Smokers: Authors' Review of Discussion," Sept. 1980, Bates 03736293–6320. The Tobacco Institute had its chief statistician write a critique; Shook, Hardy and Bacon helped Kastenbaum with this project, a fact not disclosed in the final manuscript; see Marvin A. Kastenbaum to Horace Kornegay, June 12, 1980, Bates 03736333, and for Kastenbaum's critique: Bates 03736336–6343. State Mutual responded to this and other critiques, discovering in the process that a number of other insurance companies had confirmed their general conclusions but also that Phoenix Mutual had investigated the impact of smoking on life span as early as 1910.

70. "Insurance Companies Offering Non-Smokers Plans and Discounts," 1979, Bates TIFL0537186–7189.

71. This, according to the American Council on Life Insurance Co., Bates TI46500915.

72. Robert Rosner, "Subsidizing Smokers—Something to Burn Over," *Los Angeles Times,* Nov. 17, 1988, Bates TI00261137; Gordon B. Lindsay, *Make a Killing: A Smoking Satire on Selling Cigarettes* (Bountiful, Utah: Horizon, 1997), p. 25.

73. G. E. Moore, "Smoking and Life Insurance," *British Medical Journal* 1 (1962): 1345.

74. *Current Digest* 8 (July 1963): 27, Bates TIMN0230726–0765.

75. G. E. Moore, "How to Save 40,000 Lives a Year" (Editorial), *Medical Tribune,* May 24, 1963, p. 11; compare "Challenge to Dr. Moore" and "Dr. Moore's Reply, *Medical Tribune,* June 14, 1963, p. 11, reported in Bates TIMN0230726–0765.

76. Stanley Truman Brooks, "Preliminary Report on a Critical Survey of Current Research," Nov. 20, 1953, Bates 950297104–7108.

77. Brooks to Hanmer, Dec. 24, 1953, Bates MNAT00709471–9478, pp. 2–3.

78. "Luncheon Meeting—November 5, 1953: Representatives of Industry—Yale Club," Bates 950164205–4206. Most of this meeting was devoted to Reynolds's plans for setting up "machinery for combating the propaganda which is being directed against the cigarette industry," for which Reynolds had allocated $200,000.

79. Paul M. Hahn, "Press Release" (for the American Tobacco Company), Nov. 26, 1953, MNAT00609882–9886.

80. Dwight Macdonald to Hiram Hanmer, Dec. 17, 1953, Bates 950278537–8538; Hiram Hanmer, "Memorandum on Telephone Conversation between Mr. Hanmer and Mr. Dwight Macdonald," Jan. 4, 1954, Bates 950278535.

81. Edwin F. Dakin, "Forwarding Memorandum: To Members of the Planning Committee," late Dec. 1953, Bates JH000493–0501, p. 2.

82. Engel, "Cigarettes Cause Cancer?" p. 7; H. R. Parmele to A. Riefner, July 29, 1946, Bates 92520611–0612. Milton Schur of Ecusta also attended the Nov. 5, 1953, meeting.

83. "At one time or another during those years critics have held it responsible for practically every disease of the human body. One by one these charges have been abandoned for lack of evidence"; see "A Frank Statement to Cigarette Smokers," Jan. 4, 1954, Bates HT012 7042. A Dec. 26, 1953, draft of the "Frank Statement," with corrections from another Plaza Hotel meeting of December 28, can be found at Bates 4720; and for passages proposed (but not used) by American Tobacco Chief Counsel T. J. Ross, see Bates 4711.

84. Hanmer to Miller, Oct. 8, 1953, p. 3.

85. Two of the most intelligent celebrations of smoke along these lines are Klein, *Cigarettes Are Sublime;* and Luc Sante, *No Smoking* (New York: Assouline, 2004). Ross Millhiser is cited in Kluger, *Ashes to Ashes,* p. 488. Philip Morris in its Archetype Project from 1990–91 explored the notion that new smokers could be attracted by identifying smoking as "for adults only"; Gilbert Clotaire Rapaille, a French marketing consultant with expertise in adolescent psychology, developed a series of recommendations for the company that included the following: "Make it difficult for minors to obtain cigarettes" and "Stress that smoking is dangerous [and] for people who like to take risks, who are not afraid of taboos, who take life as an adventure to prove themselves." See Carolyn Levy, "Archetype Project Summary," Aug. 20, 1991, Bates 2062145482–5496.

86. Marketing and Research Counselors, "What Have We Learned?"

87. Jonathan Kwitny, "Defending the Weed: How Embattled Group Uses Tact, Calculation to Blunt Its Opposition," *Wall Street Journal,* Jan. 24, 1972, Bates 500324162–4164.

PART III

1. Eric LeGresley, "A 'Vector Analysis' of the Tobacco Epidemic," *Bulletin of Medicus Mundi Switzerland,* no. 72 (April 1999).

CHAPTER 16

1. For "stop business tomorrow," see George Weissman's March 26, 1954, speech titled "Public Relations and Cigarette Marketing," Bates 3039590020–0025, reported in the *St. Paul Press,* March 30, 1954, Bates 1002366403–6408. For Bowling, see Kwitny, "Defending the Weed." For Bible, see his testimony in *Florida v. American Tobacco,* Aug. 21, 1997, Bates 2083493341–3364, p. 27. Bible was asked about his promise in *Minnesota v. Philip Morris* on March 2, 1998, and responded that if even one person were found to have died from smoking he would "reassess" his duties as Philip Morris CEO; see Bates BIBLEG030298, pp. 5707–9. For Gerald H. Long, see Roy McKenzie, "A Loyalist Views Tobacco's Fate," *Insight,* May 19, 1986, p. 15, Bates 515836770.

2. Paul M. Hahn's telegram of December 10, 1953, inviting the CEOs to meet at the Plaza Hotel, is at Bates 508775416. For "weighty scientific views" and "no proof": Hill & Knowlton, "Preliminary Recommendations for Cigarette Manufacturers," Dec. 24, 1953, Bates 508775406–5415.

3. "A Frank Statement to Cigarette Smokers," Jan. 4, 1954, Bates HT0127042–7042; and for an early draft, Bates 508775403–5405.

4. Fuller, Smith and Ross, "The Tobacco Industry Research Committee: A Report on Expenditures to Date and Discussion of Possible Additional Media," Jan. 15, 1954, Bates 11309839–9854. For "negro newspapers," see R. E. Allen, "Tobacco Industry Research Committee," Dec. 29, 1953, Bates 4715.

5. For "extremist attacks": Hill & Knowlton, "Statement by Timothy V. Hartnett, Chairman, Tobacco Industry Research Committee," For release not before Dec. 27, 1954, Bates 11311167–1169. For "prairie fire": "The Facts Always Win," *Cincinnati Enquirer,* Jan. 6, 1954. For modern India: Prabhat Jha et al., including R. Peto, "A Nationally Representative Case-Control Study of Smoking and Death in India," *New England Journal of Medicine* 358 (2008): 1137–47.

6. Hill & Knowlton, "Progress Report," Jan. 15, 1954, Bates 2023614849–4851; "Editorial Response in Key Cities" (Lorillard), Jan. 1954, Bates 01138883–8994.

7. The CTR's final annual report appeared on May 28, 1997; see Bates 70001394–1394. Contributions to CTR from the tobacco companies totaled $473 million from 1954 through 1998.

8. "Remarks of Dr. Leon O. Jacobson," Dec. 9, 1983, Bates 70005745–8746; emphasis added.

9. C. C. Little to T. V. Hartnett, "TIRC Research Program," July 16, 1959, Bates CTRMN004 358–4366.

10. H. R. Bentley, D. G. I. Felton, and W. W. Reid, "Report on Visit to U.S.A. and Canada, 17th April–12th May 1958," June 11, 1958, Bates TIOK 0034790–4799, p. 5.

11. ACS, *CA—Bulletin of Cancer Progress,* March–April, 1958, front inside cover and p. 71. The "sideshow" quote is from Jones Day, "Corporate Activity Project," p. 128.

12. "$82,000 Is Granted to Study Tobacco," *New York Times*, Nov. 8, 1954, Bates CORTI001 3661.

13. The Tobacco Institute was the brainchild of Edward A. Darr, president of R. J. Reynolds; see Robert K. Heimann (inferred), "Public Relations in the Field of Smoking and Health," Jan. 1963, Bates ATX110005290–5303, p. 3. Willard Greenwald at Philip Morris as early as 1938 had proposed establishing a "tobacco institute" to forge "closer and more friendly relations between the companies"; see "Memorandum of Meeting between Dr. Haag and Dr. Greenwald," Jan. 18, 1938, Bates 950200322–0323. The TI in the late 1970s moved to 1875 I Street, only four blocks from the White House. For Little's keep in his "ivory tower": Covington & Burling, "Confidential Report Prepared by TI Outside Counsel," Jan. 1963, Bates MNATPRIV00024887-4900.

14. For Brown & Williamson: Yeaman, "Implications of Battelle Hippo." For "little relevance": Rogers and Todd, "Report on Policy," p. 18. For "backwater": BATCo, "Report on Visit to U.S.A.," p. 28. For "T.I.R.C. research": Covington & Burling, "Public Relations," p. 13.

15. "Facilities of the CTR Library—June 1974," Bates 70005745–8746.

16. J. S. Campbell to Horace R. Kornegay, June 8, 1971, Bates CORTI0004683–4684.

17. The characterization of the CTR as a "shield" and a "front" is explicit in R. B. Seligman to CTR File, "Meeting in New York," Nov. 17, 1978, Bates 1003718428–8432, where we also hear, "It is extremely important that the industry continue to spend their dollars on research to show that we don't agree that the case against smoking is closed." For "Let's face it": Helmut Wakeham to J. F. Cullman III, "'Best' Program for C.T.R.," Dec. 8, 1970, Bates 1005082153–2158.

18. For the 9 volumes prepared for the Surgeon General's Advisory Committee, see Liggett & Myers Tobacco Co. and Arthur D. Little, Inc., *Current Status of Studies on Smoking and Health*, April 1, 1963. The preface and introduction are at Bates TIMN0446452–6479, and the volume on constituents and biological activity can be found at Bates LG0268863–9034. The introductory volume on epidemiology concluded that much of this work had been "unreliably conducted" and that even the "better-conducted studies" did not demonstrate a hazard warranting "a degree of public concern greater than that provided by many other common habits, not singled out for official inquiry" (pp. 2–8). For "withheld from the general public," see the unsigned document from April 1, 1963, Bates 2022969690. James D. Mold later testified that the Liggett/ADL volumes were "confidential," with access granted only on a "Need to know basis"; see his "Summary Statement" to the U.S. House of Representatives Committee on Energy and Commerce, July 1987, Bates TIMN0299685–9695.

19. For Joseph E. Bumgarner, see his deposition of Nov. 11, 1996, for *Texas v. American Tobacco Co.*, Bates Bumgarnerj111196. For "close to showing": Paul E. Brubaker for Jones, Day, Reavis & Pogue, "The R. J. Reynolds Tobacco Company's Biology Research Division: A Program Review," Dec. 15, 1985, Bates 507928501–8691. This document is a whitewash of Reynolds's biological work from the late 1960s. For the Mouse House Massacre more generally: Frank V. Tursi, Susan E. White, and Steve McQuilkin, *Lost Empire: The Fall of R. J. Reynolds Company* (Winston-Salem, NC: Winston-Salem Journal, 1999–2000). Anthony Colucci, an RJR biochemist from 1967 to 1970 and a consultant for its legal defense in the 1980s, claims that the Mouse House was closed "because Reynolds did not at that time want

to be collecting information that might be detrimental to itself. . . . Ignorance is bliss" (Kluger, *Ashes to Ashes*, p. 360).

20. "Philip Morris Research on Nicotine Pharmacology and Human Smoking Behavior," April 6, 1994, 2046819241–9265; compare the Shook, Hardy and Bacon document: "Philip Morris Behavioral Research Program," 1992, Bates 2021423403–3497.

21. William Farone, deposition for *Ironworkers v. Philip Morris*, March 1, 1999, Bates FARONEW030199, p. 1919; also Kluger, *Ashes to Ashes*, pp. 575–76.

22. Kluger, *Ashes to Ashes*, p. 576.

23. Leonard S. Zahn to Henry Ramm and Tom Hoyt, April 22, 1974, Bates ZN19604–9605. For a draft of Homburger's press release from April 8, 1974: Bates ZN19613–9613; and for his 1997 deposition on this sequence of events in *Broin v. Philip Morris:* Bates HOM BURGERF052797.

24. This "reasonable guess" is presented in Charles R. Green and Alan Rodgman, "The Tobacco Chemists' Research Conference: A Half Century Forum for Advances in Analytical Methodology of Tobacco and Its Products," June 6, 1996, Bates 525445600–5785, p. 7. A list of more than two hundred participating chemists can be found in "Tobacco Chemists Research Conference, Attendance Record, Duke University," Oct. 24, 1958, Bates 950264981–4987. The European counterpart to America's *Tobacco Science* was Germany's *Beiträge zur Tabakforschung*, established in 1961.

25. For Reynolds: Ralph L. Rowland, "Management Meeting, March 22, 1971, Rewards and Recognition," April 20, 1971, Bates 515873927–3929. For Philip Morris: W. L. Dunn to T. S. Osdene, "Proposed Study by Levy," Nov. 3, 1977, Bates 1000128680.

26. A. W. Spears to John W. Nowell, Aug. 17, 1960, Bates 01370915; Nowell to Spears, Aug. 26, 1960, Bates 01370882.

27. W. T. Hoyt to T. V. Hartnett, "Statement of F. G. Bock in Buffalo, N.Y.," Oct. 23, 1956, Bates 680911588–1589.

28. Taylor, *Smoke Ring*, pp. 18–19; Thilo Grüning, Anna B. Gilmore, and Martin McKee, "Tobacco Industry Influence on Science and Scientists in Germany," *American Journal of Public Health* 96 (2006): 20–32.

29. For "skeptical scientists": Donald K. Hoel, "Industry Research Committee Meeting," Nov. 6, 1978, Bates USX5133–5139. For "most scientists now agree": Gary D. Friedman et al., "Mortality in Middle-Aged Smokers and Nonsmokers," *New England Journal of Medicine* 300 (1979): 213–17.

30. Trial testimony of Clarence Cook Little in *Lartigue v. Reynolds*, Oct. 6, 1960, Bates 515382801–2968, p. 2818. For Little's life prior to tobacco, see Karen Rader, *Making Mice: Standardizing Animals for American Biomedical Research, 1900–1955* (Princeton: Princeton University Press, 2004).

31. For Little on fear, see his trial testimony in *Zagurski v. American Tobacco*, June 7, 1967, Bates LITTLEC060767, p. 675. For Project Truth: "Objectives," Bates 690010962–0963, attached to J. W. Burgard to R. A. Pittman, Aug. 21, 1969, Bates 1700.02. For "lynched": "Remarks of Horace Kornegay," April 20, 1970, Bates TIMN0127927–7939.

32. Others considered for the job of SAB chairman included Leon Jacobson, Clayton Loosli, R. Harrison Rigdon, and R. Lee Clark. The industry didn't contact any of the recognized leaders of the field—neither Wynder, Graham, Doll, nor Ochsner, for example, and

apparently not Hammond; see Irwin W. Tucker's deposition of July 29, 1997, Bates tucke rio72997.

33. Hueper was offered the SAB chairmanship in the spring of 1954; see my *Cancer Wars: How Politics Shapes What We Know and Don't Know about Cancer* (New York: Basic Books, 1995), pp. 110, 295 n. 61; also my "Wilhelm Hueper: Pioneer of Environmental Carcinogenesis," in *Medizingeschichte und Gesellschaftskritik: Festschrift für Gerhard Baader*, ed. Michael Hubenstorf et al. (Husum: Matthiesen Verlag, 1997), pp. 290–305. Hueper in 1959 told a Pittsburgh seminar, "I do believe cigaret smoking plays a role, either directly or indirectly, in lung cancer. But I am personally convinced it is not one of our major causative agents." See "Cigarets Get 'Reprieve' on Cancer," *Pittsburgh Press*, April 30, 1959, reported in the *Tobacco News Summary*, May 6, 1959, Bates 1005035505–5506. Hueper's 10 percent figure was, as he himself put it, a "wild guess" produced only when Geoffrey F. Todd pressured him to provide an estimate; see Todd's "Visit to U.S.A. and Canada: Report to T.M.S.C.," June 14, 1961, Bates 105367083–7098, p. 8.

34. For "safe for the industry": Hiram R. Hanmer, "Memo," March 15, 1954, Bates 950259121–9122, tid izy34foo. Charles B. Huggins's assessment of Steiner is cited in "Report of Visit to University of Chicago and Michael Reese Hospital by Irwin Tucker, Grant Clarke and H. R. Hanmer: Subject, Scientific Director for TIRC," Feb. 15, 1954, Bates 950259159–9169, p. 7.

35. Trial testimony of Clarence Cook Little in *Lartigue v. Reynolds*, Oct. 5, 1960, Bates LITTLEC100560, pp. 2715–16. Little's biographers have tended to ignore his tobacco work; the sixteen-page obituary published by Jackson Laboratory Director Earl L. Green doesn't even mention tobacco; see "Dr. Clarence Cook Little," *JAX: The Jackson Laboratory*, 19 (Winter 1971–72): 1–16, Bates 1472170–2185.

36. Typical would be Suzanne Oparil's characterization of the CTR as "a very high quality research funding organization"; see her testimony in *Engel v. Reynolds*, March 22, 1999, Bates 525526542–6664, pp. 28623–26; and in other trials at Bates 526014897–4977. John C. Burnham's 1986 disclosure for *Dewey v. Reynolds* states that the TIRC/CTR was "a respectable/commendable scientific effort" (Bates 2024941548–1551).

37. Sheldon C. Sommers, "Curriculum Vitae," Dec. 1991, Bates 2501070219–0245.

38. Sheldon C. Sommers, deposition testimony for *Galbraith v. Reynolds*, Sept. 4, 1985, Bates 505551319A-1472, p. 66.

39. Ibid., pp. 68–70.

40. See, for example, Sommers' testimony for the defense in Helsinki City Court, Jan. 31, 1991, Bates 566406564–6652.

41. "Mailing by Fisher-Stevens of 1970–71 Annual Report," Feb. 1972, Bates March 31, 1972, Bates 10399040–9040.

42. Kenneth R. Gundle, Molly J. Dingel and Barbara A. Koenig, "'To Prove This Is the Industry's Best Hope': Big Tobacco's Support of Research on the Genetics of Nicotine Addiction," *Addiction* 105 (2010): 974–83.

43. For "brush fires": J. Morrison Brady to Clarence C. Little, "TIRC Program," April 9, 1962, Bates 92520643–0644. U.S. Tobacco R&D chief W. D. Bennett in August 1974 wrote (copied) to Bantle noting that cigarette companies had built up "quite a stable of experts in these fields related to their products"; see W. D. Bennett to R. D. Harwood, Aug. 23, 1974;

and for background: Morton Mintz, "The Artful Dodgers—Did Tobacco Executives Tell the Truth about Smokeless Tobacco?" *Washington Monthly,* Oct. 1986, p. 6.

44. For Cohen: Alix M. Freedman and Laurie P. Cohen, "Smoke and Mirrors: How Cigarette Makers Keep Health Question 'Open' Year after Year," *Wall Street Journal,* Feb. 11, 1993. For Glenn, who eventually apologized for his remarks about Cohen, see John Fahs, *Cigarette Confidential: The Unfiltered Truth about the Ultimate Addiction* (New York: Berkley Books, 1996), pp. 50–52.

45. CTR applications for these six Nobel laureates can be found at Bates 50093423–3437 (Baruj Benacerraf from 1971), Bates 50234926–4967 (Stanley Cohen 1982), Bates 50177702–7727 (Harold Varmus 1984), Bates 50132484–2492 (Ferid Murad 1977), Bates 50306400–6412 (Carol Greider 1991), and Bates 40032703–2715 (Louis Ignarro 1996). Ignarro mentioned carcinogens in cigarette smoke in his 1979 application (Bates 50219035–9071), and his rejection can be found at Bates 50219026. Murad's 1977 application is apparently the only successful one to mention cigarette smoke, albeit as only one of several agents influencing cyclic guanosine monophosphate in tissues.

46. A list of all forty-three members of the TIRC/CTR's Scientific Advisory Board from 1954 through 1996 can be found in Lorraine Pollice to Ernest Pepples (Brown & Williamson), "Scientific Advisory Board Members," Oct. 18, 2000, Bates 70100464–0467.

47. Testimony of Clarence Cook Little in *Lartigue v. Reynolds,* Oct. 6, 1960, pp. 2782–83, Bates 515382801–2968. Asked whether every one of the members of the TIRC believed it was still an open question whether smoking had been shown to cause cancer, Little answered, "Every one of them believes it is an open question as to whether causation has or has not been proven" (p. 2783).

48. See David Michaels, *Doubt Is Their Product: How Industry's Assault on Science Threatens Your Health* (New York: Oxford University Press, 2008); also Oreskes and Conway, *Merchants of Doubt.*

49. Thomas J. Moran, testimony at U.S. congressional hearings on *Cigarettes and Smoking Products,* June 29, 1964, Bates 968246800–6972, p. 471.

50. Stanley Frank, "To Smoke or Not to Smoke—That Is *Still* the Question," *True Magazine,* Jan. 1968, pp. 35–36, 69–71, where Frank concluded there was "absolutely no proof that smoking causes human cancer." The story is well told in Wagner's *Cigarette Country,* pp. 176–89.

51. Clarence Cook Little, *Cancer: A Study for Laymen,* 2nd ed. (New York: American Cancer Society, 1944).

52. Testimony of Clarence Cook Little in *Lartigue v. Reynolds,* p. 2740.

53. Clarence Cook Little, deposition testimony in *Green v. American Tobacco,* Nov. 3, 1959, Bates HAHNP051960, pp. 191–92.

54. Hiram Hanmer in 1954 reassured a correspondent that failure to find carcinogens in tobacco smoke was not as widely known as it should be "because negative results are rarely published" (Hanmer to Carl A. Nau, Sept. 2, 1954, Bates 950168223–8224).

55. H. Lee Sarokin, "Opinion," *Cipollone v. Liggett,* April 21, 1988, Bates 2072420693–0725.

56. See, for example, the eighty-five-page listing in David R. Hardy (Shook, Hardy), to Frederick P. Haas et al., Oct. 6 and 25, 1966, Bates ATMXPRIV0014423–4507 and 20239 18152–8173.

57. For Saiger: "Saiger Study Involving Inclusion of Many More Variables in Statistical Analyses," Feb. 26, 1966, Bates 955008172. For SP-100: "Critique by a Panel of Experts of Statistics Relied upon by the Surgeon General's Advisory Committee," Oct. 6, 1966, Bates 955008165–8168. For Olkin: A. W. Spears to A. J. Stevens, March 1, 1976, Bates 00500240–0241; also Bates CTRSP/FILES013812–3815. Olkin was also paid at least $1,600 under Jacob and Medinger's Special Account #4, a pool of cash reserved for sensitive legal work; see Bates 955019744–9755. Compare Bates 955008065 (for SP-26), 955008099 (SP-30), 955008108 (SP-31), 955008113–8114 (SP-32), and 955008178 (SP-103).

58. Deposition of McAllister in *Blue Cross v. Philip Morris*, June 15, 2000, Bates McAllisterH061500, p. 101. A list of 106 Special Projects grantees can be found in Judge Kessler's "Amended Final Opinion," p. 135.

59. "Statement of Dr. Victor Buhler," April 24, 1969, Bates 2015039120–9130.

60. "Statement of Arthur Furst," April 24, 1969, Bates 2015039164–9171.

61. John P. Wyatt, "Statement," April 24, 1969, Bates 2015039186–9189; "Statement of Duane Carr, M.D.," April 25, 1969, Bates 2015039247–9254.

62. For "probably invalid": Statement of Theodor D. Sterling, April 24, 1969, Bates 20150 39196–9214 (and the TI press release at Bates 2015039195); and for his other work for the industry, see his "A Critical Reassessment of the Evidence Bearing on Smoking as the Cause of Lung Cancer," Sept. 1971, Bates 680143516–3625. For "exaggerated propaganda," see his "Dubious Figures Cast a Cloud over Anti-Tobacco Lobby," *Vancouver Sun*, Sept. 2, 1993, Bates 8771 5643 and 2015039272–9277; and for background: Glantz et al., *Cigarette Papers*, pp. 296–301.

63. For Grant 56-B: Alexander Holtzman to David R. Hardy, Oct. 3, 1968, Bates 10050 84784–4786. For "witness in litigation": Kessler, "Amended Final Opinion," p. 115. Hickey doesn't mention his Special Project funding in his article with Richard C. Clelland and Evelyn B. Harner, "Smoking, Birth-Weight, Development, and Pollution," *Lancet* 1 (1973): 270, Bates 955004255.

64. For "dictated by priorities": Domingo M. Aviado, "Annual Report to Shook, Hardy and Bacon," Jan. 27, 1982, Bates 94347226–7240; also his "Asbestos/Cigarette Smoking Interactions—A Review of the Medical Literature, 1882 to 1982," Oct. 5, 1983, Bates 2062 774448–4949 at 4568. For "no health hazard": Australian Tobacco Institute, "Cigarette Smoke and the Non-Smoker," March 1976, Bates 503676995–7004, p. 51. For SHB's Project No. 9: Domingo M. Aviado, "Annual Report to Shook, Hardy and Bacon," Jan. 20, 1981, Bates 94347206–7223.

65. David R. Hardy to Thomas F. Ahrensfeld et al., June 13, 1972, Bates 1005084973–4976. Mancuso had been on friendly terms with the TIRC since the 1950s, though his first application for CTR funds was not until 1972, when he asked for $328,850 to study occupational epidemiology. By July 1973, in a paper coauthored with Theodor D. Sterling, he was disputing the theory that "a single factor, smoking, is the major cause of lung cancer"; see Bates CTRSP/FILES010513/05.

66. James F. Glenn to Dr. Jacobson and CTR Staff, "Alvan R. Feinstein, MD, Yale," Feb. 2, 1988, Bates CTRSP-FILES025320. Feinstein edited the *Journal of Chronic Diseases* (1982–88) and was founding editor of the *Journal of Clinical Epidemiology* (1988–2001).

67. Timothy M . Finnegan to Ahrensfeld et al., "Alvan R. Feinstein," July 7, 1981, Bates 503654999–5000.

68. "Evidence-Based Medicine Has Come a Long Way," *BMJ* 329 (2004): 990–91.

69. Alvan R. Feinstein, "Justice, Science, and the 'Bad Guys,'" *Toxicologic Pathology* 20 (1992): 303–05.

70. Henry T. Lynch to David Stone, "Application #2352, 'Improved Scientific Methods in Clinical Epidemiology,' Alvan R. Feinstein MD," Feb. 16, 1988, Bates CTRSP/FILES025318–5319.

71. David M. Murphy to Herbert M. Wachtell, Paul Vizcarrondo Jr., and John F. Savarese, April 28, 1992, Bates 87715635–5636.

72. Kessler, "Amended Final Opinion," p. 3.

73. For "rebuts and discredits": Paul M. Hahn to John W. Hill, Feb. 5, 1958, Bates 2072420837–0841. For 536,000 copies: Tobacco Institute, "Detailed Distribution of Tobacco and Health," n.d., Bates TIMN0070595–0597. *Tobacco and Health* was also sent to 800 Reynolds "Student Representatives"; 50 copies were also sent to each of the company's 1,180 salesmen (F. G. Carter to Bowman Gray, July 9, 1958, Bates 502364141).

74. Carl Thompson to William Kloepfer Jr., "*Tobacco and Health Research* Procedural Memo," Oct. 18, 1968, Bates TIMN0071488–1491.

75. For "most important type of story": Thompson to Kloepfer, "*Tobacco and Health Research* Procedural Memo," p. 2. The Tobacco Institute in 1960 hired Group Attitudes Corporation, a subsidiary of Hill & Knowlton, to assess the medical response to the paper and found a great deal of sympathy (and that most U.S. doctors still smoked); see "Doctors' Attitudes toward *Tobacco and Health*," April 1960, Bates TIMS00029861–9910. And for doctors' responses: Bates 11291393–1394, 50014938–4938, 50077581–7582, 11278247–8247, and 50033887–3887.

76. For "controlled list": "Confidential Report: Tobacco Industry Research Committee Meeting," Nov. 8, 1957, Bates 689329566–9570. For "almost entirely": John W. Hill, "Smoking, Health and Statistics: The Story of the Tobacco Accounts," Feb. 26, 1962, Bates 98721513–1551.

77. Martin Forster et al., "The State of Knowledge Regarding Tobacco Harm, 1920–1964: Industry and Public Health Service Perspectives," Dec. 7, 2006, http://www.tobacco.org/news/243428.html; also Tobacco Industry Research Committee, "A Working Reference Catalog of Selected Scientific Papers," 1955, Bates 01138194–8288.

78. K. Michael Cummings et al., "What Scientists Funded by the Tobacco Industry Believe about the Hazards of Cigarette Smoking," *American Journal of Public Health* 81 (1991): 894–96.

79. For "one of America's foremost": "Little Dies; Researcher on Cancer," (Mamaroneck) *Daily Times,* Dec. 23, 1971, Bates 1472169. For "hobbyhorse": "Dr. Clarence Little, Cancer Researcher, Dies at 83," *New York Times,* Dec. 23, 1971, Bates 1472190.

80. For "stripped": James F. Glenn to Judith L. Swain, Oct. 20, 1998, Bates 70011788–1789. For "best that I resign": Swain to Glenn, April 13, 1998, Bates 70012088–2088.

81. See, for example, Suzanne Oparil to Harmon C. McAllister, Aug. 25, 1988, Bates 50361170–1170; and extensive correspondence at Bates 50361066 through 50361127.

82. "I became an expert on the activities of the Council of Tobacco Research when I became funded by them" (Bates 70001476–1555, p. 57). Oparil had earlier served as a witness for the Campbell Soup Co., testifying that the salt they put in soup did not cause high blood pressure.

83. Suzanne Oparil, deposition testimony for *Broin v. Philip Morris,* June 18, 1997, Bates 70001476–1555, pp. 18–35, 51–52.

84. Suzanne Oparil, deposition testimony for *Engle v. Reynolds,* July 27, 1997, Bates OPARILS072797, pp. 51, 66–68, 79–80, 84.

85. Oparil was named president of the American Society of Hypertension (ASH) on May 22, 2006, following the resignation of Jean E. Sealey, a cardiovascular biochemist at Cornell, who had called for increased disclosure of the Society's pharmaceutical ties. The ASH had been embarrassed by revelations that drug manufacturers had been giving large sums of money to the Society to broaden its definition of hypertension, thereby enlarging the number of people defined as needing medication. See Stephanie Saul, "Unease on Industry's Role in Hypertension Debate," *New York Times,* May 20, 2006; also Susan Jeffrey, "Sealey Resigns, Oparil Is in as Incoming ASH President," *HeartWire,* May 22, 2006. For "smoking does not cause hypertension": Oparil, deposition testimony for *Engle v. Reynolds,* July 27, 1997, Bates OPARILS072797, p. 72.

86. History of the American Heart Association, http://www.americanheart.org/presenter.jhtml?identifier = 10860, accessed Feb. 2009.

CHAPTER 17

1. John W. Burgard to R. A. Pittman et al., "Smoking and Health Proposal," Aug. 21, 1969, Bates 680561776–1777, and attached speech at 680561778–1786, p. 4. It is not entirely clear who spoke these "doubt is our product" lines. One copy of the speech has a marginal notation "JVB," which would be John V. Blalock, Brown & Williamson's director of public relations. Page 2 of the speech refers to "Mr. Yeaman's and John Blalock's files," however, suggesting that this part—including the "doubt is our product" passage on p. 4—was spoken by someone else. The initials "CM" are directly under JVB's on p. 1, and this is clearly Corny Muije from the marketing department, who was also presenting. Muije does not begin his remarks until page 5, however, which is one page after the "doubt is our product" remarks. The "doubt" passage therefore cannot be either Blalock or Muije and is probably spoken by John W. Burgard, the company's powerful marketing VP. For early public discussions of this memo, see "Tobacco Firm Used Doubt Ads Says FTC Secret Report," *Plain Talk* (Newport, TN), July 8, 1981, Bates 690834754; and Glantz et al., *Cigarette Papers,* pp. 188–89. John W. Burgard was named vice president for advertising at Brown & Williamson in the 1950s. At B&W he supervised Dr. I. W. ("Wally") Hughes, director of "research relative to health and outside studies," and Robert A. Sanford, director of research product and process. There are other B&W memos listing "doubt" as a "product"; see the untitled chronology listing "Doubt" as the company's "Product" in a list of "Marketing Elements," circa 1969, Bates 690010940–0945. Burgard was also the author of "History of Cigarette Advertising" up to 1953 (Bates 04238374–8433).

2. Matthew L. Myers (for the FTC), "Staff Report," May 1981, Bates 680559945.

3. Keith Richardson to R. E. Thornton (BAT Southampton), April 27, 1984, Bates 201774616–4619.

4. Brown & Williamson, *How Eminent Men of Medicine and Science Challenged the Smoking-and-Health Theory during Recent Hearings in the U.S. Congress,* 1969, Bates 80059834–

984 1. For a list of more than a hundred papers, pamphlets, films, bumper stickers, and booklets distributed by the Tobacco Institute as of 1978, see "Inventory Index," July 1978, Bates TI16581095–1103; also "Institute Publications, Smoking and Health Related, 1983–Present," Bates TI10590658–0659.

5. For a 187-page compendium of industry-friendly sound bites on tobacco and health, a veritable encyclopedia of expert ignorance, see the Tobacco Institute's "Smoking & Health Quotes Book" (intended for internal use), Nov. 1977, Bates 500504903–5089.

6. This strategy was already in place in Germany in the 1930s; for this *Paradegreise* v. *Paradeleichen* see " 'Tabakmissbrauch?' " *Reine Luft* 21 (1939): 101.

7. See, for example, Jacob Cohen and Robert K. Heimann, "Heavy Smokers with Low Mortality," *Industrial Medicine and Surgery* 31 (1962): 115–20. Raymond H. Rigdon in a letter to the editor of *Industrial Medicine and Surgery* wrote that Cohen and Heimann's study was "very difficult to refute"; this was then blown up into an American Tobacco press release (Bates 991107248–7250) and widely reported; see, for example, "New Survey Disputes Tobacco-Cancer Link," *Shreveport Times*, March 5, 1962, Bates 500034009.

8. See, for example, the Tobacco Institute's "Centuries-Old Smoking/Health Controversy Continues," *Caravan* 2 (Jan. 1968): 2–3.

9. "The Cigarette Controversy: 8 Questions and Answers," *Caravan* 3 (July 1969), Bates 507828498–8509.

10. For "creating doubt about the health charge": Fred Panzer to Horace Kornegay, "Roper Proposal," May 1, 1972, Bates TIFL0532362–2365. For "keep the controversy alive": Sharon Boyse (BAT), "Note on a Special Meeting of the UK Industry on Environmental Tobacco Smoke, London, February 17th, 1988," Bates 2063791176–1180. On the production of ignorance more generally, see my *Cancer Wars,* esp. chap. 5, and the volume edited by myself and Londa Schiebinger: *Agnotology: The Making and Unmaking of Ignorance* (Stanford: Stanford University Press, 2008).

11. "Why We're Dropping the New York Times" (AT ad), 1969, Bates 92382204. This ad was placed in at least thirty-one U.S. newspapers and magazines at a cost of $105,702; see Norman Chester to Robert K. Heimann, Sept. 5, 1969, Bates 947090322–0323.

12. Darr's letter is cited in A. H. Carrington to E. A. Darr, July 15, 1954, Bates 500718891–8892. For "direct evidence": Paul M. Hahn, "President's Letter to Our Stockholders," Feb. 4, 1958, Bates 945251644–2136, p. 10. For the words of Liggett Chairman and President Milton E. Harrington, see "Report of the Annual Meeting of Stockholders, April 27, 1965," Bates LG0154575–4587, p. 7. For Lorillard, see A. W. Spears to J. E. Bennett, "Possible Questions and Answers Pertaining to the Annual Meeting," Feb. 27, 1968, Bates 94672608–2616.

13. "Test Yourself on Tobacco/Health Issue," *Caravan* (Reynolds), May 1968, Bates 502283878. Employees are quickly informed that the correct answer is "c" in both instances.

14. "Needed: Less Heat and More Light," *Philip Morris Call News,* Aug. 1967, Bates 2051033546–3547.

15. For examples, see the *Congressional Record,* Dec. 4, 1967, pp. S17792–17815, Bates 00619074–9097.

16. R. J. Reynolds, "Internal Communications Publications," 1982, Bates 500644776–4801, p. 20.

17. For "unanswered questions": "Leading Scientist Rejects Smoking-Cancer Theories,"

RJR World, March–April 1974, Bates 502284007; "Fact and Fiction," *Caravan,* May 1968, Bates 502283877. For "no demonstrated relationship": "Smoking: Villain or Innocent Victim?" *Tobacco International Communiqué* (Reynolds Tobacco International), 5 (Nov.–Dec. 1980), p. 1, Bates 502130740–0759. For "pack a day": *Management Bulletin* (Reynolds), 9 (Aug. 5, 1957), Bates 508082205–2206. Rodgman by 1962 was worrying that his senior management was not getting valid scientific information and recommended distributing reports such as the Royal College of Physicians' *Smoking and Health* to all supervisory personnel. This, he thought, would keep them "better informed about the cigarette smoke-health problem than they would be if their main information sources were the daily newspaper, *Reader's Digest,* etc."; see his "Critical and Objective Appraisal," p. 15.

18. "Consumer Research Proposal: Employee Attitude Survey," 1982, Bates 501302435–2437.

19. "R. J. Reynolds Industries and Non-Tobacco Subsidiaries," 1980, Bates 505566775–6783, p. 5, with thanks to Jenny Pegg for discovering this document and method.

20. For "if the law . . . violence": "Los Alamos County Smoking Ordinance," Dec. 3, 1982, Bates 5705313–5317. For "campaigning": Charmian Schaller, "Tobacco Institute Poll Raising Eyebrows Here," *Los Alamos Monitor,* Dec. 15, 1982, Bates 2025684507–4509.

21. For "how to respond": *Sales Representative Training Manual,* vols. 1 and 2 (Reynolds: WLC, 1996), Bates 519810305–0853. For "complicated mathematical models": "R. J. Reynolds Issues Guide," Nov. 6, 1996, Bates 519980204–0441, pp. 3.1.1—3.1.5.

22. Philip Morris, "Jokes," 1978, Bates 2501241757–1769. Jokes of this sort were included as part of the industry's larger "Issues A–Z" pamphlet (Dec. 22, 1983, Bates 1005097556–7692). Humor is an important part of the industry's dismissal of smoking's hazards; see, for example, P. J. Hoffstrom's marvelous "Hoff 'n' Puff," *Tobacco Observer,* April 1980, Bates TIMN0121130–1141, p. 10.

23. "Issues A–Z," Dec. 22, 1983, Bates 1005097556–7692. This Philip Morris manual was periodically updated; see "Spokespersons' Guide," Oct. 1987, Bates 2503012201–2328. The Tobacco Institute developed a ninety-seven-page guide for its employees, incorporating both position statements and humor; see its "Overarching Themes/Rhetoric," 1986, Bates 0135836–5932.

24. Tobacco Institute, "College of Tobacco Knowledge," Nov. 16, 1981, Bates 690133003–3018; compare the biographies in "Student Profiles," Bates 89118698–8709; and for video from the 12th Annual Tobacco College, see http://www.archive.org/details/tobacco_car91f00.

25. "Dr. CJ Proctor—Travel/Meetings Schedule 1993–1994," Bates 500895887–5889; and "Training Schedule," Bates 500895884–5886.

26. Monique E. Muggli and Richard D. Hurt, "A Cigarette Manufacturer and a Managed Care Company Collaborate to Censor Health Information Targeted at Employees," *American Journal of Public Health* 94 (2004): 1307–11. Muggli and Hurt suggest that CIGNA's willingness to censor health information for the tobacco giant might have something to do with the fact that the insurer by 1995 held nearly $60 million in Philip Morris stock.

27. RJR Nabisco, "Annual Meeting of Shareholders," April 17, 1996, Bates 520800648–0821.

28. We shouldn't exaggerate their sophistication: a 932-page bibliography of books in Philip Morris's research library, for example, lists no works by Fritz Lickint, Germany's pre-

mier antitobacco scholar; see "Holdings of the Philip Morris Research Center Library," 1985, Bates 1002300062–0991.

29. For "couldn't be criticized": Kluger, *Ashes to Ashes*, p. 276. For "We within the industry are ignorant": W. L. Dunn to R. B. Seligman, March 21, 1980, Bates 1003289969–9970.

30. "Job Description," Sept. 1993, Bates 500895882–5883; compare 500895868–5871.

31. Randy W. Fulk, "Message from the President," http://317t.com/presmesso903.html.

32. Elizabeth M. Whelan et al., "Analysis of Coverage of Tobacco Hazards in Women's Magazines," *Journal of Public Health Policy* 2 (1981): 28–35; also her 2002 testimony before the Senate Subcommittee on Oversight: "Women's Magazines Cover Up Smoke Risks," http://www.acsh.org/healthissues/newsID.121/healthissue_detail.asp; and Kenneth E. Warner and Linda M. Goldenhar, "The Cigarette Advertising Broadcast Ban and Magazine Coverage of Smoking and Health," *Journal of Public Health Policy* 10 (1989): 32–42. For "kind of prison": Gloria Steinem, "Sex, Lies & Advertising," *Ms.* (July–Aug. 1990), cited in Bates TI51631155.

33. George Gitlitz, "Cigarette Advertising and the New York Times: An Ethical Issue That's Unfit to Print?" *New York State Journal of Medicine* 83 (1983): 1284–91.

34. "Follow-up of a Cover-up," *New York State Journal of Medicine* 85 (1985): 285–86.

35. Morton Mintz, "Parsing an Op Ed Ad in the Times," Nieman Watchdog (online), May 9, 2009; Simon Chapman, "Advocacy in Action: Extreme Corporate Makeover *interruptus*: Denormalising Tobacco Industry Corporate Schmoozing," *Tobacco Control* 13 (2004): 445–47.

36. Ruth Rosenbaum, "Cancer, Inc.," *New Times*, Nov. 25, 1977, pp. 28–43. Rosenbaum had earlier warned against the "Gestapoesque" tactics of nonsmokers: "Light up in the wrong place in Chicago and you'll be hauled into court and fined. Take a drag in a San Francisco ice cream parlor and sirens will squeal on you. Smoking in public places, once unquestioned, is now a hotly contested civil rights issue"; see her "Skirmish over Smokers' Rights," *New Times*, Dec. 10, 1976, pp. 47–53, Bates 2024272998–3004.

37. "Project Censored" website: http://www.projectcensored.org/static/1977/1977-story2.htm.

38. Frederick Panzer (TI) to Jim Peterson (Reynolds), Nov. 15, 1977, Bates 500083670–3671; Carl Jensen and Project Censored, *20 Years of Censored News* (New York: Seven Stories Press, 1997), p. 49. Rosenbaum's article was reprinted and distributed to the public through Philip Morris's Tobacco Action Program launched in 1978; see Bates 2053630241–0341.

39. Brennan Dawson on *Crossfire*, March 10, 1994, Bates TIMN0010651/0652, and the *MacNeil/Lehrer NewsHour*, April 1, 1994, Bates 515731622–1624.

40. Sharon Boyse (BAT) to the *Daily Telegraph*, June 29, 1994, Bates 500810940–0941.

41. "Baboons in Texas" (TI press release), March 12, 1982, Bates TIMN0120729–0730.

42. "The Marlboro Story: Death in the West," Sept. 9, 1976, Bates 2501188248–8260.

43. Takeshi Hirayama, "Non-Smoking Wives of Heavy Smokers Have a Higher Risk of Lung Cancer: A Study from Japan," *British Medical Journal* 282 (1981): 183–85; D. Trichopoulos et al., "Lung Cancer and Passive Smoking," *International Journal of Cancer* 27 (1981): 1–4; U.S. Department of Health and Human Services, *The Health Consequences of Involuntary Smoking: A Report of the Surgeon General* (Washington, DC: U.S. Government Printing Office, 1986); National Research Council, *Environmental Tobacco Smoke* (Washington, DC: National Academy Press, 1986); U.S. Environmental Protection Agency, *Respi-*

ratory Health Effects of Passive Smoking: Lung Cancer and Other Disorders (Washington, DC: EPA, 1992).

44. For "deep shit" and "silver bullet": Philip Morris, "Project Down Under: Conference Notes," June 24, 1987, Bates 2021502102–2134. Philip Morris here concedes that research into the ETS threat "peaks in 1984, perhaps because scientific community feels issue is resolved."

45. Monique E. Muggli, Richard Hurt, and Douglas Blanke, "Science for Hire: A Tobacco Industry Strategy to Influence Public Opinion on Secondhand Smoke," *Nicotine & Tobacco Research* 5 (2003): 303–14; also "Indoor Air Quality Association: A Proposal," 1989, Bates TCAL0475063–5071.

46. http://www.jti.com/cr/positions/cr_positions_environmental_smoke.

47. Morton Mintz, "The ACLU's Tobacco Addiction," *Progressive,* Dec. 1998, reprinted in Bates 580033285–3306.

CHAPTER 18

1. George Gallup, "Health Service Report Yet to 'Sink in' with Smokers: Little Change in Beliefs on Cigaret-Cancer Link in New Poll" (press release), Aug. 10, 1958, Bates TIMN0460 713–0714.

2. Elmo Roper and Associates, "A Study of Attitudes toward Cigarette Smoking and Different Types of Cigarettes, Volume I" (prepared for Philip Morris), Jan. 1959, Bates 10017 53936–4029.

3. George H. Gallup, *The Gallup Poll: Public Opinion 1935–71,* vol. 2 (New York: Random House, 1972), Bates 2072420455–0457; Louis Harris, "The Harris Survey," *Washington Post,* Feb. 1, 1965; National Clearinghouse for Smoking and Health, *Use of Tobacco: Practices, Attitudes, Knowledge, and Beliefs. United States—Fall 1964 and Spring 1966* (USDHEW, July 1969), Bates PA/000728, pp. 52, 68. The best summary of polls from the 1950s and early 1960s is the Gallup Organization's "Trends in Public Attitudes on the Possibility of a Health Hazard in Cigarette Smoking," March 1964, Bates 500006198-6249, p. R-4.

4. Lorillard, "Report of a Series of Depth Interviews on Cigarettes," 1956, Bates 84439158–9247.

5. "Many Doctors Link Smoking and Cancer," *Washington Daily News,* Oct. 26, 1960, Bates 1003543302–3654 at 3338.

6. Kenneth M. Colby, *A Primer for Psychotherapists* (New York: Ronald Press, 1951), p. 39; Morris Fishbein to Harris B. Parmele, June 2, 1954, Bates 89752410–2411; Medimetric Institute, "Doctors and Smoking (IV): Their Smoking Habits, Their Advice to Patients on Smoking, and Their Views on the Correlation between Cigarette Smoking and Lung Cancer" (for Hill & Knowlton for the TIRC), Oct. 1959, Bates 2072420444–0454. For "bunch of eggheads": W. A. Pennington to Edward Horrigan, Feb. 10, 1984, Bates 500638180–8181.

7. P. C. Luchsinger, "Project 6900: Physiological Studies," Oct. 25, 1966, Bates 100034 1400–1414, p. 2; Roper Research Associates (for the TI), "A Study of Public Attitudes toward Cigarette Smoking and the Tobacco Industry," July 1970, Bates 505549471–9536 at 9515; Roper Research Associates (for Philip Morris), "A Study of Cigarette Smokers' Habits and Attitudes," May 1970, Bates 1002650000–0392, pp. 9–14.

8. Roper Research Associates (for Philip Morris), "A Study of Cigarette Smokers' Habits and Attitudes in 1970," May 1970, Bates 1002650000–0392, pp. 13, 18, 39.

9. Jeffrey M. Jones, "Latest Gallup Update Shows Cigarette Smoking Near Historical Lows," July 25, 2007, http://www.gallup.com.

10. For U.S. polls: "Degree of Public Concern" (after 1972), Bates 85873496. For Britain: "60 Per Cent of British Smokers Doubt Cigarette-Health Tie, Survey Discloses," *U.S. Tobacco Journal,* Oct. 22, 1964, p. 12, reprinted in *Cigarette Tow Newsletter,* Nov. 15, 1964, p. 9, Bates 01193948–3972. For Britain 1984: Mike Daube in "Sponsorship and Sport," July 14, 1984, Bates 100198288, p. 14.

11. C. E. Hooper, Inc. (for Ted Bates & Co. and the Tobacco Institute), "Smoking Attitudes Study," Oct. 1967, Bates TIMN0003735–3760.

12. "Cigarettes Safe, Says U.S. Jury," *Charlotte Observer,* Nov. 29, 1964, reprinted in *Cigarette Tow Newsletter,* Dec. 15, 1964, Bates 80630286–0316.

13. U.S. Department of Health, Education and Welfare, *Teenage Smoking: National Patterns of Cigarette Smoking, Ages 12 through 18, in 1968 and 1970* (Rockville, MD: National Clearinghouse for Smoking and Health, 1970), Bates 508124383–4532.

14. U.S. Department of Health, Education and Welfare, *Use of Tobacco: Practices, Attitudes, Knowledge, and Beliefs* (Rockville, MD: National Clearinghouse for Smoking and Health, 1969), Bates PA/000728, pp. 727, 743.

15. Roper Organization, "A Study of Public Attitudes toward Cigarette Smoking," July 1982, Bates 1002665283–5749, pp. 3–25.

16. Louis Harris and Associates, *Prevention in America: Steps People Take—or Fail to Take—for Better Health* (Emmaus, PA: Rodale Press, 1985); Cynthia Hawkins (Philip Morris), "Prevention Index," July 11, 1984, Bates 2021561397–1398. For the Harris survey of experts: Bates TI04352082; and for the Tobacco Institute's gloss: Bates TIMN0397786.

17. Matthew L. Myers et al., *Federal Trade Commission Staff Report on the Cigarette Advertising Investigation,* esp. chap. 3, "Consumer Knowledge of the Health Hazards of Smoking" (FTC, May 1981), Bates 500630393–0440; compare also "FTC Report on Smoking Hazards," Radio TV Reports, Inc. (for the Tobacco Institute), June 25, 1981, Bates TIMN 0249208; and the exposé by Jack Anderson: "Extinguished: Report on Cigarettes," *New York Post,* June 22, 1989, Bates 2024931390. For Koop: U.S. Department of Health and Human Services, *Reducing the Health Consequences of Smoking: 25 Years of Progress. A Report of the Surgeon General* (Washington, DC: U.S. Government Printing Office, 1989), pp. 171–258.

18. "Smoking Causes Male Sexual Impotence: BMA Calls for Health Warnings," June 2, 1999, Bates 5001075295–5296; David Hammond and Carla Parkinson, "The Impact of Cigarette Package Design on Perceptions of Risk," *Journal of Public Health* 31 (2009): 345–53.

19. For "little or no harm": World Bank, *Curbing the Epidemic: Governments and the Economics of Tobacco Control* (Washington, DC: World Bank, 1999). For 2009: Yang Gonghuan, personal communication.

20. For "de-tarred": Raymond E. Scott to Reynolds, Feb. 18, 1986, Bates 505560787–0789. For design: Lynn Kozlowski et al., "Smokers Are Unaware of the Filter Vents Now on Most Cigarettes: Results of a National Survey," *Tobacco Control* 5 (1996): 265–70. Many people seem to believe tar is *added* to cigarettes, when the reality is that it is the *outcome* of burning. It is surprising how often even scholars say cigarettes "contain" tar—they do not.

21. "Kool Test Results," in Brown & Williamson's "Marketing Elements," ca. 1969, Bates 690010940–0945 at 0945.

22. For "overemphasized": Anne Duffin to William Kloepfer, June 29, 1973, Bates TIMN 0100443–0446. For showings figures: William Kloepfer to T.I. Staff, "Distribution of 'Need to Know'," Oct. 1, 1973, Bates TIMN0078203; also Bates TINY 0013656–3660 and TINY 0013545–3550. For *Answers We Seek:* Modern Talking Picture Service, "Certifications of Showing," April 30, 1982, Bates TINY0017222–7223. And for other movies see "Films at The Tobacco Institute," Feb. 1976, Bates TI16590203. Barry Palin Associates in London produced a string of similar films for the industry, with titles like *What about Smoking* (1972); *Care for a Smoke* (1975); *SAS—Cabin Air Quality* (1987); *The Science of Quality* (1988); *The Air We Breathe* (1988); *Of People and Numbers* (1989); *Why People Smoke* (1990); *Other People's Smoke* (1990); *International News* (1991); *The Courtesy of Choice* (1994); and *Good Air Quality Is Simply Good Business* (1995).

23. Jon A. Krosnick, LinChiat Chang, Steven J. Sherman, Laurie Chassin, and Clark Presson, "The Effects of Beliefs about the Health Consequences of Cigarette Smoking on Smoking Onset," *Journal of Communication* 56 (2006): S18–37.

24. The 95,000 letters preserved—almost all of which are to or from Reynolds—are only a tiny fraction of this total correspondence. By 1966, for example, Reynolds alone was getting over 35,000 letters per year in sales correspondence, plus another 5,000-odd letters handled by Public Relations; see R. D. Thompson to C. B. Wade, "Survey of Company's General Public and Consumer Correspondence Procedures," Feb. 2, 1966, Bates 500026301–6303.

25. Eloise B. Orton and Hester H. Williams to Reynolds, Oct. 16, 1954, Bates 500736528; J. C. MacDonald to Reynolds, Jan. 18, 1956, Bates 500706926–6928; J. Moore to Reynolds, May 15, 1985, Bates 505438434–8437. For the wildflower/filter idea, complete with a schematic diagram, see John R. Veillette to Walker Merryman, Aug. 1, 1989, Bates TI50240398–0399.

26. Ruth Rosander to Reynolds, Nov. 15, 1985, Bates 505563332–3333; Bucky Riley to Reynolds, Feb. 10, 1986, Bates 505563287–3289; Albert Rex to Reynolds, Dec. 6, 1985, Bates 505563316–3318; Al Rogers to Chairman of the Board, mid-August, 1986, Bates 505563272–3275; Mrs. C. M. Edwards to Reynolds, Nov. 15, 1985, Bates 505489065–9068; Miriam G. Adams (Reynolds) to C. M. Edwards, Dec. 11, 1985, Bates 505489064.

27. For "all this hooy": Lillie B. Pollack to Reynolds, May 27, 1970, Bates 500330605. For "hysterical propaganda": Foster Gunnison to Editor, *Hartford Courant,* Feb. 18, 1984, Bates 502273002 (copied to Reynolds). For "smoking does not create cancer": Martin Hunter to Consumer Relations, July 24, 2000, Bates 580103242–3362. For "vastly exaggerated": Rosalind B. Marimont to Reynolds, Aug. 29, 2000, Bates 522870033–0034. For "emotions": Frankie Hanlon to President, July 17, 2000, Bates 522752134–2136. For "treated foods": Peter Wersching to Reynolds, Aug. 4, 1997, Bates 517725173. For "theory just like Darwin's": John E. Dearing to Reynolds, Aug. 14, 1984, Bates 500621458–1460.

28. David R. Steindorf to Reynolds, Nov. 23, 1958, Bates 502393488; W. S. Koenig to Steindorf, Dec. 9, 1958, Bates 502393487; M. Vinal to Reynolds, n.d., Bates 502393634–3635; W. S. Koenig to M. Vinal, June 10, 1959, Bates 502393633.

29. See, for example, William C. Sugg to Reynolds, Jan. 27, 1964, Bates 500707039–7041.

30. Kazuhiro Ito to Reynolds, May 13, 1998, Bates 524268160. Complaint letters of this sort were typically stamped "highly confidential."

31. T. A. Porter (Reynolds) to Viola M. Wright, Jan.17, 1964, Bates 500707082; Thomas Dixon to Mrs. Herbert Nauman, Feb. 14, 1964, Bates 500706974–6975; P. T. Wilson Jr. to Sam Veatch, Jan. 24, 1964, Bates 500707052; T. A. Porter to Ralph Sanders, Jan. 29, 1964, Bates 500707023.

32. W. S. Koenig to J. L. Sipe, Feb. 28, 1964, Bates 502395317; T. A. Porter to Harold V. Moloughney, April 7, 1964, Bates 500706971; P. T. Wilson Jr. to C. W. Van Gilder, June 19, 1964, Bates 500707054; T. A. Porter to Henry M. White, June 17, 1965, Bates 500733884–3885;

33. T. K. Cahill to Paul A. Meglitsch, Oct. 16, 1973, Bates 500589318; T. K. Cahill to Anne Warhover, April 4, 1972, Bates 500670928–0929. T. A. Porter and P. T. Wilson started using the "cold fact" formula in letters from Feb. 18 and 19, 1964 (Bates 502394523, 502394288).

34. John W. Higgins to Reynolds, "Nicotine Fit," July 15, 1991, Bates 507726290–6292.

35. Carol Beattie to Reynolds, April 13, 1989, Bates 515558118–8120; first ellipsis in ·original.

36. Ruthann and William W. Kellams to Camel, Jan. 2, 1991, Bates 507717494–7495.

37. Mrs. Hall W. Grimmett to Reynolds, Sept. 9, 1986, Bates 514255569–5573.

38. Compare Pipkin to Reynolds, Jan. 8, 1968, Bates 500314401.

39. Thompson to Wade, "Survey of Company's General Public and Consumer Correspondence."

40. A search of dt:consumer letter "am addicted" retrieves 25 documents, all letters from smokers making this confession. A search of dt:consumer letter "am not addicted," by contrast, returns only 6 letters. All of the "am addicted" letters are from 1985 or later, interestingly.

41. Diane LoRusso to Reynolds, ca. June 8, 1976, Bates 500314372; compare Willis T. Maley to Reynolds, April 30, 1976, Bates 500314379.

42. Noel C. Stasiak to Reynolds, June 29, 1990, Bates 507853488.

43. Sharon Marvin to Reynolds, Oct. 15, 1999, Bates 522749715–9717.

44. Jana Clyne to Reynolds, Oct. 21, 1999, Bates 522749718–9720. Hostile correspondents were sometimes called "screamers"; see J. Restivo, "Forwarding Call Sheets for Underage Screamers," April 28, 1994, Bates 2078713415. For Philip Morris's booklet on how to deal with "screamers" and other forms of "white mail," see E. Chapman, "Direct Marketing System Procedures Manual," Nov. 1, 1993, Bates 2042007430–7606.

45. Miriam G. Adams to Annette Rodrigues, Sept. 24, 1986, Bates 505563268.

46. Miriam G. Adams, "S & H: Brief Reply (Primarily for Children)," 1985, Bates 505485325.

47. William D. Hobbs to Regna Goode, March 30, 1977, Bates 501478999–9000. For samples of Reynolds's form letters, see Miriam G. Adams to Herb Osmon, Feb. 13, 1985, Bates 505485307, and additional forms at Bates 505485311–5331.

48. Mary M. Tipple to Reynolds, Jan. 2, 1996, Bates 524108187.

49. For "organized thugs": Edward Morley to Reynolds, "Sleaze and Deceit," Jan. 6, 1996, Bates 524108189–8191. For "pleasing to kill": Meghan E. Colasanti to Disgusting Cigarette Company, Dec. 3, 1990, Bates 507726752–6756. For "murder": Irma Delisle to Reynolds, July 20, 1991, Bates 507726763–6765.

50. Corinne Martin, letter to the editor in *Time,* May 30, 1994, Bates 513614143–4147.

51. Roper Organization, "A Study of Public Attitudes toward Cigarette Smoking," July 1982, Bates 1002665283–5749, p. 31.

52. Paul Slovic, ed., *Smoking: Risk, Perception, and Policy* (Thousand Oaks, CA: Sage, 2001).

53. Kwechansky Marketing, "Project 16: English Youth" (Report to Imperial Tobacco), Oct. 18, 1977, Bates 566627826–7935.

54. W. Kip Viscusi, *Smoking: Making the Risky Decision* (New York: Oxford University Press, 1992).

55. Lydia Saad and Steve O'Brien, "The Tobacco Industry Summons Polls to the Witness Stand: A Review of Public Opinion on the Risks of Smoking," paper presented at annual meeting of the American Association for Public Opinion Research, May 15, 1998, Bates 82286394–6421. Compare also the sharp rebuke of Lacy K. Ford by Frank Newport, editor in chief of the Gallup Organization, in his letter to Ford from June 12, 1998, Bates 82286438–6441.

56. To avoid clutter I have omitted citations, which can be found by searching the industry's internal documents at http://legacy.library.ucsf.edu.

57. "Address by Addison Y. Yeaman . . . to the Tobacco Growers Information Committee, Annual Meeting, Nov. 6, 1967, Raleigh, NC," reprinted in *Congressional Record,* Dec. 4, 1967, pp. S17804–17805, Bates 00619804–9097.

58. Samuel J. Ervin, "Lung Cancer—A Disease of Unknown Cause," *Congressional Record,* Dec. 4, 1967, pp. S17792–17804, Bates 00619074–9097. Ervin also wondered how smoking could cause cancer of the lung given that stomach cancer had declined over the course of the century: "Are we to assume that smoking has cleansed the stomach while fouling the lungs?"

59. "Safer Cigarettes a Reasonable Goal," *Asheville Citizen,* Feb. 3, 1972, Bates TI55752634.

60. Abe Krash (Arnold, Fortas & Porter) to Ramm et al., May 23, 1964, Bates LG2006318–6330.

61. Richard Sobol to Ramm et al., "Consumer Survey," in Bates LG2006318–6330, p. 2.

62. Ibid., p. 4.

63. Horrigan went on to claim that "no causal link between smoking and disease" had been established; see Bates 03607523–8364, pp. 136–38, also Bates TIMN0123947–3967; and for the legal forms used to generate such comments: Bates TIMN0198492–8511 and 03013 979–3995.

64. Joan F. Cockerham (Reynolds) to Larry Stuart, Jan. 18, 1991, Bates 507726504–6504.

65. American Law Institute, *Restatement (Second) of Torts* (Philadelphia: ALI, 1964); and for background: Daniel Givelber, "Cigarette Law," *Indiana Law Journal* 73 (1998): 867–82.

66. Elizabeth Laposata, "From Strawberries to Cigarettes: How the Tobacco Industry Sabotaged the Restatement (Second) of Torts and Successfully Subverted Injured Plaintiffs' Cases for Decades," unpublished ms.

67. For ignorance of tar and nicotine numbers: "Color Perception" (Marketing Report, Brown & Williamson), 1978, Bates 774066281. American Tobacco's first mention of letting "sleeping dogs lie" with reference to carbon monoxide appears in Hanmer to Lieb, Aug. 20, 1932, Bates 950160697–0700. For "presently unaware": Brown & Williamson, "FACT: Concept Description & Potential and Marketing Plan," 1976, Bates 464702663–2685, p. 8.

68. Paul A. Eichorn to Robert Seligman, June 2, 1978, Bates 1003725613.

69. Helmut Wakeham to Dr. Seligman, Feb. 22, 1979, "Program Review—Psychology," Bates 1000017226–7227; H. David Steele to M. J. McCue, "Future Consumer Reaction to

Nicotine," Aug. 24, 1978, Bates 665043966; Federal Trade Commission, "'Tar,' Nicotine, and Carbon Monoxide of the Smoke of 1262 Varieties of Domestic Cigarettes," 1999, http://www.ftc.gov/os/1999/09/1996tnrpt.pdf.

70. Kenneth D. Ward et al., "Characteristics of U.S. Waterpipe Users: A Preliminary Report," *Nicotine & Tobacco Research* 9 (2007): 1339–46.

71. Milton E. Harrington, deposition testimony in *Cipollone v. Liggett,* May 15–16, 1985, Bates HarringtonM051685 and 051585.

72. Annual Presidential Proclamations for Cancer Control Month are available at http://www.presidency.ucsb.edu, a site organized by John T. Woolley and Gerhard Peters as part of the American Presidency Project. My thanks to Tommy Tobin for discovering and analyzing these documents.

73. For Dole: David Corn, "Bob Dole and the Tobacco Connection," *The Nation,* March 28, 1987, Bates TI02682553–2555; Glenn Frankel, "Dole's Link to Big Tobacco Aged in Years of Dealmaking," *Washington Post,* May 18, 1996; James J. Kilpatrick, "We Still Don't Know If Cigarettes Really Do Cause Cancer," Dec. 19, 1985, Bates 505562046–2051. Rush Limbaugh's radio show from April 29, 1994, is cited in "The Way Things Aren't: Rush Limbaugh Debates Reality," http://www.fair.org/index.php?page = 1895.

74. Karen Schindler, "Caravan—Consumer Relations: All in a Day's Work," March 30, 1998, Bates 527851880–1882; Jeffrey A. Kuchar, "Internal Audit Report, Marketing-Promotion Fulfillment Winston-Salem," July 22, 1997, Bates 54487258–7269.

75. "Philip Morris Customer Care Vision 2000: Defining a New Approach to Customer Relationship Management," April 2000, Bates 2082140509–0537.

76. "Statement re the 1990 Hubbard Awards" (PM), Dec. 10, 1990, Bates 2047319115; "PM Receiving Hubbard Award for Deceptive Advertising from the Center for Science in the Public Interest," Dec. 10, 1990, Bates 2046007069; Virginia Murphy to Ward A. Freese, "Mr. Charles Myers Case Number 94Co1905," July 12, 1994, Bates 2065144431–4432; and for the "awareness impact": Bates 2047532093–2181; "Marlboro Adventure Team Highlights," Oct. 29, 1993, Bates 2058211926–1927.

77. "USA DIRECT," May 7, 1998, Bates 2061708929–8935; "Marlboro Adventure Team Promotion Fulfillment and Customer Service," April 2, 1993, Bates 2062341855–1856; "Philip Morris Customer Care Vision 2000: Defining a New Approach to Customer Relationship Management," April 2000, Bates 2082140509–0537.

78. Brown & Williamson, "Records Retention Schedule," July 13, 1989, Bates 334000760–0781.

79. "Smoking and Health Issues" (Brown & Williamson), Dec. 9, 1999, Bates 206000308–0315.

80. Ibid. Brown & Williamson also compiled what might be called "complaint logs," classifying phoned-in grievances by different categories—from "Allergic Reaction" and "Burned Self" to "Chest Pain," "Chronic Illness/Death," "Cough," "Cut Self," "Headache," "Sore Throat/Burning" and "Sick/Vomit"; see "Smoking and Health Issues," Dec. 9, 1999, Bates 206000277–0307.

81. "Smoking and Health Issues" (Brown & Williamson), Dec. 9, 1999, Bates 206000308–0315.

82. For "Microscopic Mites": Joe Gagliano to Chuck Blixt, April 7, 1997, Bates 516853661.

Reynolds' email log is at "Andy Schindler's Mail Log 2000," Jan. 4, 2000, Bates 580103242–3362. Other logs are available at Bates 580103199–3226 and 580103397–3421.

83. J. F. Cullman, "Annual Report Pursuant to Section 46 of the Membership Corporation Law," Jan. 20, 1959, Bates TFAL0000001–0010; J. S. Dowdell to C. B. Wade Jr., "Consumer Correspondence," July 13, 1967, Bates 500026296–6298.

CHAPTER 19

1. Fritz Lickint, "Die Bedeutung des Tabaks für die Krebsentstehung," *Deutscher Tabakgegner* 17 (1935): 30; also his *Tabakgenuss und Gesundheit* (Hanover: Wilkens, 1936), pp. 84–85.

2. Richard Doll, "Etiology of Lung Cancer," in *Advances in Cancer Research*, vol. 3, ed. J. P. Greenstein and A. Haddow (New York: Academic, 1955), p. 26; also my *Nazi War on Cancer*, pp. 192–93, 215, 253.

3. For Roffo: "Report of Progress—Technical Research Department," B&W, Dec. 24, 1952, Bates 650200084–0095, p. 8. For Rodgman, see his letter to K. H. Hoover, Nov. 2, 1959, Bates 500945942–5945. For Wakeham, see his "Tobacco and Health—R&D Approach," Nov. 15, 1961, Bates 1005069026–9050, p. 9, and his "Tobacco and Health," Bates 100277434, p. 14.

4. Paul Koenig, *Die Entdeckung des reinen Nikotins* (Bremen: Arthur Geist, 1940), pp. 21–22 and plate 10; also my *Nazi War on Cancer*, pp. 173–247.

5. Richard Kissling, *Der Tabak im Lichte der neusten naturwissenschaftlichen Forschungen* (Berlin: Verlag von Paul Parey, 1893), p. 65; Franz K. Reckert, *Tabakwarenkunde: Der Tabak, sein Anbau und seine Verarbeitung* (Berlin: Max Schwabe Verlag, 1942), p. 31; "Fortschrittsbericht," *Chronica Nicotiana* 2, no. 1 (1941): 8. For a Philip Morris list of 100 U.S. and foreign patents, see "Denicotinization of Tobacco," Aug. 4, 1986, Bates 2025620092–0109.

6. American Tobacco Co., "Nicotine Content of Tobacco Can Be Diminished or Increased by Natural Means," Dec. 1, 1930, Bates 950298161.

7. Richard Kissling, "Method of and Apparatus for Curing Tobacco," U.S. Patent Office, June 13, 1882, Patent No. 259,553. Tobacco manufacturers have not always been honest about how much nicotine is in a cigarette. German cigarette makers in the 1930s, for example, advertised certain brands as "low nicotine" or "nicotine-free," with little or no regulatory oversight. Worries about the honesty of such claims prompted regulatory enactments, including Germany's 1939 Ordinance on Low-Nicotine and Nicotine-Free Tobacco, which required "low-nicotine" products to contain less than 0.8 percent nicotine and "nicotine-free" cigarettes to contain no more than 0.1 percent; see Wilhelm Preiss, *Verordnung über nikotinarmen und nikotinfreien Tabak* (Berlin: Von Decker, 1939). In America, too, "denicotinized" tobaccos were hardly free of nicotine. A 1928 study found that while ordinary cigarettes averaged 1.77 percent nicotine, those advertized as "denicotinized" averaged 1.28 percent—hardly a profound difference (E. M. Bailey, O. L. Nolan, and W. T. Mathis, "'Denicotinized' Tobacco," *Bulletin of the Connecticut Agricultural Experiment Station* 295 [1928]: 338–51). *JAMA* reviewed this article and commented that the difference between regular and "denicotinized" cigarettes was so slight as to constitute "a fraud on the public"; see "Denicotinized Tobacco," *JAMA* 91 (1929): 583.

8. "'Denicotea' Cigaret Holder," Sept. 17, 1941, Bates 950089928; and for a German

patent: Hans Rudolph, "Porous Materials and Process of Making," U.S. Patent Office, Sept. 29, 1942, Bates 680018801–8804.

9. For photos of asbestos particles tapped out from Kent's Micronite filter cigarettes, see Owens-Corning Testing Division to Lorillard, June 4, 1953, Bates 01057102–7119. As early as 1936 Lorillard had been informed that dusts like silica and asbestos were "known to produce fibrosis of the lungs"; see Leroy U. Gardner to W. C. Hazard, May 5, 1936, Bates 01057123–7127. Harris Parmele was also sent Hazard's warning that asbestos had been "definitely proved" to be a "disabling disease of the lungs" (Bates 01057128–7130). Parmele developed the filter—called Micronite "because it removes nicotine and tar particles as small as two tenths of a micron"—with Harold W. Knudson of Hollingsworth & Vose in East Walpole, Massachusetts; see "War-Born Filter Used to Remove Tars and Nicotine," March 19, 1952, Bates 92616335–634 and "The H & V—Kent Story," March 18, 1954, Bates 00420758–0763.

10. J. H. Heller had asked, "What is the matter with a mineral filter?"; see his letter of Dec. 26, 1953, Bates LG0220462; and for Liggett's response: F. R. Darkis to Heller, Jan. 15, 1954, Bates LG0220463–0464.

11. Testimony of James Talcott in "Cigarette and Smokeless Tobacco Products: Reports of Added Constituents and Nicotine Ratings," Jan. 30, 1997, Bates 566958219–8266; also J. A. Talcott, W. A. Thurber, and A. F. Kantor et al., "Asbestos-Associated Diseases in a Cohort of Cigarette-Filter Workers," *New England Journal of Medicine* 321 (1989): 1220–23.

12. Harris B. Parmele to Robert M. Ganger, Nov. 13, 1951, Bates 87334161.

13. Harris B. Parmele to Ernest F. Fullam, Feb. 12, 1954, Bates 94682426–2428.

14. Carl Byoir and Associates, "Cigarette with Tobacco Filter 'Goes National' " (Press release for B&W), June 22, 1960, Bates 500394514–4515.

15. For "practically the same": "Action of Cellulose Filter-Pads in Cigarettes on the Nicotine Content of the Smoke," 1935, Bates 950032937. For "better filtering agent" and "an excellent filter": "The Efficiency of Filters in Reducing the Nicotine Content of Cigaret Smoke," May 9, 1946, Bates 950051953–1957, pp. 2- 5; compare W. R. Harlan and J. M. Moseley's comment, "Tobacco itself serves as an excellent mechanical filter," in "Tobacco," *Encyclopedia of Chemical Technology,* vol. 14 (New York: Interscience, 1955), p. 260, Bates 950775523–5531, and similar remarks in documents from 1956 and 1964 at Bates 950278282–8295 and 950189096–9103.

16. H. B. Parmele to Alden James, Sept. 10, 1954, Bates 96723704; compare Parmele to A. J. Cheek, Aug. 12, 1954, Bates 96723696. American did introduce a filtered Tareyton brand in the mid-1950s, but the brand was never much of a success.

17. Ted Bates and Co., Advertising, "Viceroy Thunderbird Contest: Publicity Report" (Brown & Williamson), Nov. 18, 1955, Bates 690148121–8139.

18. The Roland Company, Inc., "Water Filters Offer Consumer Good Taste," July 1971, Bates 968027808–7810; also Bates 968027813–7815.

19. "Round, Firm, and Filtered," *Chemical and Engineering News,* April 16, 1956, pp. 1846–48.

20. Lois Mattox Miller and James Monahan, "The Facts behind Filter Tip Cigarettes," *Reader's Digest,* July 1957, pp. 33–39; and their "Wanted—*And Available*—Filter-Tips That Really Filter," *Reader's Digest,* Aug. 1957, pp. 43–49.

21. "Total Kent Sales: Fact Sheet" (Wooten Maxwell), 1970, Bates 03079517; "Hi-Fi History" (Brown & Williamson), n.d., Bates 464518657–8673.

22. Clarence W. Lieb, *Safer Smoking: What Every Smoker Should Know and Do* (New York: Exposition Press, 1953); compare his *Don't Let Smoking Kill You!* (New York: Bonus Books, 1957), p. 38; and for "our research council": Lieb to Hanmer, Aug. 22, 1932, Bates 950160696.

23. K. T. Sanderson and R. H. Blackmore (Philip Morris), "C. I. Report 36," Feb. 15, 1962, Bates 2051980038–0072, p. 21.

24. Cubebs Merit De-Nic, Next, and Benson & Hedges De-Nic were three Philip Morris low-nicotine brands dropped from production in the early 1990s, when market shares leveled off at about a quarter of one percent. See Joshua Dunsby and Lisa Bero, "A Nicotine Delivery Device without the Nicotine? Tobacco Industry Development of Low Nicotine Cigarettes," *Tobacco Control* 13 (2004): 362–69.

25. *Blatnik Report,* pp. 184–88; Lieb, *Don't Let Smoking Kill You!* pp. 94–95. On March 3, 1958, *Time* magazine reported the outrage of the House Government Operations Committee, headed by Illinois congressman William L. Dawson, who protested, "The cigarette industry has done a grave disservice to the smoking public [by] publicizing the filter-tip smoke as a health protection." Deceptions of this sort continued into subsequent decades; see Bates 968027808–7810; and for a good early critique: Ralph Lee Smith, *The Health Hucksters* (New York: Bartholomew House, 1961), pp. 116–28.

26. For "unbalanced": Hanmer to C. F. Neiley, Dec. 15, 1932, Bates 950190632. For "thermodynamic impossibility": A. E. O'Keeffe (Philip Morris) to R. N. DuPuis, "Selective Filtration," Sept. 16, 1958, Bates 1001902921–2924. Lorillard researchers similarly characterized the Aqua filter's claims to selectively reduce carbon monoxide as not just "false and misleading" but also a "theoretical impossibility"; see Alex W. Spears to C. H. Judge and A. J. Stevens, Dec. 13, 1974, Bates 00485657–5658. For "carcinogens in practically every class": Wakeham, "Tobacco and Health," p. 14.

27. For "very naïve": A. H. Roffo, "Sobre los filtros en el tabaquismo: El narguilé y el algodón como filtro del alquitrán de tabaco," *Boletín del Instituto de Medicina Experimental* 16 (1939): 255–68, translated (for litigation) as "Filters in Tobacco Addiction: Water-Pipe and Cotton as Filters for Tar in Tobacco," Bates 89742095–2099. The AMA's Chemical Laboratory in 1953 analyzed the three leading filter types—paper, asbestos, and cotton—and showed that only asbestos trapped more tar and nicotine than tobacco alone; see Walter Wolman, "A Study of Cigarettes, Cigarettes, Cigarette Smoke, and Filters," *JAMA* 152 (1953): 917–20, 1035–36; also "Filter Tips Don't Filter Much, AMA Cigaret Research Discloses," *Advertising Age,* Aug. 3, 1953, Bates 89751396–1398.

28. "The Simple Facts about a Cleaner, Finer Smoke" (1945 ad for Fleetwood Imperials), Bates 2061014830.

29. "Suggestions" (AT), 1952, Bates 950196279–6319.

30. D. M. Rowe to A. R. Stevens (AT), June 4, 1964, Bates 968191075–1078. As of 1966 companies manufacturing filters in the United States included Celanese, Eastman, Hercules, Ralston Purina, Ecusta, American Filtrona, and Schweitzer; see M. L. Reynolds and E. F. Litzinger, "Keyword Index for Filtration Studies," April 2, 1968, Bates 650206692–6693.

31. German chemists had patented the use of activated charcoal in cigarette filters in the

1930s; see Z. Brazay, "German Patent No. 607422 . . . Process for Detoxifying Tobacco Smoke by Absorbent Carbon," Dec. 27, 1934, Bates 980392203–2206.

32. M. J. Ward (Brown & Williamson), "Patent Survey—Carbon Filter," Sept. 6, 1973, Bates 650317809–7869. Hundreds of patents for filters using charcoal, some dating from the nineteenth century, are described in this document; compare Brown & Williamson's "Filters Incorporating Charcoal," May 6, 1965, Bates 680246822–6855.

33. A. W. Spears to Tore Dalhamn, Sept. 13, 1966, Bates 00105846.

34. Mrs. Ende (BAT), "Patent Survey: Cross-Flow Filters," Jan. 1974, Bates 570225722–5750.

35. Will Graham, "Lorillard '76: Options and Recommendations," March 2, 1976, Bates 01771073–1207.

36. Fred G. Bock et al., "Carcinogenic Activity of Cigarette Smoke Condensate," *JAMA* 181 (1962): 82–87.

37. Philip Morris had a "Selective Filtration Program" with Project nos. 21–2101 and 23–2101; see Andrew E. O'Keeffe to R. N. DuPuis, Oct. 14, 1958, Bates 1001902916. And for Reynolds: James D. Fredrickson, "Study of Selective Filtration," Sept. 11, 1963, Bates 504001427, and his lab notebooks at Bates 503212780–2830.

38. See Rodgman's deposition for *Arch*, Aug. 4, 1997, Bates RODGMANF080497, p. 624.

39. H. Wakeham to H. Cullman, May 4, 1962, Bates 2021656001.

40. For an early but impressive discussion, see E. W. Ashkenazi, "Survey of the Literature on Aerosol Filtration" (for Philip Morris), Dec. 19, 1958, Bates 1001802639–2790.

41. On "the merit of tobacco as a filtering agent," see Hanmer to Hahn, July 27, 1942, Bates 950198817–8818, and the attached "Literature References Concerning Tobacco as a Filtering Agent," July 27, 1942, Bates 950198819–8821. For Framingham: W. P. Castelli et al., "The Filter Cigarette and Coronary Heart Disease: The Framingham Study," *Lancet* 2 (1981): 109–13.

42. Leaf growers in the late 1950s complained that the filter fad had cut into their sales. So even though cigarette consumption grew rapidly in 1955, 1956, and 1957, sales of leaf actually dropped by more than 125 million pounds per year, saving tobacco manufacturers an estimated $65 million on leaf costs during this period. See William G. Reddan, "Editor's Forum," *Tobacco* 146 (Feb. 28, 1958): 8, Bates LG0195348–5385.

43. Thomas E. Novotny, Kristen Lum, Elizabeth Smith, Vivian Wang, and Richard Barnes, "Cigarettes Butts and the Case for an Environmental Policy on Hazardous Cigarette Waste," *International Journal of Environmental Research and Public Health* 6 (2009): 1691–1705.

44. For Darkis re filters "do not really take anything out": J. Eaves (Liggett & Myers), "Stenographic Minutes of a Conference Held at the Research Laboratory on January 21 and 22, 1952," Jan. 23, 1952, Bates LG0205897–5926, p. 265. For Ecusta's particle size research: Milton O. Schur and James C. Rickards, "The Design of Low Yield Cigarettes," *Tobacco Science* 4 (1960): 69–77, Bates 88043323–3331.

CHAPTER 20

1. Cora C. Ayers (BAT), "Project Gold Charm," Dec. 14, 1965, Bates 570342396–2416. Lorillard on May 24, 1962, announced a technique for removing "up to 90% of the phenols" from cigarette smoke (Bates 85087725). The plasticizers in question were polyethylene oxides.

2. "Cancer-Proof Cigarettes Are Here," *Science & Mechanics,* April 1968, pp. 46–48 and 75–76, Bates 1004867388–7484.

3. For threshold studies: "Subjective Irritation—Straight Inhalation," June 2, 1948, Bates 962005268–5270. For Rhoads: Kluger, *Ashes to Ashes,* p. 422. For irradiated cigars: Ronald W. Davis, "A Study of Tobacco Mold Control Using Gamma Irradiation Techniques," Jan. 29, 1968, Bates 950131716–1732 and appendixes at 1734–1743. La Corona cigars were exposed to gamma radiation (up to 1 megarad) from a cobalt 60 source at Industrial Reactor Laboratories in Plainsboro, New Jersey, for these experiments.

4. Colin L. Browne, *The Design of Cigarettes* (Charlotte, NC: Celanese Fibers Marketing Co., 1981). Browne's is one of the best introductions to cigarette design; another is Black et al., "B&W Product Knowledge Seminar."

5. For Philip Morris: C. V. Mace to R. N. DuPuis, "Brief Comments on a Program to Produce a Low Delivery Filter Cigarette with Flavor," July 24, 1958, Bates 1000305086–5087. For "evolution": "High Filtration Filters" (Lorillard), Feb. 1974, Bates 00378778–8803. Compare Helmut Wakeham to Robert P. Roper, Sept. 22, 1959: "what is wanted in a satisfying smoke is *relatively high* nicotine and low tar" (Bates 1005039423–9424); original emphasis.

6. David Kessler, *A Question of Intent: A Great American Battle with a Deadly Industry* (New York: Public Affairs, 2001), pp. 186–250; also Todd Lewan, "Brazil's Secret: Crazy Tobacco," AP, Dec. 21, 1997.

7. For Project T-0576: Imperial Tobacco Ltd., Montreal, "Work Programme: Fiscal 1986—1988," May 1985, Bates 570312400–2576 at 2502. For "attractive, useful form": Claude E. Teague Jr., "Implications and Activities Arising from Correlation of Smoke pH with Nicotine Impact, Other Smoke Qualities, and Cigarette Sales," Sept. 28, 1973, Bates 509314122–4154.

8. For "loathe to exceed": J. D. Backhurst (BAT), "A Relation between the 'Strength' of a Cigarette and the 'Extractable Nicotine' in the Smoke," Nov. 16, 1965, Bates 508102918–2941. For Project Kick: Max Häusermann (Philip Morris Europe), "Carbon Monoxide Uptake by Smokers," Jan. 3, 1974, Bates 1002645271. For "foul, rotten rubber": W. M. Henley to D. H. Piehl, "Nicotine Research," Nov. 9, 1976, Bates 509078812–8820.

9. In 1995 alone the American Association of Poison Control Centers received 7,917 reports of potentially toxic exposures to tobacco among children aged six or under, most of which were from ingesting cigarettes; see W. Lewander et al., "Ingestion of Cigarettes and Cigarette Butts by Children—Rhode Island, Jan. 1994–July 1996," *MMWR* 46 (1997): 125–28.

10. "Research Conference Southampton 1962: Smoking and Health—Policy on Research," 1962, Bates 110070785–0882. Gibb's comments are at pp. 38–39.

11. Helmut Wakeham to J. E. Lincoln, April 14, 1960, Bates 1001882378.

12. Ronald A. Tamol of Philip Morris in 1965 noted that one argument against developing a "health cigarette" would be that any such cigarette "would have to be shared with other companies"; see Bates 2078099704–9723. J. M. Moseley in 1958 reported to his superiors at American Tobacco that European manufacturers had "a tacit agreement not to trade on, or refer to, the anti-cigarette charges beyond the simple use of the word 'filter.'" See Robert K. Heimann to Alfred F. Bowden, "Verbal Report of J. M. Moseley," July 2, 1958, Bates 966015128.

13. See Reid and Ellis's discussion in "Research Conference Southampton 1962: Smoking and Health—Policy on Research," 1962, Bates 110070785–0882, pp. 40–41.

14. Bradford, Harlan, and Hanmer, "Nature of Cigarette Smoke"; W. B. Wartman, E. C. Cogbill, and E. S. Harlow, "Determination of Particulate Matter in Concentrated Aerosols," *Analytical Chemistry* 31 (1959) : 1705–9. As standardized in the 1960s, this became known as the "Cambridge Filter Method" and eventually the "FTC Method," following procedures specified by Clyde L. Ogg in his "Determination of Particulate Matter and Alkaloids (as Nicotine) in Cigarette Smoke," *Journal of the Association of Official Agricultural Chemists* 47 (1964): 356–62. Ogg, a chemist with the USDA, worked out these procedures as chair of the Analytical Methods Committee of the Tobacco Chemists Conference, a committee consisting of representatives from Liggett & Myers, Philip Morris, American Tobacco, and the Consolidated Cigar Corporation. In 1966 the FTC required that all tar and nicotine yields be reported using methods specified by Ogg and his industry colleagues.

15. For Rosenthal process: Wakeham to Cullman, March 24, 1961, Bates 1000861955. For Brunette Extra: R. Hirsbrunner, "Cigarette Development," Sept. 27–Oct. 31, 1978, Bates 2028622060–2069. For nicotine values: P. Harper (Brown & Williamson), "Project Phoenix," Jan. 28, 1987, Bates 620404055–4056.

16. Tar is not actually "in" a cigarette but rather is produced by the smoking process. I note this because I'm often asked, why do the companies add tar to cigarettes? Of course they don't: tar is not added to tobacco any more than ashes are added to a campfire. Tar is just condensed smoke minus the water (and nicotine) and is sometimes referred to as "smoke solids," "smoke condensate," or "total particulate matter."

17. Lynn T. Kozlowski, R. C. Frecker, V. Khouw, and M. A. Pope, "The Misuse of 'Less Hazardous' Cigarettes and Its Detection: Hole-Blocking of Ventilated Filters," *American Journal of Public Health* 70 (1980): 1202–03. The U.S. Surgeon General's 1988 report, *Nicotine Addiction,* cites Michael Russell et al., "Relation of Nicotine Yield of Cigarettes to Blood Nicotine Concentrations in Smokers," *British Medical Journal* 280 (1980): 972–76, as its earliest documentation of compensation; compare also R. I. Herning et al., "Puff Volume Increases When Low-Nicotine Cigarettes Are Smoked," *BMJ* 283 (1981): 187–89.

18. "The Patent Position" (BAT), Dec. 14, 1959, Bates 108069854–9855.

19. H. B. Parmele to Driscoll, Jan. 3, 1933, Bates 04355214–5217.

20. For American's experiments: J. A. Bradford, "Volatile Aldehydes in Cigarette Smoke," Feb. 7, 1933, Bates 962002433–2435. For "dilution": H. R. Hanmer to C. F. Neiley, Feb. 9, 1933, Bates 950160691–0692. For "surprising extent": C. W. Lieb to H. R. Hanmer, March 17, 1933, Bates 950160684–0688.

21. Tilley, *Reynolds Tobacco Company,* p. 503. The Rembrandt Tobacco Corp. of Canada in a series of ads from August 1959 claimed priority in its use of a porous "Multi-Venting" paper that allowed its Rembrandt cigarettes to "breathe." *Consumer Reports* in 1960 reported on the fads of "mentholation and ventilation," characterizing the latter as part of the industry's "frenzied search for methods to reduce tars and nicotine" ("Cigarettes," *Consumer Reports,* Jan. 1960, pp. 12–21, Bates 504802621–2630).

22. Edward M. Harris, "Cigarette," Patent No. 439,004, U.S. Patent Office, awarded Oct. 21, 1890.

23. A. L. Chesley to C. F. Neiley, March 9, 1927, Bates 950073013–3015.

24. C. V. Mace to L. L. Long, "Summary of Results on Ventilated Cigarettes," Oct. 25, 1955, Bates 2022204168–4174.

25. For "height of advertising prowess": David G. Felton to D. S. F. Hobson, "SPRING— the cigarette that 'air-conditions' the smoke," Sept. 4, 1959, Bates 100068231. Lorillard's brash, full-page ad in the August 18, 1959, *New York Times* can be found at Bates 100068233–8234.

26. C. N. Smyth, "Tobacco Smoke," *British Medical Journal* 1 (1959): 506–7. Some newspapers suggested that smokers could create their own ventilated cigarettes by pricking two small holes into the cigarette near the mouth end, as recommended by Smyth. One London paper claimed that a simple procedure such as this "could end the lung cancer scare"; see Roy Rutter, "Two Tiny Holes Give Safe Smoking," April 24, 1959, Bates 502393021–3022.

27. Herbert R. Bentley, "Cigarettes with Increased Porosity," March 3, 1959, Bates 105386936; emphasis added.

28. Harris B. Parmele to Robert M. Ganger, Nov. 13, 1951, Bates 87334161.

29. Lynn T. Kozlowski, R. J. O'Connor, G. A. Giovino, C. A. Whetzel, J. Pauly, and K. M. Cummings, "Maximum Yields Might Improve Public Health—If Filter Vents Were Banned: A Lesson from the History of Vented Filters," *Tobacco Control* 15 (2006): 262–66.

30. Gio B. Gori, "Low-Risk Cigarettes: A Prescription," *Science* 194 (1976): 1243–46; "Gori Gets into Another Controversy," *Cancer Letter* 4 (Aug. 1978): 1–7, Bates TIMN0142772–2775.

31. "High Filtration Filters" (Lorillard), 1973, Bates 88322091–2116.

32. For a three-hundred-page overview of ventilation "technology, history and theory," see Charles B. Altizer et al. (Philip Morris U.S.A.), "Ventilation Seminar," May 1983, Bates 2057251669–1968.

33. See the revealing "first draft" of an untitled Philip Morris report on ventilation, dated July 25, 1982, Bates 1003285784–5788.

34. "Kool Ultra and Barclay 100 Ventilation Study," June 8, 1982, Bates 505183373–3376.

35. "1982 Strategic Analysis—Product," 1982, Bates 503522357–2373.

36. Reynolds and Philip Morris both came up with "dial a filter" cigarettes in 1982, filing patents within about a month of each other. The Ecusta Paper Corporation had helped Philip Morris develop its Dial-a-Filter as part of PM's Project Data. Reynolds's test panels characterized such cigarettes as "gimmicky"; see W. F. Bultman to G. W. McKenna and J. J. Griffin, "Perspective on New Brands," June 24, 1985, Bates 505919078–9080.

37. Peter Schesslitz's words from the *Deutsche Tabakzeitung* of Oct. 28, 1940, are cited in "Der Nikotinfimmel," *Reine Luft*, 1941, p. 41. Schesslitz here also anticipates Michael Russell's famous 1971 comparison of smoking-without-nicotine to blowing bubbles, asking: "Who, upon reflection, believes that people would smoke if nicotine did not have the specific effects it does? [Without nicotine] people would be more likely to blow bubbles than to smoke" (p. 41). Russell's oft-cited comparison appears in his "Cigarette Smokng: Natural History of a Dependence Disorder," *British Journal of Medical Psychology* 44 (1971): 9.

The earliest expression of compensation I have found is from the *Nebraska Medical Journal* of 1933, where we hear that "In the process of manufacturing cigarettes where the greater percentage of nicotine had been taken out of a certain brand, it was found that the habitué consumed thrice the number of the one that had the tobacco blend in the original state"; see Henry Farrell, "The Billion Dollar Smoke," *Nebraska Medical Journal* 18 (1933): 226–28. Farrell here also traces the rise of the cigarette to "an advertising performance stealthy in the extreme, magnificent in its summons and invocation, the like and similar performance of which the world had never seen before and perhaps never will again."

38. Lynn T. Kozlowski and R. J. O'Connor, "Official Cigarette Tar Tests Are Misleading," *Lancet* 355 (2000): 2159–61.

39. Thomas R. Schori, "Smoking and Heart Rate Research Proposal," Sept. 30, 1970, Bates 1000838038–8045; also his paper with B. W. Jones, "Smoking and Aggression: A Proposal," Oct. 23, 1974, Bates 1003290519–0531. Helmut Wakeham, "R&D Presentation to the Board of Directors," Nov. 26, 1969, Bates 1000276691–6703; W. Dunn to G. Berman, "TPM Intake by Smokers," May 7, 1968, Bates 1000870189.

40. Philip Morris researcher Thomas R. Schori in 1970 cited G. Kuschinsky and R. Hotovy's research from the 1940s showing that people smoke "not in spite of, but because of nicotine"; see his "Tar, Nicotine, and Smoking Behavior: A Research Proposal," Nov. 5, 1970, Bates 1003285464–5477. Schori also cited Maurine Neuberger's 1963 *Smoke Screen* in support of the claim that smokers develop "a daily quota for nicotine." The Kuschinsky and Hotovy paper is "Über die zentral erregende Wirkung des Nicotins," *Klinische Wochenschrift* 22 (1943): 649–50.

41. For "primary reason": Bates 2020154466–4486. For "substance": Bates 517214547. For "dominant specification": Claude E. Teague Jr., "A New Type of Cigarette Delivering a Satisfying Amount of Nicotine with a Reduced 'Tar'-to-Nicotine Ratio," March 28, 1972, Bates 502987394–7403, p. 3.

42. For "vehicle": Helmut Wakeham, "Why One Smokes," Fall 1969, Bates 1003287836–7848. This document was rewritten and presented to PM's Board of Directors as "Smoker Psychology Research," Nov. 26, 1969, Bates 100273741–3771. For puffing as "injection": William L. Dunn, "Some Methods Notes on the Past Research on Cigarette Motivation," Feb. 16, 1970, Bates 1003287849. For "nicotine addicts": Bates 301083862–3865. For "nicotine seekers": Bates 501524500–4514. For "maintain a constant level": Bates 517214547–4557. For pack as "storage container": William L. Dunn, "Motives and Incentives in Cigarette Smoking," paper presented at CORESTA conference, Williamsburg, VA, Oct. 22–28, 1972, Bates 1003291922–1939.

43. William L. Dunn, ed., *Smoking Behavior: Motives and Incentives* (Washington, DC: Winston & Sons, 1973). Dunn's original (1969) plan was for a meeting "of nationally recognized authorities to discuss short term (beneficial) consequences of smoking." The original title was "The Gratification of Cigarette Smoking," which later morphed into "Conference on the Motivational Mechanisms in Cigarette Smoking." See Dunn's "Project 1600 Consumer Psychology: Annual Report," May 15, 1970, Bates 1003288243–8245; also his memo (with Myron Johnston) to P. A. Eichorn, "Accomplishments in 1969," Jan. 28, 1970, Bates 1003288492–8494.

44. For "dangerous F.D.A. implications": Dunn to Wakeham, "Jet's Money Offer," Feb. 19, 1969, Bates 1003289921–9922. For "certainly fail": Johnston (approved by Dunn), "Market Potential of a Health Cigarette," p. 5. For "primary motivation": Wakeham, "Why One Smokes."

45. Frank J. Ryan (approved by Dunn), "Bird-I: A Study of the Quit-Smoking Campaign in Greenfield, Iowa, in Conjunction with the Movie, *Cold Turkey*," March 1971, Bates 10003 48671–8751. Philip Morris employed local Girl Scouts to distribute surveys in the town and did not identify itself as the sponsor of the survey, which recipients knew only as coming from the "Product Opinion Laboratory" of Richmond, Virginia; see Bates 85873620–3621.

46. Selye's comments are on pp. 1–3 of Dunn, ed., *Smoking Behavior;* Eysenck's on pp.

121–23; Heimstra's on p. 206; Damon's on p. 221; and Hickey and Harner's on pp. 272 and 278. Erich Fromm was invited to attend but apparently refused.

47. W. Dunn, T. Schori, and J. Duggins, "Smoking Behavior: Real World Observations," March 1973, Bates 1000353356–3388.

48. W. Dunn to C. Goldsmith, "Dosage Controls," May 8, 1974, Bates 1003294972–4976.

49. Teague, "A New Type of Cigarette," p. 8.

50. R. D. Wilkie, BAT Research and Development, "Complexity of the P.A.5.A Machine and Variables Pool," June 1959, Bates 100099115–9117; Claude E. Teague, "Proposal of a New, Consumer-Oriented Business Strategy for RJR Tobacco Company," Sept. 19, 1969, Bates 5009 15701–5719, pp. 9–10. Compare BAT's 1976 forecast of "danger in the current trend of lower and lower cigarette deliveries—i.e. the smoker will be weaned away from the habit," in W. B. Fordyce to M.P.D.C. Members, "Long-Range Forecasts (1986)," June 29, 1976, Bates 110071 572–1573.

51. For Japan: Tien C. Tso (USDA), "Report of Travel to Japan, Taiwan, and Other European Countries, June 23 through August 22, 1968," Bates 968006480–6508. For Philip Morris: "1965 Cigarette," March 25, 1965, Bates 100901301. For "minimum satisfying amount": Teague, "A New Type of Cigarette," pp. 7–8. Ronald A. Tamol from Philip Morris's product design group in handwritten notes from February 1, 1965, stressed the need to determine the "minimum nicotine prop[ortion] to keep normal smokers 'hooked'"; see Bates 2078099704–9723.

52. On Hanmer: Rogers and Todd, "Report on Policy," p. 16. On "nicotine fortification": R. B. Griffith, "Report to Executive Committee," July 1, 1965, Bates 1805.01.

53. For a bibliography on lip drape and lip occlusion (ventilation), see Bates 2046816474–6478.

54. For "health filter smokers": "Annual Report, Project 1600," Nov. 18, 1966, 1003286561–6590. For "partial occlusion": William L. Dunn, "Project 1600: Consumer Psychology," June 25, 1967, Bates 1003288345–8346. For hole placement: William L. Dunn to R. B. Seligman, July 28, 1967, Bates 1000307727–7729. For "We submit": JoAnn Martin and W. L. Dunn to H. R. Wakeham and R. B. Seligman, "A Study of the Effect of Air Hole Blockage on Gross Puff Volume in Air Diluted Cigarettes," Aug. 10, 1967, Bates 1000307730–7733.

55. "Studies on Occlusion from Cenfile," n.d., Bates 2046816474–6478; Frank Ryan to William L. Dunn, "Pandora," July 29, 1982, Bates 1003285845.

56. Brown & Williamson researchers in 1983 defined "smoke elasticity" as "the potential of a cigarette, to provide the smoker with more smoke, if he draws harder"; see W. Wiethaup and W. Schneider, "Filter Effects on Smoke and Smoke Effects," July 1983, Bates 512107109–7120; also the same company's "World Wide Best Elasticity Studies," n.d., Bates B01280532–0536. In 1993 Imperial Tobacco's Montreal labs were deliberately trying to increase elasticity by increasing filter pressure drop and reducing rod pressure drop. "Gap filters" produced by on-line laser perforation were also used to augment elasticity; see Imperial Tobacco Ltd., "Progress Report, July 1993—December 1993," Bates 402415168–5194, pp. 25–26.

57. D. J. Wood, "The Design of Low Delivery Cigarettes (with Regard to Smoker Compensation)," June 28, 1977, Bates 110074887–4890.

58. Robert R. Johnson, "Cigarette with Backflow Filter Ventilation: Status Report/244," Dec. 11, 1978, Bates 680596833–6834; also his "Cigarette Filter Including Grooves in the Filter

Plug," Jan. 31, 1979, Bates 6805968116–6819, and for background: L. T. Kozlowski, N. A. Dreschel, S. D. Stellman, J. Wilkenfeld, E. B. Weiss, and M. E. Goldberg, "An Extremely Compensatible Cigarette by Design: Documentary Evidence on Industry Awareness and Reactions to the Barclay Filter Design Cheating the Tar Testing System," *Tobacco Control* 14 (2005): 64–70.

59. Barbro Goodman to Leo F. Meyer, "Marlboro—Marlboro Lights Study Delivery Data," Sept. 17, 1975, Bates 2021544486–4496. Goodman later did work examining "what might happen to deliveries to the smoker when he partially covers the dilution holes," finding that this could cause "an increased delivery to the smoker"; see Goodman to L. F. Meyer, "Effect of Reduced Dilution on Tar Delivery to a Smoker," Oct. 21, 1982, Bates 1003455000–5002.

60. David E. Creighton, "Compensation for Changed Delivery," June 27, 1978, Bates 105553905–3915.

61. Kwechansky Marketing, "Project Plus/Minus: Young People and Smoking," May 7, 1982, pp. 12–13, cited in Richard W. Pollay and Anne Lavack, "The Targeting of Youth by Cigarette Marketers: Archival Evidence on Trial," *Advances in Consumer Research* 20 (1993): 266–71.

62. For background, see A. Ramirez, "R. J. Reynolds Study of Cigarette Tar Irks an Industry Rival," *Wall Street Journal,* May 6, 1981, Bates 621007659–7666; also Lynn T. Kozlowski et al., "An Extremely Compensatible Cigarette by Design: Documentary Evidence on Industry Awareness and Reactions to the Barclay Filter Design Cheating the Tar Testing System," *Tobacco Control* 14 (2005): 64–70.

63. E. A. A. Bruell (BAT) to All No. 1s of Operating Companies, Sept. 20, 1983, Bates 105375726–5733, which also contains the Sept. 9, 1983, telex to George Weissman at Philip Morris. Original emphasis.

64. "Telephone Conversation on the Afternoon of 26th October between Mr. Bruell of BATCO and Mr. Reid of Imperial," 1983, Bates 301030946–0948.

65. For "extremely dangerous": J. B. Boder to S. C. Darrah (Philip Morris Neuchatel), Jan. 23, 1989, Bates 2023266338–6340. For BAT's promise: R. W. Pollay and T. Dewhirst, "The Dark Side of Marketing Seemingly 'Light' Cigarettes: Successful Images and Failed Fact," *Tobacco Control* 11 (2002): 18–31.

66. Kozlowski et al., "The Misuse of 'Less Hazardous' Cigarettes"; also his article with W. S. Rickert, J. C. Robinson, and N. E. Grunberg, "Have Tar and Nicotine Yields of Cigarettes Changed?" *Science* 209 (1980): 1550–51. Kozlowski became intrigued by ventilation in the fall of 1978 at the University of Pennsylvania, when he asked a young woman how she liked her "light" cigarettes and she answered, "Fine, but it's hard to keep my fingers over the little holes" (personal communication).

67. Neal L. Benowitz et al., "Smokers of Low-Yield Cigarettes Do Not Consume Less Nicotine," *New England Journal of Medicine* 309 (1983): 139–42; Claude Lenfant, "Are 'Low-Yield' Cigarettes Really Safer?" *New England Journal of Medicine* 309 (1983): 181–82.

68. Notably through the Tobacco Working Group, an ill-informed industry-NIH collaboration that lasted from 1968 through 1977; see Kluger, *Ashes to Ashes,* pp. 427–30.

69. "Smoker Compensation," April 15, 1983, Bates 501524500–4514; William L. Dunn, "Project 1600," Aug. 25, 1967, Bates 1001521213–1214. A rare but good public discussion of compensation is "Less Tar, Less Nicotine: Is That Good?" *Consumer Reports,* May 1976, pp. 274–76, Bates 968037705–7707.

70. Jonathan Samet, Written Direct testimony for *USA v. Philip Morris*, Sept. 29, 2004, Bates 20040929, pp. 164–65. For "switch to cigarettes": U.S. Department of Health and Human Services, *The Changing Cigarette: A Report of the Surgeon General* (Washington, DC: U.S. Government Printing Office, 1981), pp. v–vi. For Burns: David M. Burns, Written Direct testimony for *USA v. Philip Morris*, Feb. 15, 2005, Bates BURNSD-ER, pp. 35–56.

71. R. Fagan to H. Wakeham, "Moral Issue on FTC Tar," March 7, 1974, Bates 1000211075. BAT's Sydney Green raised similar questions: "should we 'cheat' smokers by 'cheating' League Tables? . . . . should we use our superior knowledge of our products to design them so that they give low league table positions but higher deliveries on human smoking?" ("Suggested Questions for CAC III," Aug. 26, 1977, Bates 2231.09). The company's subsequent behavior clearly indicates a decision in the affirmative.

72. R. Fagan to H. Wakeham, "Moral Issue on FTC Tar," March 7, 1974, Bates 1000211075.

73. For taxes pegged to tar levels: "Kennedy Calls for Tar Tax on Cigarettes," *Courier Journal*, Sept. 12, 1967, Bates 680278780; *Congressional Record*, Oct. 13, 1971, Bates 500020779; "Cigarette Tar Tax Act," *Congressional Record*, Jan. 18, 1973, Bates 690004964–4965. For Doll: David Appleton, "Cancer Specialist Wants High-Tar Tax," Edinburgh *Scotsman*, Dec. 4, 1982, Bates 100454636. Australian legislators debated such a tax in 1971; see Bates 2016002793. For Europe: "Maximum Tar Yield of Cigarettes," May 17, 1990, Bates 2064240706–0709; and for the Middle East: Bates 303696070–6114.

74. National Cancer Institute, *Risks Associated with Smoking Cigarettes with Low Machine-Measured Yields of Tar and Nicotine—Monograph 13* (Bethesda, MD: USDHHS, 2001), p. ii.

75. Randolph D. Smoak Jr., "AMA Commends Report Exposing Dangers of Light Cigarettes" (press release), Nov. 27, 2001.

CHAPTER 21

1. Claude E. Teague Jr., "A New Product Strategy for Circumventing Problems Arising from the Smoking-Health Controversy," Dec. 10, 1969, Bates 515864703–4705.

2. John N. Langley, "On the Reaction of Cells and of Nerve-Endings to Certain Poisons," *Journal of Physiology* 33 (1905): 374–413; Lennox M. Johnston, "Tobacco Smoking and Nicotine," *Lancet* 243 (1942): 742.

3. Harris B. Parmele to Adam Riefner, April 11, 1946, Bates 04365297–5298.

4. Harvey B. Haag in 1940 recognized that "In the smoke of cigars and in the case of some cigarettes, because of the high alkalinity of the smoke, [nicotine] probably to some extent exists in free alkaloidal form. Not investigated thoroughly, this difference might be of some practical physiologic importance because nicotine base is much more readily absorbed from mucous membranes than the various salts"; see his "Chemical and Pharmacologic Observations on Nicotine and Tobacco Smoke," *Merck Report*, Oct. 1940, Bates 9492. Parmele in 1951 noted that "two cigarettes might give rise to smoke containing the same amount of nicotine, but the absorption of this nicotine by the smoker might be radically different, dependent on other related factors, such as the degree of acidity, etc."; see Parmele to R. M. Ganger, Jan. 29, 1951, Bates 95309702–9703.

5. For "emasculated cigarette": H. R. Hanmer, "Memorandum on the Nicotine Content of Lucky Strike and Other Leading Brands of Cigarettes," April 3, 1940, p. 2. For "kiss from

one's sister": Moseley, "Second International Tobacco Congress." For sex without orgasm: Dunn, "Motives and Incentives."

6. Alix M. Freedman, "'Impact Booster': Tobacco Firm Shows How Ammonia Spurs Delivery of Nicotine," *Wall Street Journal,* Oct. 18, 1995.

7. The gas phase can be further broken down into "true gases" and "condensable vapors." According to a 1959 study by American Tobacco, true gases constituted about 409 mg/cigarette, condensable vapors about 10 mg, and the particle phase about 15 mg/cigarette. See "Composition of Cigarette Smoke," Oct. 6, 1959, Bates 962004216–4223.

8. Rodgman, "Short Explanation," p. 1.

9. A good diagram of this process can be found on the front cover of *Chemical Research in Toxicology* 14, no. 11 (Nov. 2001).

10. Backhurst at BAT R&D in 1965 reported that freebasing nicotine could result in a cigarette "with a low nicotine yield" producing "greater response than a cigarette with a high one"; see his "Relation between the 'Strength' of a Cigarette and the 'Extractable Nicotine.'"

11. Jerome E. Brooks talks about Native Americans adding alkali agents such as lime or pulverized shells to increase "the effects of tobacco as it freed the active agent, nicotine"; see his *The Mighty Leaf: Tobacco through the Centuries* (Boston: Little, Brown, 1952), pp. 16–19.

12. American Tobacco Co., "Toasting and Ultra-Violet Light Treatment of Tobacco," 1930, Bates 950296691–6704; Adolf Wenusch, *Der Tabakrauch. Seine Entstehung, Beschaffenheit und Zusammensetzung* (Bremen: Arthur Geist, 1939); Aleksandr A. Shmuk, *The Chemistry and Technology of Tobacco,* vol. 3 of his *Works, 1913–1945,* trans. from Russian (Moscow: Pishchepromizdat, 1953).

13. Claude E. Teague Jr., "Reduction of Harshness in Leaf Tobacco," April 30, 1954, Bates 504175051–5052; Shmuk, *Chemistry and Technology of Tobacco,* pp. 455–540.

14. Charles S. Philips, "Process of Treating Tobacco," U.S. Patent, Sept. 13, 1881, Bates 2026526307–6308; American Tobacco Co., "Toasting and Ultra-Violet Light Treatment of Tobacco," 1930, Bates 950296691–6704.

15. Brown & Williamson, "Cigarette Dimensions," 1993, Bates 581110529–0548. A good overview of early recon use in the United States is F. E. Van Nostran (Philip Morris), "Summary of Reconstituted Tobacco Intelligence," Feb. 20, 1962, Bates 2076277599–7617. Wakeham outlines a recipe in a note to Hugh Cullman, July 23, 1962, Bates 1000862896–2897.

16. Tilley, *Reynolds Tobacco Company,* pp. 488–94. Alan Rodgman credits Samuel Jones as the inventor of recon, though Europeans had also been doing work in this area. For patents, see "Chronology of Events: Day One Media Contact RE: Nicotine" (Reynolds), March 18, 1994, Bates 525311830–1831.

17. For "much more efficient": J. D. Hind to R. B. Seligman, "Re: Strong Chocolate Flavor in DAP-BL," Nov. 6, 1962, Bates 1000862754. For "stem soaking": Philip Morris Research Center, "Bi-Monthly Progress Report," May–June 1962, Bates 1001532315–2320. For "lemon albedo": "Project 1300: DAP-BL Process Improvements," July 5, 1963, Bates 1000826239–6245; and for process alternatives more generally: Bates 1000826367–6368. For the decision to start commercial production, see "Bi-Monthly Progress Report," July–Aug. 1963, Bates 1001532350–2353.

18. J. D. Hind and R. B. Seligman, "Tobacco Sheet Material," U.S. Patent Office, Nov. 21, 1967, Bates 2056136774–6783; A. Hyland, R. Goldstein, A. Brown, R. O'Connor, and K. M.

Cummings, "Happy Birthday Marlboro: The Cigarette Whose Taste Outlasts Its Customers," *Tobacco Control* 15 (2006): 75–77.

19. C. F. Gregory, "Observation of Free Nicotine Changes in Tobacco Smoke," Jan. 4, 1980, Bates 510000667–0670. Early ads for Merit cigarettes announced that "smoke" had been "cracked"—a remarkable coincidence given that "crack" cocaine would not appear until the early 1980s. For "Smoke Cracked" and "radical breakthrough," see Bates 2024987245–7246.

20. Robert K. Williams, "Progress during May–June on Project No. TE-5001," July 13, 1971; compare also his "Summary of Progress in 1971 on Project TE-5001," Dec. 16, 1971, Bates LG0262125–2126; and J. R. Newsome, "Progress during 1973 on Project TE 5001," Jan. 29, 1974, Bates 2073883754–2755.

21. "We are pursuing this project with the eventual goal of lowering the total nicotine present in smoke while increasing the physiological effect of the nicotine which is present, so that no physiological effect is lost on nicotine reduction"; see Robert K. Williams, "Development of a Cigarette with Increased Smoke pH," Dec. 16, 1971, Bates LG0262126.

22. Teague, "Implications and Activities."

23. RJR, "Ammonia," Draft, Aug. 9, 1982, Bates 500990999–1004; Terrell Stevenson and Robert N. Proctor, "The 'Secret' and 'Soul' of Marlboro: Philip Morris and the Origins, Spread, and Denial of Nicotine Free-Basing," *American Journal of Public Health* 98 (2008): 1184–94.

24. For "strength": Backhurst, "Relation"; for "normal impact": R. P. Newton and E. F. Litzinger, "Further Evaluations of UKELON-Treated Cigarettes," Jan. 17, 1972, Bates 650105 652–5663; "greater levels": Hawkins, McCain & Blumenthal, Inc., "Project LTS," June 20, 1977, Bates 660094371–4451; "one avenue": R. P. Newton, "Ukelon Treatment of Tobacco," 1971, Bates 1014727772–2773.

25. C. F. Gregory, "Observation of Free Nicotine Changes in Tobacco Smoke/#528," Jan. 4, 1980, Bates 510000667–0670.

26. H. C. Garrett to Larry O'Berry, "Superiority CPT/254," Oct. 24, 1989, Bates 58313 6019–6026. A list of ingredients and code names can be found in Brown & Williamson's "Additive Code Analogues," n.d., Bates 1326.01 and 1329.01. A 1972 report notes that the company's use of urea to increase impact had been "abandoned in favor of a higher impact experimental blend"; see "Research & Development Monthly Report," April 1972, Bates 620086712–6739.

27. Brown & Williamson, "Table 1—Sample Description," 1991, Bates 570360597–0601. For another set of ingredients and mixing instructions, see Brown & Williamson's "Project Cherokee," Dec. 1990, Bates 526031385–1392; and for PM's recon: Bates 1000322727.

28. Susan Braun, Information Data Search, Inc., "Ammonia Uses by Philip Morris: A Report to Brown & Williamson Tobacco Co.," May 17, 1985, Bates 681827963–8063.

29. J. S. C. Wong, "Development of a Low Alkaloid Smoking Product," Jan. 8, 1988, Bates 402373981–3993.

30. Brown & Williamson, "Woodrose B&W and Cooperative Brand Ratings," 1970, Bates 465606986–7087; Ralph Brave, "Smoked out! The Hidden History of UC Davis' 35-Year Collaboration with Big Tobacco," *Sacramento News and Review,* June 21, 2007.

31. R. Johnson, "Ammonia Tech. Conference Minutes," May 18, 1989, Bates 508104011–4164 at 4016; also "Second Annual Ammonia Technology Conference: Commercialization of Ammonia Technology," June 11–13, 1990, Bates 570353434–3770. An excellent overview

of ammoniation is Brown & Williamson's *Root Technology: A Handbook for Leaf Blenders and Product Developers,* Jan. 1991, Bates 682439026–9083.

32. J. H. Lauterbach and R. R. Johnson (Brown & Williamson), "The Project Adverb Study of Marlboro KS," Oct. 10, 1989, Bates 570244005–4027.

33. Kluger, *Ashes to Ashes,* pp. 742–47.

34. I've mentioned "folk freebasing," but it is also worth noting that some of the first nicotine gums were freebased, containing "a carbonate buffer to increase salivary pH and improve buccal absorption of nicotine." Buffered gums produced nicotine blood levels more than twice as high as unbuffered gums; see Anders Axelsson and Bo Brantmark, "The Anti-Smoking Effect of Chewing Gum with Nicotine of High and Low Bioavailability," in *Proceedings of the 3rd World Conference on Smoking and Health,* vol. 2 (Bethesda, MD: DHEW, 1977), pp. 549–59.

35. Dick Howe, "Development of Safety Protocols at the Bermuda Hundred Pilot Plant," June 29, 1988, Bates 2025619545–9603, p. 35.

36. Stephen S. Hecht, "Biochemistry, Biology and Carcinogenicity of Tobacco-Specific N-nitrosamines," *Chemical Research in Toxicology* 11 (1998): 559–603.

CHAPTER 22

1. James J. Morgan, deposition testimony in *Broin v. Philip Morris,* April 17, 1997, Bates 2063670882–0926, p. 78.

2. Trial Testimony of James J. Morgan in *Minnesota v. Philip Morris,* April 22, 1998, Bates MORGANJ042298, p. 13458, and in *Philip Morris v. R. J. Reynolds,* Oct. 15, 1974, Bates 502640001–0103.

3. For "health filter smokers": Peggy G. Martin and T. R. Schori, "Further Evaluation of Delivery Information Influence on Subjective Acceptability of a Low Delivery Cigarette," May 1976, Bates 1000363042–3061. For "alleviate": Reynolds, "Segment Summary," 1981, Bates 501984818–4823. For "less 'risky'": A. M. Heath, "Conference on Marketing Low Delivery Products," Jan. 1982, Bates 690120722–0756. For "health cigarette image": John Howley to Roy Barcell, "Kent Brand Image," Nov. 13, 1975, Bates 85002494–2499. For Project Hilton: "Excerpts from Marlboro Marketing and New Product Development Plans, Germany, 1976," Bates 2501062584–2620, p. 177. For Project Klaus, see Paul Isenring's press release from Dec. 30, 1975, Bates 2075972885–2888. The "health-oriented" reference is Bates 2501204384–4385; and "addiction" is Bates 2501204384–4385. See also "Project Gatwick," Aug. 17, 1972, Bates 100025468–5471; and N. R. L. Brown, "New Virginia Brand Projects," July 13, 1972, Bates 301003471–3479.

4. Cigarettes in the 14 to 18 mg range (Kent, Lark, Silva Thins) offered "taste with implicit health benefit," lights in the 5 to 14 mg range (Merit, Doral, Vantage) offered "taste with contemporary health benefit," and those in the 1 to 4 mg range (Now, Carlton, True) offered "explicit health benefit"; see Brown & Williamson's "Cigarette Market Product Dynamics," 1977, Bates 660000489–0490. For "throat and voice problems": Kim Joyce to Reynolds, Dec. 16, 1979, Bates 500587469. For "psychological crutch": George Weissman to Joseph F. Cullman III, Jan. 29, 1964, Bates 1005038559–8561.

5. Philip Morris marketing document, March 1992, Bates 2045726327–6349, p. 19.

6. For "dimensions of Youth": R. D. Ferris to A. Stephenson, "RE: Lights Mild Descriptors," Feb. 18, 1992, Bates 400760281. For switching to menthols: A. Grabowsky (Liggett & Myers), "Adam Package Study—Group Interviews," Nov. 17, 1970, Bates LG0113953–4002. For healthful names: Lennen & Newell, "Exploratory Study on Consumer Identification of and Association with Specific Trade Names," Nov. 1964, Bates 03361414–1486. For "health segment": Brown & Williamson's "Kool Family Overview (1978–1981)," Bates 776167302–7316.

7. Farrell Delman et al., eds., *Directory of Cigarette Brands: 1864–1988* (Princeton: Tobacco Merchants Association, 1989), Bates 282008342–8576.

8. Jerry Isaacs to Renee Simons, "Benson & Hedges Name Contest (Skinny Cigarette)," Aug. 10, 1987, Bates 2049202154.

9. G. Lyttle-Green to M. A. Bateman et al., "Project Cirrus Task Force," July 15, 1987, Bates 170321230–1234.

10. American Tobacco had started this craze in 1967 with its Silva Thins; Malibu Thins were a Brown & Williamson brand introduced that same year, followed by Empire Thins in 1968, but it is not clear whether any of these were sold as "diet cigarettes."

11. The same survey comparing superslims against Capri noted that while most perceived these as milder and having less tar, "few knew the tar levels of either product"; see Shari Teitelbaum to Carl Cohen, "Superslims Qualitative Research," Dec. 2, 1991, Bates 2041253558–3560.

12. M. J. Thun et al., "Cigarette Smoking and Changes in the Histopathology of Lung Cancer," *Journal of the National Cancer Institute* 89 (1997): 1580–86.

13. Timothy Begany, "Are Cigarette Makers Trying to Conceal Secondhand Smoke?" *RespiratoryReviews.com,* Dec. 2000; G. N. Connolly, G. D. Wayne, D. Lymperis, and M. C. Doherty, "How Cigarette Additives Are Used to Mask Environmental Tobacco Smoke," *Tobacco Control* 9 (2000): 283–91.

14. C. V. Mace (Philip Morris) to E. I. Kropa, Dec. 16, 1954, Bates 000756356.

15. James D. Fredrickson, "Communication of Invention Memorandum: Process for the Control of Tobacco Smoke," July 2, 1964, Bates 502212216–2218; also his "Communication of Invention: Process for Increasing the Volume of Tobacco and Other Materials of Biological Origin," May 31, 1967, Bates 502212221–2223.

16. Helmut Wakeham, "Presentation to Philip Morris Board, Revised Draft," Oct. 15, 1973, Bates 2022886235–6236. Reynolds's Freon-based expanded tobacco was produced in collaboration with DuPont through its Fluorocarbons Division, which drafted (with Reynolds) a denialist Q&A on potential hazards of Freon residues in smoke; see Bates 502479617–9622.

17. For Project Duerer: Philip Morris Europe (Neuchatel), "Quarterly Report," Jan. 1987, Bates 2021606791–7000. For microwaves: S. L. Merker and G. E. Stungis (Brown & Williamson), "Microwave Treatment of Cigarettes on a Making Machine," Nov. 20, 1973, Bates 680220244–0247. For cancer prevention: L. C. Jennings to M. Hansen (Philip Morris), "Expansion Testing," April 24, 1981, Bates 1003714615.

18. For Tobacco Tax Law: Vello Norman (Lorillard), "The History of Cigarettes," May 1983, Bates 81051625–81051662. For Lucky Strike: A. L. Chesley to W. J. Garvey, April 7, 1921, Bates 950298093; Tareyton Filters: "Coumarin in Main Stream Smoke of Filter Tip Tarey-

ton Cigarettes," March 26, 1956, Bates 962003063; Camels: H. R. Hanmer to J. A. Crowe, Sept. 17, 1943, Bates 950582560–2570; Tareyton Ultra Low Tar Menthols: "Cigarette Specifications," June 1981, Bates 980227878; Capri: J. E. Wickham to L. F. Meyer, "Brown and Williamson—Capri Cigarettes," Dec. 15, 1986, Bates 2020168912; Virginia Superslims: L. A. Watson to H. G. Harwood, Oct. 15, 1991, Bates 2041800353.

19. Mark Parascandola, "Lessons from the History of Tobacco Harm Reduction: The National Cancer Institute's Smoking and Health Program and the 'Less Hazardous Cigarette,'" *Nicotine and Tobacco Research* 7 (2005): 779–89.

20. "Tar reassurance" gets 458 hits on the Legacy Tobacco Documents Library; "health reassurance" gets over 1,500.

21. Kessler, "Amended Final Opinion," p. 1630.

22. "Color Perception" (Marketing Report, Brown & Williamson), 1978, Bates 77406 6281.

23. "Tobacco Giant 'Breaks Youth Code,'" *BBC News,* June 28, 2008, http://news.bbc.co .uk/2/hi/africa/7475259.stm.

CHAPTER 23

1. "Smoking and Health: Senator Proposes Federal Action," *News and Observer* (Raleigh, NC), Nov. 3, 1953, Bates 2025028780.

2. We need histories of the various industry law firms; for starters, see Mark Hansen, "Shook Hardy Smokes 'Em," *ABA Journal,* Oct. 2008; also Judge Kessler's excoriation in her "Amended Final Opinion," p. 3.

3. "Excerpts from R. J. Reynolds Tobacco Company's File on Contributions to Harvard Medical School," Jan. 15, 1972, Bates 503138609–8621A.

4. Ibid., pp. 7–10.

5. Ibid., pp. 10–13.

6. For "all six General Counsel" and "stress and not smoking": Edwin J. Jacob to W. T. Hoyt, June 27, 1968, Bates 11330520–0520, and to David R. Hardy, Feb. 2, 1967, Bates 1005 154440–4445, p. 4. For "sympathetic to our cause": David Hardy to Cyril Hetsko, Jan. 25, 1969, Bates 945369849–9850. For "squirrel monkey": "Behavioral Hypertension" (report on Barger's application), n.d., Bates HK1805041–5043. R. J. Bing, evaluating Barger, commented, "We support Dr. Barger primarily because we wanted to ride piggyback on an important project in an important institution" (Bates 50093756–3756). For "unknown" causes and "many suspects": Clifford Barger, "RJR Board Presentation," Oct. 22, 1984, Bates 503956 178–6180. For Dews on "nicotine addiction": Peter B. Dews, "Presentation Prepared by Philip Morris Outside Consultant," Sept. 28, 1994, Bates 2047097047–7060; and for hints of the points covered, see Marc S. Firestone to Peter Dews, Sept. 9, 1994, Bates 2065405848–5850.

7. A. L. Chesley to Paul M. Hahn, Jan. 23, 1931, Bates 950289552–9558.

8. Andrew W. Petre, "Summary Report of Philip Morris and Company Industrial Fellowship Nos. 11, 12," Feb. 1946, Bates 1003072220–2258; H. B. Parmele to H. S. Lukens, March 5, 1945, Bates 04365461–5462; Parmele to Riefner, Aug. 2, 1946, Bates 04365253.

9. William Esty to S. Clay Williams, April 19, 1934, Bates 507875317–5319. For "entirely without any harmful effect": Y. Henderson to H. M. Robertson, March 23, 1935, Bates

680144496. For Haggard's report to Brown & Williamson: "Report of Investigation to Determine the Physiological Effects of Menthol Derived from Smoking Kool Cigarettes," 1935, Bates 570312663–2772. For mentholating the paper: H. W. Haggard to H. M. Robertson, March 27, 1935, Bates 570312661–2662.

10. For seventy-nine medical schools, see Bates 2015002362–2375. For Philip Morris less irritating: Herbert Arkin, "An Analysis of Data on the Effect of Cigarette Smoke on the Human Throat," 1950, Bates 1003070990–1049. For headlines from April 16–18, 1955, see Bates HT0039116; and for Lorillard's citations of doubters, see Harris B. Parmele, "Petition before the Federal Trade Commission," 1958, Bates 00491221–1238. Arkin's *Current Medical Digest* paper was "Current Relationship between Human Smoking Habits and Death Rates," April 1955, pp. 37–44.

11. Richard E. Shope, "The Possible Role of Viruses in Cancer Re: Cancer Cases," Sept. 23, 1959, Bates 1005087195–7207.

12. Richard E. Shope, "Koch's Postulates and a Viral Cause of Human Cancer: Guest Editorial," *Cancer Research* 20 (1960): 1119–20, Bates 961001561–1562.

13. For "statistical judgment": "Statement of Harry S. N. Greene, MD, Before the House Committee on Interstate and Foreign Commerce on Bills Relating to Cigarette Labeling and Advertising," March 22, 1965, Bates TI19841385/2183. For the Brits on Greene: Bentley, Felton, and Reid, "Report on Visit to U.S.A. and Canada"; compare Greene's introduction to Eric Northrup's denialist *Science Looks at Smoking* (New York: Coward-McCann, 1957).

14. For "epidemiological unit": H. Wakeham to Paul D. Smith, May 21, 1969, Bates 1000321562–1564. For "information supplied": R. B. Griffith to G. W. Stokes, March 27, 1969, Bates 680226914.

15. For "which of my patients": Gary L. Huber to H. C. Roemer, Jan. 11, 1972, Bates 50313 8622–8625. For Waite's claim: Richard A. Knox, "Harvard Study Suggests Low Tar Cigarette Risk," *Boston Globe*, May 8, 1978, Bates 502405224–5225.

16. For "getting too close": Gary L. Huber, deposition testimony for *Texas v. American Tobacco*, Sept. 20, 1997, Bates HUBERG092097, p. 46; also the *Frontline* interview with Huber, http://www.pbs.org/wgbh/pages/frontline/shows/settlement/interviews/huber.html. Huber left Harvard for Kentucky in 1980 and eventually landed at the University of Texas Health Center in Tyler, where he continued to work for Shook, Hardy and Bacon, receiving about $1.7 million in research funding from the firm.

17. Some of the most sensational publicity centered on Ragnar Rylander, a Swedish toxicologist at the University of Geneva who, for decades, worked quietly for the industry as part of what Jean-Charles Rielle and Pascal Diethelm called "an unprecedented scientific fraud." Rylander sued his accusers, but a Swiss appeals court upheld Rielle and Diethelm's judgment. The "Rylander Affair" prompted the University of Geneva to bar its faculty from accepting research or consulting funds from the tobacco industry; see Alex Mauron, Alfredo Morabia, Thomas Perneger, and Thierry Rochat, "Rapport d'enguâte dans l'affaire du Pr. Ragnar Rylander Genève," Sept. 6, 2004, http://www.prevention.ch/rapryuni.pdf; and further documentation at http://www.prevention.ch/rypresse.htm.

18. For a list of Reynolds's academic collaborations in 1978, see Murray Senkus to William D. Hobbs, July 21, 1978, Bates 500259142–9153.

19. The "History" section of the Weissman School's website talks about the life of George

Weissman without mentioning his lifelong career at Philip Morris; see http://www.baruch .cuny.edu/wsas/inside_weissman/history.htm (accessed June 2010). Wills Hall's "History" website is equally silent about tobacco; see http://www.bris.ac.uk/Depts/Wills/history.htm.

20. For "no significant accumulation": "A Decade of Tobacco Research," *Journal of the Bowman Gray School of Medicine* 12 (Feb. 1954): 8–9. For the faulty disclosure: William A. Wolff, Marina A. Hawkins, and W. E. Giles, "The Spectrophotometric Estimation of Nicotine in Blood," *Journal of Biological Chemistry* 175 (1948): 825–31.

21. Horace R. Kornegay to Paul E. Lacy and Lauren V. Ackerman, March 11, 1971, Bates TIMN0081335–1337; Washington University, "News for Release," March 11, 1971, Bates TIMN0081328–1332.

22. Paul E. Lacy to David R. Hardy, Dec. 3, 1975, Bates 794002105–2109. For "foresight and generosity": Paul E. Lacy to John E. Moss, Aug. 2, 1978, Bates 680015898.

23. Lauren V. Ackerman, "Research Proposal to the Tobacco Industry on Immunologic Aspects of Cancer," Aug. 2, 1971, Bates 1005049331–9340.

24. Art Kaufman, "Tobacco Firms Helping in Fight against Cancer," *St. Louis Globe-Democrat,* June 6, 1980, Bates 2025015742–5744.

25. Joseph H. Ogura, "Application for Research Grant," Sept. 18, 1974, Bates CTRSP/ FILES013261/33.

26. For Horsfall: "Doctor Says: Smoking and Fallout Get Undue Blame for Cancer," Seattle *Post Intelligencer,* June 9, 1962, Bates 1002405384. For "we have handled it": William Ruder to James C. Bowling, June 19, 1975, Bates 2015013901. For "pro-improved tobacco": A. E. O'Keeffe to R. N. DuPuis, Oct. 4, 1955, Bates 10018131695–3696.

27. The ghosted paper is E. L. Wynder, J. R. Hebert, and G. C. Kabat, "Association of Dietary Fat and Lung Cancer," *Journal of the National Cancer Institute* 79 (1987): 631–37. For "rabid or silly antis": Philip Morris, "Environmental Tobacco Smoke," 1990, Bates 202118 1849–1850. For "insidious effect": Fields and Chapman, "Chasing Ernst L. Wynder." The industry would later use its support for Wynder as part of its defense in litigation.

28. For lawyers: David R. Hardy to Committee of Counsel, Jan. 21, 1974, Bates 202500 7864–7865. For "more on public relations": Frank G. Colby to Murray Senkus, Oct. 17, 1973, Bates 500529893. For "possible relationship": "Review of Progress: UCLA Program Project," May 1, 1975, Bates 03755366–5371. For "complex interlocking": "Progress Report for the UCLA Program," 1978, Bates 4422638–2663. Investigators included, apart from Cline, David W. Golde, Mary Territo, Robert Lehrer, Jacob Zighelboim, Robert Gale, Gregory Sarna, Peter Graze, John Wells, and John Toohey, plus sixteen postdoctoral trainees and additional collaborators from Surgical Oncology (Donald Morton), Microbiology & Immunology (John Fahey), Infectious Diseases (Lowell Young), Surgery (Paul Terasaki), and Molecular Biology (Winston Salser). For "no strong evidence": Martin J. Cline to Joseph E. Edens, April 19, 1974, Bates 680146214–6216.

29. Martin J. Cline, deposition testimony in *Broin v. Philip Morris,* May 20, 1997, Bates 516969762–9788. The flight attendants won this case, and the foundation set up with the money was used to add BAT documents to the Legacy Tobacco Documents Library.

30. James E. Enstrom to Anne Duffin, Jan. 5, 1976, Bates HK2232075–2075. For "some other factor": *Tobacco Institute Newsletter,* Nov. 25, 1974, Bates TIFL0509298–9301. Enstrom

NOTES TO PAGES 432–435   645

in his proposal stressed that Mormons' low cancer rates were "only partially explained by their smoking habits"; see Enstrom to Hockett, June 3, 1975, Bates 50207891–7892; Enstrom to John H. Kreisher, May 5, 1975, Bates 50207899–7899.

31. Anne Duffin to James E. Enstrom, Jan. 16, 1976, Bates HK2232074–2074.

32. James E. Enstrom to Richard Carchman, Jan. 15, 1997, Bates 2063654073–4073.

33. For Kessler's ruling: "Amended Final Opinion," pp. 1380–84. For "premature to conclude": James E. Enstrom and Geoffrey C. Kabat, "Environmental Tobacco Smoke and Tobacco Related Mortality in a Prospective Study of Californians, 1960–98," *BMJ* 326 (2003): 1057–61; and for criticisms: "American Cancer Society Condemns Tobacco Industry Study for Inaccurate Use of Data," May 15, 2003; and the remarkable set of *BMJ* "Rapid Responses" at Bates 3006509062–9170; also Lisa A. Bero, Stanton Glantz, and M.-K. Hong, "The Limits of Competing Interest Disclosures," *Tobacco Control* 14 (2005): 118–26.

34. Richard C. Paddock, "A Smoldering Controversy at UCLA: The School Accepts Money from Tobacco Giant Philip Morris in Its Three-Year Study of Nicotine Addiction: Teenagers and Monkeys are Part of the Research," *Los Angeles Times,* Feb. 9, 2008.

35. "Stanford Tests Hint Cigaret Smoke May Prevent Some Cancer in Mice," *San Francisco Call-Bulletin,* April 1, 1954, Bates 1005039811; compare Hanmer to Hahn, Nov. 19, 1953, Bates 950156733–6734. Griffin volunteered to represent American Tobacco at the 1954 International Cancer Congress in São Paulo, Brazil; see his letter to Hanmer, April 28, 1954, Bates 950156713–6714.

36. Final PMERP payments were made in November 2007; see Richard Izac to Anita Bacon, Nov. 9, 2007, Bates 3039515465–5465. For the decision "to not solicit or fund additional ERP research proposals" while still continuing to fund external research, see Kenneth F. Podraza to Ivana Faccini, Nov. 2, 2007, Bates 3039518420–8421. PMERP by this time had funded over 420 research proposals.

37. James Missett, deputy chief of the psychiatry service at Stanford Hospital and a member of the clinical faculty at Stanford School of Medicine, in 1998 testified for the defense in *Henley v. Philip Morris;* see Bates MISSETTJ121598, pp. 96–96. Herbert Solomon, chair of Stanford's statistics department and its first Ph.D. recipient, was designated along with twenty-six other defense witnesses to testify in *Haines v. Liggett* (in 1992); see Bates 2024929495–9496.

38. For "may improve": "Nicotine's Effect on Fatigue & Flight Performance in Drug-Naive Subjects," 1997, Bates 516764169–4177. For "positive aspects": "Objectives: Human Performance Laboratory," Bates 520016200–6211. For "nicotine enhances": Mike Johnson to Chuck Blixt, Mark Holton, and Denise Fee, "Stanford University Study," Nov. 12, 1997, Bates 520963671–3680. For the published version: Martin S. Mumenthaler, Joy L. Taylor, Ruth O'Hara, and Jerome A. Yesavage, "Influence of Nicotine on Simulator Flight Performance in Non-Smokers," *Psychopharmacology* 140 (1998): 38–41; and for peer reviews of the unpublished manuscript in Reynolds's files (!), see Bates 519972968–2972.

39. Paul Switzer, "Comments for the EPA Scientific Advisory Board EPA Review Draft: Health Effects of Passive Smoking," Nov. 5, 1990, Bates 202336136–6588 at 6512–65; and for his oral testimony on Dec. 4, 1990: Bates 515799532–9540. Other scholars paid to criticize the EPA's report included Joseph L. Fleiss of Columbia, Ragnar Rylander of the University of Gothenburg, Peter Skrabanek from Trinity College in Dublin, George Feuer of the Uni-

versity of Toronto, Alan J. Gross of the Medical University of South Carolina, Donald J. Eco-
bichon from McGill, Peter N. Lee of P. N. Lee Statistics, John W. Gorrod from the University of London, and at least fifty others; see Bates 950216620–6647.

40. Philip Morris, "Environmental Tobacco Smoke: Rush to Judgment," 1991, Bates
2022839746–9758, p. 6. And for his funding: "CIAR Funded Proposals," Jan. 18, 1996, Bates
2063654341; Paul Switzer to Clausen Ely Jr., "Invoice," Dec. 10, 1991, Bates TI10161425; Paul
Switzer, "Invoice," Feb. 1, 1996, Bates 2063610208.

41. See Timothy Lenoir, "Expert Disclosure Statement" (for *Tune v. Philip Morris*), Dec. 1,
1998, Bates 2077532085–2113; Robert E. McGinn, "Declaration" (for *Brown & Williamson
v. Regents of the University of California*), May 20, 1995, Bates 682766777–6792. Lenoir in
his carefully lawyered disclosure claimed that statistical correlations in the 1950s were regarded as "inadequate by prevailing medical and scientific standards of the time for establishing disease causation" and that when the Surgeon General finally concluded that smoking caused laryngeal cancer (in 1982) this was based on "different evidentiary standards for
establishing causality than those of the scientific research community." Lenoir also claimed
that even after this time "the causal role of smoking continued to be debated among scientific researchers" (p. 2). Lenoir's expert disclosure was not deprivileged until February of
2011; I asked him how he had become involved in litigation, and he said that Ronald Overmann from the NSF (recently retired) had put him in touch with Shook, Hardy and Bacon's
Allen Purvis, who at that time was organizing expertise for the industry (personal communication). Overmann also worked for the industry, preparing to serve as an expert witness
(1998–99) after serving as program officer for history and philosophy of science at the NSF.

42. Michael Daube (David's son), personal communication, Jan. 10, 2009.

43. For "beset by errors": "Assessment of the Medical Testimony: 1969 Cigarette Hearings, House Committee on Interstate and Foreign Commerce," 1969, Bates TI55752958–2966.
The April 15, 1969, testimony of K. Alexander Brownlee, Leo Katz, and Theodor D. Sterling
at congressional hearings on cigarette labeling and advertising can be found at Bates 2322
576–3488, pp. 750, 858–60; and Bates 1003897309–7849, pp. 930–35. Professor Katz had
earlier postulated infantile thumb sucking as just as good an explanation for lung cancer as
smoking, observing that "although you may object to a claim . . . that lung cancer is caused
by thumb-sucking, I maintain that this is precisely the nature of the supporting evidence for
the claim that lung cancer is caused by smoking"; see "Summary of Statement of Dr. Leo
Katz . . . before the Senate Committee on Commerce," March 1965, Bates 70104941–4959.

44. "Statement of Mr. Darrell Huff," U.S. Congressional Hearings on Cigarette Labeling
and Advertising, March 22, 1965, Bates 1004800682–0694.

45. The Ad Hoc Committee was a group of lawyers spun off from the Policy Committee
whose duties included maintaining the Central File (aka "Cenfile"), "a collection of every
document which can be found relating to the smoking and health controversy" (Bates
80684691–4695). The Ad Hoc Committee was also responsible for helping to locate medical witnesses and prepare testimony. Edwin Jacob from Jacob, Medinger & Finnegan supervised the Central File with financial support from all parties to the conspiracy. Responsibility for maintaining the Central File Information Center in 1971 was transferred to the
CTR, which managed "informational retrieval" and maintenance through a CTR Special
Project, organized as part of a new Information Systems division, by which means the CTR

became a crucial resource for the industry's effort to defend itself against litigation. See Kessler's "Amended Final Opinion," pp. 165–68.

46. "Congressional Preparation," Jan. 26, 1968, Bates 955007434–7439; F. P. Haas, "Memorandum," Nov. 4, 1965, Bates 502052217–2220. J. Michael Steele in his "Darrell Huff and Fifty Years of How to Lie with Statistics," *Statistical Science* 20 (2005): 205–9, ignores Huff's work for Big Tobacco in his effort to explain how Huff's became "the most widely read statistics book in the history of the world." A 1966 draft of Huff's tobacco–cancer denialist essay can be found at Bates 1005087621–7694.

47. Timothy Finnegan to William W. Shinn, "Joe Janis," Feb. 1, 1979, Bates 521030804–0805; Finnegan to Gentlemen, March 21, 1981, Bates 507731483–1484; M. H. Crohn et al., "Primary Issue," May 1980, Bates 501729943–9946.

48. See the Reynolds organization chart for Oct. 23, 1990, Bates 2026230324–0712. The Tobacco Statisticians Working Group included Anthony Springall from Imperial, Edward B. Wilkes from BAT, W. D. Rowland from Carreras Rothmans, M. R. Stevenson from Gallaher, and Manuel Bourlas from Philip Morris Europe, with lawyerly support from W. S. Paige. For the work of the subcommittee, see "Minutes of the 67th Meeting of the Statistical Sub-Committee of TRC," July 28, 1976, Bates 100210432–0438. Wolf-Dieter Heller in 1984 published a letter in *Lancet* criticizing Trichopoulos's work on secondhand smoke; the substance of the criticism had been drafted by Peter N. Lee, a long-standing consultant for the industry, but as Lee explained to BAT, the letter was "arranged to be sent from Germany through the Verband, as there was a fear I was getting rather too much exposure." See Lee, "More on Passive Smoking," Jan. 14, 1984, Bates 100203723–3737.

49. For "three independent statisticians": "Error Found in Cancer Study," *Tobacco International Communique,* June–July 1981, Bates 506642052–2067; and for the press release: Bates 503947515–7519. For press coverage: Tobacco Institute, "The Hirayama Controversy: An Analysis of Media Activity," Aug. 1981, Bates TI10080830–0953.

50. J. K. Wells (Brown & Williamson) to E. Pepples, July 24, 1981, Bates 521028146–8147.

51. Marvin A. Kastenbaum, "Epidemic by the Numbers," April 15, 1975, Bates HK0119030–9046.

52. William E. Wecker, deposition testimony in *Texas v. American Tobacco,* Sept. 26, 1997, Bates WECKERW092697, pp. 85–91.

53. R. Garrison Harvey, "Affidavit" Re Jason Budnick, July 14, 2010.

54. Donald B. Rubin, deposition testimony for *Florida v. American Tobacco,* July 9, 1997, Bates RUBIND070997, p. 26; also his testimony in *USA v. Philip Morris,* May 24, 2005, Bates RUBIND052405; and his "The Ethics of Consulting for the Tobacco Industry," *Statistical Methods in Medical Research* 11 (2002): 373–80. Rubin's opportunity to testify came through Finis Welch, an economist at Texas A&M in College Station.

55. Lynn R. LaMotte, deposition testimony in *Texas v. American Tobacco,* Sept. 27, 1997, Bates LAMOTTEL092797, pp. 41–45.

56. Wayne W. Juchatz to Samuel B. Witt III, "Dr. DiMarco," Dec. 13, 1982, Bates 505741150–1153.

57. For a list of over a hundred depositions of such experts—and these just for Philip Morris—see "Deposition Transcripts of Philip Morris Employees & Experts Taken in AG & Non-AG Cases through 4/29/99," Bates 2077744017–4036. We are very much in need of crit-

648 NOTES TO PAGES 445-451

ical histories of field-specific collaborations, including the back-scratching networks through which such contacts are maintained. One solid source is the December 2006 volume of *Tobacco Control* titled *Research on Tobacco Litigation Testimony*, edited by Stella Bialous.

58. Bernard G. Greenberg's Nov. 25, 1964, testimony for the defense in *Green v. American Tobacco* can be found at Bates GREENBERGB112564.

59. Rodney W. Nichols to Ernst Pepples, March 6, 1980, Bates 521033811–3812, cc'ed to Joshua Lederberg et al.

60. For "tremendously grateful": Joshua Lederberg to J. Paul Sticht, Aug. 17, 1979, Bates 504874151. For "carcinogenic damage": Joshua Lederberg to Ernest Pepples, Sept. 6, 1984, Bates 521033548–3549.

61. "Financial Support of Research Efforts of Rockefeller University," Sept. 11, 1975, Bates 503135598.

62. Naomi Oreskes and Erik M. Conway, "Challenging Knowledge: How Climate Science Became a Victim of the Cold War," in Proctor and Schiebinger, eds., *Agnotology*, pp. 55–89.

63. In 1982 projects supported by Reynolds's Medical Research Committee included research into blood pressure at Harvard, arteriosclerosis at the University of Washington, lung disease and necrosis at UC San Diego, cancer at the University of Colorado, immunology at the MCV, adult diabetes at the University of Pennsylvania, and "the effects of diet and stress" at four different institutions, etc.; see Frederick Seitz, "R. J. Reynolds Research Grants Program Update," May 18, 1982, Bates 515449717–9733.

64. Frederick Seitz, "R. J. Reynolds Research Grants Program Update," May 2, 1983, Bates 515449734–9764; Mark Hertsgaard, "While Washington Slept," *Vanity Fair*, April 5, 2006.

65. For "depriving people": Ernest Pepples to Joshua Lederberg, Nov. 30, 1981, Bates 521033609. For "absolute confidentiality": Ernest Pepples to Joshua Lederberg, Oct. 15, 1981, Bates 501026848. For the Manhattan visit: "Rockefeller University Faculty and Officers to Attend Meeting," April 1, 1988, Bates 506254882–4883.

66. Tobacco Institute, *Three Decades of Initiatives by a Responsible Cigarette Industry*, Nov. 29, 1988, Bates TIFL0503147–3151; E. A. Horrigan, "An Open Debate," Feb. 14, 1984, Bates TIMN0263822–3825,

67. For "not ogres": Donald K. Hoel, "Industry Research Committee Meeting," Nov. 6, 1978, Bates 2023918174–8180. For Redford Williams, see his *The Trusting Heart: Great News about Type A Behavior* (New York: Random House, 1989).

68. Brandy Fisher, "Healing Weed," *Tobacco Reporter*, May 2000, Bates 531290150–0172. Cooke's work was key in the founding of Endovasc, a publicly traded company licensed to commercialize nicotine angiogenesis. Cooke himself was an investor, as was Philip Morris. The company was eventually reduced to a penny stock amid a certain degree of "pump and dump" scandal for which the word "Endoscam" was coined.

69. "Associates for Research into the Science of Enjoyment," Sept. 1993, Bates 250409 2465–2482; "Scientists Meet in Brussels to Reflect on the Quality of Life" (ARISE press release), Sept. 28, 1993, Bates 2023128389–8390; David M. Warburton, ed., *Addiction Controversies* (London: Routledge, 1990). For a list of ARISE Associates and mission goals, see Bates 2024208105–8132 at 8115.

70. "ARISE: Information Pack," Bates 520029233–9283; compare also Bates 2050163311.

For "high priests of pleasure": David M. Warburton, "The Functions of Pleasure," Sept. 28, 1993, Bates 2023128393–8394.

71. Petra Netter, "Pleasure and Health," 1993, Bates 2023128395–8396.

72. For "alleged dangers": Timothy Evans, "Bureaucracy against Life: The Politicisation of Personal Choice," 1993, Bates 2029104023–4024. For Frank van Dun: Bates 2023128401–8402. For Luik on addiction: John C. Luik, "'I Can't Help Myself': Addiction as Ideology," *Human Psychopharmacology* 11 (1996): S21–32; also John Lepere (CECCM) to M. Arnauts et al., June 28, 1993, Bates 300544162–4191, and the online *Sourcewatch* entry on Luik. ARISE Associates were also used to fight antismoking restrictions. Philip Morris funded Jean-Pierre Dauwalder's Institute of Psychology in Lausanne, for example, to produce "third party" communications in the area of "social-political themes" like "tolerance, freedom of speech, scientific research and communication, the nanny state, health and lifestyle engineering, etc."; see the company's report for Switzerland from Oct. 12, 1992, Bates 2501362190–2203. Prof. Peter Atteslander of Augsburg was also employed for this purpose; see Dietmar Jazbinsek, "Peter Atteslander: Forschen schadet Ihrer Gesundheit," *Die Weltwoche* (2005): 47.

73. Philip Morris, "Project Cosmic: Budget/Sending Status," Feb. 1991, Bates 2023160927; Philip Morris, "Expense Elements Analysis," Feb. 19, 1991, Bates 2023160930–0931.

74. For "potentially totalitarian": Peter L. Berger, "Boston University," March 5, 1982, Bates TIMN0198603–8619; compare his interview in "What Motivates Anti-Smokers?" *Tobacco Observer,* April 1980, Bates TIMN0121130–1141. For "disturbing implication," see his statement submitted to the Labor and Human Resources Committee, U.S. Senate, on the proposed Comprehensive Smoking Prevention Education Act, March 5, 1982, Bates 2060465087–5152, pp. 271–92, and Bates TIMN0198603–8619. For "lonely zealots," see his "ETS: Ideological Issue and Cultural Syndrome," in *Clearing the Air: Perspectives on Environmental Tobacco Smoke,* ed. Robert D. Tollison (Lexington, KY: D. C. Heath, 1988), pp. 82–83, Bates 682719312–9320. For "elitist": "Excerpts from Observations by Peter L. Berger . . . after attending the Fourth World Conference on Smoking and Health in Stockholm in 1979, and the Fifth in Winnipeg," 1983, Bates TI04821555–1561. For "totalitarian encroachments": Peter L. Berger, speech of March 5, 1982, Bates 03609609–9624. For "new anti-Semitism": Peter L. Berger, "Gilgamesh on the Washington Shuttle," *Worldview,* Nov. 1977, pp. 43–45.

75. Peter L. Berger, "Furtive Smokers—And What They Tell Us about America," *Commentary,* June 1994, pp. 21–26, Bates 2078320968–0979.

76. PMERP in 2000 received 153 applications and funded 66; for a list, see "Philip Morris External Research Program Management Report," Feb. 2002, Bates 2085522647–2721.

77. http://harvest.cals.ncsu.edu/index.cfm?showpage = 293&awardid = 139.

78. Richard C. Reich, "Philip Morris Support for Agricultural Programs in Four Major Flue-Cured Tobacco States," March 27, 1987, Bates 506491092–1095.

79. Stanley Schachter to William Dunn, Dec. 26, 1972, Bates 1003290508; Schachter to Dunn, Sept. 20, 1973, Bates 1003290504.

80. "Board of Directors, Excerpt from Minutes, March 27, 1985, George Weissman—Endowment Gift," Bates 2073921336.

81. For project code names: "Potential Witnesses or Scientists Able to Help in Finding Witnesses," 1991 (est.), Bates 2028395845–5851; also "Projects Description 1991," n.d., Bates

2023856132. For Alzheimer's: "Cajal" (Philip Morris), Oct. 1990, Jan. 1991, Bates 2023856208; and John P. Blass to Ernest Pepples, Feb. 21, 1984, Bates 521033562.

82. Janine K. Cataldo, Judith J. Prochaska, and Stanton A. Glantz, "Cigarette Smoking Is a Risk Factor for Alzheimer's Disease: An Analysis Controlling for Tobacco Industry Affiliation," *Journal of Alzheimer's Disease* 19 (2010): 465–80.

83. David Spurgeon, "Canadian Universities' Links to Tobacco Industry Shown," *BMJ* 325 (2002): 734, reporting on a study by Fernand Turcotte et al.; Simon Chapman and Stan Shatenstein, "The Ethics of the Cash Register: Taking Tobacco Research Dollars," *Tobacco Control* 10 (2001): 1–2; "Cancer Professor on the Move," *Times*, March 17, 2001; J. Meikle, "Professor Quits over Tobacco Firm's £3.8m Gift to University," *Guardian*, May 18, 2001; R. Smith, "A Tainted University," *Guardian*, May 21, 2001.

84. Helmut W. Gaisch, "The European Counterpart to 'Operation Downunder': The Role of S&T PME," Feb. 21, 1988, Bates 2028343858–3860; Joaquin Barnoya and Stanton A. Glantz, "The Tobacco Industry's Worldwide ETS Consultants Project," *European Journal of Public Health*, 16 (2005): 69–77.

85. Norbert Hirschhorn, "Shameful Science: Four Decades of the German Tobacco Industry's Hidden Research on Smoking and Health," *Tobacco Control* 9 (2000): 242–47; Grüning, Gilmore, and McKee, "Tobacco Industry Influence." For a stinging critique of the German industry's corruption of "passive smoking" research, see Ferdinand Schmidt, "Symposium war ein Skandal," *Die Neue Ärztliche*, May 14, 1987, Bates TI10010556–0559. For Germany's Institute for Heart Research: http://member.globalink.org/nimi/26673.

86. Jones Day uses the "stable of experts" metaphor with regard to experts organized by the industry's Special Trial Issues Committee (STIC); see Jones Day, "Corporate Activity Project," p. 327; and for STIC activities: King and Spalding to Brown & Williamson, April 7, 1992, Bates 689103258–3437.

87. "Potential Witnesses or Scientists Able to Help in Finding Witnesses," 1991 (est.), Bates 2028395845–5851.

88. Deborah E. Barnes and Lisa A. Bero, "Why Review Articles on the Health Effects of Passive Smoking Reach Different Conclusions," *JAMA* 279 (1998): 1566–70.

89. "Transcript of E-chat with Dr. Sharon Boyse, Director of Scientific Issues, B&W, June 6, 2000," Bates 2083483332–3340, corrected for punctuation.

CHAPTER 24

1. Marc Edell, "Cigarette Litigation: The Second Wave," *Tort and Insurance Law* 22 (1986): 90–103.

2. An excellent history of mechanization can be found in Walford's 1979 "Development of Cigarette Technology." For brand histories, see "Salem," 1994, Bates 513912600–2610; and AT's "Lucky Strike," 1916, Bates 544010006–0032. For the CTR, see W. T. Hoyt, "Excerpt from History of the Council for Tobacco Research—U.S.A., Inc.," 1984, Bates 92743050–3070. For filters, see "Hi-Fi History" (Brown & Williamson), n.d., Bates 464518657–8673. An excellent history of menthols is Jack R. Reid (Lorillard), "A History of Mentholated Cigarettes: 'This Spud's for You,'" *47th Tobacco Chemists Research Conference*, Oct. 23, 1993, Bates 2057 764407–4420. A superb review of the history of tobacco chemistry can be found in Vello

Norman (Lorillard), "Changes in Smoke Chemistry of Modern Day Cigarettes," 1976, Bates 503853939–3975. A short (and deceptive) history of the idea that smoking was killing 300,000 people per year in the United States can be found in the Tobacco Institute's "Two Days in May," May 1978, Bates PA/000776. For a Tobacco Institute bibliography of historiography, see "Tobacco History Bibliography," April 1976, Bates 502111718–1722. For the history of CORESTA, an international organization created by the French tobacco monopoly (SEITA), see "25 Years of International Cooperation in the Service of Scientific and Technical Research in Connection with Tobacco (1956–1982)," 1982, Bates 510648213–8235. For history for litigation, see Jones, Day, Reavis and Pogue, "RJR Research and Development Activities: Fact Team Memorandum," Dec. 31, 1985, Bates 515871651–1912; also "The Tobacco Institute: A Brief History," Feb. 7, 1997, Bates TINY0001751–1755. For medical science history, see the 300-page anonymous review for Philip Morris: "The Incidence and Etiology of Bronchiogenic Carcinoma—A Review of Literature," 1953, Bates 2025017820–7880, 2025017881–7923, and 2025017924–8049. For brand reviews, see American Tobacco's "Pall Mall Advertising 1919–1950, Pall Mall Brand Review 1975–1983," n.d., Bates 970227411–7465; also "RJR—History—Winston," Oct. 26, 2000, Bates 522901708–1731. For chronologies, see A. L. Fritschler, "Chronology of Important Events in the Cigarette Labeling Controversy," 1972, Bates TIMN0082916–2928; also the "Partial Chronology of Tobacco-Related Political, Scientific, and Media Events between 1962 and 1968" prepared by Brown & Williamson, n.d., Bates 1007.01. Historians have occasionally entertained the industry by delivering speeches at colloquia; Spencer Weart on April 25, 1979, presented an "Evening Seminar" at Philip Morris's headquarters with the nicely ironic title "Prostituted Physics"; see P. A. Eichorn, "Evening Seminars," Oct. 19, 1978, Bates 100076148.

3. Lawrence M. Hughes, "R. J. Reynolds and Its First 50 Years with 'Old Joe' Camel," *Sales Management,* Nov. 1, 1963, Bates 500627570–7577; Silvette, Larson, and Haag, "Medical Uses of Tobacco, Past and Present," *Virginia Medical Monthly* 85 (1958): 472–84.

4. Jerome E. Brooks, *Tobacco: Its History Illustrated by the Books, Manuscripts and Engravings in the Library of George Arents, Jr.,* 5 vols. (1937–52; Reprint Mansfied Centre: Maurizio Martino & Krown and Spellman, 1999). The first of these volumes cost $75 in 1938—at that time an enormous sum.

5. T. K. Cahill to George Schramek, May 21, 1975, Bates 502101534–1535.

6. William Kloepfer to J. C. B. Ehringhaus, Dec. 28, 1977, Bates TI07711315. Robicsek, a cardiopulmonary surgeon at the Sanger Institute in Charlotte, North Carolina, declares tobacco "a universal necessity without which man is now very reluctant to live" (*Smoking Gods,* p. 202). Industry fronts have often published histories of smoking; see, for example, Sean Gabb's *Smoking and Its Enemies: A Short History of 500 Years of the Use and Prohibition of Tobacco,* published in the early 1990s by the London-based Freedom Organisation for the Right to Enjoy Smoking Tobacco (FOREST).

7. Brady to Little, "TIRC Program." For CBS television: "Discussion with Dr. John F. W. King and Dr. Milton B. Rosenblatt," April 5, 1962, Bates 01141415. For "colossal blunder": "Statement of Dr. Milton B. Rosenblatt before the Parliamentary Committee on Health, Welfare and Social Affairs," May 22, 1969, Bates 696000551–0568; and for video: TI06600187.

8. "Statement of Robert Casad Hockett," May 9, 1983, Bates 680574120–4415, p. 329. The archives contain an unpublished manuscript by Rosenblatt (prepared for Philip Morris)

chronicling the recognition of lung diseases such as emphysema and cancer; see "Cancer of the Lung: Collected Reprints," n.d., Bates 1005102574–2607.

9. Joseph Robert's books include *The Tobacco Kingdom: Plantation, Market and Factory in Virginia and North Carolina* (Durham: Duke University Press, 1938) and *The Story of Tobacco in America* (New York: Knopf, 1949); and for one of his speeches, see "General Program: 22nd Tobacco Chemists' Research Conference," Oct. 18, 1968, Bates 500980060–0090. Nannie M. Tilley's two main books are *The Bright-Tobacco Industry* (Chapel Hill: University of North Carolina Press, 1948) and *Reynolds Tobacco Company* (1985). For Jerome E. Brooks's "authorized unpublished history," see his "The Philip Morris Century," ca. 1978, Bates 96746624–6648. For BAT's "History Project," see Mair Davies and Augustus Muir, "Report on B.A.T. History Project, Folio Two," 1972, Bates 406110072–0185.

10. "The News," *Brandstand: Viewing the World of Cigarette Collecting,* June–July 1980, p. 3.

11. Cox, *The Global Cigarette.*

12. B. W. E. Alford, *W. D. & H. O. Wills and the Development of the U.K. Tobacco Industry, 1786–1965* (London: Methuen, 1973); Brian M. Du Toit, *Ecusta and the Legacy of Harry H. Straus* (Baltimore: PublishAmerica, 2007); W. Twiston Davies, *Fifty Years of Progress: An Account of the African Organisation of the Imperial Tobacco Company, 1907–1957* (Bristol: Imperial Tobacco Co., 1958); Sue V. Dickinson, *The First Sixty Years: A History of the Imperial Tobacco Company* (Bristol: Imperial Tobacco Co., 1965). Apart from Tilley's, other official histories include Heimann, *Americans and Tobacco;* the anonymous Brown and Williamson Tobacco Corp., *The First Hundred Years, 1893–1993* (Louisville, KY: Brown & Williamson Tobacco Corp., 1993); Mark W. Rien and Gustaf N. Dorén, *Das neue Tabago Buch* (Hamburg: Reemtsma, 1985); and Laurie Dennett, "B.A.T. Industries: An Historical Note" (BAT, 1987), Bates 202032484–2513. A history of the U.S. Tobacco Co. can be found in the *U.S. Tobacco Review* 2 (First Quarter 1986), Bates TIWA 004069–4093; compare also Jack Jones, *Cigarettes—Liverpool 5—The Story of the Liverpool Branch of British American Tobacco Company Ltd* (BAT, ca. 1972). There are many handsomely illustrated histories of tobacco in Japanese, most of which are published by Japan Tobacco International.

13. For "network": "Chronology and Development of Project Cosmic," 1988, Bates 2023919844–9846; for "papers suitable": David Harley to Kenneth S. Houghton, Dec. 1, 1987, Bates 2001260154–0158; for Columbus quincentenary: Harley, "Project Report," Aug. 1990, Bates 2022884760; for article: David Harley, "The Beginnings of the Tobacco Controversy: Puritanism, James I, and the Royal Physicians," *Bulletin of the History of Medicine* 67 (1993): 28–50; for paid handsomely: Philip Morris, "R&D Outside Contractor Expenditures from 1984 through 1997," Aug. 12, 1997, Bates 2063665351–5372. John E. Sauer, Burnham's colleague at Ohio State, was paid $10,312 in Cosmic monies to explore "why people smoke."

14. For Musto's $300,000: "Project Cosmic: Proposals, Contracts and Progress Reports," Nov. 20, 1990, Bates 2023160937–0941. For Burnham on the industry's response as "timely and appropriate": "Cipollone v. Liggett Group, Inc.," March 20, 1987, Bates 92497061–7064.

15. "Musto, Yale University," Nov. 20, 1990, Bates 2022884770; Gina Kolata, "Temperance: An Old Cycle Repeats Itself," *New York Times,* Jan. 1, 1991; also Sam Nelson to Jack Nelson, July 13, 1992, Bates 2023919842–9843.

16. Leon E. Rosenberg to Daniel M. Ennis, Sept. 9, 1988, Bates 2022884774.

17. Jon Wiener, "Big Tobacco and the Historians," *The Nation*, March 15, 2010.

18. Colin Talley, Howard I. Kushner, and Claire E. Sterk, "Lung Cancer, Chronic Disease Epidemiology, and Medicine, 1948–1964," *Journal of the History of Medicine* 59 (2004): 329–74. Allan Brandt reviewed Talley et al.'s manuscript prior to publication and was shocked to see its conclusion that the "controversy" over smoking and health prior to 1964 was "reasonable and perhaps necessary to advance the science of chronic disease epidemiology." Concerned that the authors might have been taking tobacco money, Brandt asked the editor to request a formal disclosure, which resulted in the authors revealing that Talley and Kushner had both been consulting for Johnson, Tyler and Purvis, a Washington, D.C., law firm specializing in "recruiting and developing expert witnesses for the defense in tobacco industry lawsuits" (ibid.; personal communication).

19. Annamaria Baba et al., including Lisa Bero, "Legislating 'Sound Science': The Role of the Tobacco Industry," *American Journal of Public Health* 95 (2005): S20–27; Wallace Ravven, "Unprecedented Industry-backed Laws Limit Public Safety, Study Shows," *Medical News Today*, July 22, 2005, reporting on Baba et al.'s study. For "tool to clobber" (citing Rena Steinzor): Rick Weiss, " 'Data Quality' Law Is Nemesis of Regulation," *Washington Post*, Aug. 16, 2004.

20. J. Michael Jordan (outside counsel for Reynolds from Womble, Carlyle, Sandridge, & Rice) to S&H Attorneys, April 29, 1988, Bates 2583.

21. Brandt, *Cigarette Century*, pp. 319–99.

22. King & Spalding to Brown & Williamson, "Special Trial Issues Committee (STIC)," April 7, 1992, Bates 689103258–3437. STIC compiled an elaborate "witness inventory" with scholars assigned to particular "responsible lawyers"; see Bates 682718560–8599.

23. Allen R. Purvis to Donald F. Miles, "California Awareness Sources—'The Grapevine,' " July 29, 1986, Bates 2025033473. Purvis here described PHR Associates as a "consulting group of public historians."

24. "Manual for Historic Awareness Coding Project," April 26, 1986, Bates 515873086–3207; compare Bates 682718560–8599. Tobacco industry attorneys in 1986 described the "key-stone" of their defense as "the endlessly detailed factual specifics of who the plaintiff is" to counter the abstract knowledge of judges and juries that smokers have been "led to their doom" by advertising and industry PR"; see the 1986 "Training Materials for Counsel in Smoking & Health Litigation," Bates 282012884–3316.

25. Kyriakoudes, "Historians' Testimony," p. iv107.

26. See my "Everyone Knew"; also Bates 2048242640 for "everybody knew, nobody knows."

27. John Burnham, "Medical Historians and the Tobacco Industry," *Lancet* 364 (2004): 838; also my response on this same page. Historians working for the industry were often told not to talk about their work; see the "Manual for Historic Awareness Coding Project," April 26, 1986, Bates 515873086–3207.

28. Cassandra Tate was invited to work for Reynolds in the 1990s but refused, not wanting to compromise her integrity. Many other historians—probably dozens—have refused offers of work from the industry.

29. http://www.yale.edu/history/faculty/musto.html; accessed Nov. 1, 2006.

30. See again my "Everyone Knew But No One Had Proof."

31. The American Thoracic Society implemented such a policy in 1995 for its *American*

Journal of Respiratory and Critical Care Medicine and the *American Journal of Respiratory Cell and Molecular Biology.* Similar policies were subsequently established for the *Journal of Health Psychology,* the *British Journal of Cancer,* and a number of other scholarly publications. *PLOS Medicine*—part of the open-access Public Library of Science—in February 2010 announced that it would no longer publish articles financed by the tobacco industry.

32. See, for example, the deposition of Paul Robert Dommel for *Mississippi Tobacco Litigation,* March 14, 1997, Bates dommelp031497. Dommel, a political scientist, was hired to investigate and testify on the history of tobacco regulation.

33. Jeffrey E. Harris, "Expert's Report on the State of the Art," Aug. 1, 1985, Bates 2023082166–2250.

34. Deposition of Kenneth Ludmerer in *Harvey v. Lummus,* May 13, 2002, pp. 146–48. For "helped erase": Deposition of Kenneth Ludmerer in *USA v. Philip Morris,* Aug. 8, 2002, Bates LudmererK080802.

35. Deposition of Kenneth Ludmerer in *Cipollone v. Liggett,* March 25–26, 1991, Bates LudmererK032591 and 032691. For "setting boundaries": Trial testimony of Kenneth Ludmerer in *Anderson v. American Tobacco,* June 12, 2000, Bates LudmererK061200. For "out of my area": Deposition of Kenneth Ludmerer in *USA v. Philip Morris,* Aug. 8, 2002, Bates LudmererK080802.

36. Janet L. Johnson to State-of-the-Art Subcommittee, "Witness Development," July 26, 1988, Bates 2048245281–5297.

37. Ibid., pp. 2–3.

38. Ibid., p. 7.

39. Ibid.

40. Expert reports submitted by defense attorneys sometimes contain near-identical passages, suggesting the helping hand of attorneys in their drafting. An alternative explanation given by Michael E. Parrish, a persistent witness for the defense, is that "Good historians think alike." See Theodore A. Wilson, "Affidavit," April 19, 1997, Bates WILSONT041997ER; Michael Parrish, "Affidavit," Dec. 5, 1996, Bates PARRISHM120596ER, pp. 2–3; and Parrish's deposition for *Barnes v. American,* Sept. 30, 1997, Bates 519731625–2175, p. 40. Parrish later revised his explanation for the similarity, stating that Wilson had "obviously stolen" from his report; see his cross-examination by David Golub in *Izzarelli v. Reynolds,* May 11, 2010, pp. 1894–98.

41. "Daily Clip Report," Bates 20000717.

42. We can also ask, what is the impact on public health of legal verdicts against the cigarette industry? Americans smoke about 340 billion cigarettes per year, for which they pay about $80 billion. A $1 million verdict against the industry, if passed on to consumers in the form of higher prices, would mean an increase in the total paid for cigarettes (in the United States) from $80 billion to $80.001 billion—or one part in 80,000. So a $1 million verdict would cause consumption to fall by (340 billion cigs. × .4) / 80,000 = about 2 million cigarettes. One person dies for every million cigarettes smoked—which means that a million-dollar verdict against the industry will prevent two people from dying of smoking. Litigating against the industry can and does save lives, functioning as a kind of (inefficient) tax. Modest increases in taxes of course are far more effective: a tax sufficient to force an increase in the price of cigarettes by 10 percent, for example, would cause a reduction in the number

of cigarettes smoked by 4 percent, which would be .04 × 340 billion = 14 billion cigarettes per year. A tax of this (modest) magnitude would save 14,000 lives per year.

43. "The Cigarette Consumer" (Philip Morris), March 20, 1984, Bates 2500002189–2207.

44. The U.S. case is dramatic, but historians from all over the world have worked for the industry. In Australia, Geoffrey Hawker of Macquarie University in 1994 drafted a report for the Tobacco Institute of Australia, claiming that addiction and other health harms from smoking have long been "popular knowledge"; see Geoffrey Hawker, "An Historical Analysis of the Tobacco Growing and Manufacturing Industries," May 1994, Bates 2504203370–3397. In Finland Professor Pertti Haapala has testified for the defense in cigarette litigation, following this same "common knowledge" script; see Heikki T. Hiilamo, "The Impact of Strategic Funding by the Tobacco Industry of Medical Expert Witnesses Appearing for the Defence in the Aho Finnish Product Liability Case," *Addiction* 102 (2007): 979–88. Canadian historians have also joined this parade: Jacques Lacoursière of Quebec, David H. Flaherty of the University of Western Ontario, and Robert John Perrins of Acadia University in Nova Scotia have all worked for the defense in tobacco litigation, e.g., *Létourneau v. Imperial Tobacco* and *Conseil québécois sur le tabac et la santé v. JTI-Macdonald*. Judith Fyfe, a New Zealand historian, was paid for more than twenty thousand hours of work for the defense in *Janice Pou v. British American Tobacco*, convincing the court that the health risks of smoking were "common knowledge" in 1968 when the plaintiff began smoking. See Kate Tokeley, "Case Note: *Pou v. British American Tobacco (NZ) Ltd*—A Comprehensive Win for the New Zealand Tobacco Industry," *Waikato Law Review* 14 (2006): 136–44.

PART IV

1. Chip Jones, "Philip Morris Finds Culprit," *Richmond Times-Dispatch,* June 21, 1995, Bates 2054406322–6223.

2. Caitlin Francke, "$2 million Award in Smoking Lawsuit," *Baltimore Sun,* April 30, 1999.

3. David Tijernina sued Philip Morris et al. (including Hoechst Celanese), claiming that cellulose acetate fibers were lodging in the bodily tissues of smokers; see J. L. Pauly et al., "Cigarettes with Defective Filters Marketed for 40 Years: What Philip Morris Never Told Smokers," *Tobacco Control* 11 (2002): i51–61. D. G. Felton and J. A. Sykes, "A Study of the Sand and Iron Balance during Cigarette Manufacture," March 13, 1958, Bates 654035770–5800.

4. Illeg. to QA Team, Feb. 21, 1998, Bates 524268171–8172.

5. John S. McBride to Reynolds, June 21, 1998, Bates 524268198–8200.

6. Patricia West to Reynolds, July 24, 1998, Bates 524268218–8219.

7. For "bug spray": Ray Campbell to Reynolds, June 20, 1998, Bates 524268185–8186; "blinding headache": Debbie Phillips to Reynolds, June 30, 1998, Bates 524268189–8190; worms: Lori Murch to Forsyth Tobacco Products, July 18, 1998, Bates 524268226–8227; smoking while driving: Donald E. Crawford to Quality Assurance, July 28, 1998, Bates 524268246–8248; stick inside cigarette: Tina Rendeiro to Camel, July 19, 1998, Bates 524268235–8238; "Fire Falls Out": "Case Comments," Jan. 26, 1996, Bates 519102721–2760.

8. "Domestic & T.I. Complaints, March 1995" (Reynolds), Bates 513052274–2316.

9. Ginger Coe to Marshall Hughes, Dec. 2, 1999, Bates 522749727–9728.

10. P. H. Leake to C. C. Kern, "Consumer Complaints by Type for Filter Cigarettes," Feb. 24, 1984, Bates 965044915–4917; A. F. Press to P. H. Leake, "Wormy Complaints," Feb. 14, 1989, Bates 967015635–5636.

CHAPTER 25

1. In 1972 Brown & Williamson researchers found certain "volatile components in the solvents used to seal cellophane" being transferred to the cigarettes; see T. D. Bakker, "Woodrose Final Report: Viceroy 84 Cellophane Solvent Test," Sept. 20, 1972, Bates 670610337–0340.

2. A solid exception is Clive Bates, Martin Jarvis, and Gregory Connolly, "Tobacco Additives: Cigarette Engineering and Nicotine Addiction," July 14, 1999, http://old.ash.org.uk/html/regulation/html/additives.html.

3. For a list of additives prepared for litigation, see Brown & Williamson's "Pesticides and Potentially Hazardous Additives," April 1996, Bates 1327.01. For "most potent": Peter Waltz to Helmut Wakeham, Sept. 25, 1963, Bates 1000825946–5951.

4. F. Roth, "Chronic Arsenicism and Cancers among Vineyard Workers in the Moselle Valley," *Zeitschrift für Krebsforschung* 61 (1956): 287–319.

5. Henry Ford, *The Case against the Little White Slaver* (Detroit: H. Ford, 1916), pp. 18–19. For Lorillard: "Arsenic in Plain Havana Blossom," May 7, 1932, Bates 04358853–8858. R. E. Remington was one of the first to draw attention to the presence of arsenic in tobacco (up to 30 ppm in pipe and chewing tobacco); see his "A Hitherto Unsuspected Source of Arsenic in Human Environment," *Journal of the American Chemical Society* 49 (1927): 1410–15; compare C. R. Gross and O. A. Nelson, "Arsenic in Tobacco Smoke," *American Journal of Public Health* 24 (1934): 36–42.

6. "Lead and Arsenic Poisoning from Tobacco," *Consumers Research Bulletin,* Feb. 1936, pp. 4–5, Bates 80690949–0951; "Lead Foil Use Banned on Cigarette Packs," April 7, 1942, Bates 950229584.

7. J. H. Weber, "Arsenic in Cigarettes," Oct. 9, 1956, Bates HK0551017–1020. William E. Smith of NYU entertained the arsenic idea; Smith spoke with American Tobacco President Paul Hahn about this in the spring of 1950, and Hanmer sent Smith some of his data, which indicated .19 mg of arsenic in the mainstream smoke per hundred cigarettes. Hanmer justified this by noting that the Federal Security Agency in 1940 had raised its permissible levels of arsenic in food to 1.625 mg/pound. Assuming .19 mg/100 cigarettes you would have to smoke 850 cigarettes to inhale the same quantity of arsenic allowed in a pound of food. Hanmer produced this bizarre justification in a letter to Smith of June 2, 1950, Bates MNAT00587093–7094.

8. For an overview from the tobacco man's point of view, see Davis and Nielsen's *Tobacco,* pp. 183–264; compare also Patricia A. McDaniel, Gina Solomon, and Ruth E. Malone, "The Tobacco Industry and Pesticide Regulations," *Environmental Health Perspectives* 113 (2005): 1659–65.

9. Davis and Nielsen, *Tobacco,* p. 241.

10. Philip Morris Europe, "Quarterly Report," Oct.–Dec. 1987, Bates 2021606791–7000, p. 39.

11. S. R. Evelyn (BAT), "The Transfer and Pyrolysis of Maleic Hydrazide," Dec. 10, 1965, Bates 105417095–7131.

12. U.S. General Accounting Office, *Pesticides on Tobacco: Federal Activities to Assess Risks and Monitor Residues* (Washington, DC: U.S. GAO, 2003); Rachel Carson, *Silent Spring* (Boston: Houghton Mifflin, 1962), pp. 58–59.

13. See "Kabat Tobacco Protector: International Status Report," April 26, 1991, Bates 2024113486–3488.

14. George Lindahl to Bob McCuen, April 8, 1992, Bates 2024113495–3497, which contains a proposal that the tobacco companies "lobby Brussels to exclude tobacco from the requirement for MRL's [Maximum Residue Levels]."

15. A BAT "Glossary of Code Names and Trade Names" from 1955, listing also suppliers and prices, can be found at Bates 104508972–9067; recipes from 1944 can be found at Bates 102640297–0494; and other code translations can be found at Bates 100666548–6640 and 104682812–3252. Bates 100645335–5357 gives first known date of use for many BAT ingredients.

16. For bitter: "Chemical and Sensory Aspects of Tobacco Flavor," Bates 523400800–0850, pp. 170–71. For fecal: Bates 507054616–4620 and 2505475760.

17. D. M. Frank and T. F. Riehl, "Cigarettes with Recognizable Flavors: A Review," May 10, 1972, Bates 621618728–8737.

18. M. D. Rosenberg to T. S. Osdene, July 27, 1978, Bates 1000761824.

19. "Flavoring Roundup: A Pinch of This, a Touch of That," *Tobacco Reporter*, Sept. 1979, Bates TIMN0221652–1656.

20. K. N. Walker (Brown & Williamson), "Analysis of the Top Flavorings on Kent Deluxe 100's," July 26, 1990, Bates 583209556–9560.

21. "Additive Code Analogues," n.d., Bates 1326.01.

22. Brown & Williamson, "Pesticides and Potentially Hazardous Additives."

23. Marvin K. Cook (MacAndrews & Forbes), "The Use of Licorice and Other Flavoring Material in Tobacco," April 10, 1975, Bates 4480111–0124.

24. Covington & Burling, "Sorted by Ingredient," Feb. 24, 1992, Bates 566602856–2891.

25. For Reynolds: E. H. Harwood, "Tonka Beans—Coumarin," Oct. 13, 1930, Bates 502322068. For Georgia swamps: Jim Mintz, "Low Tar, High Risk," *Mother Jones*, Feb.–March 1983, pp. 54–56, Bates 4429831–9833; also Ken Cummins, "Additive Adds Mystery to Risk of Smoking," (Jacksonville, FL) *Times Union*, Jan. 12, 1983, Bates 4436328–6334; and Bates 4644242–4269. For Now and Carlton: Alan F. Rodgman to Sam B. Witt, "Coumarin," Sept. 29, 1981, Bates 500540923–0926.

26. For preemptive research: George Cooper to Hugo Cunliffe-Owen, April 29, 1935, Bates 680144480. For Yale: Batten, Barton, Durstine and Osborn (for Brown & Williamson), "Notes from the Haggard-Henderson Report," May 23, 1935, Bates 680144479.

27. For "mildly carcinogenic" and "direct allegation": BAT, "Additives Guidance Panel," Jan. 25, 1967, Bates 500012793–2796.

28. For "good starter products": D. V. Cantrell to I. D. Macdonald, Feb. 17, 1987, Bates 621079918–9921. For "poison go down easier": Phillip Gardiner and Pamela I. Clark, "Menthol Cigarettes: Moving toward a Broader Definition of Harm," *Nicotine and Tobacco Research* 12 (2010): S85–S93.

29. For Robinson: Stephanie Saul, "Black Group Turns Away from Bill on Smoking," *New York Times,* May 30, 2008.

30. Tobacco Products Scientific Advisory Committee, FDA, *Menthol Cigarettes and Public Health,* March 23, 2011, http://www.fda.gov/downloads/Advisory Committees/Com mitteesMeetingMaterials/TobaccoProductsScientificAdvisoryCommittee/UCM247689.pdf.

31. Brown & Williamson, "Justification and Framework of an R&D Program," May 14, 1985, Bates 512001187–1197.

32. John A. Brown of Thiele-Engdahl on Feb. 13, 1987, wrote to Mike Collins of Ecusta: "Our suppliers certify, all of the talcs used in our products, are free of detectable amounts of asbestos or other fibrous asbestiform minerals" (Bates 506522602, from Reynolds's files).

33. G. A. Reid, "BTC Status Review Notes," July 28, 1993, Bates 400448808–8826.

34. Jerry E. Bishop, "Safer Smokes? Researchers Step up Broad Drive to Develop Less Harmful Cigarets: Cabbage Cigarets Still Smell," *Wall Street Journal,* March, 9, 1964, Bates 01194377, reporting on the work of Fred G. Bock and his colleagues.

35. For cocoa cigars: D. A. Cuenot, "Les succédanés du Tabac," *Journal d'Agriculture tropicale* 14 (1967): 191–252, translated as "The Substitutes for Tobacco," Bates 502525374–5447. For Cytrel: P. N. Gauvin to F. E. Resnik, "Status of Project Abstract," Aug. 16, 1971, Bates 10007 19190; also Philip Morris's "Reference Book on Nontobacco Smoking Materials," March 21, 1975, Bates 1003057028–7061. For a list of dozens of tobacco substitutes, organic and inorganic, along with a chronology of reconstituted tobacco, see M. A. Manzelli to P. A. Eichorn, "Identification of Reconstituted Tobacco," March 9, 1971, Bates 1000017833–7847.

36. Taylor, *Smoke Ring,* pp. 95–96.

37. Sydney J. Green, "C.A.C. II—Salamander: S & H Item 1. Developments in Scientific Field 1976/77," April 18, 1977, Bates 110069825–9829; compare W. King, R. Borland, and M. Christie, "Way-out Developments at BATCO," *Tobacco Control* 12 (2003): 107–8.

38. For YOMARON: BAT, "This seems to 'clear' Yomaron," 1960, Bates 100197794. For "more desirable additives": BAT, "Additives Guidance Panel," Jan. 25, 1967, Bates 500012793–2796.

39. BAT, "Additives Guidance Panel," Jan. 25, 1967, Bates 500012793–2796, p. 3.

40. "We used only additives that were approved by the FDA as food additives" (Murray Senkus, deposition in *Richardson v. Philip Morris,* Oct. 12–13, 1998, Bates 519199093–9773).

CHAPTER 26

1. The best history of radioactivity in cigarette smoke is Brianna Rego, "The Polonium Brief: A History of Cancer, Radiation, and the Tobacco Industry," *Isis* 101 (2009): 453–84.

2. D. K. Mulvany, "Lung Cancer and Smoking," *Lancet* 2 (1953): 205–6; also his "Radioactivity of Tobacco and Lung Cancer," *Lancet* 1 (1954): 980; Richard Doll, "Etiology of Lung Cancer," in *Advances in Cancer Research,* vol. 3, ed. J. P. Greenstein and A. Haddow (New York: Academic, 1955), p. 26. V. C. Runeckles's letter appeared in *Nature* 191 (1961): 322; compare his more detailed report for Imperial Tobacco: "Natural Radioactivity in Tobacco and Tobacco Smoke," Nov. 21, 1960, Bates 402402263–2277; also F. W. Spiers and R. D. Passey, "Radioactivity of Tobacco and Lung Cancer," *Lancet* 2 (1953): 1259–60. For "Physical Properties": Tobacco Manufacturers' Standing Committee, "Library Classification and Subject

Index," Dec. 1959, Bates 105386404–6480, p. 27. For lighter flints: Robert B. Rice to Reynolds, Jan. 11, 1959, Bates 502393229–3230; W. T. Hoyt to Robert B. Rice, Jan. 16, 1959, Bates 502393226.

3. Edward P. Radford and Vilma R. Hunt, "Polonium 210: A Volatile Radioelement in Cigarettes," *Science* 143 (1964): 247–49.

4. "Polonium Threat a 'Scare Tactic,' According to Tobacco Industry" (Tucson) *Star,* Aug. 22, 1982; compare "Cancer Link Is Probed in 'Radioactive' Smoke" (Lexington, KY) *Herald,* April 11, 1975. Tobacco makers compiled bibliographies on polonium; see the 976-page "Personal Copy of Dr. Alan Rodgman," ca. 1974, Bates 510992591–3561 at 3335.

5. See, for example, Freddy Homburger to H. B. Parmele (for Lorillard), April 6, 1964, Bates 80004655–4656; Rego, "Polonium Brief," pp. 459–60.

6. T. C. Tso, Naomi Harley, and L. T. Alexander, "Source of Lead-210 and Polonium-210 in Tobacco," *Science* 153 (1966): 880–82; T. C. Tso, N. A. Hallden, and L. T. Alexander, "Radium-226 and Polonium-210 in Leaf Tobacco and Tobacco Soil," *Science* 146 (1964): 1043–45; L. P. Gregory, "Polonium-210 in Leaf Tobacco from Four Countries," *Science* 150 (1965): 74–76.

7. J. Marmorstein, "Lung Cancer: Is the Increasing Incidence Due to Radioactive Polonium in Cigarettes?" *Southern Medical Journal* 79 (1986): 145–50.

8. G. Segura to A. Bavley, "Polonium in Tobacco and Smoke," Oct. 27, 1964, Bates 1001896688–6689.

9. Robert C. Hockett to CTR committee, Aug. 29, 1967, Bates BBAT021859–1862.

10. Edward Martell, "Radioactivity of Tobacco Trichomes and Insoluble Cigarette Smoke Particles," *Nature* 249 (1974): 215–17.

11. For washing: R. W. Jenkins (Philip Morris), "Nuclear and Radiochemistry of Smoke," June 7, 1977, Bates 1001925327–5328. For "Three Mile Marlboro": J. L. Charles to R. B. Seligman, Nov. 14, 1980, Bates 1000016574–6576. *Mother Jones* used this "Three Mile Marlboro" expression in a December 1980 exposé of radioactivity in smoke.

12. R. D. Carpenter to H. Wakeham and R. B. Seligman, "Polonium in Tobacco," Dec. 16, 1965, Bates 1001881339.

13. T. S. Osdene to R. B. Seligman, "Quarterly Report—Research," Sept. 26, 1980, Bates 1000085865–5867.

14. Charles W. Nystrom to Alan Rodgman, "Comments on the Stauffer Patent," March 5, 1982, Bates 504970288. For "proper disposal": R. W. Jenkins to Tom Goodale, March 15, 1985, Bates 2012615307–5308. For "appeared and disappeared": Alan Rodgman to Roy E. Morse, "Stauffer Patent," March 8, 1982, Bates 501522602.

15. Arthur J. Flynn, "Senior Field Manager's Report," Feb. 1982, Bates 670915637.

16. Miriam G. Adams to Alan Rodgman, "Consumer Inquiry," April 4, 1985, Bates 504974165–4167.

17. Paul A. Eichorn to Robert B. Seligman, June 2, 1978, Bates 1003725613; Rego, "Polonium Brief," p. 476. The suppressed paper in question, by Robert W. Jenkins et al., titled "Naturally Occurring ^{222}Radon Daughters in Tobacco and Smoke Condensate," can be found at Bates 1003725619–5644.

18. Monique E. Muggli, Jon O. Ebbert, Channing Robertson, and Richard D. Hurt, "Waking a Sleeping Giant: The Tobacco Industry's Response to the Polonium-210 Issue," *Ameri-*

can *Journal of Public Health* 98 (2008): 1– 8; and for my opinion piece: "Puffing on Polonium," *New York Times,* Dec. 1, 2006.

CHAPTER 27

1. See "Cigarette Butts Toxic to Marine Life," May 1, 2009, http://newscenter.sdsu.edu/sdsu_newscenter/news.aspx?s = 71209.

2. "Sydney to Butt out Smoking Litterbugs," *RJRI News Report,* June 10, 1996, Bates 531456669–6681.

3. Kelly D. Brownell and Thomas R. Frieden, "Ounces of Prevention—The Public Policy Case for Taxes on Sugared Beverages," *New England Journal of Medicine* 360 (2009): 1805–8.

4. Novotny et al., "Cigarettes Butts and the Case for an Environmental Policy."

5. W. M. Abbitt, a U.S. congressman from Virginia, cited this passage in his statement presented to the congressional *Hearings on Cigarette Labeling and Advertising,* April 15, 1969, Bates TI19842450–0288, p. 61. The original is from an article by Frank B. Snodgrass in the *United States Tobacco Journal,* Dec. 26, 1968.

6. Two of the plagiarists were U.S. congressmen from North Carolina: Walter B. Jones ("Tobacco's Positive Contributions," *Tarheel Wheels,* Aug. 1970, Bates TI08881881) and Wilmer D. Mizell (Statement to the House Committee on Interstate and Foreign Commerce, April 15, 1969, Bates TI19842450–0288, p. 43). Very similar passages appear in a statement presented by Fred S. Royster before this same House Committee (TI19842450–0288, p. 657) and in a speech by Tobacco Institute Vice President Edward F. Ragland from January 13, 1970 (Bates TIMN0122731–2742). The facts in question also appear in Hill & Knowlton's "Some Facts about Tobacco," Dec. 1968, Bates 1005038509–8512.

7. These numbers are derived from data from the Bureau of Economic Standards and the EIOLCA website: http://www.eiolca.net/cgi-bin/dft/use.pl, with thanks to Christopher Weber.

8. Jeanette W. Chung and David O. Meltzer, "Estimate of the Carbon Footprint of the US Health Care Sector," *JAMA* 302 (2009): 1970–72.

9. Helmut J. Geist, "Global Assessment of Deforestation Related to Tobacco Farming," *Tobacco Control* 8 (1999): 18–28.

10. For 5.3 million hectares: Michele Barry, "The Influence of the U.S. Tobacco Industry on the Health, Economy and Environment of Developing Countries," *New England Journal of Medicine* 324 (1991): 917–20. For the Ilyushin-18: *Sunday Telegraph,* Feb. 27, 1983.

11. John R. Hall, *Fire in the U.S. and Canada* (Quincy, MA: National Fire Protection Association, 2005), http://www.nfpa.org/assets/files/PDF/osuscanada.pdf.

CHAPTER 28

1. Yeaman, "Implications of Battelle Hippo," p. 4.

2. For "appropriate levels" (referencing Gio Gori), see Murray Senkus to J. F. Hind, "Update on the Smoking and Health Issue and Smoking Satisfaction," Nov. 17, 1977, Bates 5018 77091–7108. For representations in court, see the opening statement of Stephanie Parker,

Esq., in *Sherman v. Reynolds*, April 22, 2009, plus the occasional testimony of David Townsend, James Figlar, or Peter Lipowitz.

3. "A Report on Little Cigars," *Consumer Reports*, Oct. 1959, p. 512, Bates 03357555–7560.

4. Jones Day, "Corporate Activity Project," pp. 218–22. Reynolds had also experimented with a palladium cigarette, with the metal incorporated into the filter rather than the tobacco. Page 244 of this document reveals, "We know (although plaintiffs do not at this point) of Reynolds' aborted work with a palladium cigarette of its own." Kluger has a good account of Liggett's palladium misadventure in his *Ashes to Ashes*, pp. 455–61.

5. Carter's remarks were made at the Wilson tobacco market in North Carolina on Aug. 4, 1978; see "MacNeil/Lehrer Report," Aug. 17, 1978, Bates 511287193. For 200,000 ounces: J. Bowen Ross to Jack Africk, "Brief Summary of Project XA," Jan. 16, 1979, Bates 528810268–0271. For Mold and legal fears: Jones Day, "Corporate Activity Project," pp. 30–31, 232. A history of Liggett's effort to identify and eliminate carcinogens from tobacco smoke can be found in J. H. Greer to Charles J. Kensler, Jan. 9, 1979, Bates LG0147750–7757.

6. James D. Mold was the first former industry scientist to testify on behalf of plaintiffs in tobacco litigation. His testimony is refreshingly honest, admitting, for example, that Wynder's skin-painting studies "more or less confirmed the epidemiologic studies . . . studies that had already taken place in humans, if you will, with the conventional cigarettes." Mold had concluded that cigarettes were causing cancer prior even to the 1964 Surgeon General's report but also expressed his view that corporate management "didn't want to believe this, professed not to believe it"; see Jones Day, "Corporate Activity Project," pp. 232–47; and for "clobber," see Mold's deposition testimony for *Cipollone v. Liggett*, Jan. 11, 1988, Bates MOLDJo11188, p. 83.

7. "Liggett Responds to Press Report on New Tobacco Research," *LiggettGram*, Sept. 26, 1978, Bates LG0165916. This press release was widely reported; see Bates LG0165917–5923 and LG0203357. For "first cigarette maker" and "wrong substance": Jones Day, "Corporate Activity Project," pp. 238–39.

8. The query was from Marc Edell, cross-examining Liggett President K. V. Dey for *Cipollone* (1988), Bates 968272665–2792, p. 2301; compare Jones Day, "Corporate Activity Project," p. 242.

9. R. D. Latshaw (Philip Morris) to file, "Merrell Dow Pharmaceutical Meeting," July 21, 1982, Bates 2023799798; T. S. Osdene (Philip Morris) to W. W. McDowell, "Merrell Dow Smoking Cessation Newsletter," Jan. 4, 1982, Bates 2021539712.

10. R. D. Latshaw to A. J. Kay, "Suspension of Dow Purchases," May 7, 1984, Bates 20237 99799–9800; R. D. Latshaw, "Dow-Nicorette Meeting," Oct. 25, 1984, Bates 2023799801–9802.

11. R. D. Latshaw to A. J. Kay, "Dow-Nicorette Situation," Sept. 6, 1985, Bates 20237 99796–9797; R. D. Latshaw to File, "January 18 Conference Call," Jan. 22, 1985, Bates 20237 99803.

12. Frank Cotignola (Philip Morris) to Distribution, "Nicotine Patch Industry Volume Analysis," April 27, 1992, Bates 2040573092–3093; Richard Barth (CIBA-Geigy), "Groundrules," Feb. 24, 1992, Bates 2056525521; L. Sykes to Distribution, March 13, 1992, Bates 2056 525519.

13. "Cigarettes," *Consumer Reports*, Jan. 1960, pp. 15–18, Bates 03357518–7525; Bhavna

Shamasunder and Lisa Bero, "Financial Ties and Conflicts of Interest between Pharmaceutical and Tobacco Companies," *JAMA* 288 (2002): 738–44.

14. Furniture makers actually petitioned the CPSC to require cigarette makers to make fire-safe cigarettes prior to forcing furniture makers to make fire-safe upholstery. The CPSC refused, claiming lack of jurisdiction.

15. Sekap in Greece in 1997 introduced a cigarette with a hemoglobin "Biofilter" that "can be regarded as an artificial lung"; see Chris Glass, "A 'SAFER' Cigarette? Controversial Filter Appears on Cigarettes in Greece," *Tobacco Reporter*, Feb. 1998, Bates 522877797–7801.

16. Direct Testimony of David E. Townsend for *Karbiwnyk v. Reynolds*, Oct. 21, 1997, Bates 518834338–4355, pp. 2914–21, 2943. Townsend here claimed that the scientific community "doesn't walk in long steps, it never does," meaning that interests shift and researchers move on to new topics. This is perhaps more typical of science in a corrupted, lawyerly, context. Genuine science does in fact walk in long steps; there is an effort to integrate small work with deeper traditions and the larger edifice of scientific truth-making. The industry's scientists, by contrast, were very much traveling firemen, putting out local fires and only rarely building up long-standing evidentiary traditions, especially when it came to smoking and health. Professional skeptics and corruptionists, one might say.

17. For "very elegant": "Scientific Affairs," May 1985, Bates 506890621–0653. For "very industrial": Mike Dixon (BAT) to Graham Read, "Flavour Profiling—Eclipse v. Premier," June 6, 1996, Bates 623800148–0155. For "grave": Bates 2060533075–3076.

18. For crack pipe: E. Cone and J. Henningfield, "Premier 'Smokeless Cigarettes' Can Be Used to Deliver Crack," *JAMA* 261 (1989): 41. For "spoon": Reynolds, "Possible 'Must Airs' on Crack Issues," Dec. 15, 1988, Bates 515788076–8078, with thanks to William White for alerting me to this document. For "efficient system": Mario Perez-Reyes to Sam Simmons, Jan. 31, 1989, Bates 511477676–7677. For crack "puffing" baboons: Perez-Reyes to Simmons, March 2, 1989, Bates 511477538–7539. For baboon compensation: Walter R. Rogers, "First Draft Report on Pilot Experiment on Crack Puffing by Baboons via Premier," Feb. 9, 1989, Bates 515787997–8001.

19. W. L. Dunn, "On the Smoking Baboons in Texas," April 15, 1976, Bates 1005127701–7704.

20. For "will be painful": Frank J. Ryan to W. L. Dunn, "Proposed Research Project: Smoking and Anxiety," Dec. 23, 1969, Bates 1003287893–7897; compare Frank Ryan, "Shock I, II, III, and IV," and "Shock V," in "Consumer Psychology," Oct. 16, 1971, and Feb. 15, 1972, Bates 1003288445 and 1003288443. For "fear of shock": W. L. Dunn to P. A. Eichorn, "Quarterly Report—Projects 1600 and 2102," Oct. 5, 1972, Bates 2046516231–6233. Ryan by September 1971 was using "a loud noise in place of [electric] shock as a threat to students" given the "increasing difficulty" of finding human subjects (Bates 2022147792–7794). Compare also Patricia A. McDaniel, Gina Solomon, and Ruth E. Malone, "The Ethics of Industry Experimentation Using Employees: The Case of Taste-Testing Pesticide-Treated Tobacco," *American Journal of Public Health* 96 (2007): 37–46.

21. Arnold M. Katz to Frank E. Young, Nov. 1, 1988, Bates 506920864.

22. "Project Advance," 1984, Bates 2020045324–5325; "Alternative Smoking Devices and New Products," n.d., Bates 2079071197–1211; Gauvin to Meyer, June 1, 1984, Bates 1002801162–1163.

23. Glenn Collins, "A Cigarette Holder Burns One Puff at a Time," *New York Times,* Oct. 23, 1997, Bates 138011392–1393.

24. http://revver.com/video/587560/vapir-one-vaporizer/.

25. Robert N. DuPuis, acting as Special Technical Consultant for the Consolidated Cigar Corporation, in 1973 defended cigars as "a less hazardous form of smoking than cigarettes, whose principal ingredient is flue-cured tobacco." DuPuis went on to say that cigars were less hazardous given that (1) "The fermentation process destroys most of the sugar in the tobacco"; and (2) "The smoke from fermented cigar tobacco is neutral to alkaline, whereas the smoke from the popular American cigarettes is acidic." Crucial for smokers of Dutch Treat cigars was that smoke from such cigars was "unpleasant to inhale" and therefore "not inhaled to the same extent as American cigarette smoke." See his "Statement" before the Committee on Interstate and Foreign Commerce, U.S. House of Representatives, May 22, 1973, Bates 1000244835–4840.

26. For "if they get cigarettes": Philip Morris Corporate Affairs, "Talking Points—FET Week Participants," Aug. 1994, Bates 2048619009–9013. For rally at the Capitol: Chris Donohue to Beat FET Week Task Force, Feb. 2, 1994, Bates 2062341171–1173. For Oscar Mayer: Joan Cryan and John C. Lenzi to Robert A. Eckert (Oscar Mayer), April 8, 1994, Bates 2078845705.

27. One Philip Morris study found users of PM snus averaging only 4 nanograms per milliliter of nicotine in their blood, compared to 18 ng/ml for smokers. Users of Swedish snus, by contrast, achieved blood nicotine levels of about 15 ng/ml—more like that of smokers. See Jonathan Foulds and Helena Furberg, "Is Low-Nicotine Marlboro Snus Really Snus?" *Harm Reduction Journal* 5 (2008): 9.

28. The European Union banned the sale of snus in 1992, though an exception was made for Sweden when it entered the Union (in 1995) in a tilt to its long-standing use in Scandinavia. Hong Kong, Ireland, New Zealand, and Israel had all banned smokeless tobacco products by 1987, and Australia followed suit in 1991.

29. Gregory N. Connolly et al., "Unintentional Child Poisonings through Ingestion of Conventional and Novel Tobacco Products," *Pediatrics* 125 (2010): 896–99; Duff Wilson, "Flavored Tobacco Pellets Are Denounced as a Lure to Young Users," *New York Times,* April 19, 2010.

CHAPTER 29

1. Zeman's claim was based on research conducted by the Czech arm of Philip Morris, which in 2000 hired Arthur D. Little to calculate the money saved for the Czech state by premature deaths from tobacco. The report concluded that the 21.5 billion koruna saved by early deaths outweighed the 15.6 billion koruna lost from medical bills, absenteeism, and lost income taxes (not paid because the smokers were dead). Zeman in a March 2001 trip to India commented that since heavy smokers die young, "it is not necessary to pay them pensions." See Kate Swoger, "Report Says Smoking Has Benefits," *Prague Post,* June 27, 2001.

2. Rene Scull, Vice President, Philip Morris Asia, "The Tobacco Industry in the Asia/Pacific Region up to the Year 2000," Dec. 1985, Bates 2044448375–8401, p. 22.

3. Elizabeth Davies, "Bollywood Fumes at Smoking Ban," *Independent,* June 2, 2005. For

the WHO report, see http://www.youtube.com/watch?v = s1rFQfIOnhA. For the older history of tobacco in India, see Cox, *Global Cigarette,* pp. 202–37.

4. K. Srinath Reddy and Prakash C. Gupta, eds., *Report on Tobacco Control in India* (New Delhi: Ministry of Health, 2004), http://www.mohfw.nic.in/Tobacco%20control%20in%20 India_(10%20Dec%2004)_PDF.pdf.

5. Jha et al., with Peto, "A Nationally Representative Case-Control Study of Smoking and Death in India."

6. Riyadi Suparno, "RMI Expands into Tobacco Industry," *Jakarta Post,* Dec. 15, 2009.

7. http://www.gallup.com/poll/28432/smoking-rates-around-world-how-americans-compare.aspx; Omar Shafey, Michael Eriksen, Hana Ross, and Judith Mackay, *Tobacco Atlas,* 3d ed. (Atlanta: ACS, 2009).

8. Britain's Tobacco Manufacturers Association (TMA) has undergone several name changes since its establishment as the Tobacco Manufacturers Standing Committee in 1956: the name was changed to Tobacco Research Council in 1963 and then to Tobacco Advisory Council in 1978. The present name was adopted in 1994.

9. For "unanimous agreement": Philip Morris, "Smoking: Social Unacceptability Issue," June 1976, Bates 2025025481–5494. For "open to debate": W. D. & H. O. Wills (Australia), "A Review of and Recommendations on Passive Smoking and Social Acceptability of Smoking," July 1976, Bates 2025025461–5480.

10. For "unite with common targets": "ICOSI: International Committee on Smoking Issues," April 1979, Bates 1003717317–7330. For "legal position": Peter M. Wilson (Gallaher) to Principal Board Members of INFOTAB and CECCM, "Legal Clearance of Documents," Jan. 14, 1991, Bates 2023237649–7650; also Kessler's "Amended Final Opinion," pp. 172–209.

11. For "domino effect": R. A. Garrett to Hugh Cullman, Dec. 3, 1976, Bates 2025025290–5291; Hugh Cullman to Files, Dec. 3, 1976, Bates 2025025286; also Bates 2025025347–5348 and 2025025347–5348. For speaking "with one voice": "Position Paper," April 28, 1977, Bates 2501024572–4575. For "Smoker Reassurance": "Operation Berkshire," April 15, 1977, Bates 2501024570. Much of this collaboration was first exposed by Neil Francey and Simon Chapman in "'Operation Berkshire': The International Tobacco Companies' Conspiracy," *British Medical Journal* 321 (2000): 371–74.

12. For "discreetly": "Working Party on the Social Acceptability of Smoking Issue," late June 1977, Bates 2025025295–5300. For "defensive research": BATCo's files from a March 1978 meeting in Australia, Bates 321588692–8692. For "considerable ability to delay": W. D. & H. O. Wills, "Review of and Recommendations on Passive Smoking." And for background: Patricia A. McDaniel, Gina Intinarelli, and Ruth E. Malone, "Tobacco Industry Issues Management Organizations: Creating a Global Corporate Network to Undermine Public Health," *Global Health* 4 (2008): 2.

13. For "Resist and roll back": "Proposal for the Organisation of the Whitecoat Project," Feb. 22, 1988, Bates 2501474262–4265. For the Latin Project: Ernesto M. Sebrie et al., "Tobacco Industry Dominating National Tobacco Policy Making in Argentina, 1966–2005," Center for Tobacco Control Research and Education, http://repositories.cdlib.org/cgi/view content.cgi?article = 1051&context = ctcre.

14. Brandt, *Cigarette Century,* pp. 458–68. William Ecenbarger describes how Senator Jesse Helms in the mid-1980s used the Office of the U.S. Trade Representative to open up

Asian tobacco markets; see his "America's New Merchants of Death," *Readers Digest,* April 1993, pp. 50–57.

15. Speech by Judith McKay, 1987, Bates 980170160–0167.

CHAPTER 30

1. Joanna E. Cohen et al., "Political Ideology and Tobacco Control," *Tobacco Control* 9 (2000): 263–67.

2. Geoffrey Fong et al., "The Near-Universal Experience of Regret among Smokers in Four Countries," *Nicotine and Tobacco Research* 6 (2004): S341–51.

3. A 2010 Google search of "laws prohibiting" turned up, in order (eliminating duplicates), prohibitions of the following: on-the-job discrimination, sexual abuse, tobacco sales to minors, phone use while driving, discrimination against people with disabilities, smoking in stand-alone bars, firearms, Internet purchase of California wines, false medical claims, smoking in private worksites, sex discrimination, criticism of agricultural products, piranhas, discrimination based on criminal conviction, discrimination against gays, racial discrimination, driving while stoned, marriage based on genetics, sale of alcohol to minors, assisted suicide, and so forth.

4. R. Rosell et al., "The Eel Fishery in Lough Neagh, Northern Ireland—An Example of Sustainable Management?" *Fisheries Management and Ecology* 12 (2005): 377–85.

SELECTED BIBLIOGRAPHY

Action on Smoking and Health. *Tobacco Explained: The Truth about the Tobacco Industry . . . in Its Own Words.* London: ASH, 1998.

Adler, Isaac. *Primary Malignant Growths of the Lungs and Bronchi: A Pathological and Clinical Study.* London: Longmans, Green, 1912.

Air Resources Board, State of California. "Proposed Identification of Environmental Tobacco Smoke as a Toxic Air Contaminant." June 24, 2005. http://www.arb.ca.gov/regact/ets2006/ets2006.htm.

Altizer, Charles B., et al. (Philip Morris). "Ventilation Seminar." May 1983. Bates 2057251669–1968.

American Tobacco Co., Research Laboratory. "Memorandum on A. Alleged Effects of Smoking B. Improvement of Cigarette Tobaccos with Special Reference to Irritation." Jan. 4, 1943. Bates 950291224–1339.

Auerbach, Oscar, et al. "Changes in the Bronchial Epithelium in Relation to Smoking and Cancer of the Lung." *New England Journal of Medicine* 256 (1957): 97–104.

Backhurst, J. D. (BAT). "A Relation between the 'Strength' of a Cigarette and the 'Extractable Nicotine' in the Smoke." Nov. 16, 1965. Bates 508102918–2941.

Barnes, Deborah E., and Lisa A. Bero. "Why Review Articles on the Health Effects of Passive Smoking Reach Different Conclusions." *JAMA* 279 (1998): 1566–70.

BATCo. "Report on Visit to U.S.A., May 1973." 1973. Bates 100226995–7033.

Benowitz, Neal L., and Jack E. Henningfield. "Establishing a Nicotine Threshold for Addiction: The Implications for Tobacco Regulation." *New England Journal of Medicine* 331 (1994): 123–25.

Benowitz, Neal L., et al. "Smokers of Low-Yield Cigarettes Do Not Consume Less Nicotine." *New England Journal of Medicine* 309 (1983): 139–42.

Bentley, Herbert R., D. G. I. Felton, and W. W. Reid. "Report on Visit to U.S.A. and Canada, 17th April—12th May 1958" (for BAT). June 11, 1958. Bates TIOK 0034790–4799.

Berger, Peter L. "Gilgamesh on the Washington Shuttle." *Worldview*, Nov. 1977, 43–45.

Black, R., et al. "B&W Product Knowledge Seminar Spring 1990." 1990. Bates 505304459–4647.

Blum, Alan. "Candy Cigarettes." *New England Journal of Medicine* 302 (1980): 972.

———, ed. *The Cigarette Underworld*. Secaucus: Lyle Stuart, 1985.

———. Tobacco Industry Sponsorship of Sports: A Growing Dependency." Paper presented to the Surgeon General and Interagency Committee on Smoking and Health. Oct. 27, 1988. Bates 980171240–1336.

———. "Tobacco in Sport: An Endless Addiction?" *Tobacco Control* 14 (2005): 1–2.

Bradford, J. A., W. R. Harlan, and H. R. Hanmer. "Nature of Cigaret Smoke: Technic of Experimental Smoking." *Industrial and Engineering Chemistry* 28 (1936): 836–39.

Brady, J. Morrison, to Clarence Cook Little. "TIRC Program." April 9, 1962. Bates 92520643–0644.

Brandt, Allan M. "The Cigarette, Risk, and American Culture." *Daedalus* (Fall 1990): 155–76.

———. *The Cigarette Century: The Rise, Fall, and Deadly Persistence of the Product That Defined America*. New York: Basic Books, 2007.

Brave, Ralph. "Smoked Out! The Hidden History of UC Davis' 35-Year Collaboration with Big Tobacco." *Sacramento News and Review*, June 21, 2007.

Brooks, Jerome E. *The Mighty Leaf: Tobacco through the Centuries*. Boston: Little, Brown, 1952.

———. *Tobacco: Its History Illustrated by the Books & Manuscripts in the Library of George Arents*. 5 vols. (1937–52). Reprint. Mansfield Centre: Maurizio Martino & Krown & Spellman, 1999.

Brosch, Anton. "Theoretische und experimentelle Untersuchungen zur Pathogenesis und Histogenesis der malignen Geschwülste." *Virchows Archiv für pathologische Anatomie und Physiologie* 162 (1900): 32–84.

Brown, Janet C. (Chadbourne & Parke). "Research Liaison Committee." Nov. 19, 1977. Bates USX4981730–1769.

Brown & Williamson. "Pesticides and Potentially Hazardous Additives." April 1996. Bates 1327.01.

———. *Root Technology: A Handbook for Leaf Blenders and Product Developers*. Jan. 1991. Bates 682435026–9803.

Browne, Colin L. *The Design of Cigarettes*. Charlotte: Celanese Fibers Marketing Co., 1981.

Burns, David M., Jacqueline M. Major, Thomas G. Shanks, Michael J. Thun, and Jonathan M. Samet. "Smoking Lower Yield Cigarettes and Disease Risks." In the NCI's *Risks Associated with Smoking Cigarettes with Low Machine-Measured Yields of Tar and Nicotine. Smoking and Tobacco Control—Monograph 13*, 65–158. Bethesda, MD: USDHHS, 2001.

Burrough, Bryan, and John Helyar. *Barbarians at the Gate: The Fall of RJR Nabisco*. New York: Harper and Row, 1990.

Callard, Cynthia, Dave Thompson, and Neil Collishaw, *Curing the Addiction to Profits: A Supply-Side Approach to Phasing Out Tobacco*. Ottawa: Canadian Centre for Policy Alternatives, 2005.

Carroll, William W., and H. J. Rand. "A Fluorospectrographic Indication of Carcinogens in Cigarette Papers." March 17, 1952. Bates 950166333–6336.

Chapman, Simon. *Public Health Advocacy and Tobacco Control: Making Smoking History.* London: Blackwell, 2007.

Cochran, Sherman. *Big Business in China: Sino-Foreign Rivalry in the Cigarette Industry, 1890–1930.* Cambridge, MA: Harvard University Press, 1990.

Cohn, Gary. "Confusion, Paranoia Have Crippled UK Tobacco Research Institute." *Herald-Leader,* April 5, 1981. Bates 680147142–7172.

Cox, Howard. *The Global Cigarette: Origins and Evolution of British American Tobacco, 1880–1945.* Oxford: Oxford University Press, 2000.

Creuzburg, M. Richard. "Die Tabakmaschinenindustrie." *Chronica Nicotiana* 1, no. 2 (1940): 30–53.

Cummings, K. Michael, et al. "What Scientists Funded by the Tobacco Industry Believe about the Hazards of Cigarette Smoking." *American Journal of Public Health* 81 (1991): 894–96.

Cunningham, Rob. *Smoke and Mirrors: The Canadian Tobacco War.* Ottawa: International Development Research Centre, 1996.

Dakin, Edwin F. (Hill & Knowlton). "Forwarding Memorandum: To Members of the Planning Committee." Late Dec. 1953. Bates JH000493–0501.

Darkis, Frederick R. (Liggett), to W. A. Blount. Feb. 4, 1954. Bates LG0090704–0708.

Davis, D. Layten, and Mark T. Nielsen, eds. *Tobacco: Production, Chemistry and Technology.* Oxford: Blackwell, 1999.

Diehl, Harold S. *Tobacco and Your Health: The Smoking Controversy.* New York: McGraw-Hill, 1969.

Doll, Richard, and A. Bradford Hill. "Smoking and Carcinoma of the Lung. Preliminary Report." *British Medical Journal* 2 (1950): 739–48.

———. "A Study of the Aetiology of Carcinoma of the Lung." *British Medical Journal* 2 (1952): 1271–86.

———. "The Mortality of Doctors in Relation to their Smoking Habits." *British Medical Journal* 1 (1954): 1451–55.

Donner Foundation. *Index to Literature of Experimental Cancer Research 1900 to 1935.* Philadelphia: Donner Foundation, 1948.

Dunn, William L. (Philip Morris). "Motives and Incentives in Cigarette Smoking." Paper presented at CORESTA conference, Williamsburg, VA, Oct. 22–28, 1972. Bates 1003291922–1939.

———, ed. *Smoking Behavior: Motives and Incentives.* Washington, DC: Winston & Sons, 1973.

Eaves, Jean P. "Stenographic Minutes of a Conference Held at the Research Laboratory on January 21 and 22, 1952." Jan. 23, 1952. Bates lg0205897–5926.

Ecenbarger, William. "America's New Merchants of Death." *Readers Digest,* April 1993, 50–57.

Ellis, Charles (BAT). "Meeting in London with Dr. Haselbach." Nov. 15, 1961. Bates 301083862–3865.

———. "The Effects of Smoking: Proposal for Further Research Contracts with Battelle." Feb. 13, 1962. Bates 301083820–3835.

Fahs, John. *Cigarette Confidential: The Unfiltered Truth about the Ultimate Addiction.* New York: Berkley Books, 1996.

False and Misleading Advertising (Filter-Tip Cigarettes). Hearings before a Subcommittee of the Committee on Government Operations, House of Representatives, 85th Cong., July 18–26, 1957. Washington, DC: U.S. Government Printing Office, 1957. [Referenced as the *Blatnik Report.*]

Fields, Nicole, and Simon Chapman. "Chasing Ernst L. Wynder: 40 Years of Philip Morris's Efforts to Influence a Leading Scientist." *Journal of Epidemiology and Community Health* 57 (2003): 571–78.

Fischer, Paul M., et al. "Brand Logo Recognition by Children Aged 3 to 6 Years: Mickey Mouse and Old Joe the Camel." *JAMA* 266 (1991): 3145–48.

Fishel, David B. (Reynolds). "Performance Planning System." 1982. Bates 500624802–4827.

Forster, Martin, et al. "The State of Knowledge Regarding Tobacco Harm, 1920–1964: Industry and Public Health Service Perspectives." Dec. 7, 2006. http://www.tobacco.org/news/243428.html.

Freedman, Alix M. "'Impact Booster': Tobacco Firm Shows How Ammonia Spurs Delivery of Nicotine." *Wall Street Journal,* Oct. 18, 1995.

Freedman, Alix M., and Laurie P. Cohen. "Smoke and Mirrors: How Cigarette Makers Keep Health Question 'Open' Year after Year." *Wall Street Journal,* Feb. 11, 1993.

Frieden, Thomas R., and Michael R. Bloomberg. "How to Prevent 100 Million Deaths from Tobacco." *Lancet* 369 (2007): 1758–61.

Gardiner, Phillip S. "The African Americanization of Menthol Cigarette Use in the United States." *Nicotine & Tobacco Research* 6 (2004): S55–65.

Gardner, Martha N., and Allan M. Brandt. "'The Doctors' Choice Is America's Choice': The Physician in US Cigarette Advertisements, 1930–1953." *American Journal of Public Health* 96 (2006): 222–32.

Glantz, Stanton A., and Michael E. Begay. "Tobacco Industry Campaign Contributions Are Affecting Tobacco Control Policymaking in California." *JAMA* 272 (1994): 1176–82.

Glantz, Stanton A., John Slade, Lisa A. Bero, Peter Hanauer, and Deborah E. Barnes. *The Cigarette Papers.* Berkeley: University of California Press, 1996.

Goodman, Jordan. *Tobacco in History: The Cultures of Dependence.* London: Routledge, 1993.

Gori, Gio B., and F. G. Boch, eds. *A Safe Cigarette?* Cold Spring Harbor: Cold Spring Harbor Laboratory, 1983.

Green, Charles R., and Alan Rodgman (Reynolds). "The Tobacco Chemists' Research Conference: A Half Century Forum for Advances in Analytical Methodology of Tobacco and Its Products." June 6, 1996. Bates 525445600–5785.

Greenwald, Willard F. (Philip Morris), to Officers and Members of the Board of Trustees of the American Medical Association. Ca. Nov. 1950. Bates 1003080067–0080.

Grüning, Thilo, Anna B. Gilmore, and Martin McKee. "Tobacco Industry Influence on Science and Scientists in Germany." *American Journal of Public Health* 96 (2006): 20–32.

Gundle, Kenneth R., Molly J. Dingel, and Barbara A. Koenig. "'To Prove This Is the Industry's Best Hope': Big Tobacco's Support of Research on the Genetics of Nicotine Addiction," *Addiction* 105 (2010): 974–83.

Hanmer, Hiram R. (American Tobacco), to Clarence W. Lieb. March 17, 1933. Bates 950160 684–0688.

Hanmer, Hiram R., to Paul M. Hahn. "Memorandum on Alleged Causative Relation between Cigarette Smoke and Bronchiogenic Carcinoma." Sept. 15, 1950. Bates 950218815–8825.

Hanmer, Hiram R., to Preston L. Fowler. May 16, 1951. Bates MNNAT00730744–0746.

Hanmer, Hiram R., to Preston L. Fowler. Feb. 26, 1953. Bates 950164328–4333.

Hanmer, Hiram R. "Observations Concerning Individuals Participating in the Meetings" (of Nov. 5, 1953, at NYU). n.d. Bates MNAT00688881–8886.

———. "Meeting, 9 A.M., November 5, 1953, Sloan-Kettering Institute." Nov. 17, 1953. Bates 950167411–7415.

Harlow E. S., to H. R. Hanmer. "The Importance of Biological Research." Feb. 3, 1941. Bates 0060250848–0852.

Heimann, Robert K. (American Tobacco). *Tobacco and Americans*. New York: McGraw-Hill, 1960.

———. "Public Relations in the Field of Smoking and Health." Jan. 1963. Bates ATX11000 5290–5303.

Hilton, Matthew. *Smoking in British Popular Culture*. Manchester: Manchester University Press, 2000.

Hilts, Philip J. *Smokescreen: The Truth behind the Tobacco Industry Cover-Up*. Reading: Addison-Wesley, 1996.

Hirayama, Takeshi. "Non-Smoking Wives of Heavy Smokers Have a Higher Risk of Lung Cancer: A Study from Japan." *British Medical Journal* 282 (1981): 183–85.

Hirschhorn, N., Stella Aguinaga Bialous, and Stan Shatenstein. "The Philip Morris External Research Program: Results from the First Round of Projects." *Tobacco Control* 15 (2006): 267–69.

Hobbs, Marcus E. "Notes on Trip to New York University." Jan. 28, 1953. Bates 950164340–4343.

Hoffmann, Dietrich, and Ilse Hoffmann. "The Changing Cigarette: 1950–1995." *Journal of Toxicology and Environmental Health* 50 (1997): 307–64.

Hu, Teh-wei, Zhengzhong Mao, Jian Shi, and Wendong Chen. *Tobacco Taxation and Its Potential Impact in China*. Paris: International Union against Tuberculosis and Lung Disease, 2008.

Hueper, Wilhelm C. "The Cigarette Theory of Lung Cancer." *Current Medical Digest*, Oct. 1954, pp. 35–39.

Huismann, R. G. J. P. "Tabak und Lungenkrebs." *Chronica Nicotiana* 4 (May–June 1943): 7–19; 4 (July–Aug. 1943): 5–15.

Iida, Kaori, and Robert N. Proctor. "Learning from Philip Morris: Japan Tobacco's Strategies Regarding Evidence of Tobacco Health Harms as Revealed in Internal Documents from the American Tobacco Industry." *Lancet* 363 (2004): 1820–24.

Jha, Prabhat, and Frank J. Chaloupka, eds. *Tobacco Control in Developing Countries*. New York: Oxford University Press, 2000.

Jha, Prabhat, et al., with R. Peto. "A Nationally Representative Case-Control Study of Smoking and Death in India." *New England Journal of Medicine* 358 (2008): 1137–47.

Johnson, Janet L. (Arnold and Porter), to State-of-the-Art Subcommittee. "Witness Development." July 26, 1988. Bates 2048245281–5297.

Johnston, Lennox. "Tobacco Smoking and Nicotine." *Lancet* 243 (1942): 742.

———. *The Disease of Tobacco Smoking and Its Cure.* London: Christopher Johnson, 1957.

Johnston, Myron E. (Philip Morris). "Market Potential of a Health Cigarette." June 1966. Bates 1001913853–3878.

Jones, Day, Reavis & Pogue. "Management and Legal Supervision and Control of R&D Activities." Dec. 31, 1985. Bates 519198732–8819.

———. "RJR Research and Development Activities: Fact Team Memorandum." Dec. 31, 1985. Bates 515871651–1912.

———. "Total Tar and Nicotine Reduction." Dec. 31, 1985. Bates 515871937–2066.

———. "Corporate Activity Project" (for RJR). Nov. 17, 1986. Bates 681879254–9715.

———. "Dr. Claude E. Teague, Jr., Deposition Preparation." Oct. 16, 1990. Bates 515873224–3304.

Joossens, Luk, and Martin Raw. "Cigarette Smuggling in Europe, Who Really Benefits?" *Tobacco Control* 7 (1998): 66–71.

Kessler, David. *A Question of Intent: A Great American Battle with a Deadly Industry.* New York: Public Affairs, 2001.

Kessler, Gladys. "Amended Final Opinion." In *USA v. Philip Morris et al.*, Sept. 8, 2006. http://www.usdoj.gov/civil/cases/tobacco2/amended%20opinion.pdf.

King & Spalding to Brown & Williamson. "Special Trial Issues Committee (STIC)." April 7, 1992. Bates 689103258–3437.

Kirkpatrick, Miles W. "Statistical Supplement to Federal Trade Commission Report to Congress Pursuant to the Public Health Cigarette Smoking Act." Dec. 31, 1970. Bates 01152315–2329.

Klein, Jonathan D., and Steve St. Clair. "Do Candy Cigarettes Encourage Young People to Smoke?" *British Medical Journal* 321 (2000): 362–65.

Klein, Richard. *Cigarettes Are Sublime.* Durham: Duke University Press, 1995.

Kluger, Richard. *Ashes to Ashes: America's Hundred-Year Cigarette War, the Public Health, and the Unabashed Triumph of Philip Morris.* New York: Knopf, 1996.

Kornegay, Horace R. "Tobacco Institute Annual Meeting." Jan. 10, 1980. Bates TIMN 0066632–6640.

Korstad, Robert R. *Civil Rights Unionism: Tobacco Workers and the Struggle for Democracy in the Mid-Twentieth-Century South.* Chapel Hill: University of North Carolina Press, 2003.

Kozlowski, Lynn T., R. C. Frecker, V. Khouw, and M. A. Pope. "The Misuse of 'Less Hazardous' Cigarettes and Its Detection: Hole-Blocking of Ventilated Filters." *American Journal of Public Health* 70 (1980): 1202–3.

Kozlowski, Lynn T., R. J. O'Connor, G. A. Giovino, C. A. Whetzel, J. Pauly, and K. M. Cummings. "Maximum Yields Might Improve Public Health—If Filter Vents Were Banned: A Lesson from the History of Vented Filters." *Tobacco Control* 15 (2006): 262–66.

Kozlowski, Lynn T., W. S. Rickert, J. C. Robinson, and N. E. Grunberg. "Have Tar and Nicotine Yields of Cigarettes Changed?" *Science* 209 (1980): 1550–51.

Kwitny, Jonathan. "Defending the Weed: How Embattled Group Uses Tact, Calculation to Blunt Its Opposition." *Wall Street Journal,* Jan. 24, 1972. Bates 500324162–4164.

Kyriakoudes, Louis M. "The Grand Ole Opry and Big Tobacco: Radio Scripts from the Files of the R. J. Reynolds Tobacco Company, 1948 to 1959." *Southern Cultures* 12 (2006): 76–89.

———. "Historians' Testimony on 'Common Knowledge' of the Risks of Tobacco Use: A Review and Analysis of Experts Testifying on Behalf of Cigarette Manufacturers in Civil Litigation." *Tobacco Control* 15 (2006): iv107–16.

Larson, Paul S., Harvey B. Haag, and H. Silvette. *Tobacco: Experimental and Clinical Studies: A Comprehensive Account of the World Literature.* Baltimore: Williams and Wilkins, 1961.

Lauterbach, J. H., and R. R. Johnson (Brown & Williamson). "The Project Adverb Study of Marlboro KS." Oct. 10, 1989. Bates 570244005–4027.

LeGresley, Eric. "A 'Vector Analysis' of the Tobacco Epidemic." *Bulletin of Medicus Mundi Switzerland,* no. 72 (April 1999).

Levin, Morton L., et al. "Cancer and Tobacco Smoking: A Preliminary Report." *JAMA* 143 (1950): 336–38.

Levy, Carolyn. "Archetype Project Summary." Aug. 20, 1991. Bates 2062145482–5496.

Lickint, Fritz. "Tabak und Tabakrauch als ätiologischer Factor des Carcinoms." *Zeitschrift für Krebsforschung* 30 (1929): 349–65.

———. *Tabak und Organismus: Handbuch der gesamten Tabakkunde.* Stuttgart: Hippokrates, 1939.

———. *Ätiologie und Prophylaxe des Lungenkrebses.* Dresden: Steinkopff, 1953.

Lieb, Clarence W. *Safer Smoking: What Every Smoker Should Know and Do.* New York: Exposition Press, 1953.

———. *Don't Let Smoking Kill You!* New York: Bonus Books, 1957.

"Liggett Responds to Press Report on New Tobacco Research." *LiggettGram* 4, no. 30 (Sept. 26, 1978). Bates LG0165916.

Lindsay, Gordon B. *Make a Killing: A Smoking Satire on Selling Cigarettes.* Bountiful, Utah: Horizon, 1997.

Little, Clarence Cook. *Report of the Scientific Director.* New York: Tobacco Industry Research Committee, 1957.

Lombard, Herbert L., and Carl R. Doering. "Cancer Studies in Massachusetts." *New England Journal of Medicine* 198 (1928): 481–87.

Longo, William E., Mark W. Rigler, and John Slade. "Crocidolite Asbestos Fibers in Smoke from Original Kent Cigarettes." *Cancer Research* 55 (1995): 2232–35.

Lorenz, Egon, Harold L. Stewart, John H. Daniel, and Clifford V. Nelson. "The Effects of Breathing Tobacco Smoke on Strain A Mice." *Cancer Research* 3 (1943): 123–24.

Lum, Kristen L., Jonathan R. Polansky, Robert K. Jackler, and Stanton A. Glantz. "Signed, Sealed, and Delivered: Big Tobacco in Hollywood, 1927–1951." *Tobacco Control* 17 (2008): 313–23.

Marketing and Research Counselors, Inc. "What Have We Learned from People? A Conceptual Summarization of 18 Focus Group Interviews on the Subject of Smoking" (for Ted Bates Advertising for Brown & Williamson). May 26, 1975. Bates 680559454–9490.

"Master Summary for B&W Subjective Document Review." 1989. Bates 1000.01.

McDaniel, Patricia A., Gina Intinarelli, and Ruth E. Malone. "Tobacco Industry Issues Management Organizations: Creating a Global Corporate Network to Undermine Public Health." *Globalization and Health* 4 (2008): 2.

McKeown, Frank E. "Kool Family Utopian Objectives, 1979–1985." Aug. 15, 1978. Bates 680562156–2169.

Mertens, Victor E. "Zigarettenrauch eine Ursache des Lungenkrebses? (Eine Anregung)." *Zeitschrift für Krebsforschung* 32 (1930): 82–91.

Michaels, David. *Doubt Is Their Product: How Industry's Assault on Science Threatens Your Health.* New York: Oxford University Press, 2008.

Moseley, John M. (American Tobacco). "Second International Tobacco Congress, Brussels, Belgium, and Visit to Research Institutes and Cigarette Factories in Central Europe for the Period June 5 to July 2, 1958." July 1958. Bates 950158605–8664.

Muggli, Monique, Jean L. Forster, Richard D. Hurt, and James L. Repace. "The Smoke You Don't See: Uncovering Tobacco Industry Scientific Strategies Aimed against Environmental Tobacco Smoke Policies." *American Journal of Public Health* 91 (2001): 1419–23.

Muggli, Monique E., and Richard D. Hurt. "A Cigarette Manufacturer and a Managed Care Company Collaborate to Censor Health Information Targeted at Employees." *American Journal of Public Health* 94 (2004): 1307–11.

Müller, Franz H. "Tabakmissbrauch und Lungencarcinom." *Zeitschrift für Krebsforschung* 49 (1939): 57–85.

Mulvey, Kathryn, Mary Assunta, and Konstantin Krasovsky, et al., for INFACT. *Global Aggression: The Case for World Standards and Bold US Action Challenging Philip Morris and RJR Nabisco.* New York: Apex Press, 1998.

Myers, Matthew L., et al. *Federal Trade Commission Staff Report on the Cigarette Advertising Investigation.* FTC, May 1981.

National Cancer Institute. *Changes in Cigarette-Related Disease Risks and Their Implication for Prevention and Control—Monograph 8.* Bethesda, MD: USDHHS, 1996.

———. *Risks Associated with Smoking Cigarettes with Low Machine-Measured Yields of Tar and Nicotine. Smoking and Tobacco Control—Monograph 13.* Bethesda, MD: USDHHS, 2001.

———. *The Role of the Media in Promoting and Reducing Tobacco Use—Monograph 19.* Bethesda, MD: USDHHS, 2008.

Neuberger, Maurine B. *Smoke Screen: Tobacco and the Public Welfare.* Englewood Cliffs, NJ: Prentice-Hall, 1963.

Norman, Vello (Lorillard). "The History of Cigarettes." May 1983. Bates 81051625–1662.

Novotny, Thomas E., Kristen Lum, Elizabeth Smith, Vivian Wang, and Richard Barnes. "Cigarettes Butts and the Case for an Environmental Policy on Hazardous Cigarette Waste." *International Journal of Environmental Research and Public Health* 6 (2009): 1691–1705.

Ochsner, Alton. *Smoking and Cancer: A Doctor's Report.* New York: Julian Messner, 1954.

Oreskes, Naomi, and Erik M. Conway. *Merchants of Doubt.* New York: Bloomsbury Press, 2010.

Pearl, Raymond. "Tobacco Smoking and Longevity." *Science* 87 (1938): 216–17.

Peng, Yali. "Smoke and Power: The Political Economy of Chinese Tobacco." Ph.D. diss., University of Oregon, 1997.

Philip Morris. "Project Down Under: Conference Notes." June 24, 1987. Bates 2021502102–2134.

Pollay, Richard W. "Propaganda, Puffing and the Public Interest." *Public Relations Review* 16 (1990): 39–54.

———. *A Scientific Smoke Screen: A Documentary History of Public Relations Efforts for and by the Tobacco Industry Research Council (TIRC), 1954–1958.* Vancouver: History of Advertising Archives, 1990.

Pollock, David. *Denial & Delay: The Political History of Smoking and Health, 1951–1964.* London: Action on Smoking and Health, 1999.

Proctor, Robert N. *Cancer Wars: How Politics Shapes What We Know and Don't Know about Cancer.* New York: Basic Books, 1995.

———. *The Nazi War on Cancer.* Princeton: Princeton University Press, 1999.

———. "Tobacco and the Global Lung Cancer Epidemic." *Nature Reviews Cancer* 1 (2001): 82–86.

———. "The Global Smoking Epidemic: A History and Status Report." *Clinical Lung Cancer* 5 (2004): 371–76.

———. "Should Medical Historians Be Working for the Tobacco Industry?" *Lancet* 383 (2004): 1174–75.

———. "Angel H. Roffo: The Forgotten Father of Experimental Tobacco Carcinogenesis." *Bulletin of the World Health Organization* 84 (2006): 494–95.

———. "'Everyone Knew But No One Had Proof': Tobacco Industry Use of Medical History Expertise in US Courts, 1990–2002." *Tobacco Control* 15 (2006): iv117–25.

Radford, Edward P., and Vilma R. Hunt. "Polonium 210: A Volatile Radioelement in Cigarettes." *Science* 143 (1964): 247–49.

Rego, Brianna. "The Polonium Brief: A History of Cancer, Radiation, and the Tobacco Industry." *Isis* 101 (2009): 453–84.

Rien, Mark W., and Gustaf N. Dorén. *Das neue Tabago Buch.* Hamburg: Reemtsma, 1985.

R. J. Reynolds. "Project Scum." Dec. 12, 1995. Bates 518021121–1129.

Robicsek, Francis. *The Smoking Gods: Tobacco in Maya Art, History, and Religion.* Norman: University of Oklahoma Press, 1978.

Rodgman, Alan (Reynolds). "A Critical and Objective Appraisal of the Smoking and Health Problem." Sept. 12, 1962. Bates 504822823–2846.

———. "A Short Explanation and Analysis of Method of Measuring 'Tar and Nicotine' in Cigarette Smoke." Jan. 22, 1965. Bates 501013245–3255.

Roffo, Angel H. "Leucoplasia tabáquica experimental." *Boletín del Instituto de Medicina Experimental* 7 (1930): 130–44.

———. "Durch Tabak beim Kaninchen entwickeltes Carcinom." *Zeitschrift für Krebsforschung* 33 (1931): 321.

———. "El tabaco como cancerígeno." *Boletín del Instituto de Medicina Experimental* 42 (1936): 287–336.

———. "Krebserzeugendes Benzpyren gewonnen aus Tabakteer." *Zeitschrift für Krebsforschung* 49 (1939): 588–97.

———. "Tabak und Krebs." *Reine Luft* 21 (1939): 123–25.

———. "Krebserzeugende Einheit der verschiedenen Tabakteere." *Deutsche medizinische Wochenschrift* 65 (1939): 963–67.

———. "Krebserzeugende Tabakwirkung." *Monatsschrift für Krebsbekämpfung* 8 (1940): 97–102.

Rogers, Phillip J., and Geoffrey F. Todd. "Report on Policy Aspects of the Smoking and Health Situation in U.S.A." Oct. 15, 1964. Bates 1003119099–9135.

Russell, M. A. Hamilton. "Cigarette Smoking: Natural History of a Dependence Disorder." *British Journal of Medical Psychology* 44 (1971): 1–16.

Saad, Lydia, and Steve O'Brien (Gallup Organization). "The Tobacco Industry Summons Polls to the Witness Stand: A Review of Public Opinion on the Risks of Smoking." Prepared for Annual Meeting of American Association for Public Opinion Research, St. Louis, May 15, 1998. Bates 82286394–6421.

Sante, Luc. *No Smoking.* New York: Assouline, 2004.

Schairer, Eberhard, and Erich Schöniger. "Lungenkrebs und Tabakverbrauch." *Zeitschrift für Krebsforschung* 54 (1943): 261–69.

Schapiro, Mark. "Big Tobacco." *The Nation,* May 6, 2002. http://www.thenation.com/doc/20020506/schapiro.

Schesslitz, Peter. "Tabak und Krebs." From *Deutsche Tabak-Zeitung.* Reprint. *Reine Luft* 23 (1941): 39.

Schick, Suzaynn, and Stanton Glantz. "Scientific Analysis of Second-Hand Smoke by the Tobacco Industry, 1929–1972." *Nicotine & Tobacco Research* 7 (2005): 591–612.

Seldes, George. *Lords of the Press.* New York: Julian Messner, 1938.

———. "Tobacco Shortens Life." *In Fact,* Jan. 13, 1941, pp. 1–5; Jan. 27, 1941, pp. 3–4.

———. "US to Force Europe to Take $911,100,000 in Tobacco, Only 2 Billions in Food in ERP Plan." *In Fact,* March 22, 1948, pp. 1–3.

Seligman, Robert B. (Philip Morris), to CTR File. "Meeting in New York." Nov. 17, 1978. Bates 1003718428–8432.

Shafey, Omar, Michael Eriksen, Hana Ross, and Judith Mackay. *Tobacco Atlas.* 3rd ed. Atlanta: American Cancer Society, 2009.

Shmuk, Aleksandr A. *The Chemistry and Technology of Tobacco.* Vol. 3 of his *Works, 1913–1945.* Trans. from the Russian. Moscow: Pishchepromizdat, 1953.

"Sloan-Kettering Institute—Cigarette Paper Tars." n.d. (March 1952). Bates MNAT00587275.

Slovic, Paul, ed. *Smoking: Risk, Perception, and Policy.* Thousand Oaks: Sage, 2001.

Smith, R. C. "The Magazines' Smoking Habit." *Columbia Journalism Review* 16 (1978): 29–31.

Solomon, Alisa. "The Other Nicotine Addiction." *Village Voice,* Oct. 18, 1994, 4–5. Bates 2041128423–8548.

Stevenson, Terrell, and Robert N. Proctor. "The 'Secret' and 'Soul' of Marlboro: Philip Morris and the Origins, Spread, and Denial of Nicotine Free-Basing." *American Journal of Public Health* 98 (2008): 1184–94.

Tate, Cassandra. *Cigarette Wars: The Triumph of the Little White Slaver.* New York: Oxford University Press, 1999.

Taylor, Peter R. *The Smoke Ring: Tobacco, Money, and Multinational Politics.* New York: Pantheon, 1984.

Teague, Claude E., Jr. (Reynolds). "Survey of Cancer Research, with Emphasis upon Possible Carcinogens from Tobacco." Feb. 2, 1953. Bates 504184895–4923 and 504184873–4894.

———. "A New Type of Cigarette Delivering a Satisfying Amount of Nicotine with a Reduced 'Tar'-to-Nicotine Ratio." March 28, 1972. Bates 502987394–7403.

———. "The Nature of the Tobacco Business and the Crucial Role of Nicotine Therein." April 14, 1972. Bates 83570661–0670.

———. "Some Thoughts about New Brands of Cigarettes for the Youth Market." Feb. 2, 1973. Bates 502987357–7368.

———. "Implications and Activities Arising from Correlation of Smoke pH with Nicotine Impact, Other Smoke Qualities, and Cigarette Sales." Sept. 28, 1973. Bates 509314122–4154.

Teague, Claude E., Jr., to Gabriel R. DiMarco. "Nordine Study." Dec. 1, 1982. Bates 500898255–8257.

Tennant, Richard B. *The American Cigarette Industry: A Study in Economic Analysis and Public Policy.* New Haven: Yale University Press, 1950.

Thompson, R. D., to C. B. Wade Jr. "Survey of Company's General Public and Consumer Correspondence Procedures." Feb. 2, 1966. Bates 500026301–6303.

Tilley, Nannie May. *The Bright-Tobacco Industry, 1860–1929.* Chapel Hill: University of North Carolina Press, 1948.

———. *The R. J. Reynolds Tobacco Company.* Chapel Hill: University of North Carolina Press, 1985.

Tobacco Industry Research Committee. *A Scientific Perspective on the Cigarette Controversy.* April 14, 1954. Bates 961008056–8076.

Todd, Geoffrey F. (Imperial Tobacco). "Visit to U.S.A. and Canada: Report to T.M.S.C." June 14, 1961. Bates 105367083–7098.

———. "Smoking and Health: The Present Position in the U.K. and How It Came About." 1963. Bates 1000215063–5085.

"Training Materials for Counsel in Smoking & Health Litigation." 1986. Bates 282012884–3316.

Tucker, Charles A. "1975 Marketing Plans Presentation, Hilton Head" (presented to RJRI Board of Directors). Sept. 30, 1974. Bates 501421310–1335.

Tursi, Frank V., Susan E. White, and Steve McQuilkin. *Lost Empire: The Fall of R. J. Reynolds Tobacco Company.* Winston-Salem: Winston-Salem Journal, 2000.

U.S. Department of Health and Human Services. *Nicotine Addiction: A Report of the Surgeon General.* Washington, DC: U.S. Government Printing Office, 1988.

———. *Reducing the Health Consequences of Smoking: 25 Years of Progress.* Washington, DC: U.S. Government Printing Office, 1989.

U.S. Department of Health, Education, and Welfare. *Smoking and Health. Report of the Advisory Committee of the Surgeon General.* Washington, DC: U.S. Government Printing Office, 1964.

Wagner, Susan. *Cigarette Country: Tobacco in American History and Politics.* New York: Praeger, 1971.

Wakeham, Helmut (Philip Morris). "Tobacco and Health—R&D Approach." Nov. 15, 1961. Bates 1005069026–9050.

———. "Why One Smokes" (draft). Fall 1969. Bates 1003287836–7848.

———. "Presentation to Philip Morris Board, Revised Draft." Oct. 15, 1973. Bates 202288 6235–6236.

Wakeham, Helmut, to Joseph F. Cullman III. " 'Best' Program for C.T.R." Dec. 8, 1970. Bates 2022200161–0163.

Walford, Pat (Philip Morris). "The Development of Cigarette Technology." Feb. 28, 1979. Bates 1000774237–4245.

Ward, M. J. (Brown & Williamson). "Patent Survey—Carbon Filter." Sept. 6, 1973. Bates 6503 17809–7869.

Warner, Kenneth E. *Selling Smoke: Cigarette Advertising and Public Health.* Washington, DC: APHA, 1986.

———. "Tobacco Industry Scientific Advisors: Serving Society or Selling Cigarettes?" *American Journal of Public Health* 81 (1991): 839–42.

W. D. & H. O. Wills (Australia). "A Review of and Recommendations on Passive Smoking and Social Acceptability of Smoking." July 1976. Bates 2025025461–5480.

Weiss, Francis J. (Sugar Research Foundation, for R. J. Reynolds). "Tobacco and Sugar." Oct. 1950. Bates 502477793–7881.

Wenusch, Adolf. *Der Tabakrauch. Seine Entstehung, Beschaffenheit und Zusammensetzung.* Bremen: Arthur Geist Verlag, 1939.

Whelan, Elizabeth. *A Smoking Gun: How the American Tobacco Industry Gets Away with Murder.* Philadelphia: George F. Stickley, 1984.

White, Colin. "Research on Smoking and Lung Cancer: A Landmark in the History of Chronic Disease Epidemiology." *Yale Journal of Biology and Medicine* 63 (1990): 29–46.

White, Larry C. *The Smoking Business.* Melbourne: Schwartz, 1988.

Whiteside, Thomas. *Selling Death: Cigarette Advertising and Public Health.* New York: Liveright, 1971.

Wiener, Jon. "Big Tobacco and the Historians." *The Nation,* March 15, 2010.

Wilner, Norwood S. *The Criminal Negligence of the Cigarette Industry and How Its Customers Have Paid with Their Lives.* Jacksonville: n.p., n.d. Bates 321923052–3110.

World Bank. *Curbing the Epidemic: Governments and the Economics of Tobacco Control.* Washington, DC: World Bank, 1999.

World Health Organization. *Tobacco or Health: A Global Status Report.* Geneva: WHO, 1997.

———. *Framework Convention on Tobacco Control.* Geneva: WHO, 2003.

———. *MPOWER: WHO Report on the Global Tobacco Epidemic.* Geneva: WHO, 2008.

Wynder, Ernst L., and Evarts A. Graham. "Tobacco Smoking as a Possible Etiologic Factor in Bronchiogenic Carcinoma: A Study of 684 Proven Cases." *JAMA* 143 (1950): 329–36.

Wynder, Ernst L., Evarts A. Graham, and Adele B. Croninger. "Experimental Production of Carcinoma with Cigarette Tar." *Cancer Research* 13 (1953): 855–66.

Yach, Derek, and Stella Aguinaga Bialous. "Junking Science to Promote Tobacco." *American Journal of Public Health* 91 (2001): 1745–48.

Yeaman, Addison (Brown & Williamson). "Implications of Battelle Hippo I & II and the Griffith Filter." July 17, 1963. Bates 435.

FILMOGRAPHY

One in 20 Thousand. With Norr and Ochsner. American Temperance Society, 1950s.
Cancer by the Carton. With Norr and Ochsner. American Temperance Society, 1950s.
Cold Turkey. Directed by Norman Lear. United Artists, 1971.
Smoking and Health: The Need to Know. Tobacco Institute, 1972.
Smoking and Health: The Answers We Seek. Tobacco Institute, 1975.
Death in the West. Directed by Peter R. Taylor. Thames, 1976.
Frontline: Inside the Tobacco Deal. PBS, 1998.
Making a Killing: Philip Morris, Kraft, and Global Tobacco Addiction. Directed by Kelly Anderson and Tami Gold. INFACT, 2000.
Bright Leaves. Directed by Ross McElwee. 2003.
Thank You for Smoking. Directed by Jason Reitman, based on a book by Christopher Buckley. 2005.

WEBOGRAPHY

http://lane.stanford.edu/tobacco/index.html. [Best site for tobacco ads, especially ads with a medical theme.]
http://legacy.library.ucsf.edu. [UCSF's legacy documents; the best resource for searching the industry's formerly secret archives.]
http://tobacco.neu.edu/. [Tobacco Products Liability Project—news reports on litigation.]
http://www.ash.org. [Website of ASH, "America's first antismoking and non-smokers' rights organization."]
http://www.euro-cig.com/gallery.php?id_cap = 90. [Sex appeal in advertising images.]
http://smokefreemovies.ucsf.edu. [Smoke-free movies.]
http://www.smoke-free.ca/documents/Manipulation1.htm. [Neil E. Collishaw's history of Imperial Tobacco for Physicians for a Smoke-Free Canada.]
http://www.tobacco.org/. [Tobacco news and information organized by Gene Borio and Michael Tacelosky.]
http://www.tobaccofreekids.org/. [Matthew Myers's Tobacco-Free Kids website.]
http://www.tobaccovideos.com. [Tobacco videos organized by brand.]
http://www.trinketsandtrash.org/. [A collection of "Artifacts of the Tobacco Epidemic," principally tobacco ads, organized by John Slade.]
http://www.who.int/fctc/en/index.html. [World Health Organization's Framework Convention on Tobacco Control.]
https://www.stanford.edu/group/tobaccoprv/cgi-bin/wordpress/. [Cigarette Citadels, locating tobacco factories throughout the world. Piloted by the Stanford anthropologist Matthew Kohrman.]

acceptable rebellion   Expression used by R. J. Reynolds to describe the youth appeal of its Camel brand, identified also as "slightly anti-establishment." As in "I want to stand out and make a point. Not too much, though." Allied terms include *maverick, rogue,* and *James Dean.*

accommodation   Key element in the 1980s–2000s efforts to thwart smoke-free legislation, following the demonstration of health harms from secondhand smoke. Prominent in the industry's global Courtesy of Choice campaign, in which the idea was that smokers and non-smokers should be able to live and eat in harmony, with both having a right to enjoy the common air of restaurants and hotels. The professed goal was to avoid "American-style ostracism" of smokers. "Fair accommodation of smokers" was also a key element in the industry's Operation Down Under and Operation Rainmaker.

alleged   Qualifier required whenever talking about carcinogens or other dangers of smoking. The word appears in more than one hundred thousand documents preserved in the industry's formerly secret archives now online at http://legacy.library.ucsf.edu. Teague at Reynolds, for example, talked about the need to eliminate "alleged health hazards" from cigarettes; nonburning cigarettes were supposed to reduce "the alleged risks to other people's health," etc.

alternate filler   Inert materials used to replace some of the tobacco in cigarettes, especially in the 1970s and 1980s. These typically contained non-combustible materials such as calcium carbonate, silica, glass, or

681

even asbestos. The idea was that cigarettes stuffed with "non-smoking materials" (NSMs) would reduce tar yields when smoked.

ammonia technology
Technique by which ammonia was added to freebase the nicotine in cigarette smoke (by raising the pH, increasing the alkaloid's "impact"). Philip Morris's development of ammonia technology in the early 1960s helped make Marlboro the world's most popular cigarette. Similar techniques were later developed to freebase street cocaine ("crack").

annoyance
Term used by the industry to describe the effect of smoking on non-smokers. Secondhand smoke was "annoying"—rather than, say, *carcinogenic*—with the proper comparison being to a baby crying on an airplane or having to sit next to someone with body odor or strong perfume, etc.

Antis
Industry term for "anti-tobacco activists." Health advocates are characterized as "anti-smoker" to obscure the fact they are actually pro–public health and, in this sense, "pro-smoker." Compare *screamers*.

biological activity
The most common industry euphemism for cancer or precancerous growth. Term is used (for example) to designate the abnormal cellular proliferation produced when tobacco tars are applied to the shaved backs of experimental mice, as in "estimated biological activity" or "EBA." Sometimes referred to as "Ames activity," "activity," or "mouse numbers." Compare also RAN-1 and RAN-2.

BORSTAL
BAT code word from the late 1950s (used in internal corporate records) for *benzpyrene,* a polycyclic aromatic hydrocarbon found in cigarette smoke by Roffo in the 1930s and widely blamed for the carcinogenic powers of cigarette smoke in the 1940s and 1950s. "Borstal" was originally a British term for a home for juvenile delinquents.

brand stretching
Expression used to designate the marketing of tobacco through non-tobacco vehicles such as Marlboro Country Stores or Marlboro Classics (clothing) or Benson & Hedges Bistros. Other terms for this practice include "indirect advertising," "trademark diversification," "alibi advertising," "parallel communications," "logo licensing," "image transfer advertising," and "below the line advertising." The point in most instances is to circumvent bans on more traditional forms of advertising.

casing
Liquids sprayed onto tobacco sheet in the course of cigarette manufacturing. Casing materials typically include flavorants such as licorice, sugar, and coumarin but also moistening agents such

diethylene glycol and oxidants such as potassium citrate. And freebasing agents such as urea or ammonia.

Central File
Also referred to as "Cenfile" or "Tobacco Litigation File." Central repository of smoking and health documents maintained as index cards in the 1950s and computerized from the 1960s on. Contained 96,558 documents as of 1984.

Committee of Counsel
Also known as the "Policy Committee of Lawyers" or "the Secret Six," the powerful group of lawyers from the six largest U.S. tobacco firms—American Tobacco, Philip Morris, Lorillard, Brown & Williamson, Liggett & Myers, and R. J. Reynolds—formed in 1958 to control tobacco and health policy.

common knowledge
Industry legal term of art used to claim that everyone has always known about the hazards of tobacco, so people have only themselves to blame for whatever illnesses they contract. Also called "universal awareness." Contrast *open controversy.*

compensation
Term designating the fact that when smokers switch to a lower-yield cigarette they will often "compensate" by inhaling more deeply, holding the smoke longer in their lungs, smoking more cigarettes or more puffs per cigarette, smoking farther down on the butt, covering ventilation holes, or otherwise altering their behavior to obtain more nicotine (consciously or unconsciously). Compensation, also known as "titration," "quota mechanism," or "accommodation," is the principal reason lower-yield or "light" cigarettes are no safer than regulars. See also *elasticity, lipping behavior,* and *ventilation.*

conversion
R. J. Reynolds term for convincing a target smoker to shift from a competitor's brand to its own. Thereafter the problem becomes "retention."

DIET
Acronym for "dry ice expanded tobacco," a technique developed in the early 1970s involving application of extreme cold to tobacco leaves, causing them to "puff up" or "swell." Light cigarettes are generally made from expanded tobacco, which is why cigarettes today contain less tobacco than their pre-1960s counterparts. Light cigarettes are "light" in the same way that cotton candy might be considered a low-cal form of candy (falsely, in other words).

D.N.P. (duty not paid)
Tobacco industry euphemism for smuggling, also referred to as "transit trade," "general trade (GT)," "parallel market," "second channel," "border trade," "re-export" or "back door transactions," "special" or "opportunistic" markets or customers, "contraband," "black" or "gray" markets, etc., as in BAT's description of its 555 International brand: "IED shipments were mainly

to Indonesia (as legal imports), and to Hong Kong and Singapore for the Duty Free/Transit trade." BAT affiliates in the 1990s described D.N.P. as a market "segment."

document retention policy

Document destruction policy.

elasticity

Notion that cigarettes can be designed to allow smokers to control tar and nicotine yields, according to how they are smoked. Ventilation holes, for example, were placed where they could be covered up by the smoker's lips or fingers, allowing more smoke to enter the mouth and lungs. Elasticity was deliberately built into cigarettes so that smokers of low-yield brands could obtain higher "satisfaction." See also *compensation, lipping behavior,* and *ventilation.*

ETS

Environmental Tobacco Smoke, a term of art used by the industry to pretty up "secondhand" or "involuntary" smoke, smoke produced by "passive" smoking.

expanded tobacco

Leaf that has been "puffed up," or expanded, to increase its filling power. Expanded tobacco is less dense, which means a cigarette can be filled with less mass. One of the principal means by which "low tar" and "light" cigarettes are made to deliver less tar on automatic smoking machines and one reason cigarettes weigh significantly less than they used to. See also *DIET.*

FUBYAS

R. J. Reynolds acronym for "First Usual Brand Young Adult Smokers" or "First Unbranded Young Smokers." Camel makers used this term when designing strategies for marketing to teenagers, distinguishing (on a scale from conformist to nonconformist) Goody Goodies, Preps, GQs, DISCOs, Rockers, Party Parties, Punkers, and Burnouts.

full flavor

Industry term for "high tar" or "regular" (vs. low-tar or light) cigarettes. There are many acronyms, for example, FFLT (full flavor low tar). Manufacturers typically wanted as much "flavor" with as little tar as possible, but this was not generally possible.

gentlemen's agreement

Informal agreement reached by leaders of the U.S. tobacco industry in the 1950s not to compete on health effects. Many companies cheated on this agreement, seeking competitive advantages in the realm of "health reassurance."

grasstops

Friends of influential people (U.S. senators and representatives, for example) whom the tobacco industry would approach to exercise influence. Elaborate computerized records were kept of "grasstops networks"; a senator might have thirty, forty, or even more "grasstops" contacted by "field action teams" for purposes of influencing policy (Rep. David Obey of Wisconsin had 33; Rep. Collin C. Peterson of Minnesota had 42, etc.). Also referred to as "influencers."

healthy buildings

Construct designed to indicate that buildings can be engineered to be smoker-friendly, by increasing ventilation rather than by limiting smoking. Institutionalized with the establishment of Healthy Buildings International, an industry front to combat efforts to stop indoor smoking. Later spawned comparable terms of art such as "healthy forests" (= extensive logging).

irritation

Catchall term for whatever might be wrong with a cigarette, used to diminish or trivialize dangers. Occupying a flexible middle ground between "taste" and "cancer," irritation was something the industry could seek to reduce as purely a matter of ensuring satisfaction while simultaneously hoping this would help to reduce carcinogenicity. Irritation was the most common explanation for why a particular chemical or physical act caused cancer (prior to the mutation theory); so the industry could research "irritation" and defend this as an effort to provide customer satisfaction. The conflation had both legal and PR value, since a test of an additive or smoke constituent in, say, a rabbit's eye could be defended as either a "taste test" (to avoid irritation) or a test to determine pathologic potency. The industry's solution to "irritation" was to make cigarettes "mild." Compare *annoyance*.

learners

One of a number of terms applied to young people just beginning to smoke, along with "starters," "new smokers," "pre-smokers," "initial triers," etc. Claude Teague at Reynolds distinguished "pre-smokers," "learning smokers," and "confirmed smokers" in a 1973 memo complaining about being "unfairly constrained from directly promoting cigarettes to the youth market" and stressing the need for "new brands designed to be particularly attractive to the young smoker." Compare *FUBYAS* and *restarters*.

lipping behavior

Philip Morris term from the 1960s referring to the unconscious covering of ventilation holes by the lips, allowing smokers to obtain more tar and nicotine than predicted from measurements derived from smoking robots. Also known as "lip occlusion" and "lip drape."

"more research"

Less action; a reason for delay. As in "We need more research."

mouse carcinogens

Term used by the industry when referring to animal experiments indicating a cancer hazard. So "mouse carcinogens" have been found in tobacco smoke but are not indicative of a human danger. Potencies revealed by animal experiments were sometimes referred to as "mouse numbers."

niche opportunities   Expression used by Philip Morris in discussions of how to target "African Americans, Hispanics, Asians, Gays," etc.; also referred to as "niche markets" or "audiences."

nicotine stains   Term invented to replace "tar stains" or "coal tar stains" in the 1930s, when coal tar was found to cause cancer. The new term—used mainly to describe discolorations on smokers' fingers—was introduced to divert attention from the fact that stains of this sort contained cancer-causing tars. The industry would later dispute the presence even of tars in tobacco smoke. See *tar*.

open controversy   A main pillar in the doubt-mongering project, the idea here was that no one has ever been able to *prove* that tobacco is hazardous; the controversy remains "open" and in need of "more research." Paired with "common knowledge" in the industry's legal defense strategy.

privileging   Industry technique by which scientific documents or other sensitive papers are produced for discussion with industry lawyers in order to protect them under the guise of attorney-client privilege. Tens of thousands of documents have been protected from subpoena by this process.

prohibition   Always bad. Tobacco's defenders use this term—along with "abolition" and "abolitionists"—to denigrate any and all efforts to curtail tobacco use. The move is to associate health advocacy with puritanical intolerance, and specifically the unpopular ban on the sale of alcohol in the United States circa 1919–33. The industry's ridicule of "abolitionists" is curious, given the implied reference to opposing slavery, but the denigration seems to work by calling up a kind of oppositional zealotry or fanaticism, odious by virtue of its antiquarian taint.

RAN-1, RAN-2   R. J. Reynolds abbreviation for "reduced Ames numbers," referencing the bacterial bioassay developed by Bruce Ames, a Berkeley biochemist, in the mid-1970s. A cigarette with "reduced Ames numbers" was one that generated smoke with a lowered mutagenic potential or "biological activity" (cancer-causing capacity) via use of low-nitrogen blends or washed stems, for example.

reconstituted tobacco   Cigarette ingredient made from tobacco waste by a papermaking process. Recon was used to economize on inputs (by using more of the whole tobacco leaf) but also to fine-tune the chemical composition of cigarette filler ("precision manufacture"). Known inside Philip Morris as "blended leaf" or "BL," and elsewhere as "R.T." or "tobacco sheet." Reynolds referred to it—and the process by which it was made—as "G-7."

replacement smokers	Industry term for the young smokers needed to "replace" those who die from illnesses caused by tobacco. Expression appears in Reynolds, Lorillard, Philip Morris, and Brown & Williamson documents.
restarters	Brown & Williamson term for people who have quit and then begin smoking again. An important market target, along with "starters" ("learners") and "switchers" (people who switch from one brand to another or from regulars to lights).
risk factor	Preferred euphemism for cancer-causing agents or activities. The companies have never liked talk of tobacco "causing" cancer but in the 1990s started admitting smoking could be "a risk factor" for various ailments. Similar expressions are used with reference to dangerous persons, as in "it cannot be excluded that [Adlkofer] will become a risk factor for the industry." Risk can also imply profit, as if smoking were a kind of investment. More honest would be "less lethal" or "less deadly."
safer cigarette	Used to imply that conventional cigarettes are already "safe."
satisfaction	Euphemism for nicotine, as in BAT's claim that "B&H smokers have a preference for slightly higher initial satisfaction." Satisfaction is to nicotine as taste is to tar. Nicotine is defended as a "taste element," when it is actually kept in cigarettes to maintain addiction. Also referred to as "impact."
screamers	Philip Morris term for people who protest receiving cigarette solicitations via direct mail. Millions of such solicitations are sent out annually, and some end up going to people who are underage or have already died from smoking. Philip Morris distinguishes screamers "soft" and "hard": "soft" screamers are simply people who request being removed from such lists, whereas "hard" screamers (also known as "mass mob screamers") include direct mail targets who are underage or otherwise troublesome from a legal point of view.
sick building syndrome (SBS)	Concept created by Gray Robertson of Healthy Buildings International—a tobacco industry front—to distract from the hazards of secondhand smoke in indoor spaces. The idea was that buildings suffering from indoor air pollution (from carpet fumes and the like) could be healed by proper ventilation—rather than bans on smoking. SBS becomes a centerpiece of tobacco industry effort to minimize and/or deny the reality of harms caused by breathing indoor smoke.
statistics	Generally suspect, or "mere." Invectives against statistics appear by the thousands in tobacco industry propaganda. Darrell Huff, author of *How to Lie with Statistics* (1954), was employed by the

industry to present confounding testimony before the U.S. Congress in the 1960s.

tar

The wet, gooey substance that blackens smokers' lungs. Called "coal tar" for a time in the 1930s, changed to "nicotine stains" or just "tar" (in quotes) when coal tar was found to cause cancer. Clarence C. Little advised against its use ("most undesirable") given its connotations for "the lay mind." American Tobacco's chief of research in 1957 preferred "resins," adding that "it is quite possible that they are beneficial in a physiological sense, since they may adsorb, enclose and dilute the irritants such as acids and aldehydes. Certainly, from the standpoint of flavor, taste and palatability, they are an essential ingredient of cigarette smoke." Closely related terms include "smoke solids," "total particulate matter," "dry particular matter," and "condensed phase" smoke constituents. See also *nicotine stains*.

taste

The principal advertised virtue of smoking but also an industry euphemism for tar (vs. nicotine = "satisfaction"). Compare *satisfaction*.

transit

Industry code word for smuggling, as in "Opportunities for legal imports need to be fully investigated before we seek transit opportunities." Smuggling was also known within the industry as "Duty Not Paid"; see *D.N.P.*

unattractive side effects

Brown & Williamson's characterization of lung and heart maladies caused by smoking, from 1963.

ventilation

Also referred to as "dilution," "shunting," "freshing," "air suction," or "smoke bypass." A technique to lower machine-measured tar and nicotine deliveries by cutting tiny slits in the mouth end of a cigarette. Ventilation slits were strategically placed so that while smoking robots would record lower yields, smokers could cover them to obtain their requisite dosages ("self-titration"). "Ventilation" was also a term used to distract from cigarettes as a cause of indoor air pollution: rooms had not "too much smoke" but rather "too little ventilation."

virile market

Term for military and/or macho market targets. "Virile females" included female soldiers but also "NASCAR girls."

weaning

Big Tobacco term for withdrawal from nicotine—smoking cessation—and something to be feared. Tobacco companies worry that if nicotine levels drop significantly below some threshold level, smokers will be "weaned" from the habit.

wordsmithing

Strategic use of language to advance the industry's legal or PR agenda. Reynolds lawyers in 1985 used "wordsmithing" to characterize their client's efforts to "to minimize the risk of statements [in internal research reports] that are misleading or incorrect because of poor or imprecise wording." Chemists at the company were advised "to refrain from discussing potential biological activity and to refer only to 'alleged' carcinogens."

young adults   A euphemism for teenagers, a principal target of many marketing efforts. When cigarette manufacturers are stung by charges of marketing to teens, they can always claim to be targeting "young adults." Many acronyms: YAS (young adult smokers), FUBYAS, etc. A Brown & Williamson memo from 1975 advised its marketing agents henceforth to use the term "young adult smoker" or "young adult smoking market" rather than "young smokers" or "youth market." The Ngram for "young adult smokers" indicates a much broader cultural use of this expression after 1975.

ZEPHYR   In classical mythology a mild and propitious early summer breeze; in the late 1950s a BAT code word for cancer. Internal company documents talk about statistical studies demonstrating a causal relationship "between ZEPHYR and tobacco smoking, particularly cigarette smoking." Compare *BORSTAL.*

TIMELINE OF GLOBAL TOBACCO MERGERS
AND ACQUISITIONS (SELECTED)

Year	Purchase	Price ($ millions)
<1900	American Tobacco buys 250 tobacco makers, forming a global monopoly	$ n.a.
1901	American Tobacco buys Ogden in Britain	$ n.a.
1901	Imperial Tobacco formed from merger of H. O. Wills and 12 other British firms	$ n.a.
1902	British American Tobacco Co. formed with purchase of Imperial by American Tobacco	$ n.a.
1904	Japanese Imperial Tobacco Monopoly established	$ n.a.
1911	Duke empire broken up into American Tobacco, Reynolds, Liggett, and Lorillard	$ n.a.
1914	BAT buys the Souza Co. in Brazil	$???
1925	BAT acquires overseas business of Ardath Tobacco (State Express brand)	$???
1927	BAT buys Brown & Williamson	$???
1929	Carreras buys John Sinclair Ltd of Newcastle-upon-Tyne	$???
1932	BAT acquires Haus Bergmann Cigaretten-Fabriken in Dresden	$???
1932	Imperial buys controlling stake in Gallaher	$???
1934	Philip Morris buys assets of Continental Tobacco Co.	$???
1944	Philip Morris buys Axton-Fisher facilities in Louisville (Fleetwoods and Spud)	$???

1945–60	BAT assets expropriated in Indonesia, Pakistan, and Egypt	$ n.a.
1949	BAT loses Chinese market with Communist Revolution	$ n.a.
1954	Philip Morris acquires U.S. rights to Benson & Hedges	$???
1958	Carreras (Black Cat, Craven A) merges with Rothmans of Pall Mall in England	$???
1961	Augustinus, Fabrikker, and Obel merge to form Scandinavian Tobacco Co	$???
1962	Benson & Hedges (Canada) acquires Tabacofina of Canada	$???
1963	Philip Morris acquires Switzerland's Fabriques de Tabac Réunies	$???
1964	Gallaher acquires 25% share in Dutch firm Theodorus Niemeyer	$ 3
1964	Lorillard acquires 50% stake in Hong Kong's United Tobacco Co.	$ 2
1968	Liggett buys Austin, Nichols & Co. (Wild Turkey, Campari, Metaxa)	$???
1968	Loews Theatres buys Lorillard Tobacco	$ 450
1968	American Tobacco buys Gallaher, takes full control in 1975	$???
1972	Rothmans International formed from merger of several British tobacco companies	$???
1977	BAT acquires Lorillard's international business (Kent, True, etc.)	$???
1978	Philip Morris buys Liggett's international division	$ 108
1980	Tchibo, the coffee maker, acquires stake in Reemtsma (Davidoff and West cigs.)	$???
1983	Liggett & Myers bought by Grand Metropolitan	$ 575
1986	Liggett & Myers sold to Robert E. Gillis and Bennett S. LeBow (Brooke Partners)	$ 137
1986	Imperial Group acquired by Hanson Trust Plc	£2,500
1989	BAT acquires W.D. and H.O. Wills (Australia)	$???
1990	Philip Morris buys VZ Dresden, in Germany (F6, Juwel, Karo brands)	$???
1990	Liggett changes name to Brooke Group, diversifies into sports and entertainment	$ n.a.
1992	Philip Morris Int'l acquires controlling stake in Czech Republic Tabak, SA	$???
1992	Reynolds acquires Satoraljaujhely cigarette factory in Hungary	$???
1990s	Reemtsma buys Mocne brand from Polish state tobacco monopoly	$???
1992	RJR buys Petro plant in St. Petersburg	$???
1992	Japan Tobacco buys Manchester Tobacco of England	$???
1992	BAT acquires Hungary's Pecs Tobacco Factory (Pecsi Dohanygyar)	$???

1993	BAT acquires global rights to Lucky Strike in brand swap with American Brands	$???
1994	Reynolds buys candy and cookie venture in Kazakhstan to make cigarettes	$ 100
1994	BAT's Brown & Williamson acquires American Tobacco Company	$1000
1995	BAT buys Uzbekistan's tobacco monopoly, invests in Poland	$???
1995	BAT buys 65% of state-run tobacco factory in Augustow, forming BAT Polska	$???
1996	Philip Morris buys one-third of Cracow's Zakłady Przemysłu Tytoniowego (Poland)	$ 227
1996	Reynolds buys stake in Tanzanian Cigarette Corp	$ 55
1997	Swedish Match buys Reynolds's Finnish cigar-making facilities	$???
1997	BAT buys Cigarerra La Moderna, Mexico's biggest cigarette manufacturer	$???
1997	Rizla sold to Imperial Tobacco	$???
1997	Reynolds sells Satoraljaujhely cigarette factory to Continental Tobacco Group	$???
1998	Imperial acquires a 90% interest in Reemtsma (Davidoff, West, Stuyvesant)	$5,100
1999	BAT buys controlling share in Imasco	$17,300
1999	French and Spanish monopolies merge (SEITA + Tabacalera), creating Altadis	$???
1999	BAT buys Rothmans International (Dunhill) from Richemont of South Africa	$???
1999	Japan Tobacco buys RJR Nabisco's international rights to Camel, Winston, etc.	$7,800
1999	Reemtsma acquires majority share in Cambodia's Paradise Tobacco Co.	$???
1999	Austria Tabak buys cigarette division of Swedish Match	$???
2000	BAT buys PT Rothmans of Pall Mall Indonesia	$???
2000	BAT sells Rothmans' Canadian interests, forming Imperial Tobacco Canada	$???
2000	Gallaher buys Russian cigarette maker Liggett-Ducat from Vector Group	$ 390
2001	Imperial acquires controlling share in sub-Saharan manufacturer Tobaccor	£ 179
2001	Gallaher buys Austria Tabak (state monopoly)	£1.1 billion = $1,600

2001	Houchens buys Commonwealth Brands	$1,900
2001	BAT invests in North Korea's state-owned Korea Sogyong Trading Corporation	$ 7
2003	BAT acquires stake in Rwanda's TabaRwanda, forming BAT Rwanda	$ 2
2003	Imperial Tobacco completes purchase of Reemtsma Cigarettenfabriken	£3,500
2002	Reynolds buys Santa Fe Natural Tobacco Co. (American Spirit brand)	$ 340
2003	BAT buys Tabacalera Nacional (Peru)	$ 37
2003	BAT buys Ente Tabacchi Italiani (Italy's tobacco monopoly)	$ 3
2003	BAT buys Serbia's Vranje Tobacco Industry	$ 111
2003	BAT sells its Burmese factory, acquired in 1999	$???
2003	Philip Morris buys Nis Tobacco Industry (Serbia)	$ 660
2003	Moroccan government sells 80% stake in Regie des Tabacs to Altadis	$1,530
2003	Altria Group established as parent company of Philip Morris USA	$ n.a.
2004	Reynolds buys B&W, forming Reynolds American; BAT has 42% share	$4,200
2005	Gallaher buys Cita Tabacos de Canarias from Altadis	$ 104
2005	Philip Morris International buys controlling stake in Sampoerna, maker of clove cigarettes	$5,200
2005	Philip Morris International buys Colombia's Compañía Colombiana de Tabaco SA	$ 300
2006	Japan Tobacco International buys Senta Tobacco Industry (Serbia)	$ 36
2006	Reynolds buys Conwood, maker of Kodiak & Grizzly chewing tobacco	$3,500
2006	Japan Tobacco, maker of Mild Seven, buys Gallaher, maker of Silk Cut	$15,000
2007	Imperial Tobacco buys Commonwealth Brands (USA Gold and Sonoma)	$1,900
2007	Philip Morris International increases stake in Pakistan's Lakson Tobacco to 90%	$ 600
2007	Altria buys John Middleton, Inc., makers of Black & Mild cigars	$2,900
2008	Imperial Tobacco buys Altadis (Gauloises Blondes, Gitanes, cigars)	$22,400
2008	BAT buys TEKEL, Turkey's tobacco and alcohol monopoly	$1,720
2008	BAT Plc buys cigarette and snus operations of Skandinavisk Tobakskompagni	$4,100
2008	Altria Group spins off Philip Morris International as a separate company	$ n.a.

2008	Philip Morris International buys Rothmans Inc., the Canadian cigarette maker	$ 1,950
2009	Altria Group buys UST, makers of Skoal and Copenhagen smokeless brands	$11,700
2009	BAT buys Indonesia's PT Bentoel International Investama	$ 494
2009	Philip Morris buys Swedish Match AB's South African unit	$ 224
2009	JTI buys Tribac Leaf, Ltd, with operations in Malawi, Zambia, China, and India	$???
2009	Philip Morris International buys Productora Tabacalera de Colombia, Protabaco Ltd.	$ 452
2009	Reynolds buys Niconovum, a Swedish maker of nicotine gums, sprays, and pouche	$ 43
2010	Philip Morris Philippines merges with Fortune Tobacco to form PMFTC Inc.	$ n.a.

N.B.: A chronology of Philip Morris mergers and acquisitions up to 1973 can be found at http://www.sourcewatch.org/index.php?title = History_of_Philip_Morris.

TIMELINE OF TOBACCO INDUSTRY DIVERSIFICATION INTO CANDY, FOOD, ALCOHOL, AND OTHER PRODUCTS (SELECTED)

1962   BAT acquires manufacturers of paper and pulp, perfumes and fragrances

1962   Reynolds buys Pacific Hawaiian, makers of Hawaiian Punch, for $40 million

1963   Philip Morris buys Clark Brothers Chewing Gum

1964   BAT buys Tonibell, an ice-cream manufacturer

1964   Liggett & Myers buys Allen Products, makers of Alpo dog food, for $15 million

1965   Lorillard acquires Golden Nugget Candy Co. and Usen Products Co.

1965   BAT acquires Lenthèric, Ltd, cosmetics

1966   Lorillard acquires Reed Candy

1966   American Tobacco buys Sunshine Biscuits and James Beam Distilling

1966   Liggett & Myers buys Paddington Corp (J&B Scotch Whiskey, Izmira Vodka) and Carillon Importers (Grand Marnier and Bombay Gin)

1967   BAT acquires Yardley Perfume and National Oats (popcorn, grits)

1967   Liggett, via Allen Products, establishes Irradco, a food-irradiation business

1969   Liggett & Myers buys Ready Foods

1969   Philip Morris buys Miller Beer from W. R. Grace for $130 million

1969   Reynolds acquires McLean Industries (global shipping and trucking)

1970   Imperial Tobacco (U.K.) buys animal feed business of Associated British Foods

1972   BAT buys controlling interest in Kohl's Corp. (food and drug stores)

1973   BAT acquires Saks Fifth Avenue in New York and Argos in U.K.

1973   BAT buys Gimbels, parent company of Saks, for $200 million

1978   BAT Industries buys NCR's Appleton Papers Division for $280 million

1978	Philip Morris buys Seven-Up for $514 million, later sells it to Pepsi
1979	Reynolds buys Del Monte Corp. for $619 million
1980	Reemtsma, Germany's leading cigarette manufacturer, is bought by Tchibo Coffee
1982	Reynolds acquire Heublein, Inc., makers of A1 Steak Sauce
1982	BATUS buys Marshall Field's
1983	Rothmans acquires interest in Cartier Monde (jewelry, watches)
1984	Reynolds buys Canada Dry, spins off Sea-Land Corporation
1984	BAT buys Eagle Star financial services
1984	Malaysian Tobacco Co. buys a 35% share in Teguh Insurance Co.
1985	BAT moves into the insurance business with its purchase of Allied Dunbar
1985	Philip Morris buys General Foods for $5.6 billion
1985	Reynolds acquires Nabisco for $4.9 billion, forming RJR Nabisco, Inc.
1985	BAT divests its perfume and cosmetics holdings (British American Cosmetics)
1986	Hanson Trust buys Imperial; spins off beer business, hotels, and frozen foods
1988	BAT buys Farmer's Insurance, making it the largest insurer in the U.K.
1988	Philip Morris buys Kraft Foods for $12.9 billion
1990	BAT sells Marshall Field's, Saks, Breuners, and Ivey
1993	Philip Morris buys Nabisco's North American cold cereal operations
1997	BAT merges with Zurich Insurance, tobacco business spun off as BAT Plc
1997	Japan Tobacco acquires food operations of Asahi Chemical
1998	BAT buys Ken Tyrrell's Formula One team (for #30 million) to form British American Racing (1999)
1998	BAT divests its financial services
2000	Philip Morris buys Nabisco Holdings for $14.9 billion
2002	BAT buys rights to five Warner Bros. films, organizes cinema tour in Nigeria
2002	Philip Morris sells Miller Beer to South African Breweries for $5.5 billion
2007	Altria (Philip Morris) sells its Kraft Foods shares to Altria stockholders
2008	Altria Group acquires Ste. Michelle Wine Estates with purchase of UST

ACKNOWLEDGMENTS

I could not have written this book without access to the seventy-plus million pages of documents released by the tobacco industry in response to subpoenas. I would therefore like to thank those many trial attorneys who have fought to bring these racketeers to justice. Lawyers do not always have good reputations, but I have been impressed by the courage and stamina of attorneys fighting the good fight: Madelyn Chaber, Michael V. Ciresi, Richard A. Daynard, Marc Edell, Phil Gerson, C. K. Hoffler, Russell Kinner, Ron Motley, Matthew Myers, William H. Ogle, Gary Paige, Stanley Rosenblatt, Robert Shields, Rod Smith, Mike Withey, and their diligent staffers. These and many others have stood up bravely against one of the world's most powerful polluters, and in some cases managed to bring them to a modicum of justice. The history of the law firms working on both sides of such trials has yet to be written—the industry's side is truly terra incognita—and I look forward to seeing scholars explore this territory.

I am also indebted to those many Herculean scholars who have labored to expose the misdeeds of Big Tobacco. Crucial here, just to name a few, are Mary Assunta, Deborah Barnes, Lisa Bero, Stella Bialous, Alan Blum, Allan Brandt, Simon Chapman, Greg Connolly, Michael Cummings, Rob Cunningham, Stanton Glantz, Norbert Hirschhorn, Richard Hurt, Rob Jackler, Luk Joossens, Matthew Kohrman, Louis Kyriakoudes, Anne Landman, Pamela Ling, Judith Mackay, Ruth Malone, Monique Muggli, Kathryn Mulvey, Naomi Oreskes, Rick Pollay, Channing Robertson, Suzaynn Schick, and Stan Shatenstein. I would also like to thank those precious few industry "insiders" who, at great risk to themselves, have helped to break the iron chains of secrecy surrounding this business: William Farone, Victor J. DeNoble, Paul C. Mele, James D. Mold, Ian Uydess, Jeffrey Wigand, and Merrell Williams.

Collectively, these right-minded attorneys, scholars, and whistle-blowers have saved many lives. We also are fortunate to have dedicated, policy-oriented bodies like Action on Smoking and Health, the American Legacy Foundation, Americans for Nonsmokers' Rights, Doctors Ought to Care, SmokeFreeMovies, the Campaign for Tobacco–Free Kids, the World Congress on Tobacco or Health, and the State of California's Air Resources Board and Tobacco Control Program, all actively engaged in clean air advocacy. That battle is far from over; there is much to be done. Philanthropic bodies are also starting to make important contributions, notably the Bloomberg Initiative to Reduce Tobacco Use and the Bill and Melinda Gates Foundation. Governments have often been slow to act to reduce the tobacco toll, which is why grassroots efforts are so vital.

The Legacy Tobacco Documents Library represents an unparalleled historical treasure, and one barely probed by historians. I have colleagues who work on slavery; the archives contain over 2,400 documents referencing that topic. I have colleagues who work on China; China appears in over 100,000 documents. "Surgeon General" appears in 414,000, and "cancer" in nearly two million documents. And new documents—including now some 8,000 videos—are constantly being added. Equally important is the opportunity recently opened up to explore the *rhetorical microstructure* of the archives. Prior to computerization, it would have taken many lifetimes to go through such a large body of documents and gather up all usages of words such as "alleged," "castoreum," or "propaganda." With full text searchability online, however—thanks to optical character recognition—this can now be done in a matter of seconds, and by anyone with an Internet connection.

We can only search what has been turned over by the companies, of course— and that limitation is profound—but the archives do make it harder for ideas once captured to be lost. And optical character recognition works like an enormous magnet, allowing the tiniest of rhetorical needles to be found even in large archival haystacks. History is rendered transparent in ways not previous possible. Many of my colleagues used to labor in secret for the industry, for example, and some presumably still do. The archives make it harder to keep such work secret, however, and therefore facilitate a certain degree of accountability. In the Internet age it is harder to hide in the shadows.

It would be wrong, though, to imagine that the archives have entirely transformed our understanding of Big Tobacco. Observers with keen eyes and a probing mind have long known about the duplicity of the cartel and its desperation to harvest the young. Fritz Lickint recognized this in the 1930s, as did George Seldes in the 1940s, Alton Ochsner in the 1950s, Maurine Neuberger in the 1960s, and legions more from the 1970s onward. Details of the conspiracy even today remain hidden, but that there *was* such a conspiracy was evident to anyone who compared the industry's propaganda against brute realities. Prior even to the release of the documents, dozens of exposés captured most of the crucial facts: Maurine Neuberger's *Smoke*

Screen, Peter Taylor's *Smoke Ring,* Larry C. White's *Merchants of Death,* and the many works of Fritz Lickint or Alan Blum or people affiliated with Action on Smoking or Health (ASH) and the like. Subsequent histories have filled in the picture: Stanton Glantz's *Cigarette Papers,* Richard Kluger's *Ashes to Ashes,* David Kessler's *Question of Intent,* Allan Brandt's *Cigarette Century,* Simon Chapman's *Public Health Advocacy,* just to name a few. Crucial here has also been the long-standing web presence of groups like ASH and GLOBALink and the many probing scholarly exposés in journals like *Tobacco Control* and the *American Journal of Public Health.*

I probably would not have written this book if three of my four grandparents had not died from smoking: one cancer, one emphysema, one heart attack. Witnessing suffering is often a prompt for seeking answers, if not for finding solace. Most of the people reading this book will have relatives who have succumbed to Lady Nicotine; indeed it is probably the rare person who has not, though they may not know it.

One reason I decided to write this book—about a decade ago—was my surprise to find that many people were swallowing the industry's line that the tobacco "problem" had been "solved." Even worse was this notion—spread by cigarette makers themselves—that the industry had finally "come clean," reformed itself, admitted the errors of its ways.

Nothing could be further from the truth. Few people appreciate the scale on which cigarettes are smoked and how shallow are the industry's concessions. It is true that some ground has been conceded—that smoking can cause disease, for example—but the most important facts have never been admitted. We never hear a tobacco manufacturer admit that millions of people die every year from smoking, or that advertising causes people to smoke, or that for fifty-odd years the companies labored night and day to manufacture doubt. Or that young people have been targeted—and continue to be targeted. Some of the companies now begrudge that secondhand smoke can kill, but none will admit that the victims number in the tens of thousands per year in the United States alone, with an order of magnitude more worldwide. The industry won't admit that most of the world's cigarette deaths lie in the future, or that nicotine is as addictive as heroin or cocaine. Or that addiction deeply compromises a smoker's freedom of choice. The companies never admit that their best customers come from the least fortunate parts of society, people who are often least able to understand or to escape their addiction. There is no admission that cigarette makers lied for decades about the dangers of smoking and that the deception continues in the form of brands sold as "light" or "mild" or their color-coded counterparts. There is no admission that filters are fraudulent, or that the cigarettes sold today are as deadly as any ever sold in the past. History is, in a sense, the industry's worst enemy: they don't want anyone comparing what they now say (and do) to what they so often said (and did) in the past. They don't want to be held accountable. Anyone who thinks there is a "new Philip Morris" should read a few of the transcripts from any of our recent "tobacco and health" trials, where blaming the victim is alive and well as a strategy for exculpation.

I should also say that I am thankful for the detailed and insightful comments on early drafts of this book by Richard Barnes, Iain Boal, Elizabeth Borgwardt, Mike Daube, DeWitt Durham, William Frable, Stanton Glantz, Ray Goldstein, David Hollinger, Phyra McCandless, Jennifer Morris, Mark Parascandola, John Proctor (my brother), David Rosner, Jonathan Samet, Steven Schroeder, Elizabeth A. Smith, Eugenia Somers (my mom), and Elizabeth Watkins. To my editors, Hannah Love and Sheila Berg, I must express a debt of thanks for tolerating my prolix prose. And a thanks to my companions at CASBS up on the hill.

I would also like to thank two colleagues—Allan Brandt and Louis Kyriakoudes—for their acumen and insight. Both of these distinguished historians know what it is like to be on the receiving end of the industry's legal fury, a story that some day will require a separate telling (Jon Wiener makes a good first start in his 2010 account, "Big Tobacco and the Historians," for the *Nation*). Suffice it here to say I owe a debt of gratitude to the judiciary of the state of Florida, which barred the tobacco industry from gaining access to an early draft of the present book (which had been subpoenaed). I should also thank Lauren Schoenthaler in Stanford University's Office of the General Counsel for helping me to protect my First Amendment rights.

Last but not least, I would like to thank those many cigarette industry lawyers with whom I have sparred over the past dozen-odd years. Being deposed is not always a pleasant experience, but it can help sharpen one's ideas—and can even open up opportunities to reverse engineer anxieties. Several of the lines of inquiry explored in this book were first proposed to me (inadvertently, perhaps) by attorneys working for the defense in litigation. I am particularly grateful in this regard to William Allinder, David Bernick, Annie Chuang, Jeffrey L. Furr, Roger Geary, Theodore Grossman, Stephen J. Kaczynski, Frank P. Kelly, Elizabeth P. Kessler, Paul D. Koethe, Christine Lawson, Kenneth J. Reilly, Bruce Sheffler, and Douglas B. Smith, all esquires for the tobacco trade.

Most people have no idea how much energy has been marshaled in defense of this, the world's deadliest business enterprise. Critics of the industry, even with mountains of truth on their side, remain as Davids against the tobacco Goliath. Sometimes, though, even a small stone can work wonders.

INDEX

abortions, spontaneous, caused by smoking, 5, 272

Academia Nicotiana Internationalis, 543

"acceptable rebellion," 78–80, 582n3, 681

Accommodation Program (Philip Morris), 70, 104, 573n44, 681

Accord cigarette (Philip Morris brand), 190, 521, 530–31

acid-base balance, crucial role of, in cigarette smoke, 33–34, 177, 392–96, 400

Ackerman, Lauren V. (Professor of Pathology, Washington University), 428, 588n8

acrolein, 174–76, 210–16, 353, 422, 490

Action on Smoking and Health (ASH), 314, 700–701

activated charcoal, as filter material, 344–46, 629n31

Adams, Miriam G. (Manager, Public Relations Consumer Correspondence, Reynolds), 324, 511

addiction: cigarettes vs. alcohol, 5–6, 557; cigarettes vs. opiates, 50, 161, 237, 302, 695n37; Columbus on, 18; "common knowledge," 655n44; Dole denies, 335; as "an ideology," 451; not impossible to overcome, 451; industry regards as "fortunate," 250, 537; nicotine levels sufficient to create, 380; Roper poll on, 326; "second addiction" (to taxes), 28, 49–55; Seevers on, 236–37; Shook Hardy recognizes as "potent weapon," 236; smokers abhor, 10,

311; smokers become painfully familiar with, 323–27, 333, 624n40; Surgeon General fails to recognize, 236; Teague admits, 196–97; "third addiction," 55; tobacco industry admits, 238, 250, 375–76, 564n9; tobacco industry denies, 295, 301–2, 43; trivialized, 291, 301, 335, 406; Mark Twain jokes about, 391, 473. *See also* baboons; compensation; nicotine

additives: appetite suppressants, 504; bronchial dilators, 3, 501; burn accelerants, 371, 502; castoreum, 495, Chemosol, 358; chlorophyll, 213, 352; in cigarette paper, 501–02; cloves, 542; cocoa and cocoa butter, 494–95, 497, 501–04, 658n35; code names for, 401–3, 495, 504, 639n26; hemoglobin, 527; humectants, 42, 175; impact boosters, 315, 391, 402; licorice, 2–3, 33, 495, 497–98; mechanization requires, 42–43; no obligation to study health impact of, 494; Parmesan cheese, 354; "potentially hazardous," 497; tonnages used, 497–98, 501; unregulated, 3, 149, 496. *See also* ammoniation and ammonia technology; chocolate; freebasing; glycerine; menthol; sugar

Ad Hoc Committee, 437, 646n45

Adlkofer, Friedrich (German industry scientist), 439, 687

Admiral cigarettes, 62

advertising of cigarettes: advertorials, 112; alibi ads and branding, 117, 211–17, 228, 230, 264, 682; billboard, 62; causes kids to start

irritation, 402; key to competing with Philip Morris, 402; Reynolds adopts, 400; as "soul of Marlboro," 403; by urea, 403; W.D. & H.O. Wills explores, 402. *See also* diammonium phosphate; freebasing; ROOT technology; UKELON

animal abuse and cruelty, 218, 223, 433, 528–30

Archetype Project, 609n85

Arenco-Decouflé, 40, 554

Arents, George, library of, 466, 475

ARISE, 450–52, 649n72

Arnold & Porter LLP (tobacco industry law firm), 331, 472–77, 672

arsenic, 13, 175, 177, 210, 214–15, 229, 240–42, 340, 353–54, 490–93, 600n18, 656nn5,7

Arthur D. Little Corporation (contract research facility): admits filters "do not really take anything out," 355; calculates money saved by cigarette death, 663n1; denialist non-chalance, 611n18; huge staff, 595n37; paid by Liggett to identify carcinogens in smoke, 186, 230, 236; palladium fiasco, 523–24; verifies Wynder's experiments, 239–40, 263, 524, 595n37. *See also* Charles J. Kensler

asbestos: factories (for Kent's Micronite filters), 344; in Kent cigarettes, 344, 486, 628n9; from ceiling insulation, 486; surgical masks made from, 345. *See also* Hollingsworth & Vose; Kent cigarettes

Aschenbrenner, Helmuth (German tobacco apologist), 168, 589n17

Ashe, Arthur (tennis champion), 579n22

ashtrays: "active," 138; in airplanes and cars, 136; available in Second Life, 141; in computers, 136; on eBay, 143; Kyriakoudes on, 136, 564n10; made by children, 7, 137; miniature and toy, 138–39; patents for, 137; portable, 138, 163, 516; used to shore up smoking's social acceptability, 138; word coined, 136

Astel, Karl (President, University of Jena, Germany), 160–63, 169

Athlete brand cigarettes, 131

Atlas vs. Hercules, 536

Audubon Society, 114

Auerbach, Oscar (Chief of Laboratory Services, VA Hospital, East Orange, NJ), 188, 229, 596n44, 603n9

Austern, H. Thomas (Covington & Burling attorney), 332, 445

Australia: anti-butt movement, 515; DEG

prohibited, 505; electronic cigarettes banned, 532; freebasing at W.D. & H.O. Wills, 402; health question "open to debate," 543–44; impact of sponsorships, 107, 115; industry's "high degree of access to government," 545; monetary value of advertising in, 99–100; Philip Morris sponsorships, 106; plain packaging mandate, 132, 547; smoke-free universities, 427; smokeless banned in, 663; Smoking and Health Research Foundation, 455; sports sponsored, 92–100, 106–7, 578n10; tar tax debated, 637n73; Tobacco Institute of, 655n44; Wool Research Laboratory researches sheep's wool filters, 354

automatic smoking machines: yield deceptive data, 9, 372–73, 387, 412; first developed in Germany, 591n6; Imperial's Slave Smoker, 383; Philip Morris's Human Smoker Simulator, 383

Avatar (film), 66

Aviado, Domingo M. (Professor of Pharmacology, University of Pennsylvania, and CTR Special Projects operative), 279–80, 615n64

Axton-Fisher Tobacco Company, 131, 350, 498, 691, Fig. 20

baboons forced to smoke crack cocaine, 529–30, 447, 529

Baisha Tobacco Co., 116

Bakery, Confectionery, Tobacco Workers, and Grain Millers International Union, 299

bald men, lung cancer rare in, 283–84

ballet, industry sponsorship of, 120

Bantle, Louis (President, U.S. Tobacco Co.), 108, 581n44, 613n43

Barclay cigarettes (Brown & Williamson brand), 431

Barclay squabble, 372–73, 383–85

Barger, A. Clifford (Professor of Medicine, Harvard University), 420

Barnes, Deborah (co-author, *Cigarette Papers*), 457, 462–63, 650n88

Barron's magazine, 48

Baryshnikov, Mikhail (Artistic Director, American Ballet Theatre), 65

baseball: cards, 60, 88–89; cigarette testimonials, 72, 88; players dying from tobacco, 67, 536–37; smokeless fashions, 536; sponsored by tobacco companies, 62, 89–90, 106; team-brand identities, 90. *See also* Ty Cobb; Babe Ruth; Honus Wagner

ing, 127–28; Bristol brand in Sri Lanka, 83; buys Farmer's Insurance, 698; calculates benefit of sponsorships, 99–100; cigarettes introduced into China and Korea using film, 62–63; code names for additives, 495; corporate history, 468; diversifies, 697–98; INTERBAT, 139; Lucky Strike Leisure Wear, 128; needs larger bag to carry cash, 390; Neverfail BlackBerry network, 143; organizes smuggling ring, 54; and particulate filth, 502; pleads not guilty, 111; ponders spiking cigarettes with etorphine, 504; smuggling operations, 53–54; Southampton laboratories, 266, 361, 383; sponsors Philharmonia, 121; sponsors sports, 109, 580n41, 581n46; targets German drivers, 114; on TIRC, 261; tonnage of cocoa butter added to cigarettes, 501; trivializes addiction, 301–02. *See also* BORSTAL; Nobleza-Piccardo; ZEPHYR

Brooks, Jerome E. (American tobacco historian), 466–468, 570n3, 638n11, 651n4, 652n9, 668

Brooks, Stanley Truman (malacologist hired by American Tobacco), 248–249, 609n76

Brown & Williamson Tobacco Corporation: admits nicotine is addictive, 564n9; on "all-tobacco filter," 345; agnometrics, 315; bankrolls University of Kentucky, 425; Barclay Lights Ultra Thins, 410; breaks into majors with Kool, 58; in business of "selling nicotine, an addictive drug," 238; on candy cigarettes as "not too bad an advertisement," 71–75; on cigarette-ashtray "fit," 138; cigarette additives, 496–97; cigarettes "brought to trial by lynch law," 2, 268; collaboration with DNA Plant Technology, 361; contest for college students, 346; on CTR as public relations gesture, 262; on color coding for health reassurance, 417; on disease as "unattractive side effect," 529; disputes secondhand smoke hazard, 457; "Doubt is our product" memo, 289–90; on free nicotine and freebasing, 400–03; funds Gio Gori, 370; gives Paul Newman a car, 64; investigates Philip Morris's ammonia usage, 402; isolates benzopyrene in cigarette smoke, 230, 340, 587n3; Kool Jazz Festivals, 122–23; Lederberg's appreciation of, 446; on menthol brands as "good starter products," 499; military markets, 86; phone logs, 336–37, Fig. 30; Project BIG BOY, 85–86; Project Truth, 268; on Roffo, 340; ROOT Technol-

ogy, 403; sampling at ice fishing festivals, 112; on smoking as "entrance ticket" to adult society, 78; Rockefeller University's gratitude, 446; Special Markets Department, 86; sponsorship of sports, 62, 104–106; Sylvester Stallone paid to smoke in films, 63; strategic plan for Kools, 122; targets blacks, 122; telemarketing, 336; use of UKELON, 401; Viceroy strategy targets "young starters," 76; "worse than Hitler," 337. *See also* Barclay squabble; Kool; Reynolds; Viceroy; Addison Yeaman

Brownlee, K. Alexander (Special Projects statistician), 277–278, 436, 646n43

Brownshirts (Nazi Stormtroopers), 41, 51, 131

Buerger's Disease, 5

Buffett, Warren (American investment guru), 4, 42

Buhler, Victor (President, College of American Pathologists), 277–78

Bulletin of the History of Medicine, 467, 469, Fig. 33

Bumgarner, Joseph E., 264

Bunn, Douglas (Master of Hickstead), 106

Burgard, John W. (Marketing VP, Brown & Williamson): "Doubt is our product," 289–92, 617n1; history of advertising, 617n711

Burke, Arthur W., Jr. (Professor of Pharmacology, Medical College of Virginia), 187–88, 596n44

burley tobacco: absorbs sugars and flavorings, 33; in "American blend" cigarettes, 33–34; chocolate taste, 398, 400; farmers, 453; high-nicotine, 349, 364; high pH, 396; low sugar, 33; Teague tries to lower free nicotine in, 396

burn accelerants, 502

Burnett, Leo (advertising agency), 246, 608n65

Burnham, John C. (Professor of History, Ohio State), 445, 469–70, 475–6, 478, 613n36, 652n13, 653n27

Burns, David M. (Professor of Medicine, UC San Diego), 386, 388

Burns, George (cigar-smoking comedian), 305, 337

buttlegging. *See* smuggling

Cahill, Tim K. ("cold facts Cahill," Reynolds), 320

Califano, Joseph A., Jr. (Secretary of Health, Education, and Welfare, Carter Administration), 239, 607n60

Charlie's Paradise Bar and Country Club, 118–19

Chemosol, 358–59

Chesley, A. L. (Chief Chemist, American Tobacco Co.), 149, 421

Chesterfield cigarettes (Liggett & Myers brand): "pure as the water you drink," 67; baseball stars plug, 88–89, 578n3; "salutes the Yanks," 89; sponsors music, radio and television shows, 90. *See also* Liggett & Myers

chewing tobacco: air-cured burley leaf used in, 33; arsenic in, 491, 656n5; commonly used in collegiate sports, 536; freebasing of, with lime, 396; in India, 542; mouth cancer caused by, 160; nitrosamines in, 537; revived, 536; spittoons for, 137; sports sponsored by, 108

China: 15 vs. 15 million, 456; army owns cigarette factories, 51; cigarettes introduced into, by BAT, 62; cigarette brands in, 130, 540; cigarette consumption, 51, 540–41; confounds imagination, 541; coveted by transnationals, 541; deaths from smoking, 5, 51; Deng Xiaoping encouraged smoking, 540; factories abuse Chinese life and symbols, 129–30; fingered by "Buck" Duke, 541; as global cigarette superpower, 541; half of all physicians still smoke, 540; herbal brands, 490; ignorance of tobacco harms, 314–15; Liu Xiang's cigarette endorsements, 116; Marlboro Chinese Football League, 108–9; new opium war in, 546; opposition to graphic warnings, 130; Panda brand, 538, 541; Philip Morris penetrates, 109, 541; schools used to promote cigarettes, 130; smoking will disappear from, 456; sports sponsorships, 76, 108–9, 116; tax revenue from cigarettes, 50, 540–41; third of world's cigarettes now smoked in, 540; in tobacco archives, 700; Tobacco Museum in Shanghai, 466; tricks used to circumvent ad bans, 129; Yunnan Hongta Group, 109; Zhengzhou Tobacco Research Institute, 456. *See also* Chunghwa cigarettes

China National Tobacco Corporation (CNTC), 51, 540

chocolate: added to cigarettes, 495–97; chocolate cigarettes, 71–73, 503; flavor notes from ammoniation, 398–99

"choice," ideology of, 557

cholanthrene, 197, 212, 598n14

Chronica Nicotiana, 164–68

Chunghwa cigarettes (Shanghai Tobacco Co. brand), 109, 129

CIBA-Geigy, 526

Cigarette Butt Advisory Committee, 515

cigarette butt waste: Astel condemns, 163; a billion kilograms discarded every year, 355, 514; gathered and re-rolled, 514; idea for generating wildflowers from, 317; kills fish, 514–15; Novotny on, 515; Philip Morris on, 514; Singapore and Sydney strict on, 515; staining patterns on, 384; as toxic trash, 513–15

cigarette cards and silks, 59–60, 64, 88–89, 134, 165

Cigarette Citadels, 679

cigarette design: amateur, 317; illusions key to, 390, 486, 527; ash color altered, 486; billions spent on, 3–4, 265, 486; companies deny having manipulated, 416; doesn't get much attention, 3; elasticity key to, 381; gimmick, 363; hopes for an Einstein of, 358; nicotine crucial in 375, 379; not entirely cynical, 353–54; popular ignorance of, 315; ventilation important in, 374. *See also* ammonia and ammoniation; compensation; filters and filtration; nicotine; ventilation

cigarette filters. *See* filters and filtration

cigarette giveaways. *See* sampling

cigarette lighters: Art Nouveau, 37; blamed for cancer epidemic, 13, 210, 215, 337; built into in artificial limbs, 135; built into cars, 135; built into computers, 136; carved, 45, 134; CPSC has power to regulate, 526; crucial to success of cigarette, 36; history of, 37–38; Kiddiecraft miniature, 139; leaded gasoline used in, 177, 491; Marlboro, 119, 142; radioactivity in flints, 507; squander resources, 516; Zippo, 37–38

cigarette making machines: Bonsack's, 39–40; British, 41; Italian, 41, 554, 567n9; French, 41; Hauni 43, Fig. 6; Nazi government bans certain, 41; Philip Morris uses Molins, 42; should be taxed or banned, 553; Susini & Sons, 42; trounce Lily Lavender, "Queen of the hand-rollers," 39. *See also* Bonsack; Hauni; G.D (Generate Differences)

Cigarette Pack Collectors Association, 468

cigarette packs: as cameras, radios, amplifiers, etc., 138; for your dollhouse, 138, Fig. 22; as miniature mobile ads, 129, 132, 550; in power walls, 132

confirms work of, 239; British reproduce work of, 242, 607n55; champions high-nicotine cigarettes, 394, 403; compromised by taking tobacco money, 429–30; Cuzin in France impressed by, 241; early funding by industry, 201–5, 600n10; epidemiology, 152, 227; Frank Statement criticizes, 258; Germans rebuff, 243; Greene dismisses, 424; Hanmer tries to discredit or "get rid of," 205–06, 248–49, 600nn13,15; ignored in TIRC's first "white paper," 195; as industry ally, 430; industry's tracking of, 192, 208, 215–16; Lanza on, 206; mouse painting experiments, 148, 159, 192; makes fuss about phenols, 363; Mold on, 661n6; on presumptive evidence, 231; predicted to convert "more and more doctors," 608n18; proposes testing paper tars, 211; as *Roffo nouveau*, 206; Schur at Ecusta tries to influence, 215–16; Teeter conveys confidential correspondence to American Tobacco, 192

Y-1 (genetically-engineered tobacco plants), 361
Yale University: happy to have tobacco funding, 470; scholars working for cigarette companies, 280–81, 422, 424, 438, 499; Philip Morris Chair in Marketing, 453. *See also* Alvan R. Feinstein; David F. Musto; Leon E. Rosenberg
Yang, Gonghuan (Deputy Director, CDC of China), 315
Yeaman, Addison Y. (Vice President and General Counsel, Brown & Williamson): admits "nicotine is addictive," 564n9; on candy

cigarettes as "not too bad an advertisement," 71–72; vitriol in *Congressional Record*, 329–30
Yeutter, Clayton (U.S. Trade Representative, Reagan administration), 546
Young American Corporation, 336
youth marketing: by BAT, 114; by Brown & Williamson, 78–79; in Canada, 76; in China, 76; early history of, 75; expressions for, 75–81; facilitated by access to vending machines, 135–36; in Germany, 114–15; in Holland, 76; by Lorillard, 78, 112; by Philip Morris, 76, 88, 118–19; by Reynolds, 75–81, 120, 575n66; Roper on, 76; of smokeless, 108; Teague encourages, 80, 400; tempting by forbidding fruit, 1; as "typo," 575n67; "young adult smokers" (euphemism), 689; youthening, Reynolds efforts at, 60. *See also* "acceptable rebellion"; candy cigarettes; Joe Camel
YouTube, 62, 141–3, 585n23, 664n3
"You've Come a Long Way, Baby" (Virginia Slims slogan and film), 87, 102, 127
Yunnan Tobacco Institute (Yuxi, China), 541

Zahn, Leonard S. (Public Relations consultant), 264–65
Zeman Milos (Prime Minister, Czech Republic), 540, 663n1
ZEPHYR (code word for "cancer"), 689
Zhengzhou Tobacco Research Institute, 456
Zippo lighter, 37–38
Zodiac, 62. *See also* secret projects
zombie, festering logic, 275

TEX
10/12.5 Minion Pro

DISPLAY
Minion Pro

COMPOSITOR
Integrated Composition Systems

PRINTER AND BINDER
Thomson-Shore, Inc.